Evidence-Based Treatments for Trauma Related Disorders in Children and Adolescents

Markus A. Landolt • Marylène Cloitre
Ulrich Schnyder
Editors

Evidence-Based Treatments for Trauma Related Disorders in Children and Adolescents

Springer

Editors
Markus A. Landolt
Department of Psychosomatics
and Psychiatry
University Children's Hospital
University of Zurich
Zurich
Switzerland

Ulrich Schnyder
Department of Psychiatry
and Psychotherapy
University Hospital Zurich
Zurich
Switzerland

Marylène Cloitre
Division of Dissemination and Training
National Center for PTSD
Palo Alto, CA
USA

Psychiatry and Behavioral Sciences
Stanford University
Palo Alto, CA
USA

ISBN 978-3-319-46136-6   ISBN 978-3-319-46138-0 (eBook)
DOI 10.1007/978-3-319-46138-0

Library of Congress Control Number: 2017930960

© Springer International Publishing Switzerland 2017
This work is subject to copyright. All rights are reserved by the Publisher, whether the whole or part of the material is concerned, specifically the rights of translation, reprinting, reuse of illustrations, recitation, broadcasting, reproduction on microfilms or in any other physical way, and transmission or information storage and retrieval, electronic adaptation, computer software, or by similar or dissimilar methodology now known or hereafter developed.
The use of general descriptive names, registered names, trademarks, service marks, etc. in this publication does not imply, even in the absence of a specific statement, that such names are exempt from the relevant protective laws and regulations and therefore free for general use.
The publisher, the authors and the editors are safe to assume that the advice and information in this book are believed to be true and accurate at the date of publication. Neither the publisher nor the authors or the editors give a warranty, express or implied, with respect to the material contained herein or for any errors or omissions that may have been made.

Printed on acid-free paper

This Springer imprint is published by Springer Nature
The registered company is Springer International Publishing AG
The registered company address is: Gewerbestrasse 11, 6330 Cham, Switzerland

Preface

This book is the result of many years of collaboration among the editors and the contributing authors, and it is designed to be the standard handbook of treatment of trauma-related disorders in children and adolescents. It has been written for clinical psychologists, psychiatrists, psychotherapists, and other clinicians who want to understand more about traumatic stress in children and the treatment of its mental health consequences. In contrast to other books which present single approaches, this volume gives an in-depth overview of all the currently available treatment approaches that are either evidence-based or at least evidence-supported. We hope that our book will stimulate further dissemination of these treatments in clinical practice all over the world.

We would like to thank the many people who helped to write this book. First of all, we are very grateful to all the wonderful authors of the chapters, of whom many are among the leading clinicians and researchers in their fields. Not only did the authors submit their manuscripts in a timely fashion, they were also very responsive to our editorial feedback and suggestions. We also thank Springer International for giving us the opportunity to publish this book and for the support throughout the publishing process.

But most of all, we thank all the children, adolescents, and their families who shared their stories with us and taught us so much about childhood trauma and how to overcome its repercussions. This book is dedicated to them.

Zurich, Switzerland	Markus A. Landolt
Palo Alto, CA, USA	Marylène Cloitre
Zurich, Switzerland	Ulrich Schnyder

Contents

Part I Basics

1 **The Diagnostic Spectrum of Trauma-Related Disorders in Children and Adolescents** 3
Lutz Goldbeck and Tine K. Jensen

2 **Epidemiology of Trauma and Trauma-Related Disorders in Children and Adolescents** 29
Shaminka Gunaratnam and Eva Alisic

3 **Childhood Trauma as a Public Health Issue** 49
Hilary K. Lambert, Rosemary Meza, Prerna Martin, Eliot Fearey, and Katie A. McLaughlin

4 **Applying Evidence-Based Assessment to Childhood Trauma and Bereavement: Concepts, Principles, and Practices**............ 67
Christopher M. Layne, Julie B. Kaplow, and Eric A. Youngstrom

5 **Psychological and Biological Theories of Child and Adolescent Traumatic Stress Disorders** 97
Julian D. Ford and Carolyn A. Greene

Part II Interventions

6 **Preventative Early Intervention for Children and Adolescents Exposed to Trauma**.. 121
Alexandra C. De Young and Justin A. Kenardy

7 **The Child and Family Traumatic Stress Intervention**............. 145
Carrie Epstein, Hilary Hahn, Steven Berkowitz, and Steven Marans

8 **Trauma-Focused Cognitive Behavioral Therapy**................. 167
Matthew D. Kliethermes, Kate Drewry, and Rachel Wamser-Nanney

9 **Cognitive Therapy for PTSD in Children and Adolescents** 187
Sean Perrin, Eleanor Leigh, Patrick Smith, William Yule, Anke Ehlers, and David M. Clark

10	Prolonged Exposure Therapy for Adolescents with PTSD: Emotional Processing of Traumatic Experiences................ 209
	Sandy Capaldi, Laurie J. Zandberg, and Edna B. Foa
11	Narrative Exposure Therapy for Children and Adolescents (KIDNET)... 227
	Maggie Schauer, Frank Neuner, and Thomas Elbert
12	STAIR Narrative Therapy for Adolescents 251
	Omar G. Gudiño, Skyler Leonard, Allison A. Stiles, Jennifer F. Havens, and Marylène Cloitre
13	Eye Movement Desensitization and Reprocessing Therapy (EMDR).. 273
	Francine Shapiro, Debra Wesselmann, and Liesbeth Mevissen
14	Attachment, Self-Regulation, and Competency (ARC)............ 299
	Margaret E. Blaustein and Kristine M. Kinniburgh
15	Child-Parent Psychotherapy: An Evidence-Based Treatment for Infants and Young Children............................. 321
	Vilma Reyes, Barclay Jane Stone, Miriam Hernandez Dimmler, and Alicia F. Lieberman
16	Parent-Child Interaction Therapy 341
	Robin H. Gurwitch, Erica Pearl Messer, and Beverly W. Funderburk
17	Trauma Systems Therapy for Children and Adolescents 363
	Adam Brown, Christina Laitner, and Glenn Saxe
18	Pharmacological Treatment for Children and Adolescents with Trauma-Related Disorders 385
	Julia Huemer, Michael Greenberg, and Hans Steiner

Part III Settings

19	Interventions in Medical Settings 405
	Meghan L. Marsac, Aimee K. Hildenbrand, and Nancy Kassam-Adams
20	Trauma-Informed Care in Inpatient and Residential Settings...... 427
	Jennifer F. Havens and Mollie Marr
21	Juvenile Justice and Forensic Settings: The TARGET Approach 445
	Julian D. Ford
22	School-Based Interventions 465
	Thormod Idsoe, Atle Dyregrov, and Kari Dyregrov

23 **Treating and Preventing Psychological Trauma of Children and Adolescents in Post-Conflict Settings**................. 483
Anselm Crombach, Sarah Wilker, Katharin Hermenau, Elizabeth Wieling, and Tobias Hecker

Part IV Summary and Conclusions

24 **How to Treat Children and Adolescents with Trauma-Related Disorders**... 507
Markus A. Landolt, Marylène Cloitre, and Ulrich Schnyder

Introduction

Background

Exposure to potentially traumatic events such as physical maltreatment, sexual abuse, injury, natural disasters, war, and terrorism is far more prevalent among children and adolescents than many of us might expect. Studies all over the world have shown that more than half of the child and adolescent population will have experienced one or more potentially traumatic events by the time they reach adulthood (Copeland et al. 2007; Landolt et al. 2013; McLaughlin et al. 2013). In countries with on-going wars, in post-conflict areas, and in regions affected by large-scale natural disasters or chronic community violence, these figures are even higher (e.g., Karsberg and Elklit 2012). Depending on various risk factors a significant proportion of children exposed to such events go on to develop trauma-related psychological disorders such as posttraumatic stress disorder (Alisic et al. 2014).

Research has shown that exposure to trauma – especially when it occurs at a young age and when chronic – and suffering from trauma-related disorders can be associated with significant deterioration of mental and physical health across the lifespan (e.g., Kessler et al. 2010; McLaughlin et al. 2012). Consequently, childhood trauma and its effects are nowadays a major public health issue across the globe. Prevention of trauma is the most important measure to reduce the number of trauma-exposed children and the prevalence of trauma-related disorders. Unfortunately, even the best measures will never prevent all children from experiencing exposure to trauma. To avoid long-term consequences for the individual as well as society, it is crucial to identify traumatized children as early as possible and to treat them with effective methods as soon as possible.

In the last two decades, many treatment approaches have been developed for children and adolescents who suffer from trauma-related disorders. Some of these approaches have been studied with regard to their effectiveness, and many of them have not or not yet. Today, the number of published books and articles describing specific treatment methods for children is so large that it is extremely difficult for a clinician to get an overview without feeling overwhelmed. Which are evidence-based or at least evidence-informed treatment methods and which are not? How do the different treatment approaches work? Are they useful for all ages and all types of trauma-related disorders? In other words, while there is a huge literature on treatment of child trauma, there is, to date, no comprehensive overview of the different treatment approaches which would allow a clinician to answer some of the above questions. As clinical psychologists, psychiatrists, psychotherapists, and other professionals working with traumatized children and adolescents in various settings, we need a handbook on the treatment of trauma-related disorders in which different empirically supported methods are presented and discussed. Such a clinical guide can, of course, never replace formal training in a specific treatment method but can provide an in-depth description of different approaches and their supporting evidence. Based on this information, the individual clinician can then select and complete formal training in those methods that are most appropriate for their work setting and the population they treat.

When we began planning this book, it was our vision to fill this gap and to bring together as many leaders in the field as possible to present the current evidence-based and promising evidence-informed treatment approaches for trauma-related disorders in children and adolescents. In addition, it seemed important to provide a big picture framework regarding childhood trauma as a public health issue and recognition that the types of treatments that are effective and their delivery are likely to differ in different settings. Now, with this book written, we are confident that this goal has been reached. This volume gives a comprehensive overview of basic concepts for understanding trauma in childhood and adolescence and of current knowledge on the treatment of trauma-related disorders in youth. It is our hope that it will stimulate dissemination of evidence-based treatments among practitioners, since many children with trauma-related disorders are still not treated appropriately or at all.

Content of This Book

Part I ("Basics") of this book provides the background and the basic concepts for understanding trauma in childhood and adolescence. The first chapter presents the diagnostic spectrum of trauma-related disorders in children and adolescents with reference to DSM-5 and the soon to be published ICD-11. Chapter 2 gives a comprehensive overview of epidemiological findings on trauma exposure and trauma-related disorders in youth. Chapter 3 discusses the public health issues that go along with the considerably high numbers of children who are exposed to trauma and who suffer from posttraumatic stress disorder or other trauma-related disorders. Chapter 4 presents concepts, principles, and standardized practices of evidence-based assessment of trauma-related disorders in youth. In the last chapter of this first part of this book, an overview of the current psychological and biological theories of traumatic stress disorders in children and adolescents is given (Chap. 5).

Part II ("Interventions") contains 13 chapters and is the core part of this book. It presents the currently available and empirically supported psychological treatments for children and adolescents with trauma-related disorders. We are very pleased that most of these chapters are authored by the developers of these treatments. The first chapter of this part gives an overview of the current state of early interventions (Chap. 6), followed by a chapter on the Child Family Traumatic Stress Intervention (CFTSI) which is the early intervention approach with the best evidence to date in children (Chap. 7). Evidence-based and empirically supported treatment approaches, including some new approaches to treat children with complex trauma, are presented next: Trauma-Focused Cognitive-Behavioral Therapy (TF-CBT; Chap. 8), Cognitive Therapy (CT; Chap. 9), Prolonged Exposure Therapy for Adolescents (PE-A; Chap. 10), Narrative Exposure Therapy for Children and Adolescents (KIDNET; Chap. 11), Skills Training in Affective and Interpersonal Regulation (STAIR) plus Narrative Therapy – Adolescent Version (SNT-A; Chap. 12), Eye Movement Desensitization and Reprocessing Therapy (EMDR; Chap. 13), Attachment, Self-Regulation, and Competency (ARC) Therapy (Chap. 14), Child-Parent Psychotherapy (CPT; Chap. 15), Parent-Child Interaction Therapy (PCIT; Chap. 16), and Trauma Systems Therapy (TST; Chap. 17). The section ends with an overview of pharmacological treatments for trauma-related disorders in children and adolescents (Chap. 18). To provide some consistency across treatment approaches, the chapters in this second part of this book are structured in a similar way: first, authors present the theoretical underpinnings of their approach; second, the clinical application of the treatment approach is described step by step and illustrated by one or several case presentations; third, the authors discuss clinical challenges that can be met when applying the treatment; and fourth, current evidence of the efficacy of the treatment approach is presented.

Part III of this book contains five chapters that cover special treatment settings that are relevant for children and adolescents with trauma-related disorders, such as medical settings (Chap. 19), residential and psychiatric inpatient care (Chap. 20), juvenile justice and forensic settings (Chap. 21), schools (Chap. 22), and post-conflict regions (Chap. 23).

In the final chapter, we summarize the current state of knowledge on treatment of trauma-related disorders in children and adolescents and describe commonalities and differences between different treatment methods. Also, current shortcomings and limitations are discussed. This book ends with current challenges in the treatment of children with trauma-related disorders and an outlook to the future.

Taken together, this book provides the reader with up-to-date information on basic principles of trauma in children, in-depth information about specific empirically supported treatment approaches, and special treatment settings. We hope this book will be useful for the practicing clinician as well as a good reference source for those in university and clinical training programs.

References

Alisic E, Zalta AK, van Wesel F, Larsen SE, Hafstad GS, Hassanpour K, Smid GE (2014) PTSD rates in trauma-exposed children and adolescents: a meta-analysis. Br J Psychiatr 204:335–340. doi:10.1192/bjp.bp.113.131227

Copeland WE, Keller G, Angold A, Costello EJ (2007) Traumatic events and posttraumatic stress in childhood. Arch Gen Psychiatr 64:577–584. doi: 10.1001/archpsyc.64.5.577

Karsberg SH, Elklit A (2012) Victimization and PTSD in a Rural Kenyan youth sample. Clin Pract Epidemiol Mental Health 8:91–101. doi:10.2174/1745017901208010091

Kessler RC, McLaughlin KA, Green JG, Gruber MJ, Sampson NA, Zaslavsky AM, Aguilar-Gaxiola S, Alhamzawi AO, Alonso J, Angermeyer M, Benjet C, Bromet E, Chatterji S, de Girolamo G, Demyttenaere K, Fayyad J, Florescu S, Gal G, Gureje O, Haro JM, Hu CY, Karam EG, Kawakami N, Lee S, Lépine JP, Ormel J, Posada-Villa J, Sagar R, Tsang A, Ustün TB, Vassilev S, Viana MC, Williams DR (2010) Childhood adversities and adult psychopathology in the WHO World Mental Health Surveys. Br J Psychiatry J Ment Sci 197(5):378–385. doi: 10.1192/bjp.bp.110.080499

Landolt MA, Schnyder U, Maier T, Schoenbucher V, Mohler-Kuo M (2013) Trauma exposure and posttraumatic stress disorder in adolescents: a national survey in Switzerland. J Trauma Stress 26(2):209–216. doi:10.1002/jts.21794

McLaughlin KA, Green JG, Gruber MJ, Sampson NA, Zaslavsky AM, Kessler RC (2012) Childhood adversities and first onset of psychiatric disorders in a national sample of US adolescents. Arch Gen Psychiatry 69(11):1151–1160. doi: 10.1001/archgenpsychiatry.2011.2277

McLaughlin KA, Koenen KC, Hill ED, Petukhova M, Sampson NA, Zaslavsky AM, Kessler RC (2013) Trauma exposure and posttraumatic stress disorder in a national sample of adolescents. J Am Acad Child Adolesc Psychiatry 52(8):815–830. doi:10.1016/j.jaac.2013.05.011

Part I

Basics

The Diagnostic Spectrum of Trauma-Related Disorders in Children and Adolescents

Lutz Goldbeck and Tine K. Jensen

1.1 Introduction

The recognition that children and adolescents may suffer after trauma, not quite unlike adults, is relatively new. In fact when Lenore Terr published her papers on the consequences of the Chowchilla school bus kidnapping (Terr 1983), the scientific community and clinicians were reluctant to believe that the children displayed significant problems resembling posttraumatic stress (Benedek 1985; Garmezy and Rutter 1985). Benedek (1985) reflects on whether it all in all is difficult for professionals and adults to face the fact that children's exposure to trauma, especially when caused by adults, may indeed lead to long-lasting suffering that may impair children's development in devastating ways. There is now a growing body of evidence that young children and adolescents can develop mental health problems after trauma, and studies are seeking to document the differential effects of trauma on children and their development (Straussner and Calnan 2014; Teicher and Samson 2016).

1.2 Developmental Aspects of Trauma-Related Reactions

> Ellen (1 year), Peter (4 years), Niklas (10 years), and Susan (17 years) are siblings and have grown up in a family with violence and abuse. They are now all living in a foster home. Although they have grown up in the same family, their experiences are quite different, and at the time of the foster home placement, their symptoms appeared differently. Ellen cried a lot and was difficult to soothe. Peter had frequent temper tantrums, had difficulty playing with other children at preschool, and seemed distrustful to his foster parents. Niklas refused to go to school. He did not like his math teacher because he reminded him of his dad, and he felt scared when approaching him. He also had medically unexplained stomach aches. Right before the placement into foster care, he started wetting his bed at night. Susan was described as thoughtful and taking care of her siblings. She went to school every day, and her homework had to be perfect or else she feared everyone would understand she's crazy. Recently her foster mother observed some unexplainable cuts on her arm. Susan does not have many friends and stays home most of the time.

Trauma experienced in childhood is considered to be particularly harmful because the experiences may interfere with the child's development. At least two fundamental developmental processes are negatively affected by childhood trauma: neurodevelopment (such as the development of the brain and nervous system) and psychosocial development (such as personality formation, moral development, social relationships) (Putnam 2006). The symptoms after trauma may manifest themselves differently for children of different age groups, and developmental considerations should be taken into account when we try to understand the effects of trauma.

What may be considered to be developmentally abnormal is very much dependent on how old the child is. In fact, many symptoms typically described as reactions to trauma may be considered developmentally appropriate and normative behaviors for certain age groups, such as sleep disruption in toddlers, restricted concentration or attention span, and temper tantrums (De Young et al. 2011; Scheeringa et al. 2003). Clinginess and signs of discomfort at separation from a parent is, for instance, viewed upon very differently if the child is 4 or 14 years old. The younger the child is, the less specific symptoms may be. For very young children, various forms of dysregulation, for example, excessive and persistent crying, may be the only observable sign of traumatic distress.

For *toddlers and preschool children*, separation anxiety, phobic reactions, temper tantrums, enuresis, hyperactivity, and sleep disturbances have been reported after trauma exposure (La Greca 2007; Norris et al. 2002; Scheeringa et al. 2012). Feelings of helplessness and perceptions of continued danger may be expressed, and a loss of previously acquired developmental skills may be seen. Children may want to sleep in their parents' bed or not want to play outside alone. Disruptions in play activities, different forms of social withdrawal, and increased negative emotional states may be observed. Traumatized children often have difficulties regulating emotions, and their attachment to caregivers may be undermined by a sense of insecurity.

In *school-aged children* oppositional behavior, hyperactivity, and social problems are often seen. After experiencing trauma, they may exhibit excessive concern for their own or others' safety and seem anxious. Because school-age children often reflect over their own responsibility for what happened, they may struggle more with feelings of guilt and shame than younger children. Stress-reactive somatic complaints such as stomach and headaches have also been reported. High rates of depression have been found both among traumatized preadolescents and adolescents, and teachers have reported concentration problems and learning difficulties (Goenjian et al. 1995; Yule and Udwin 1991).

As children grow into *adolescence*, they face a range of new developmental demands such as forming their identity, establishing relations with peers, and developing independence from parents. Experiencing trauma may impede these developmental goals. For instance, studies after the earthquake in Armenia found that adolescents exhibited chronic separation anxiety disorder delaying the development of independence from parents (Goenjian et al. 1995). Adolescents may be more self-conscious about their emotional responses and be afraid of being labeled as different from peers. This may lead to withdrawal from friends and family (Pynoos et al. 1999). Difficulty at school has been reported, and traumatized adolescents are more at risk for failing a grade or being suspended from school than other youth (Lipschitz et al. 1999; Nooner et al. 2012). Self-injury, suicidal ideation, reckless behavior, and substance abuse are more typical for adolescents than younger youth (De Bellis 2001; Nooner et al. 2012; Pynoos et al. 2009; Schmid et al. 2013). Youth may express thoughts of revenge and changes in their perceptions of the world (Pynoos et al. 1999). Also, psychosis has been found to be predicted by serious childhood trauma (Kelleher et al. 2013).

Children do not always possess the verbal or cognitive ability to express their symptoms or stress. Because symptoms vary in the degree to which they can be observed, underreporting of symptoms can occur for internalizing relative to externalizing symptoms. For instance, the externalizing symptoms commonly associated with ADHD and anxiety disorder may be more observable to adults than the internalized symptoms of PTSD, and therefore, clinicians may rather target these disorders and overlook the PTSD symptoms (Cohen and Scheeringa 2009). Therefore, the temporal relationship between exposure to traumatic events and the manifestation of symptom clusters needs to be examined closely when diagnosing children. New symptoms or clear exacerbations after traumatic experiences may often be good indicators for the associations between symptoms and trauma.

1.3   Classification in the DSM-5 and the ICD-11

Based on an evaluation of empirical research (Friedman 2013), the classification of trauma- and stressor-related disorders (TSRD) was revised for the fifth revision of the Diagnostic and Statistical Manual of Mental Disorders (DSM-5) (2013) with two major changes. First, DSM-PTSD is located in a separate category "trauma- and stressor-related disorders" rather than as previously conceptualized as an anxiety disorder. Second, DSM-5 includes developmentally modified diagnostic criteria and a specific algorithm for the diagnosis of PTSD in preschool children. The International Classification of Diseases (ICD) is currently under revision, and the release of the ICD-11 is announced for 2018. The proposal of a working group of the World Health Organization (WHO) for the 11th edition of the ICD follows a strategy of clinical utility and brevity of the new diagnostic criteria for "disorders specifically associated with stress." The main components of the proposal are the restriction of the PTSD criteria to six core symptoms (Brewin 2013; Maercker et al. 2013b; Maercker et al. 2013a) and the introduction of two new disorders called complex PTSD (CPTSD) and prolonged grief disorder (PGD). However, while symptom presentations according to age or developmental phase have been proposed, field studies of the proposed new criteria have not yet included children and adolescents. Thus, the consideration of developmental aspects and the validity of these diagnostic categories and criteria for children and adolescents are still limited.

When comparing DSM-5 and ICD-11, both systems have similarities, but also significant differences (see Table 1.1). Both manuals include the child-specific attachment disorders, which are per definition closely related to childhood adversity due to severe failure of the caregivers. Beyond attachment disorders, the remaining diagnostic constructs in both classification systems are independent of age and developmental status, with the exception of the new preschool PTSD subtype in the DSM-5. Convergence between DSM-5 and ICD-11 can also be seen in the distinction between traumatic and nontraumatic experiences as triggers for symptoms, with corresponding discrimination between PTSD and adjustment disorders.

Table 1.1 Trauma- and stressor-related disorders (TSRD) as defined in the DSM-5 and disorders specifically associated with stress proposed for the ICD-11

DSM-5 category	DSM-5 code	Proposed ICD-11 category	ICD-11 code
Acute stress disorder	308.3	(*Non-disorder phenomena*: acute stress reaction)	–
Adjustment disorders	309.x	Adjustment disorders	7B23

Posttraumatic stress disorder
  With dissociative symptoms
  With delayed expression
  PTSD for children <6 years
	309.81	Traumatic stress disorders
		  Posttraumatic stress disorder
		  Complex posttraumatic stress disorder
			7B20
			7B21

		Prolonged grief disorder	7B22
Reactive attachment disorder	313.89	Reactive attachment disorder	7B24
Disinhibited social engagement disorder	313.89	Disinhibited social engagement disorder	7B25
Other specified TSRD	309.89	Other specified disorders specifically associated with stress	7B2Y
Unspecified TSRD	309.9	Unspecified disorders specifically associated with stress	7B2Z

DSM-5 and ICD-11 show fundamental differences regarding three other diagnoses. While DSM-5 is comprised of an expanded version of DSM-IV PTSD, ICD-11 has formulated two PTSD diagnoses that discriminate between a three-cluster fear-based PTSD diagnosis and a complex PTSD diagnosis, which includes three additional symptom clusters related to disturbances in affect, self-identity, and relationships. Second, prolonged grief disorder (PGD) is a category of its own in the ICD-11, while PGD is not included in DSM-5. A third difference between DSM-5 and ICD-11 is the consideration of stress symptoms within the first 4 weeks. According to DSM-5, a separate disorder acute stress disorder (ASD) is restricted to 4 weeks after the event, whereas ICD-11 explicitly normalizes acute stress reactions within the first days and weeks after a traumatic event. Both classification systems provide rather consistent minimum time intervals for the diagnosis of a PTSD with 4 weeks (DSM-5) or "at least several weeks" (ICD-11).

In the following sections, the main diagnostic categories and their subtypes will be described and discussed regarding their applicability with children and adolescents.

1.4 Acute Stress

> Alicia is 5 years old when she and her mother were in a serious car accident where two people were killed. The days after the accident, she would repeatedly take all her brother's play cars and pile them on top of each other. She would then take a basketball and throw the ball on all the cars so they scattered around the room and say "Now you're all dead!" She was reluctant to sleep in her own bed and woke up several nights with scary dreams. In the first 2 weeks, she refused to go to preschool and would not sit in any cars. Slowly she accepted to sit in a car if someone sat in the backseat with her. Her nightmares receded and her normal play behavior resumed.

In the DSM-5 acute stress disorder (ASD) refers to the reactions that occur in people immediately and up to 1 month after experiencing a traumatic event. In the proposed ICD-11, the comparable term is acute stress reaction (ASR). The constructs are conceptualized very differently in the two systems as ASR is not defined as a mental disorder, whereas ASD is. For ASR the symptoms are defined broadly and include shock and confusion. The symptom clusters of ASD resemble those of PTSD with added attention to dissociative features.

There seems to be consensus that there is a need to differentiate between short-term and long-term symptom development after exposure to trauma. However, some scholars have argued that ASD is most applicable to single incident traumas since it may be difficult to specify an index trauma in cases of ongoing chronic trauma such as in ongoing child sexual abuse (Kassam-Adams and Winston 2004).

1.4.1 Acute Stress Disorder in the DSM-5

The symptoms for ASD resemble those in PTSD with the core symptoms being intrusion, negative mood, dissociation, avoidance, and arousal (see Table 1.2). The developmental modifications are also similar to those for PTSD, where change in play may be an indicator of PTSD and where it is not expected that children are able to report trauma content of nightmares. For both adults and children, 9 of the 14 symptoms are required for a diagnosis. There is a concern that this requirement may lead to an underdiagnosing of many children who present with significant impairment after trauma. A meta-analysis based on data from 15 youth studies from four countries showed that children and adolescents do experience several acute symptoms after trauma, and on average approximately 40 % of the children experienced severe impairment. However, when using a threshold of eight symptoms (i.e., one less than in the DSM-5), only about 12 % met diagnostic criteria. Lowering the

Table 1.2 Acute stress disorder in DSM-5 (*with modifications for children in italics*) and acute stress reactions as proposed for ICD-11

DSM-5 (code 308.3)			ICD-11(code 7B26)	
A	*Exposed to* death/threatened death, serious injury or sexual violation in one or more ways Directly experienced Witnessed Learning of such events occurring to close other person		A	*Exposed to* threat
B	*Presence of at least nine of:*		B	Transient emotional, somatic cognitive, or behavioral symptoms
Intrusion symptoms	1. Recurrent, involuntary, and intrusive distressing memories of the traumatic event(s). *Note: In children, repetitive play may occur in which themes or aspects of the traumatic event(s) are expressed* 2. Recurrent distressing dreams in which the content and/or affect of the dream are related to the event(s). *Note: In children, there may be frightening dreams without recognizable content* 3. Dissociative reactions (e.g., flashbacks) in which the individual feels or acts as if the traumatic event(s) were recurring. (Such reactions may occur on a continuum, with the most extreme expression being a complete loss of awareness of present surroundings.) *Note: In children, trauma-specific reenactment may occur in play* 4. Intense or prolonged psychological distress or marked physiological reactions in response to internal or external cues that symbolize or resemble an aspect of the traumatic event(s)		C	Normal response to severe stressor

1 The Diagnostic Spectrum of Trauma-Related Disorders in Children and Adolescents

Table 1.2 (continued)

DSM-5 (code 308.3)		ICD-11 (code 7B26)	
Negative mood	5. Persistent inability to experience positive emotions (e.g., inability to experience happiness, satisfaction, or loving feelings)		
Dissociative symptoms	6. An altered sense of the reality of one's surroundings or oneself (e.g., seeing oneself from another's perspective, being in a daze, time slowing) 7. Inability to remember an important aspect of the traumatic event(s) (typically due to dissociative amnesia and not to other factors such as head injury, alcohol, or drugs)		
Avoidance symptoms	8. Efforts to avoid distressing memories, thoughts, or feelings about or closely associated with the traumatic event(s) 9. Efforts to avoid external reminders (people, places, conversations, activities, objects, situations) that arouse distressing memories, thoughts, or feelings about or closely associated with the traumatic event(s)		
Arousal symptoms	10. Sleep disturbance (e.g., difficulty falling or staying asleep, restless sleep) 11. Irritable behavior and angry outbursts (with little or no provocation), typically expressed as verbal or physical aggression toward people or objects 12. Hypervigilance 13. Problems with concentration 14. Exaggerated startle response		
C. Duration	Symptoms in criterion B 3 days to 1 month after trauma exposure *Note:* symptoms typically begin immediately after the trauma, but persistence for at least 3 days and up to a month is needed to meet disorder criteria	D E	Symptoms appear within days Symptoms subside within 1 week or after removal of stressor
D. Impairment	The disturbance causes clinically significant distress or impairment in social, occupational, or other important areas of functioning	F	Symptoms do not meet criteria for mental disorder
E.	The disturbance is not attributable to the physiological effects of a substance (e.g., medication or alcohol) or another medical condition (e.g., mild traumatic brain injury) and is not better explained by brief psychotic disorder		

threshold to three or four improved sensitivity and at the same time maintained specificity (Kassam-Adams et al. 2012). When assessing children's need for early interventions, clinicians need to be aware that many children may experience acute distress and impairment even though they may not fulfill the diagnostic requirements for ASD.

1.4.2 Acute Stress Reaction in the ICD-11

Since there is no strict minimum time limit for diagnosing PTSD in the proposed ICD-11, the PTSD diagnosis can be used in the early aftermath of a traumatic event, provided the symptoms are severe enough and cause impairment. Hence, it has been argued that there is no need for an acute stress diagnosis. However, since it may be helpful to have a category describing transient subclinical reactions after an acute stressful event, the ICD-11 workgroup has suggested that acute stress reaction be placed as a condition that does not relate to diseases or disorders but which nonetheless may warrant psychosocial interventions. The proposed ICD-11 description of ASR refers thus to the development of transient emotional, cognitive, somatic, and behavioral symptoms in response to an exceptional stressor involving exposure to an event or situation of an extremely threatening or horrific nature (Maercker et al. 2013c). Some of the proposed symptoms are feeling as if one were in a daze, feeling confused, sadness, anxiety, anger, despair, overactivity, stupor, and social withdrawal as well as physiological signs of anxiety such as rapid heartbeat, sweating, and flushing. The symptoms appear within hours to days of the impact and subside within about a week after exposure, or following removal from the threatening situation. To our knowledge no developmental considerations are noted other than the ones mentioned related to PTSD.

1.5 Posttraumatic Stress Disorder

> Fredric is 11 years old. He and his mom have just moved after living in an abusive relationship to Fredric's father. Fredric's father would beat his mom and call her ugly names. This happened mostly after Fredric was in bed but he could hear the fighting. On one occasion he went to intervene and his father slapped him and said it was his entire fault. Fredric is happy they moved but he misses his friends. He has nightmares and becomes very frightened when he sees men that remind him of his dad. He does not like talking about his dad or seeing ambulances because it reminds him of when his mom was sent to the hospital. He feels everything is his fault and he must be a bad person since his dad slapped him. He has difficulty concentrating in school and feels restless all the time.

Since its inclusion in the DSM-III in 1980, there is an ongoing controversy around the definition of PTSD. Although PTSD is well accepted as a distinct mental disorder, the need and definition of the trauma event criterion A, the specificity, and the minimum number and range of required symptoms are continuously discussed. Divergent definitions in the DSM-5 and the ICD-11 reflect different conceptualizations of the disorder. Although there is sufficient evidence that children and adolescents can develop PTSD as defined for adults, there is an ongoing discussion about the need to modify the diagnostic criteria for minors, e.g., by lowering the diagnostic threshold or by adjusting the symptom description to the child's developmental level.

Regarding the criterion A defining the traumatic event(s), the DSM-5 provides a more explicit definition compared to the ICD-11. According to the DSM-5, a traumatic event is characterized by exposure to actual or threatened death, serious injury, or sexual violence in one of the following ways:

- Directly experiencing the event(s).
- Witnessing, in person, the event(s) as it occurred to others.
- Learning that the traumatic event(s) occurred to a close family member or close friend. In cases of actual or threatened death of a family member or friend, the event(s) must have been violent or accidental.

A fourth way, which does not apply for youth, refers to professionals or first responders. In contrast to the DSM-5, some of the authors of the ICD-11 propose to rely on symptoms rather than exposure (Brewin et al. 2009) and simply define trauma as "extremely threatening or horrifying event(s)." This leaves room for defining traumatic events as perceived by the individual.

Differences in the range and number of symptoms emerge when comparing the DSM-5 and the proposed ICD-11 criteria of PTSD (see Tables 1.3). The authors of the DSM-5 decided to reconceptualize PTSD broadly to include posttraumatic anhedonic, dysphoric, externalizing, and dissociative clinical presentations along

Table 1.3 Variation of the clinical manifestation of DSM-5 posttraumatic stress symptoms in children >6 years and adolescents (for symptoms in preschool children see Table 1.4)

B	Reexperiencing	B1 distressing memories: Repetitive play may occur in which themes or aspects of the traumatic event(s) are expressed B2 distressing dreams: In children trauma-specific content of nightmares may not be recognizable B3 dissociative reactions: In children, trauma-specific reenactment may occur in play
C	Avoidance	School-age children may show reduced participation in new activities Adolescents may be reluctant to pursue developmental opportunities (e.g., dating, driving) In addition to avoidance, children may become preoccupied with reminders
D	Cognitions and mood	In young children, due to limitations in expressing thoughts or labeling emotions, primarily mood changes In adolescents, negative cognitions may refer to themselves (e.g., as a coward) or to social undesirability among peers, and they may lose aspirations for the future
E	Hyperarousal	E1: In children irritable or aggressive behavior can interfere with peer relationships and school behavior E2: In children and adolescents, reckless behavior may lead to (self-)destructive, thrill-seeking, or high-risk behavior, including the risk for accidental injury to self or others

with the original fear-based anxiety disorder (Friedman 2014). Altogether 20 single symptoms are grouped into four symptom clusters based on initial analyses (Elhai and Palmieri 2011). In contrast, the authors of the ICD-11 challenged the complexity of the construct (Galatzer-Levy and Bryant 2013) and defined six symptoms of PTSD, two per each dimension reexperiencing, avoidance, and perceived threat, with an emphasis on intrusive recollections as the cardinal symptom (Brewin et al. 2009; Maercker et al. 2013b).

Both major classification systems refer to child-specific modifications of the diagnostic criteria, but only the DSM-5 explicitly includes a subtype for preschool children. In contrast to the adult literature, the concern regarding children has been lack of sensitivity rather than lack of specificity (Cohen and Scheeringa 2009; Carrion et al. 2002; Stein et al. 1997), i.e., diagnoses among children are seen as under-recognized due to internalizing symptoms that are not reported. Some of the symptoms identified in adults such as dissociative flashbacks or negative expectations of self/the world are developmentally inappropriate for young children, making it more difficult for them to reach criteria for diagnosis. Research with children showed that they may develop different reactions at the time of exposure to a traumatic event and in the manner in which they present intrusive symptoms. As children may present insufficient avoidance symptoms, they may not qualify for a diagnosis, although they have clear intrusive symptoms and hyperarousal symptoms with significant impairment (Smith et al. 2009). Therefore, a substantial body of the child literature recommends to use alternative diagnostic criteria and an alternative algorithm for the diagnosis of PTSD in children (Meiser-Stedman et al. 2008; Scheeringa et al. 2003; see also below). The DSM-5 maintained the previous recommendations of the DSM-IV to consider child-specific symptom manifestations (see Table 1.3).

1.5.1 PTSD According to the DSM-5

The definition of PTSD in the fifth revision of the DSM underwent major changes. Due to insufficient empirical support, the previous A2 criterion of peritraumatic fear, horror, or helplessness was removed from the DSM-5. The range of symptoms was substantially extended in the DSM-5. The reexperiencing cluster mainly remained unchanged, whereas the avoidance cluster now contains avoidance of internal and external trauma reminders only. A new symptom cluster referring to negative alterations in cognitions and mood was introduced, including emotional numbing that was previously combined with avoidance. Thus, the DSM-5 does now acknowledge the evidence for dysfunctional cognitions closely associated with the development and maintenance of PTSD, such as overgeneralized negative expectations and distorted causal attributions of the traumatic events. The new cluster D also includes trauma-related alterations of mood and emotions, which have to be distinguished from preexisting depressive symptoms. Reckless and/or self-destructive behavior was introduced as additional hyperarousal symptom. Within the range of now 20 symptoms describing PTSD, there is room to capture the clinical picture of those individuals with a more complex clinical presentation of their disorder. Additionally, the new DSM-5 subtype PTSD with dissociative symptoms allows specifying whether there are additional symptoms of depersonalization, e.g., detachment from others, or derealization, e.g., experiences of unreality of surroundings.

After the release of the new proposed DSM-5 criteria, a handful of empirical studies have been conducted, but very few of these have used child and adolescent samples. At least one study comparing the DSM-IV with the DSM-5 in a sample of traumatized adolescents and young adults has shown that the PTSD prevalence does not differ significantly whether using DSM-IV or DSM-5 and that the four factor structure of the DSM-5 fits the data well (Hafstad et al. 2014). New studies are however suggesting that a seven-factor structure of intrusion, avoidance, negative affect, anhedonia, externalizing behavior, anxious arousal, and dysphoric arousal may be more fitting, showing just how complex and multifaceted children's responses to trauma may be (Liu et al. 2016).

The DSM-IV TR included modifications of the diagnostic criteria for PTSD in children 6 years and older, which have been retained in the DSM-5 (for details, see Table 1.3):

- Intrusive memories may occur as repetitive play in which themes or aspects of the traumatic event(s) are expressed.
- Frightening dreams after the trauma may lack trauma-specific content.
- Dissociative reactions (e.g., flashbacks) may occur in play as trauma-specific reenactment.

An extended proposal for developmental modifications of PTSD symptom criteria (Pynoos et al. 2009) was not approved by the authors of the DSM-5. However, primarily based on the empirical work of Michael Scheeringa and coauthors, who defined an alternative algorithm for diagnosing PTSD in preschool children (Scheeringa et al. 1995; Scheeringa et al. 2003; Scheeringa et al. 2011), the DSM-5 included a preschool subtype of PTSD with modified diagnostic criteria for children 6 years and younger (see Table 1.4). Multiple studies supported the usefulness of the alternative criteria to identify young children with clinically significant impairment due to exposure to traumatic events. A major difference compared to the PTSD for children >6 years is that the symptom clusters avoidance and negative alterations in cognitions and mood are combined into one, with at least one required symptom out of six symptoms. Thus, according to the preschool criteria, children with at least 4 out of 16 posttraumatic stress symptoms and with clinically significant impairment can qualify for the diagnosis.

1.5.2 PTSD According to the ICD-11

The main objectives of the ICD-11 working group was to specify PTSD, to reduce comorbidity, to overcome the overuse of the diagnosis as having been criticized due

Table 1.4 PTSD in preschool children <6 years according to the DSM-5 (*developmental modifications in italics*)

A	Exposure	Directly experiencing the traumatic event(s)
		Witnessing, in person, the event(s) as it occurred to others, *especially primary caregivers*
		Learning that the traumatic event(s) occurred *to a parent or caregiving figure*
B	Reexperiencing	At least one of
		Intrusive memories (*may not necessarily appear distressing and may be expressed as play reenactment*)
		Recurrent distressing dreams (*it may not be possible to ascertain that the frightening content is related to the traumatic event*)
		Flashbacks (*such trauma-specific reenactment may occur in play*)
		Distress to reminders
		Physiological reactivity
C	Avoidance and negative alterations in cognitions[a]	At least one of
		Avoidance of activities, places, or physical reminders
		Avoidance of or efforts to avoid people, conversations, or interpersonal situations
		Negative emotional states
		Diminished interest (including constriction of play)
		Socially withdrawn behavior
		Emotional numbing
D	Hyperarousal	At least two of
		Irritable behavior and angry outbursts (*including extreme temper tantrums*)
		Hypervigilance
		Startle response
		Concentration problems
		Sleep problems
E	Duration	Duration >1 month
F	Impairment	Significant distress or impairment *in relationships with parents, siblings, peers, or other caregivers or with school behavior*

[a]This symptom cluster also covers emotions and mood

to a low threshold to diagnosis in the ICD-10 at least for adults (Brewin et al. 2009), and to provide simple criteria which can easily be utilized by nonspecialized clinicians. The proposed core criteria (see Table 1.5) comprise at least one of two reexperiencing symptoms (flashbacks and/or nightmares), at least one of two avoidance symptoms (avoidance of internal and/or external reminders), and at least one of two hyperarousal symptoms (hypervigilance and/or startle response), now summarized as perceived threat. Thus, in contrast to the DSM-5, the ICD-11 PTSD does not consider trauma-related alterations of cognitions and mood as part of the disorder. Rather, a more complex spectrum of trauma-related symptoms is defined as complex posttraumatic stress disorder, which goes beyond the six core symptoms of PTSD and includes a range of additional emotional and behavioral symptoms.

Table 1.5 Posttraumatic stress disorder definitions in DSM-5 (age >6 years) and proposed for ICD-11 (all ages)

	DSM-5 (code 309.81)			ICD-11 traumatic stress disorders		
				PTSD (code 7B20)		Complex PTSD (code 7B21)
A	Exposed to threatened death, serious injury or sexual violence Experienced/witnessed threat to life or sexual violence Learning events occur to close other person		A	Exposed to extremely threatening or horrifying event or series of events	A	Exposed to extremely threatening or horrifying event or series of events
B	Reexperiencing (at least one of)		1.	Reexperiencing (at least one of)	1.	Reexperiencing (at least one of)
B1	Intrusive memories		(a)	Vivid intrusive memories	(a)	Vivid intrusive memories
B2	Nightmares		(b)	Nightmares	(b)	Nightmares
B3	Flashbacks					
B4	Distress to reminders					
B5	Physiological reactivity					
C	Avoidance (at least one of)		2.	Avoidance (at least one of)	2.	Avoidance (at least one of)
C1	Thoughts and feelings		(a)	Thoughts and memories	(a)	Thoughts and memories
C2	Situations		(b)	Activities or situations	(b)	Activities or situations
D	Negative alterations in cognitions/mood (at least three of)					
D1	Dissociative amnesia					
D2	Negative expectations of self/world					
D3	Distorted blame					
D4	Negative emotional state					
D5	Diminished interest					
D6	Emotional numbing					
E	Hyperarousal (at least two of)		3.	Perceived threat (at least one of)	3.	Perceived threat (at least one of)
E1	Irritability and angry outbursts					
E2	Reckless/self-destructive behavior					
E3	Hypervigilance		(a)	Hypervigilance	(a)	Hypervigilance
E4	Startle response		(b)	Startle response	(b)	Startle response
E5	Concentration deficits					
E6	Sleep problems					

Table 1.5 (continued)

DSM-5 (code 309.81)	ICD-11 traumatic stress disorders		
		4.	*Affect dysregulation*
		(a)	Sensitivity
		(b)	Hypo or hyper activation
		5.	*Negative self-concept*
		(a)	Worthless, failure, defeated
		(b)	Shame, guilt
		6.	*Disturbances in relationships*
		(a)	Avoid relationships
		(b)	Distant or cutoff
F	Duration: >1 month after trauma	Duration: at least several weeks	Duration: at least several weeks
G	Significant impairment	Significant impairment	Significant impairment
Specifier: with dissociative symptoms			
Specifier: with delayed expression			

1.5.2.1 Proposed definition of PTSD for the ICD-11 (Maercker et al. 2013b)

> "Post-traumatic stress disorder (PTSD) is a disorder that may develop following exposure to an extremely threatening or horrific event or series of events characterized by reexperiencing the traumatic event or events in the present in the form of vivid intrusive memories, flashbacks, or nightmares, typically accompanied by strong and overwhelming emotions such as fear or horror, and strong physical sensations, avoidance of thoughts and memories of the event or events, or avoidance of activities, situations, or people reminiscent of the event or events, and persistent perceptions of heightened current threat, for example as indicated by hypervigilance or an enhanced startle reaction to stimuli such as unexpected noises. The symptoms must last for at least several weeks and cause significant impairment in functioning."

The authors of the ICD-11 proposal briefly comment on the need to consider age-related symptom presentations for children and adolescents (Maercker et al. 2013b). The developmental modifications proposed for ICD-11 PTSD (First et al. 2015) include disorganization, agitation, temper tantrums, clinging, excessive crying, social withdrawal, separation anxiety, distrust, trauma-specific reenactments

1 The Diagnostic Spectrum of Trauma-Related Disorders in Children and Adolescents

such as repetitive play or drawings, frightening dreams without clear content or night terrors, sense of foreshortened future, and impulsivity. For adolescents, they note that self-injurious or risky behaviors are frequent.

Concerns regarding the restrictive definition of PTSD in the ICD-11 have been expressed based on studies describing significantly lower prevalence rates in adults compared with both the ICD-10 and DSM-5 (Wisco et al. 2016) and in children and adolescents compared to the ICD-10 and DSM-IV (Haravouori et al. 2016; Sachser and Goldbeck 2016). Among adolescent and young adult survivors of school shootings, Haravouori et al. (2016) found support rather for a two-factor model of ICD-11 PTSD with reexperiencing and avoidance as one factor than for the three-factor solution as proposed by the authors of the ICD-11. The still pending precise symptom definitions of the proposed criteria will probably have an impact upon the prevalence rates among children and adolescents when using ICD-11 criteria.

1.5.3 ICD-11 Complex PTSD

> Aisha was 14 years old when she flew from Somalia. Both her parents were killed and she grew up most of her life with her grandmother. Her father was very violent and hit Aisha, her siblings, and her mother. Aisha can remember always feeling frightened when her father was at home. Her mother was very depressed and had difficulty caring for her children when they were young. Aisha and her sister were forced to prostitution by their grandmother after their parents died. They later fled to Kenya where they were placed in a refugee camp. There Aisha experienced new episodes of rape and violence. She was finally able to seek asylum in a European country. Aisha has serious sleep disturbances due to recurrent nightmares. She has flashbacks from her abuse. She avoids things that remind her of the beatings from her father and she tries to avoid thinking about what has happened. She is experienced as "dreamy" and "distant," and the staff where she lives thinks she dissociates when reminded of her past. She has difficulty paying attention in school and startles easily. She says she does not deserve to live because of the shameful things that have happened to her. She feels as if she is a bad person that deserves bad things happening to her, and she feels extremely guilty for not being able to protect her younger sister from abuse. She isolates herself from other adults and peers.

The ICD-11 group has proposed to include complex PTSD for the first time as a diagnostic entity. The definition of the trauma criterion explicitly refers to, e.g., repeated traumatic experiences during childhood such as domestic violence or sexual and physical abuse as a risk factor but not as a requirement. CPTSD requires the symptoms of PTSD, as well as symptoms of affective dysregulation, negative self-concept, and interpersonal difficulties (see Table 1.5). There are currently six studies supporting the validity of ICD-11 complex PTSD in adults (Cloitre et al. 2013;

Elklit et al. 2014). However, so far there are only a limited number of studies evaluating ICD-11 complex PTSD in children and adolescents. One study on adolescents and young adults supports the ICD-11 proposal to differentiate between PTSD and CPTSD (Perkonigg et al. 2016).

> **Definition of Complex Posttraumatic Stress Disorder as Proposed for the ICD-11 (Maercker et al. 2013b)**
> Complex posttraumatic stress disorder (Complex PTSD) is a disorder that may develop following exposure to an event or series of events of an extreme and prolonged or repetitive nature that is experienced as extremely threatening or horrific and from which escape is difficult or impossible (e.g., torture, slavery, genocide campaigns, prolonged domestic violence, repeated childhood sexual, or physical abuse).
>
> The disorder is characterized by the core symptoms of PTSD, that is, all diagnostic requirements for PTSD have been met at some point during the course of the disorder.
>
> In addition, complex PTSD is characterized by:
>
> 1. Severe and pervasive problems in affect regulation
> 2. Persistent beliefs about oneself as diminished, defeated, or worthless, accompanied by deep and pervasive feelings of shame, guilt, or failure related to the stressor
> 3. Persistent difficulties in sustaining relationships and in feeling close to others
>
> The disturbance causes significant impairment in personal, family, social, educational, occupational, or other important areas of functioning.

The authors of the ICD-11 proposal mention a range of non-specific symptom presentations of CPTSD in children and adolescents, such as regressive and/or aggressive behavior in children or substance abuse and risky behavior in adolescents (Maercker et al. 2013b). There will be specific proposed developmental modifications for ICD-11 CPTSD and they are as follows: "Among children, the core symptoms of PTSD may differ in that re-experiencing symptoms can be observed in trauma-specific re-enactments such as repetitive play, while emotion regulation and interpersonal difficulties may be observed in regressive and/or aggressive behaviours towards self or others. In adolescence, substance use, risky behaviours (unsafe sex, unsafe driving), and aggressive behaviours may be particularly evident as expressions of emotion regulation and interpersonal difficulties"(Cloitre 2016).

Operational symptom criteria or instruments to assess CPTSD in children and adolescents have not yet been developed but are expected when the ICD-11 is released in 2018. Initial empirical approaches to complex PTSD in youth have utilized a range of generic measures of internalizing and externalizing symptoms, such as the Child Behavior Checklist or the Child Depression Inventory to assess the proposed CPTSD symptoms. However, these instruments have limited sensitivity and specificity for trauma, as they do not temporally relate symptoms to the traumatic experiences. Difficulties to diagnose CPTSD comprise, for instance, the differentiation from normal developmental problems such as exacerbated temper tantrums in toddlers, or mood swings in adolescents, or mood disorders in children such as dysphoria or depression from posttraumatic affective dysregulation.

There is an ongoing controversy about the need and utility of a new complex PTSD disorder. Proponents refer to the studies showing that there are distinct PTSD and CPTSD classes with different symptom profiles across the six cores plus six additional symptoms. Opponents argue that those complex symptom manifestations are rather representing a more severe PTSD with a broader range of symptoms than a different disorder (Resick et al. 2012). Moreover, similarly to the non-specific symptoms in the DSM-5 PTSD difficulties in determining the temporal relatedness of the additional symptoms with the traumatic event(s) may occur. Differential indications for treatment are not yet clear. Case series of trauma-focused cognitive behavioral therapy with youth have shown its effectiveness also in children and adolescents who have symptoms similar to those proposed for complex PTSD (Cohen et al. 2012). The authors recommend to expand and adapt the treatment as needed for complex trauma populations. Next step following the final formulation of CPTSD for children will be to determine whether different diagnoses will improve treatment development, selection, and outcome.

1.5.4 Comorbidity with PTSD

Across all ages, individuals with PTSD show high rates of comorbid symptoms, such as depression, anxiety, substance abuse, dissociation, dysphoria, or aggressive behavior (Keane and Kaloupek 1997). Alterations in social functions are frequent. Thus, the presence of comorbidity is not a flaw of the classification system in general or of PTSD specifically. Multi-morbidity is especially prevalent after prolonged or repeated exposure to severe stressors from which separation is not possible (Cloitre et al. 2009). Especially multiple adverse experiences during childhood, such as sexual and physical abuse, witnessing severe domestic violence, or child soldiering, have been shown to be associated with a broad range of internalizing and externalizing symptoms, often persisting into adulthood. A key feature of this type of prolonged interpersonal traumatization is the inability of the individual to escape from a perpetrator, which clearly is the typical situation of children who are abused by their caregivers (Herman 1992). When the source of trauma and fear also is an attachment figure, the child is left with little help to regulate emotions and create meaning out of the situation.

A group of authors who had proposed a developmental trauma disorder (DTD) diagnosis for children and adolescents in DSM-5 (van der Kolk et al. 2009) worry that children who have been chronically and repeatedly traumatized, abused, and/or neglected may not be diagnosed with PTSD because their symptoms are not detected or are not seen as a consequence of trauma and thus may receive potentially misleading diagnoses with the risk of receiving inappropriate interventions, such as medications for ADHD or psychotic disorders. DTD was proposed to include symptoms of affective and physiological dysregulation, attentional and behavioral dysregulation, and self- and relational dysregulation together with at least partial symptoms of PTSD. Clinicians working with children indicated in an international survey that the DTD criteria had clinical utility, and they were discriminable from PTSD and other internalizing and externalizing diagnoses (Ford et al. 2013). However, due to insufficient empirical support for the DTD construct at the time of revision of the classification system, the authors of the DSM-5 declined to include this disorder.

1.6 Attachment Disorders

> Peter is 3 years old. He was placed in foster care when he was 2 years old after being abandoned by his mother. When social services arrived at the home, Peter was sitting in his bed, and he did not respond to the social workers' attempt to make contact. His foster parents report that they find it difficult to bond with Peter. He does not seek comfort when he hurts himself, and he avoids any form of physical contact with them.

Absence of adequate caregiving in childhood is the common diagnostic requirement of both reactive attachment disorder and disinhibited social engagement disorder. They represent either rather internalizing or primarily externalizing symptom patterns that can be observed in children following severe social neglect. These disorders cannot be observed in adults, but they may be precursors of other chronic mental disorders in later life, such as conduct disorders or personality disorders. Former research based on observations in institutional care referred to these symptoms in hospitalized children also as hospitalization or anaclitic depression (Spitz 1945). More recently, in a follow-up observational study of former Romanian orphans, Rutter and colleagues (Roy et al. 2004; Rutter and Sonuga-Barke 2010) described persisting developmental and functional problems, among them, attachment problems. Attachment disorders were implemented in previous versions of the DSM and the ICD and are maintained unchanged in the DSM-5 and in the ICD-10. Both classification systems use quite similar definitions.

1.6.1 Reactive Attachment Disorder

Reactive attachment behavior reflects the lack of opportunity in young children to have basic emotional and social needs met and to form stable and selective relationships. It is characterized by deficits in requesting reactions and responding to caregivers, especially when distressed. Reactive attachment disorders refer to the failure of caregivers to meet the child-specific needs of having a secure relational basis (for detailed diagnostic criteria see Table 1.6).

Table 1.6 Definitions of reactive attachment disorder in the DSM-5 and the ICD-11

DSM-5	ICD-11
A. A consistent pattern of inhibited, emotionally withdrawn behavior toward adult caregivers, manifested by 　1. Rare or minimal seeking comfort when distressed 　2. Rare or minimal responding to comfort when distressed	Grossly abnormal attachment behaviors in early childhood, occurring in the context of a history of grossly inadequate child care (e.g., severe neglect, maltreatment, institutional deprivation). Even when an adequate primary caregiver is newly available, the child does not turn to the primary caregiver for comfort, support, and nurture, rarely displays security-seeking behaviors toward any adult, and does not respond when comfort is offered. Reactive attachment disorder can only be diagnosed in children, and features of the disorder develop within the first 5 years of life
B. A persistent social and emotional disturbance characterized by at least two of the following 　1. Minimal social and emotional responsiveness to others 　2. Limited positive affect 　3. Episodes of unexplained irritability, sadness, or fearfulness even during nonthreatening interactions with caregivers	
C. The child has experienced a pattern of extremes of insufficient care as evidenced by at least one of the following 　1. Social neglect or deprivation (lack of having basic emotional needs for comfort, stimulation, and affection met) 　2. Repeated changes of primary caregivers (limited opportunities to form stable attachments, e.g., frequent changes in foster care) 　3. Rearing in unusual settings (limited opportunities to form selective attachments, e.g., institutional care with high child-caregiver ratios)	
D. C is presumed responsible for A	
E. No autism	
F. Manifestation before age 5	
Specify: 　Persistent (>12 months) 　Severe (all symptoms high)	

1.6.2 Disinhibited Social Engagement Disorder

> Sara is 4 years old. Her mother has a long history of depression and was diagnosed with a postnatal depression after Sara was born. Sara's father suffers from alcohol dependence and has intermittent contact with Sara and her mother. Sara's preschool teachers are concerned because Sara runs up to other children's parents that she has never met before to give them hugs, and she often kisses them on the mouth. She also sits in their car and says she wants to go home with them. Parents have complained and don't want their children to be with Sara.

Table 1.7 Definitions of disinhibited social engagement disorder in the DSM-5 and the ICD-11

DSM-5	ICD-11
A. Actively approaching and interacting with unfamiliar adults, at least two of the following 1. Reduced or absent reticence 2. Overly familiar verbal or physical behavior 3. Diminished or absent checking back with adult caregiver when venturing away 4. Willingness to go off with unfamiliar adult	Grossly abnormal social behavior, occurring in the context of a history of grossly inadequate child care (e.g., severe neglect, institutional deprivation). The child approaches adults indiscriminately, lacks reticence to approach, will go away with unfamiliar adults, and exhibits overly familiar behavior toward strangers. Disinhibited social engagement disorder can only be diagnosed in children, and features of the disorder develop within the first 5 years of life
B. Behavior as described in A is not restricted to impulsivity (as in ADHD)	
C. The child has experienced a pattern of extremes and insufficient care (same details as in reactive attachment disorder)	
D. C is presumed responsible for A	
E. Developmental age >9 months	

The disinhibited social engagement disorder is also restricted to children. It describes a pattern of inappropriate, non-discriminant familiar social behavior when approaching adults, regardless whether they may be strangers or known to the child (see Table 1.7).

1.7 Prolonged Grief Disorder

> Paul was 13 when his twin brother committed suicide. Paul was the only other person at home and he was the person who found him. His brother was still alive at the time and Paul called the ambulance while he tried to keep his twin brother alive. Several months after the death, Paul still wakes up in the morning and plans to run into his brother's room like he always did and tell him to wake up. He just can't accept his brother is dead. He feels a part of him is gone and that life will never be the same. He thinks constantly about his brother and all the things they did together, but he avoids going to places they went to before he died and he changed schools. He has recurrent memories of the suicide and blames himself for not being able to save his brother's life. He avoids friends they had together and he is sure everyone blames him for what happened. He has trouble concentrating and is failing school.

Although there is much controversy in the field about how to define and understand certain grief responses, there is agreement that some children and adolescents will experience loss in the context of trauma or losses that they struggle to overcome (Kaplow et al. 2012; Nader and Salloum 2011). Particularly the loss of adult attachment figures is thought to be devastating for children. Common reactions to loss in children are symptoms of depression, anxiety, and PTSD, in addition to behavioral problems, substance abuse and somatic complaints. Studies indicate a shift from more anxiety-related symptoms for younger children to depressive symptoms in adolescents (Kaplow et al. 2012).

Children's adjustment after loss is closely related to their caretaking environment and how these facilitate mourning. On one hand, because of this close relationship between children's loss experiences and available social support, child researchers have argued that maladaptive grief could be placed within the adjustment disorders (Kaplow et al. 2012). On the other hand, adult bereavement researchers have argued for a separate bereavement-related disorder and refer to studies showing that many bereaved persons experience prolonged grief (Prigerson et al. 2009), or complicated grief (Shear 2011). Also some studies of bereaved children and adolescents complement the adult studies suggesting that prolonged grief represents some distinct features that separate them from PTSD or depression (Melhem et al. 2013; Melhem et al. 2007; Spuij et al. 2012). Such grief refers to intense yearning that persists longer than 6 months, difficulty accepting the death, anger over the loss, a diminished sense of one's identity, feeling that life is empty, and problems in engaging in new relations or activities. However, because of an overriding concern among the DSM-5 work group for pathologizing grief responses and on the basis of insufficient evidence to justify it as a separate diagnosis, it was transferred to the appendix.

In contrast to DSM-5, prolonged grief disorder is proposed as a new disorder in ICD-11. Prolonged grief refers to the persistence of grief that is longer than the normal grieving period in the culture the person belongs to and when symptoms interfere with one's capacity to function. The symptoms are related to severe and enduring yearning or longing for the deceased or a preoccupation with the deceased. The following associated features are mentioned: difficulty accepting the death, feelings of loss of a part of oneself, anger, guilt or blame, and difficulties in engaging in social activities due to the loss (Maercker et al. 2013b). The proposal will include the following developmental considerations: in children the loss of a primary attachment figure (e.g., parent, caregiver) may compound the grief response because the loss of caregiver compounds the sense of loss. Yearning may be expressed in play and behavior, including behaviors that involve separation themes.

> Proposed ICD-11 criteria for prolonged grief disorder
>
> 1. Experienced bereavement of close other person.
> 2. Severe yearning/emotional pain persisting for greater than 6 months since death.
> 3. Grief impedes normal functioning.
> 4. Grief reaction is beyond normative cultural/religious context. Associated features may include preoccupation with circumstances of death, bitterness about death, guilt, blame, difficulty accepting loss, reduced sense of self, oscillating between preoccupation and avoidance, difficulty progressing with activities or friendships, withdrawal, perception that life is meaningless, and emotional numbing.

1.8 Summary and Outlook

The current classification systems regarding trauma- and stressor-related diagnoses provide only few but nonetheless important categories exclusively considered for children and adolescents. Preschool PTSD as defined in the DSM-5, reactive attachment disorder, and disinhibited social disengagement disorder were defined for children who have experienced either traumatic events, persistent and serious failure of their caregivers, or interruptions of care respectively. In contrast, acute stress disorder, posttraumatic stress disorder beyond 6 years, and the recently defined prolonged grief disorder were created as diagnostic categories for adults and need some developmental adaptations when applied to children and adolescents. This leaves clinicians working with children with the challenge to observe behavioral equivalents of internal states, e.g., repetitive play or reenactment instead of flashbacks. It is especially urgent to adapt the adult-oriented diagnostic criteria for infants, toddlers, and preschool children and to consider the crucial role of their primary caregivers in helping them to cope with traumatic and stressful events and situations. As a guideline in child and adolescent psychotraumatology, it can be recommended to evaluate the impairment of functioning and development due to significant stress symptoms rather than the completeness of the full spectrum of symptoms as required for adults. So far, the DSM-5 provides some hints and examples for developmental modifications of diagnostic criteria of ASD and PTSD, whereas the proposed developmental modifications for the ICD-11 CPTSD and prolonged grief disorder will be studied and refined over time.

Whereas the DSM is the most influential classification system in research, the ICD becomes increasingly important worldwide as a diagnostic tool for clinicians. In many countries reimbursement of treatments is dependent of a diagnosis according to ICD. As we have to recognize growing inconsistencies between the definitions of trauma- and stressor-related disorders in the DSM versus the ICD, it is necessary to provide a clear reference to one of the major classification systems when reporting diagnoses. The classification systems have limited overlap between diagnostic categories despite the same diagnostic label. Due to different diagnostic thresholds for DSM-5 and ICD-11, decisions about treatment for individuals will not be managed by the same standards. Whereas researchers may rather prefer to use the DSM, clinicians may not have a choice to use DSM as an alternative classification system to the ICD. Due to the clinical importance of the ICD, it will be crucial to provide greater child-specific amendments in the future to guide clinicians when applying the new ICD-11 criteria to children and adolescents.

Consequences of the newly revised or proposed criteria for PTSD, complex PTSD, and prolonged grief disorder for the diagnosis of children and adolescents and for the prevalence of trauma- and stressor-related disorders in youth are not yet clear. Access of trauma-exposed children and adolescents to early trauma-focused interventions is extremely important as the detrimental effects of childhood adversities into adulthood are one of the major public health issues. Therefore, the detection of children and adolescents in need for treatment requires appropriate and sensitive diagnostic criteria and thresholds. The effects of changes of the diagnostic criteria should be tested in field studies with children and adolescents before the implementation of new versions. New diagnoses or new subtypes of diagnoses may be introduced if there is evidence that they require different treatments than the already established ones.

Whether the new classifications of PTSD according to the DSM-5 and ICD-11 with or without dissociation or complex PTSD according to ICD-11 will be useful diagnoses for traumatized children and adolescents is currently an open question due to the limited literature. The development or revisions of now outdated assessment instruments are necessary to capture the new formulations of PTSD. For non-specialized clinicians comprehensive diagnostic entities with 12 symptoms such as in the ICD-11 complex PTSD or 20 symptoms such as in the DSM-5 PTSD may appear too difficult, especially if modifications of criteria for children are needed. Therefore, it will be important to investigate the feasibility and utility of the six-item PTSD as proposed for the ICD-11 in children and adolescents.

More epidemiological and clinical research with trauma- and stressor-exposed children and adolescents is needed to determine the validity of the current and the newly proposed diagnostic criteria across different age groups and across different trauma types. Empirical approaches and especially thorough behavioral observations across youth populations that have been exposed to different potentially traumatic or stressful events at different ages may help to better determine and differentiate acute and chronic patterns of trauma- and stressor-related symptoms and their clinical significance in children and adolescents. Given their high adaptability and neuronal plasticity, future diagnostic categories for children and adolescents may need to consider repeated assessments over periods of adaptation rather than one comprehensive clinical evaluation at only one time point. The course of symptoms over time may be more important to indicate interventions than single assessments. More emphasis has to be put onto the development of operational diagnostic criteria for children and adolescents and age-appropriate assessment instruments. No classification systems can fully capture the range of human response, and diagnosing children and adolescents requires careful consideration of developmental and environmental aspects of the child's life.

References

American Psychiatric Association (2013) Diagnostic and statistical manual of mental disorders, 5 edn. American Psychiatric Publishing, Arlington

Benedek E (1985) Children and psychic trauma: a brief review of contemporary thinking. In: Eth S, Pynoos RS (eds) Posttraumatic stress disorder in children. American Psychiatric Press, Washington, DC, pp. 3–16

Brewin CR (2013) "I wouldn't start from here"–an alternative perspective on PTSD from the ICD-11: comment on Friedman (2013). J Trauma Stress 26:557–559

Brewin CR, Lanius RA, Novac A, Schnyder U, Galea S (2009) Reformulating PTSD for DSM-V: life after criterion A. J Trauma Stress 22:366–373

Carrion VG, Weems CF, Ray R, Reiss AL (2002) Toward an empirical definition of pediatric PTSD: the phenomenology of PTSD symptoms in youth. J Am Acad Child Adolesc Psychiatry 41:166–173

Cloitre M (2016) Personal communication

Cloitre M, Stolbach BC, Herman JL, Kolk BV, Pynoos R, Wang J et al (2009) A developmental approach to complex PTSD: childhood and adult cumulative trauma as predictors of symptom complexity. J Trauma Stress 22(5):399–408

Cloitre M, Garvert DW, Brewin CR, Bryant RA, Maercker A (2013) Evidence for proposed ICD-11 PTSD and complex PTSD: a latent profile analysis. Eur J Psychotraumatol 2013 May 15; 4. doi: 10.3402/ejpt.v4i0.207064.

Cohen JA, Scheeringa MS (2009) Post-traumatic stress disorder diagnosis in children: challenges and promises. Dialogues Clin Neurosci 11:91–99

Cohen J, Mannarino A, Kliethermen M, Murray L (2012) Trauma-focused CBT for youth with complex PTSD. Child Abuse Negl 36:528–541

De Bellis MD (2001) Developmental traumatology: the psychobiological development of maltreated children and its implications for research, treatment, and policy. Dev Psychopathol 13:539–564

De Young AC, Kenardy JA, Cobham VE (2011) Diagnosis of posttraumatic stress disorder in preschool children. J Clin Child Adolesc Psychol 40:375–384

Elhai JD, Palmieri PA (2011) The factor structure of posttraumatic stress disorder: a literature update, critique of methodology, and agenda for future research. J Anxiety Disord 25:849–854

Elklit A, Hyland P, Shevlin M (2014) Evidence of symptom profiles consistent with posttraumatic stress disorder and complex posttraumatic stress disorder in different trauma samples. Eur J Psychotraumatol 5

First MB, Reed GM, Hyman SE, Saxena S (2015) The development of the ICD-11 clinical descriptions and diagnostic guidelines for mental and behavioural disorders. World Psychiatry 14:82–90

Ford JD, Grasso D, Greene C, Levine J, Spinazzola J, van der Kolk B (2013) Clinical significance of a proposed developmental trauma disorder diagnosis: results of an international survey of clinicians. J Clin Psychiatry 74:841–849

Friedman MJ (2013) Finalizing PTSD in DSM-5: getting here from there and where to go next. J Trauma Stress 26:548–556

Friedman MJ (2014) Literature on DSM-5 and ICD-11. PTSD Res Q Adv Sci Promot Under Traum Stress 25:1–10

Galatzer-Levy IR, Bryant RA (2013) 636,120 ways to have posttraumatic stress disorder. Perspect Psychol Sci 8:651–662

Garmezy N, Rutter M (1985) Acute reactions to stress. In: Rutter M, Hersov L (eds) Child and adolescent psychiatry: modern approaches, 2 edn. Blackwell, Oxford, pp. 152–176

Goenjian AK, Pynoos RS, Steinberg AM, Najarian LM, Asarnow JR, Karayan I et al (1995) Psychiatric comorbidity in children after the 1988 earthquake in Armenia. J Am Acad Child Adolesc Psychiatry 34:1174–1184

Hafstad GS, Dyb G, Jensen TK, Steinberg AM, Pynoos RS (2014) PTSD prevalence and symptom structure of DSM-5 criteria in adolescents and young adults surviving the 2011 shooting in Norway. J Affect Disord 169:40–46

Haravouori H, Kviiuusu O, Suomalainen L, Marttunen M (2016) An evaluation of ICD-11 post-traumatic stress disorder criteria in two samples of adolescents and young adults exposed to mass shootings: factor analysis and comparisons to ICD-10 and DSM-IV. BMC Psychiatry 16:140

Herman JL (1992) Complex PTSD: a syndrome in survivors of prolonged and repeated trauma. J Trauma Stress 5:377–391

Kaplow JB, Layne CM, Pynoos RS, Cohen JA, Lieberman A (2012) DSM-V diagnostic criteria for bereavement-related disorders in children and adolescents: developmental considerations. Psychiatry 75:243–266

Kassam-Adams N, Winston FK (2004) Predicting child PTSD: the relationship between acute stress disorder and PTSD in injured children. J Am Acad Child Adolesc Psychiatry 43:403–411

Kassam-Adams N, Palmieri PA, Rork K, Delahanty DL, Kenardy J, Kohser KL et al (2012) Acute stress symptoms in children: results from an international data archive. J Am Acad Child Adolesc Psychiatry 51:812–820

Keane TM, Kaloupek DG (1997) Comorbid psychiatric disorders in PTSD. Implications for research. Ann N Y Acad Sci 821:24–34

Kelleher I, Keeley H, Corcoran P, Ramsay H, Wasserman C, Carli V et al (2013) Childhood trauma and psychosis in a prospective cohort study: cause, effect, and directionality. Am J Psychiatry 170:734–741

La Greca AM (2007) Posttraumatic stress disorder in children. In: Fink G (ed) Encyclopedia of stress, 2 edn. Academic Press, New York, pp. 145–149

Lipschitz DS, Winegar RK, Hartnick E, Foote B, Southwick SM (1999) Posttraumatic stress disorder in hospitalized adolescents: psychiatric comorbidity and clinical correlates. J Am Acad Child Adolesc Psychiatry 38:385–392

Liu L, Wang L, Cao C, Qing Y, Armour C (2016) Testing the dimensional structure of DSM-5 posttraumatic stress disorder symptoms in a nonclinical trauma-exposed adolescent sample. J Child Psychol Psychiatry 57:204–212

Maercker A, Brewin CR, Bryant RA, Cloitre M, Reed GM, van Ommeren M et al (2013a) Proposals for mental disorders specifically associated with stress in the International Classification of Disease-11. Lancet 11. doi:10.1016/S0140-6736(12)62191-6

Maercker A, Brewin CR, Bryant RA, Cloitre M, van Ommeren M, Jones LM et al (2013b) Diagnosis and classification of disorders specifically associated with stress: proposals for ICD-11. World Psychiatry 12:198–206

Meiser-Stedman R, Smith P, Glucksman E, Yule W, Dalgleish T (2008) The posttraumatic stress disorder diagnosis in preschool- and elementary school-age children exposed to motor vehicle accidents. Am J Psychiatry 165:1326–1337

Melhem NM, Moritz G, Walker M, Shear MK, Brent D (2007) Phenomenology and correlates of complicated grief in children and adolescents. J Am Acad Child Adolesc Psychiatry 46:493–499

Melhem NM, Porta G, Walker PM, Brent DA (2013) Identifying prolonged grief reactions in children: dimensional and diagnostic approaches. J Am Acad Child Adolesc Psychiatry 52:599–607

Nader K, Salloum A (2011) Complicated grief reactions in children and adolescents. J Child Adolesc Trauma 4:233–257

Nooner KB, Linares LO, Batinjane J, Kramer RA, Silva R, Cloitre M (2012) Factors related to posttraumatic stress disorder in adolescence. Trauma Violence Abuse 13:153–166

Norris FH, Friedman MJ, Watson PJ (2002) 60,000 disaster victims speak: part II. Summary and implications of the disaster mental health research. Psychiatry 65:240–260

Perkonigg A, Hofler M, Cloitre M, Wittchen HU, Trautmann S, Maercker A (2016) Evidence for two different ICD-11 posttraumatic stress disorders in a community sample of adolescents and young adults. Eur Arch Psychiatry Clin Neurosci 266:317–328

Prigerson HG, Horowitz MJ, Jacobs SC, Parkes CM, Aslan M, Goodkin K et al (2009) Prolonged grief disorder: psychometric validation of criteria proposed for DSM-V and ICD-11. PLoS Med 6:e1000121

Putnam FW (2006) The impact of trauma on child development. Juv Fam Court J 52:1–11

Pynoos RS, Steinberg AM, Piacentini JC (1999) A developmental psychopathology model of childhood traumatic stress and intersection with anxiety disorders. Biol Psychiatry 46:1542–1554

Pynoos RS, Steinberg AM, Layne CM, Briggs EC, Ostrowski SA, Fairbank JA (2009) DSM-V PTSD diagnostic criteria for children and adolescents: a developmental perspective and recommendations. J Trauma Stress 22:391–398

Resick PA, Bovin MJ, Calloway AL, Dick AM, King MW, Mitchell KS et al (2012) A critical evaluation of the complex PTSD literature: implications for DSM-5. J Trauma Stress 25:241–251

Roy P, Rutter M, Pickles A (2004) Institutional care: associations between overactivity and lack of selectivity in social relationships. J Child Psychol Psychiatry 45(4):866–873

Rutter M, Sonuga-Barke EJ (2010) X. Conclusions: overview of findings from the era study, inferences, and research implications. Monogr Soc Res Child Dev 75:212–229

Sachser C, Goldbeck L (2016) Consequences of the diagnostic criteria proposed for the ICD-11 on the prevalence of PTSD in children and adolescents. J Trauma Stress 29:120–123

Scheeringa MS, Zeanah CH, Drell MJ, Larrieu JA (1995) Two approaches to the diagnosis of posttraumatic stress disorder in infancy and early childhood. J Am Acad Child Adolesc Psychiatry 34:191–200

Scheeringa M, Zeanah C, Myers L, Putnam F (2003) New findings on alternative criteria for PTSD in preschool children. J Am Acad Child Adolesc Psychiatry 42:561–570

Scheeringa MS, Zeanah CH, Cohen JA (2011) PTSD in children and adolescents: toward an empirically based algorithm. Depress Anxiety 28:770–782

Scheeringa MS, Myers L, Putnam FW, Zeanah CH (2012) Diagnosing PTSD in early childhood: an empirical assessment of four approaches. J Trauma Stress 25:359–367

Schmid M, Petermann F, Fegert JM (2013) Developmental trauma disorder: pros and cons of including formal criteria in the psychiatric diagnostic systems. BMC Psychiatry 13:3

Shear MK (2011) Bereavement and the DSM5. Omega (Westport) 64:101–118

Smith P, Perrin S, Yule W, Clark DM (2009) Post traumatic stress disorder: cognitive therapy with children and young people. Routledge Chapman & Hall, East Sussex

Spitz RA (1945) Hospitalism: an inquiry into the genesis of psychiatric conditions in early childhood. Psychoanal Study Child 1:53–74

Spuij M, Reitz E, Prinzie P, Stikkelbroek Y, de RC, Boelen PA (2012) Distinctiveness of symptoms of prolonged grief, depression, and post-traumatic stress in bereaved children and adolescents. Eur Child Adolesc Psychiatry 21:673–679

Stein MB, Walker JR, Hazen AL, Forde DR (1997) Full and partial posttraumatic stress disorder: findings from a community survey. Am J Psychiatry 154:1114–1119

Straussner SLA, Calnan AJ (2014) Trauma through the life cycle: a review of current literature. Clin Soc Work J 42:323–335

Teicher MH, Samson JA (2016) Annual research review: enduring neurobiological effects of childhood abuse and neglect. J Child Psychol Psychiatry 57(3):241–266

Terr LC (1983) Chowchilla revisited: the effects of psychic trauma four years after a school-bus kidnapping. Am J Psychiatry 140:1543–1550

van der Kolk B, Pynoos R, Cicchetti D, Cloitre M (2009) [Developmental trauma disorder: towards a rational diagnosis for chronically traumatized children]. Prax Kinderpsychol Kinderpsychiatr. 2009;58:572–586. German.

Wisco BE, Miller MW, Wolf EJ, Kilpatrick D, Resnick HS, Badour CL et al (2016) The impact of proposed changes to ICD-11 on estimates of PTSD prevalence and comorbidity. Psychiatry Res 240:226–233

Yule W, Udwin O (1991) Screening child survivors for post-traumatic stress disorders: experiences from the 'Jupiter' sinking. Br J Clin Psychol 30:131–138

Epidemiology of Trauma and Trauma-Related Disorders in Children and Adolescents

Shaminka Gunaratnam and Eva Alisic

How many children and adolescents are exposed to potentially traumatic events (PTEs)? Is exposure a random phenomenon or can we identify specific risk factors? Similarly, how many and which children and adolescents develop trauma-related disorders? The present chapter gives an overview of the current evidence base regarding exposure to PTEs, acute stress disorder (ASD), post-traumatic stress disorder (PTSD) and related predictors. The updated PTSD criteria in the *Diagnostic and Statistical Manual of Mental Disorders* (5th ed.; *DSM-5*; American Psychiatric Association [APA] 2013) include mood and cognitive symptoms and a new preschool subtype which will likely increase prevalence rates of these disorders for preschool-aged children compared to the *DSM-IV* (APA 2000). In general, only a small proportion of children and adolescents faced with a similar type of exposure develop high levels of symptoms or disorders. Therefore, consideration of potential demographic, biological, cognitive and family or environment predictors are important to help guide prevention, screening, assessment and intervention efforts. We also discuss methodological differences among studies that may affect empirical findings.

2.1 Exposure to Potentially Traumatic Events

2.1.1 Estimates of Exposure

Exposure to PTEs is common in children and adolescents. By the time young people reach their 18th birthday, many have faced the loss of a loved one, a serious accident, violence or other type of trauma. General population studies in the

---

S. Gunaratnam • E. Alisic (✉)
Trauma Recovery Lab, Monash University Accident Research Centre, Melbourne, Australia
e-mail: shaminka.gunaratnam@monash.edu; eva.alisic@monash.edu

USA have found particularly high rates of exposure. For example, Copeland et al. (2007) reported that 68 % of adolescents in a large population sample had been exposed, about half of whom reported two or more events. These findings are similar to a recent study by McLaughlin et al. (2013) in which 62 % of over 6,000 American adolescents reported exposure. Again, about half of the exposed adolescents had been confronted with more than one event. Both American studies used the *DSM-IV* A1 criterion of objective exposure. A recent population study with Swiss adolescents reported around 56 % of adolescents reported at least one PTE (Landolt et al. 2013), a figure that is akin to US samples, likely due to a large proportion of migrants in the Swiss study. Most population studies focus on adolescents: population studies among primary school children are fairly rare. One such study in the Netherlands reported an exposure rate of 15 % (Alisic et al. 2008), suggesting that trauma is also a common experience in earlier childhood.

Studies that assessed exposure beyond *DSM-IV* A1 criterion events, including experiences such as divorce of parents and bullying, found high rates among young people. In Denmark, 78 % of a student sample reported exposure to at least one distressing or traumatic event (Elklit and Frandsen 2014; N=1088, age range=15–20 years), with approximately 60 % of the exposed students reporting two or more. Similar and even higher rates were reported for adolescents in Malaysia (78 %; Ghazali et al. 2014), Greenland (86 %; Karsberg et al. 2012) and Kenya (95 %; Karsberg and Elklit 2012).

In sum, around one in two adolescents report lifetime exposure to at least one PTE according to *DSM-IV*, with lower figures reported for younger children. However, a greater emphasis on developing nations in the literature is warranted. For example, 87 % of the peer-reviewed articles on traumatic stress published in 2012 regarded high-income countries and 51 % of all papers described studies in the USA (Fodor et al. 2014). By contrast, trauma exposure in developing nations tends to be substantially more common compared to developed countries (e.g. Karsberg and Elklit 2012), lending weight to the importance of these oft-overlooked nations. Refugee youth are a particularly under-researched heterogeneous minority. The next few paragraphs discuss specific types of events that children and adolescents are exposed to.

2.1.1.1 Exposure to the Sudden Loss of a Loved One

In the studies among adolescents in the USA (McLaughlin et al. 2013) and Switzerland (Landolt et al. 2013) and the study among primary school children in the Netherlands (Alisic et al. 2008), the most frequently reported trauma was the sudden loss of a loved one. In particular, the death of a parent or a sibling is one of the most stressful life events that a child or adolescent can experience (Melhem et al. 2011). In the study by McLaughlin et al. (2013), 28 % of the sample lost a loved one. Strictly speaking, not all of the deaths would meet the *DSM-5* stressor criteria, since some of these may not have been sudden or violent (but instead, after a long period of illness).

2.1.1.2 Exposure to Injury

Serious accidental injury is the global leading cause of death in the 10–19-year-old age bracket (World Health Organization (WHO) 2014). As is often mentioned, this is only the "tip of the iceberg", with millions of children who are not fatally but seriously injured every year. Injuries in children most commonly occur due to motor vehicle accidents, drowning, burns and falls (WHO 2014). Motor vehicle accidents tend to be some of the most common PTEs overall (Elklit and Frandsen 2014; Ghazali et al. 2014).

While not all injuries would be considered serious or traumatic, those that warrant a hospital visit longer than 24 hours are often placed into this category (e.g. Olsson et al. 2008). Nevertheless, children may also experience trauma symptoms following an event that leads to an emergency department visit without subsequent hospitalisation (Bryant et al. 2004). For example, involvement in a motor vehicle accident without serious injury can be traumatic due to the perceived threat to life (Meiser-Stedman et al. 2008). In addition, invasive medical procedures are relatively common and may be experienced as traumatic, particularly when life-threatening (Marsac et al. 2014).

2.1.1.3 Exposure to Violence

Rates of exposure to violence are likely underestimated due to under-reporting of physical and especially sexual trauma (Saunders and Adams 2014). With this in mind, witnessing and experiencing violence and abuse are probably fairly common (Elklit and Frandsen 2014; Mohler-Kuo et al. 2014). Finkelhor et al. (2015) found that of 4000 US children and adolescents, 1.4 % had been sexually assaulted, 5 % had been physically abused, 15.2 % had suffered any type of maltreatment and 24.5 % had witnessed violence in the past year. Given that assault and abuse exposure increases with age (Finkelhor et al. 2015; Saunders and Adams 2014), the large age range in this study may have diluted findings for the adolescent age group. Relatively little is known about prevalence in different countries, which is likely to vary as for young females (aged 15–19 years), rates of physical or sexual intimate partner violence were 36.6 % in Johannesburg, South Africa, 32.8 % in Ibadan, Nigeria, 27.7 % in Baltimore, USA, 19.4 % in Delhi, India and 10.2 % in Shanghai, China (Decker et al. 2014). Considering contact or non-contact sexual abuse alone, a Swiss population study with adolescents showed that 40.2 % of girls and 17.2 % of boys reported at least one incident (Mohler-Kuo et al. 2014), highlighting its high frequency among adolescents, particularly females.

2.1.1.4 Exposure to Mass Trauma

Rates of exposure to natural disasters, terrorism and war differ from other forms of trauma as they are location specific. In many cases, countries with the fewest resources are hit the hardest (Neuner et al. 2006).While it is apparent that exposure to disaster, terrorism and mass conflict depend on geography and proximity to an event, mass trauma research often arises from high-income countries that are less prone to these disasters compared to low- and middle-income countries. In the

USA, rates of exposure to disasters ranged from 11.1 (Copeland et al. 2007) to 14.8 % (McLaughlin et al. 2013) in the general population. By contrast, the 2010 earthquake in Haiti was labelled "acute on chronic trauma", given the existing systemic issues in the country and high rates of pre-existing trauma exposure (Gabrielli et al. 2014). Research in low- and middle-income countries post-trauma tends to lack baseline data, making population estimates of trauma exposure difficult to determine.

2.1.2 Predictors of Exposure

2.1.2.1 Demographic Predictors

Exposure to trauma is related to age. Older children and adolescents have had more time available for PTEs to occur (Copeland et al. 2007; Finkelhor et al. 2009) than younger children. In addition, mobility (Haller and Chassin 2012), sexual activity and in some cases risk taking (Forgey and Bursch 2013) increase with age, leading to a greater likelihood of trauma exposure. However, the type of PTEs experienced may differ across stages of development. For example, burn injuries are more prevalent in younger children (Stoddard et al. 2006), while risk of sexual trauma is higher for older children (Finkelhor et al. 2015).

It is unclear whether, overall, boys are more exposed to trauma than girls. While several recent studies have found such an effect (Elklit and Frandsen 2014; Haller and Chassin 2012; Karsberg and Elklit 2012; c.f. Karsberg et al. 2012), a few did not (Ghazali et al. 2014; Landolt et al. 2013; Salazar et al. 2013). However, there appear to be differences according to the type of trauma. Particularly, boys are more likely to be exposed to non-sexual violence (Atwoli et al. 2014; Finkelhor et al. 2015; Karsberg and Elklit 2012; McLaughlin et al. 2013; Salazar et al. 2013; Zona and Milan 2011) and accidental injury (e.g. Landolt et al. 2013; McLaughlin et al. 2013). The reason may be higher levels of externalising behaviour in boys compared to girls (Lalloo et al. 2003). For sexual trauma, the opposite gender difference has been found (e.g. Finkelhor et al. 2015; Landolt et al. 2013; McLaughlin et al. 2013; Salazar et al. 2013).

As mentioned above, while trauma occurs everywhere, exposure rates are related to geography. Within countries, differences in trauma exposure may be better explained by demographic characteristics such as minority status, nativity, parental education, poverty and justice system involvement than ethnicity per se (e.g. Landolt et al. 2013; McLaughlin et al. 2013; Milan et al. 2013).

2.1.2.2 Behavioural Predictors

Intuitively, children who engage in more externalising behaviour put themselves at greater risk of accidents (Lalloo et al. 2003). Additionally, poor sleep in young children may precipitate externalising behaviour and subsequent injury (Owens et al. 2005). More generally, behaviour disorders have been linked to a higher likelihood of trauma exposure in US adolescents (McLaughlin et al. 2013). Behaviour problems may have differing consequences in boys and girls (e.g. Haller and Chassin

2012; Zona and Milan 2011). For example, in males, but not females, internalising symptoms were protective against assaultive violence exposure (Haller and Chassin 2012). The authors suggested that socially withdrawn males may be less likely to engage in aggressive behaviour or to expose themselves to others engaging in such behaviour, thereby protecting them from violent trauma exposure to some extent.

2.1.2.3 Family and Social Environment Predictors

Poverty and the home environment can set a backdrop upon which trauma exposure is more likely. In lower socio-economic status (SES) households, there is often less supervision of children and consequently higher risk of trauma exposure (e.g. Morrongiello and House 2004). The mental health of family members and past parenting problems can also confer risk of trauma exposure (Copeland et al. 2007), and physical and sexual abuse often occur within the home environment (Landolt et al. 2013). Externalising problems are also more common in lower SES and single-/step-parent households (Lalloo et al. 2003; Landolt et al. 2013; McLaughlin 2013).

Looking at children and adolescents' broader context, belonging to a "deviant" peer group, may increase the risk of violence exposure in adolescents (Milan et al. 2013). In another study on environmental factors, physical and sexual abuse was highest in street children compared to households and orphanages, (Atwoli et al. 2014) as a lack of permanent address and safe place to sleep may leave these children more vulnerable. Living in the city may confer risk for particular traumas like assault-related injury (Irie et al. 2012), physical violence, robbery and being threatened with a weapon (Elklit and Frandsen 2014). Importantly, prior exposure to violence can predict future violence exposure, as one type of violence exposure increases the chances of experiencing other types of violence (Finkelhor et al. 2015; Milan et al. 2013).

2.1.3 Methodological Considerations

While it is clear that a substantial proportion of young people are exposed to (potential) trauma during their childhood, the risk of exposure is difficult to disentangle from definitions of what constitutes a PTE, assessment methodology and sample characteristics. Some studies used definitions of trauma that were broader than the *DSM-5* stipulates (e.g. Karsberg et al. 2012 included divorce and unplanned pregnancy). Therefore, comparisons across countries and studies are to be made with caution. As mentioned earlier, the geographical location of a study makes a difference, in terms of rates of exposure and potential predictors. In addition, the extent to which exposure is measured appears to play a role. For example, Copeland et al. (2007) reported substantially higher rates of exposure based on repeated assessments with the adolescents in their sample, than they would have based on a single assessment. The same is likely to apply to children.

Study methodology may also influence outcomes in other ways. For example, it is common for parents to report on trauma exposure on behalf of their young children. However, parent and child reports can conflict and may be subject to memory failures, mental health of the informant or a lack of knowledge, for example, if the primary caregiver was not present during exposure (Finkelhor et al. 2015). This effect may be more pronounced as a child ages (Saunders and Adams 2014). In self-report of exposure on the other hand, some memories may not be adequately salient to be recalled over time, or distressing memories may even be repressed (Finkelhor et al. 2009) or recalled more easily. Mandatory reporting of abuse by professionals in many countries may decrease willingness to disclose violence and abuse to researchers and clinicians (Copeland et al. 2007). In addition, cultural understandings of what constitutes trauma, in particular violence, may affect reporting (Saunders and Adams 2014). Finally, there is a need to replicate studies across a number of different regions and trauma types to gain a broader picture of trauma exposure across the globe.

2.2 Acute Stress Disorder

2.2.1 Prevalence Estimates of Acute Stress Disorder

Acute stress disorder (ASD) is the main trauma-related disorder diagnosed in the almost immediate aftermath of exposure. It signifies the experience of severe stress reactions in the first few weeks after the trauma. Our knowledge of ASD among children and adolescents is relatively limited, since research on this trauma-related disorder is not as plentiful as research on PTSD. According to *DSM-5* it requires identification and assessment of survivors within a month after exposure, which is not always feasible, either because the trauma is not detected (e.g. in the case of violence) or because the resources are not available (e.g. after a mass-scale trauma). The majority of currently available studies are hospital-based and regard injury, sometimes in the context of a natural disaster or abuse. Most are based on the *DSM-IV* criteria. Overall, ASD rates among exposed children and adolescents appear to vary from about 5 % (e.g. Ellis et al. 2009) to around 50 % (e.g. Liu et al. 2010). Dalgleish et al. (2008) combined the data of 367 road accident survivors (6–17 years old) and found that 9 % of them met criteria for ASD, with a further 23 % meeting criteria for subthreshold ASD. The most robust evidence comes from aggregated data from 15 studies involving 1,645 children and adolescents in four high-income countries (USA, Australia, UK and Switzerland; Kassam-Adams et al. 2012). The authors studied the proposed *DSM-5* criteria and found that 41 % of the children and adolescents reported clinically relevant impairment. Each ASD symptom was endorsed by 14–51 % of the sample. While the *DSM-5* eventually required nine symptoms for ASD criteria to be met, at the time of the study this was eight symptoms. This requirement was met by 12 % of the children and adolescents. It did not predict concurrent impairment very well. The authors found that requiring only three to four symptoms substantially improved sensitivity while maintaining moderate specificity.

2.2.2 Predictors of Acute Stress Disorder

2.2.2.1 Demographic Predictors

Age, gender and ethnicity are easily identifiable characteristics that would be useful in identifying youth in need of intervention and treatment in the direct aftermath of trauma. However, demographic characteristics have produced mixed results in predicting ASD, and because only a small number of studies have been conducted so far, conclusions are somewhat hard to reach.

Concerning age, some studies have found that young children have an elevated risk of ASD (Doron-LaMarca et al. 2010; Le Brocque et al. 2010; Saxe et al. 2005a) and may have more severe ASD (McKinnon et al. 2008). Le Brocque et al. (2010) found that younger children were more likely to have high levels of symptoms immediately post-trauma but recovered quickly. Still, other studies have not found evidence of age as a predictor of acute stress (e.g. Bryant et al. 2004; Daviss et al. 2000; Haag et al. 2015; Ostrowski et al. 2011).

Whenever a gender difference in ASD has been found, girls have been at higher risk than boys (Bryant et al. 2004; Doron-LaMarca et al. 2010; Haag et al. 2015; Holbrook et al. 2005; Karabekiroglu et al. 2008; Liu et al. 2010). Yet, it remains unclear what factors may interact with female gender to produce these findings in some studies and not others (e.g. Daviss et al. 2000; Ellis et al. 2009).

Ethnicity has not been studied as extensively as age or gender. So far, there is a lack of support for the role of race or ethnicity in predicting ASD (e.g. Ostrowski et al. 2011). Further, with respect to SES, parental income has not predicted acute stress either (Ostrowski et al. 2011).

2.2.2.2 Exposure Characteristics as Predictors

There is some evidence to suggest a "dose-response relationship" whereby a greater extent of exposure is related to higher risk of acute trauma symptoms. For example, after an earthquake ASD was more common in bereaved children and those whose residence had been damaged, compared to those who did not suffer a loss or were further away from the earthquake (Demir et al. 2010). It has further been suggested that disasters in less well-resourced areas are generally more traumatic due to a lack of infrastructure and therefore greater secondary traumas, death and general distress (Demir et al. 2010).

Injury characteristics may predict ASD in children. For example, among those exposed to a motor vehicle accident, children with injuries who sought medical assistance were at a greater risk of ASD than those who did not (Winston et al. 2005). Additionally, experiencing pain following injury predicted ASD symptoms in children (McKinnon et al. 2008; Saxe et al. 2005a). Yet, injury severity itself does not appear to predict ASD (Bryant et al. 2004; Daviss et al. 2000; Haag et al. 2015; Ostrowski et al. 2011) nor does hospitalisation after a motor vehicle accident (Bryant et al. 2004). For children with burns, burn size was a risk factor for ASD only by its association with increased parental ASD and elevated heart rate (Saxe et al. 2005b).

ASD appears more likely in violently injured youth compared to those with unintentional injuries or medical illnesses (Hamrin et al. 2004; Holbrook et al. 2005; c.f. Meiser-Stedman et al. 2005). These findings lend support to the idea that intentional traumas are more difficult to cope with than unintentional traumas.

2.2.2.3 Cognitive and Emotion-Related Predictors

ASD has been associated with negative cognitive appraisals about the experienced trauma and perceived threat of serious injury (Ellis et al. 2009). Specifically, ASD is more likely when the child perceives that they are going to die during the trauma (Ellis et al. 2009; Holbrook et al. 2005) or that they are vulnerable to consequent harm (Salmon et al. 2007). The role of cognitions may differ depending on age (Salmon et al. 2007) and injury type. For children with burns, a positive body image despite the injury was a protective factor (Saxe et al. 2005b). Data-driven processing of the perceptual and physical aspects of the trauma, self-reported memory quality and peri-traumatic fear was also associated with ASD in injured children (McKinnon et al. 2008). In addition, peri-traumatic guilt has predicted ASD in children following motor vehicle accidents (Haag et al. 2015).

2.2.2.4 Biological Predictors

Biological predictors of ASD have only been studied sporadically. Elevated heart rate appears to be a risk factor for ASD in children with burns (Saxe et al. 2005b), and average heart rate mediated the relationship between burn size and ASD symptoms (Stoddard et al. 2006).

2.2.2.5 Behavioural Predictors

Pre-existing internalising and externalising behaviours may precipitate acute stress following an injury (Daviss et al. 2000). However, in another study, only higher pre-injury externalising scores predicted initial trauma symptoms in injured children and adolescents, while internalising scores did not (Doron-LaMarca et al. 2010). In the latter study, gender interacted with behaviour such that females with higher externalising scores experienced more symptoms than males with externalising behaviours (Doron-LaMarca et al. 2010).

2.2.2.6 Family and Social Environment Predictors

Caregiver and general family stress have presented as a risk factor for child ASD following injury (Daviss et al. 2000; Haag et al. 2015; Saxe et al. 2005a, b). In a study of survivors of assaults and motor vehicle accidents, both parental depression and parental worrying were associated with child acute trauma symptoms (Meiser-Stedman et al. 2006). While social support more broadly has been found to be protective against PTSD in children (Langley et al. 2013), it does not appear to hinder initial ASD development (Ellis et al. 2009); potentially, social support takes some time to have an effect post-trauma.

2.2.3 Methodological Considerations

Parent and child reports of ASD symptoms can differ (Kassam-Adams et al. 2006; Meiser-Stedman et al. 2007, 2008), with internal experiences and symptoms likely being more difficult for parents to estimate (Doron-LaMarca et al. 2010; c.f. Meiser-Stedman et al. 2007). Given the finding that parental ASD and child ASD are related, it is possible that parents with ASD rate their child's symptoms as more severe (Daviss et al. 2000; Haag et al. 2015) or, conversely, normalise acute responses (Meiser-Stedman et al. 2007). Therefore, studies involving both parent and child reports are likely to elicit more accurate estimates of the child's acute response to trauma.

As mentioned before, the study of ASD in children and adolescents is relatively new. Early studies did not use proper screening measures for children as they had not yet been developed (e.g. Hamrin et al. 2004) and some have used PTSD criteria within 1 month of the trauma (e.g. Karabekiroglu et al. 2008; Ostrowski et al. 2011). Despite ASD criteria being present in *DSM-IV* and *DSM-5*, studies have used varying combinations of "subthreshold" symptomatology to derive a measure of general acute stress (e.g. Meiser-Stedman et al. 2005). Particularly, criticism of the dissociative criterion led studies to use a variety of definitions of ASD. Now that dissociation is no longer a necessary criterion, the new *DSM-5* criteria may unite these definitions (see Chap. 1).

2.3 Post-traumatic Stress Disorder

2.3.1 Prevalence Estimates of Post-traumatic Stress Disorder

Post-traumatic stress disorder (PTSD) is the predominant mental health problem taken into consideration after trauma exposure in children and adolescents. Rates of PTSD among youth who have been confronted with a PTE have varied considerably in previous studies. The most robust information on the conditional risk for PTSD after trauma among children and adolescents comes from a meta-analysis that combines information of studies among 3,563 children who had been assessed with well-established diagnostic interviews. The overall rate of PTSD was 16 % (Alisic et al. 2014). Children and adolescents do not randomly experience posttraumatic stress after exposure: specific groups of children appear to be more at risk than others (Alisic et al. 2011; Cox et al. 2008; Kahana et al. 2006; Trickey et al. 2012).

2.3.2 Predictors of Post-traumatic Stress Disorder

2.3.2.1 Demographic Predictors
Gender differences have been reported quite consistently for PTSD, with higher prevalence rates for girls than boys (e.g. Elklit and Frandsen 2014; Haller and Chassin 2012; Karabekiroglu et al. 2008; Karsberg and Elklit 2012; Landolt et al.

2013; Lavi et al. 2013; McLaughlin et al. 2013). There have been a few exceptions, where no gender differences were found (e.g. Ghazali et al. 2014; Milan et al. 2013), but, overall, meta-analyses indicate a gender difference with girls being more prone to PTSD than boys (Alisic et al. 2011, 2014; Cox et al. 2008; Trickey et al. 2012). Despite the consistency, the effect sizes of this overall gender difference tend to be rather small. There has been some suggestion that certain types of trauma may affect males and females differently (Elklit and Frandsen 2014; Landolt et al. 2013) but that, overall, PTSD rates are higher for females.

Regarding age, the findings are inconsistent. There is some evidence to suggest that PTSD prevalence increases with age, with one study finding significantly more lifetime subclinical PTSD in adolescence than in childhood (Copeland et al. 2007). A review by Nooner et al. (2012) also suggested that adolescents are generally at greater risk of PTSD than children. However, this result may be an artefact of applying *DSM-IV* criteria to young children, whose verbal abilities are unlikely to enable detection of some symptoms (Friedman 2013). Meta-analyses have found no or relatively small effects for age as a predictor of posttraumatic stress (Alisic et al. 2011; Cox et al. 2008; Kahana et al. 2006; Trickey et al. 2012). Even though there may be no observable age effect in PTSD rates or posttraumatic stress severity scores, it is likely that symptom patterns differ across various developmental stages. For example, younger children may show more behavioural disturbances, while adolescents may express more guilt and shame (Scheeringa et al. 2011).

Concerning race and minority status, these appear to predict overall risk for PTSD or rates of posttraumatic stress to a negligible or small extent (Alisic et al. 2011; Trickey et al. 2012). Like with age however, it is possible that ethnicity is related to posttraumatic stress in specific circumstances. For example, African-American adolescents in Chicago were more likely to be exposed to violence but less likely to develop PTSD than their White or Latino counterparts, highlighting a possible influence of ethnicity in this population (Milan et al. 2013).

Socio-economic status (SES) may predict PTSD but is rarely studied and yielded zero or small effect sizes in meta-analyses so far (Alisic et al. 2011; Kahana et al. 2006; Trickey et al. 2012). As an example, markers of SES in Kenyan adolescents, like parental education, number of meals per day and household resources, did not predict posttraumatic stress (Karsberg and Elklit 2012). Although, in Greenland, fathers' limited education did predict posttraumatic stress in adolescents (Karsberg et al. 2012).

2.3.2.2 Exposure Characteristics as Predictors

Children are more likely to develop PTSD following an interpersonal compared to a non-interpersonal trauma. In a recent meta-analysis, the pooled PTSD rate after interpersonal trauma was 25 % (with a 95 % confidence interval of 17–36 %), versus 10 % after non-interpersonal trauma (with a 95 % confidence interval of 6–15 %; Alisic et al. 2014). Within both types of exposure, further differences may exist. For example, adolescents who experienced violence perpetrated by a parent were more likely to develop PTSD than those exposed to other types of violence (Milan et al. 2013). Both groups of events may also have differential outcomes for witnesses and direct victims. Following motor vehicle accidents, witnesses reported less internalising symptoms compared to those involved in the accident (Tierens et al. 2012). Conversely, Bayarri Fernàndez et al. (2011) found that children who were witnesses, perpetrators or direct victims of violence were all similarly affected.

Objective ratings of trauma severity, like injury severity or amount of exposure, have shown limited predictive value (e.g. Lavi et al. 2013). In prospective studies among injured children, injury severity failed to predict subsequent posttraumatic stress (Alisic et al. 2011). In a meta-analysis of cross-sectional studies including a range of indications of trauma severity, a moderate effect was found (Trickey et al. 2012). However, this effect showed substantial heterogeneity that could not be explained within the available models; we do not yet know under which circumstances or in what way trauma severity may predict posttraumatic stress.

2.3.2.3 Prior Exposure as a Predictor

Prior trauma exposure has predicted PTSD in US adolescents (McLaughlin et al. 2013) and is a robust predictor of posttraumatic stress following an accident (Cox et al. 2008). A study on mental health in children in New Orleans 15 months after Hurricane Katrina found that gender, social support and lifetime trauma exposure, but not hurricane exposure, significantly predicted PTSD. Lifetime trauma exposure was the strongest predictor (Langley et al. 2013). Likewise, previous violence exposure has been linked to an increased likelihood of PTSD (Salloum et al. 2011). Generally, as the number of PTEs increases, poor psychiatric outcomes increase as well, providing evidence for a "dose-response" relationship (Copeland et al. 2007; Catani et al. 2008; Karsberg and Elklit 2012; Karsberg et al. 2012; Salazar et al. 2013). This has particular relevance for refugees who have often experienced multiple traumas, leading to high reported prevalence of posttraumatic stress symptoms (PTSS) in these populations (Neuner et al. 2004). As for many predictors, also in this case, there are exceptions. A study on Hurricane Gustav showed that children who had endured prior exposure to violence and Hurricane Katrina did not experience an elevation in PTSS following exposure to Hurricane Gustav (Salloum et al. 2011). The authors suggested that either posttraumatic stress levels had reached a threshold or Hurricane Gustav was not as traumatic as previous PTEs and therefore did not worsen PTSS.

2.3.2.4 Psychiatric History as a Predictor

ASD has emerged as a strong predictor of long-term PTSD among children and adolescents (Alisic et al. 2011; Kahana et al. 2006). Nevertheless, ASD has not predicted PTSD as well as was hoped; children with ASD do not all continue to develop PTSD, and not all children who develop PTSD had ASD first. Le Brocque et al. (2010) propose that some children with ASD may follow a "recovery" trajectory, where initial symptoms dissipate, while others follow a "chronic" trajectory, who continue to suffer long-term symptoms. Thus far, the *DSM-IV* criteria have not adequately differentiated these groups. However, alternative criteria for ASD requiring less symptoms have emerged in the literature and are better predictors of PTSD than *DSM-IV* ASD in young (2–6 years; Meiser-Stedman et al. 2008) and older children (7–13 years; Bryant et al. 2007) exposed to motor vehicle accidents and/or injuries. As alternate definitions of ASD often did not necessitate dissociative symptoms, these criteria may be more akin to the current *DSM-5* criteria for ASD. In adult samples, the *DSM-5* criteria have improved prediction of PTSD from ASD (Bryant et al. 2015); this may also be the case for children and adolescents.

More generally, meta-analyses have revealed that prior psychopathology is a robust predictor of PTSD following an accident (Cox et al. 2008) and depression and anxiety are moderate predictors of PTSD in children (Alisic et al. 2011; Kahana et al. 2006). In single studies, a history of anxiety (Copeland et al. 2007) and prior internalising disorders (McLaughlin et al. 2013) also significantly predicted PTSD in US children and adolescents.

2.3.2.5 Biological Predictors

So far, relatively little empirical knowledge is available regarding biological correlates and predictors of posttraumatic stress in children and adolescents. Of these variables, fluctuations in cortisol, heart rate, norepinephrine levels and interleukin-6 have been studied most frequently to determine their relationship with PTSD (Kirsch et al. 2011). Contrary to research conducted in adults, not low but high cortisol levels appear to be related to PTSD in children (Pervanidou 2008). More specifically, elevated post-trauma evening salivary cortisol levels and morning interleukin-6 predicted PTSD in children 6 months later (Pervanidou et al. 2007). Elevated heart rate immediately following a PTE has also predicted PTSS 6 weeks and 6 months later (e.g. Neuner et al. 2006) yet has yielded small effect sizes in meta-analyses (Alisic et al. 2011) and may be moderated by parental PTSS (Nugent et al. 2007). In addition, higher post-trauma norepinephrine has predicted PTSS in children (Kirsch et al. 2011).

2.3.2.6 Cognitive Predictors

Both peri-trauma and post-trauma cognitive factors appear to predict PTSD in children. Although the number of underlying studies is still fairly small, perceived life threat during or in the direct aftermath of a PTE appears to predict PTSD to a moderate to strong extent (Kahana et al. 2006; Meiser-Stedman et al. 2009; Trickey et al. 2012). Following motor vehicle accidents and assault, cognitions regarding "permanent and disturbing change" seem to affect PTSD symptoms (Meiser-Stedman et al. 2009). More in general, posttraumatic thought suppression has been strongly related to PTSD, although, again, the number of studies involved is small (Trickey et al. 2012). A recent study has underlined the potential strength of rumination in predicting PTSD in children and adolescents (Meiser-Stedman et al. 2014). There is also some evidence to suggest an effect of IQ or academic performance, albeit with small to medium effect sizes (Trickey et al. 2012).

2.3.2.7 Behavioural Predictors

High externalising and internalising behaviour puts children and adolescents at greater risk of consequent trauma symptoms, whether acutely or long term. Specifically, injured children with greater externalising and internalising traits were significantly more likely to belong to "recovery" or "chronic" trajectories, than the "resilient" trajectory, that do not develop PTSS (Le Brocque et al. 2010). In a longitudinal study with urban adolescents, Zona and Milan (2011) found that violence exposure itself increased internalising and externalising symptoms, as well as PTSD and dissociative symptoms. Therefore, this relationship may be multifaceted, with trauma exposure increasing behavioural symptoms, which increase posttraumatic stress in tandem. However, the substantial overlap between, in particular internalising, behavioural symptoms and posttraumatic stress is potentially blurring these findings.

2.3.2.8 Family and Social Environment Predictors

Parental posttraumatic stress has emerged as a strong predictor of child posttraumatic stress (Alisic et al. 2011; Cox et al. 2008; Landolt et al. 2012). In fact, initial traumatic stress symptoms in children have also predicted PTSS in parents (Stowman et al. 2015), highlighting the bidirectional nature of the relationship (cf. Scheeringa and Zeanah 2001). Poor family functioning in general has been associated with child posttraumatic stress (Trickey et al. 2012), and separation from family has predicted PTSS in resettled refugee youth (McGregor et al. 2015). Social support more broadly can be protective against PTSD for children and adolescents (e.g. Langley et al. 2013), and low levels of social support are a moderately strong predictor of PTSD in children (Trickey et al. 2012). However, social support is a complex relational construct, and potential resources for social support may not be utilised post-trauma for fear of being misunderstood or overburdening others (Thoresen et al. 2014).

2.3.3 Methodological Considerations

As in ASD, reporting of PTSD in children may be over- or underestimated by parents and nursing staff (Daviss et al. 2000). Prediction of PTSD in older children may be improved by the use of child instead of parent reports (Meiser-Stedman et al. 2007) or combined child and parent reports, which show even greater predictive ability than either type alone (Meiser-Stedman et al. 2008). Furthermore, the timing of reports is an important consideration. Several studies have assessed lifetime trauma exposure with current PTSD, and post-trauma assessment timing differs across studies and types of samples (Cox et al. 2008). For example, ill youth were often examined years after their trauma and had significantly lower rates of PTSD compared to injured youth, who were examined within months of the trauma (Kahana et al. 2006). Rates of PTSD in injured youth might decrease with time and eventually be comparable to that of ill youth (Kahana et al. 2006). Variables of interest are often examined in cross-sectional studies, making causal relationships difficult to establish, and a general lack of consistency in how predictors are examined makes comparisons between studies difficult (Alisic et al. 2011; Kahana et al. 2006).

> **Conclusion**
> Exposure to potential trauma is common in childhood. Some types of exposure, such as the sudden loss of loved ones, happen everywhere including in the safest parts of the world. Others, such as disaster and war, are more tied to specific locations and are more prevalent in low and middle-income than high-income countries. For many parts of the world, we have relatively little knowledge of exposure,

especially among children under 13 years of age. The most important factors to keep in mind as predictors of exposure are prior exposure, age (older children have faced more trauma), gender with respect to specific types of trauma (e.g. accidents for boys, sexual trauma for girls), externalising behaviour and stressors in the home environment.

Relatively little is known about ASD among children and adolescents. The best estimate of how many children develop ASD according to the *DSM-IV* criteria is 9 % (with a further 23 % of exposed children showing subthreshold levels of ASD; Dalgleish et al. 2008). Especially the dissociation symptom appeared to be problematic in diagnosis of ASD. The current *DSM-5* criteria no longer require dissociation as a necessary criterion, and it is likely that prediction of PTSD from ASD will improve with the current criteria. In terms of predictors of ASD, the findings remain inconclusive as well. At this point, the extent of exposure (although not severity of an injury), the intentionality of the trauma, peri-traumatic cognitions, emotions and processing, externalising behaviour and parental depression and worrying have shown some effect and merit further investigation.

Finally, PTSD is experienced by a substantial minority of children and adolescents exposed to trauma. The best estimate of overall average PTSD rates after exposure is 16 % (Alisic et al. 2014). Factors that are more closely linked to the trauma – and generally take more effort to measure – such as acute stress, cognitive appraisals and family or social support and the interpersonal or non-interpersonal nature of the exposure appear to be more powerful predictors of PTSD than demographic characteristics such as age, ethnicity and gender (although some gender effect has been found). There is substantial methodological variation between studies, in particular with regard to time points of detection of trauma-related disorders, which make comparisons across studies and trauma types less than straightforward. However, some patterns are emerging. In particular, cognitive and family or social support factors appear to merit further investigation.

Rather than static conditions, trauma-related disorders and symptom levels appear to show dynamic patterns. We are only just starting to understand what exposure and recovery trajectories in children and adolescents look like. In the future, we will hopefully be able to understand and predict these trajectories much more adequately.

Highlights
Prevalence
Trauma exposure is relatively common in childhood and adolescence
By contrast, a small proportion of trauma-exposed children develop acute stress disorder (ASD) or post-traumatic stress disorder (PTSD)
Not all who develop ASD develop PTSD, and vice versa
Predictors
Females are at a greater risk of some types of trauma (e.g. sexual)
Younger children may be at a greater risk of ASD

Highlights
Generally the perceived severity of the trauma (e.g. intentionality, risk of death) is more predictive of consequent trauma symptoms than the objective severity
Life stress may precipitate both exposure and consequent trauma symptoms
Behaviour problems have been bidirectionally linked to trauma exposure and disorders
Children who have been exposed to multiple traumas may be predisposed to experiencing trauma symptoms and even subsequent trauma
Social support may be one of the most important protective factors against PTSD

References

Alisic E, van der Schoot TA, van Ginkel JR, Kleber RJ (2008) Trauma exposure in primary school children: who is at risk? J Child Adolesc Trauma 1(3):263–269

Alisic E, Jongmans MJ, van Wesel F, Kleber RJ (2011) Building child trauma theory from longitudinal studies: a meta-analysis. Clin Psychol Rev 31(5):736–747. doi:10.1016/j.cpr.2011.03.001

Alisic E, Zalta AK, Van Wesel F, Larsen SE, Hafstad GS, Hassanpour K, Smid GE (2014) Rates of post-traumatic stress disorder in trauma-exposed children and adolescents: meta-analysis. Br J Psychiatry 204(5):335–340. doi:10.1192/bjp.bp.113.131227

American Psychiatric Association (2000) Diagnostic and statistical manual of mental disorders, 4th edn, text rev. Washington, DC, American Psychiatric Association

American Psychiatric Association (2013) Diagnostic and statistical manual of mental disorders, 5th edn. Washington, DC, American Psychiatric Association

Atwoli L, Ayuku D, Hogan J, Koech J, Vreeman RC, Ayaya S, Braitstein P (2014) Impact of domestic care environment on trauma and posttraumatic stress disorder among orphans in Western Kenya. PLoS One 9(3). doi:10.1371/journal.pone.0089937

Bayarri Fernàndez E, Ezpeleta L, Granero R, de la Osa N, Domènech JM (2011) Degree of exposure to domestic violence, psychopathology, and functional impairment in children and adolescents. J Interpers Violence 26(6):1215–1231

Bryant RA, Creamer M, O'Donnell M, Silove D, McFarlane AC, Forbes D (2015) A comparison of the capacity of DSM-IV and DSM-5 acute stress disorder definitions to predict posttraumatic stress disorder and related disorders. J Clin Psychiatry 76(4):391–397. doi:10.4088/JCP.13m08731

Bryant B, Mayou R, Wiggs L, Ehlers A, Stores G (2004) Psychological consequences of road traffic accidents for children and their mothers. Psychol Med 34(02):335–346

Bryant RA, Salmon K, Sinclair E, Davidson P (2007) The relationship between acute stress disorder and posttraumatic stress disorder in injured children. J Trauma Stress 20(6):1075–1079. doi:10.1002/jts.20282

Catani C, Jacob N, Schauer E, Kohila M, Neuner F (2008) Family violence, war, and natural disasters: a study of the effect of extreme stress on children's mental health in Sri Lanka. BMC Psychiatry 8:33–42. doi:10.1186/1471-244X-8-33

Copeland WE, Keeler G, Angold A, Costello EJ (2007) Traumatic events and posttraumatic stress in childhood. Arch Gen Psychiatry 64(5):577–584

Cox CM, Kenardy JA, Hendrikz JK (2008) A meta-analysis of risk factors that predict psychopathology following accidental trauma. J Spec Pediatr Nurs 13(2):98–110

Dalgleish T, Meiser-Stedman R, Kassam-Adams N, Ehlers A, Winston F, Smith P, Bryant B, Mayou RA, Yule W (2008) Predictive validity of acute stress disorder in children and adolescents. Br J Psychiatry 192(5):392–393. doi:10.1192/bjp.bp.107.040451

Daviss W, Racusin R, Fleischer A, Mooney D, Ford JD, McHugo GJ (2000) Acute stress disorder symptomatology during hospitalization for pediatric injury. J Am Acad Child Adolesc Psychiatry 39(5):569–575. 10.1097/00004583-200005000-00010

Decker MR, Peitzmeier S, Olumide A, Acharya R, Ojengbede O, Covarrubias L, Gao E, Cheng Y, Delany-Moretlwe S, Brahmbhatt H (2014) Prevalence and health impact of intimate partner violence and non-partner sexual violence among female adolescents aged 15-19 years in vulnerable urban environments: a multi-country study. J Adolesc Health 55(6):S58–S67. doi: 10.1016/j.jadohealth.2014.08.022

Demir T, Demir DE, Alkas L, Copur M, Dogangun B, Kayaalp L (2010) Some clinical characteristics of children who survived the Marmara earthquakes. Eur Child Adolesc Psychiatry 19(2):125–133. doi:10.1007/s00787-009-0048-1

Doron-LaMarca S, Vogt DS, King DW, King LA, Saxe GN (2010) Pretrauma problems, prior stressor exposure, and gender as predictors of change in posttraumatic stress symptoms among physically injured children and adolescents. J Consult Clin Psychol 78(6):781

Elklit A, Frandsen L (2014) Trauma exposure and posttraumatic stress among Danish adolescents. J Trauma Stress Dis Treat 4:2

Ellis AA, Nixon RD, Williamson P (2009) The effects of social support and negative appraisals on acute stress symptoms and depression in children and adolescents. Br J Clin Psychol 48(Pt 4):347–361. doi:10.1348/014466508X401894

Finkelhor D, Ormrod RK, Turner HA (2009) Lifetime assessment of poly-victimization in a national sample of children and youth. Child Abuse Negl 33(7):403–411. doi:10.1016/j.chiabu.2008.09.012

Finkelhor D, Turner HA, Shattuck A, Hamby SL (2015) Prevalence of childhood exposure to violence, crime, and abuse: results from the national survey of children's exposure to violence. JAMA Pediatr. doi:10.1001/jamapediatrics.2015.0676

Fodor KE, Unterhitzenberger J, Chou CY, Kartal D, Leistner S, Milosavljevic M, Nocon A, Soler L, White J, Yoo S (2014) Is traumatic stress research global? A bibliometric analysis. Eur J Psychotraumatol 5. doi: 10.3402/ejpt.v5.23269

Forgey M, Bursch B (2013) Assessment and management of pediatric iatrogenic medical trauma. Curr Psychiatry Rep 15(2):1–9. doi:10.1007/s11920-012-0340-5

Friedman MJ (2013) Finalizing PTSD in DSM-5: getting here from there and where to go next. J Trauma Stress 26(5):548–556. doi:10.1002/jts.21840

Gabrielli J, Gill M, Koester LS, Borntrager C (2014) Psychological perspectives on 'acute on chronic' trauma in children: implications of the 2010 earthquake in Haiti. Child Soc 28(6):438–450. doi:10.1111/chso.12010

Ghazali SR, Elklit A, Balang RV, Sultan M, Kana K (2014) Preliminary findings on lifetime trauma prevalence and PTSD symptoms among adolescents in Sarawak Malaysia. Asian J Psychiatr 11:45–49. doi: 10.1016/j.ajp.2014.05.008

Haag AC, Zehnder D, Landolt MA (2015) Guilt is associated with acute stress symptoms in children after road traffic accidents. Eur J Psychotraumatol 6. doi: 10.3402/ejpt.v6.29074

Haller M, Chassin L (2012) A test of adolescent internalizing and externalizing symptoms as prospective predictors of type of trauma exposure and posttraumatic stress disorder. J Trauma Stress 25(6):691–699. doi:10.1002/jts.21751

Hamrin V, Jonker B, Scahill L (2004) Acute stress disorder symptoms in gunshot-injured youth. J Child Adolesc Psychiatr Nurs 17(4):161–172. Retrieved from http://www.ncbi.nlm.nih.gov/pubmed/15742797

Holbrook TL, Hoyt DB, Coimbra R, Potenza B, Sise M, Anderson JP (2005) High rates of acute stress disorder impact quality-of-life outcomes in injured adolescents: mechanism and gender predict acute stress disorder risk. J Trauma Acute Care Surg 59(5):1126–1130. Retrieved from http://www.ncbi.nlm.nih.gov/pubmed/16385290

Irie F, Lang J, Kaltner M, Le Brocque R, Kenardy J (2012) Effects of gender, indigenous status and remoteness to health services on the occurrence of assault-related injuries in children and adolescents. Injury 43(11):1873–1880. doi:10.1016/j.injury.2012.07.183

Kahana SY, Feeny NC, Youngstrom EA, Drotar D (2006) Posttraumatic stress in youth experiencing illnesses and injuries: an exploratory meta-analysis. Traumatology 12(2):148–161. doi: 10.1177/1534765606294562

Karabekiroglu K, Akbas S, Tasdemir GN, Karakurt MN (2008) Post-traumatic stress symptoms in adolescents after two murders in a school: a controlled follow-up study. Int J Psychiatry Med 38(4):407–424. doi:10.2190/PM.38.4.b

Karsberg SH, Elklit A (2012) Victimization and PTSD in a Rural Kenyan youth sample. Clin Pract Epidemiol Ment Health 8:91–101. doi:10.2174/1745017901208010091

Karsberg SH, Lasgaard M, Elklit A (2012) Victimisation and PTSD in a Greenlandic youth sample. Int J Circumpolar Health 71(1). doi:10.3402/ijch.v71i0.18378

Kassam-Adams N, Garcia-Espana JF, Miller VA, & Winston F (2006) Parent-child agreement regarding children's acute stress: The role of parent acute stress reactions. J Am Acad Child Adolesc Psychiatry 45(12):1485–1493.

Kassam-Adams N, Palmieri PA, Rork K, Delahanty DL, Kenardy J, Kohser KL, Landolt MA, Le Brocque R, Marsac ML, Meiser-Stedman R, Nixon RD, Bui E, McGrath C (2012) Acute stress symptoms in children: results from an international data archive. J Am Acad Child Adolesc Psychiatry 51(8):812–820. doi:10.1016/j.jaac.2012.05.013

Kirsch V, Wilhelm FH, Goldbeck L (2011) Psychophysiological characteristics of PTSD in children and adolescents: a review of the literature. J Trauma Stress 24(2):146–154. doi:10.1002/jts.20620

Lalloo R, Sheiham A, Nazroo JY (2003) Behavioural characteristics and accidents: findings from the health survey for England, 1997. Accid Anal Prev 35(5):661–667

Landolt MA, Schnyder U, Maier T, Schoenbucher V, Mohler-Kuo M (2013) Trauma exposure and posttraumatic stress disorder in adolescents: a national survey in Switzerland. J Trauma Stress 26(2):209–216. doi:10.1002/jts.21794

Landolt MA, Ystrom E, Sennhauser FH, Gnehm HE, Vollrath ME (2012) The mutual prospective influence of child and parental post-traumatic stress symptoms in pediatric patients. J Child Psychol Psychiatry 53:767–774. doi:10.1111/j.1469-7610.2011.02520.x

Langley AK, Cohen JA, Mannarino AP, Jaycox LH, Schonlau M, Scott M et al (2013) Trauma exposure and mental health problems among school children 15 months post-Hurricane Katrina. J Child Adolesc Trauma 6(3):143–156

Lavi T, Green O, Dekel R (2013) The contribution of personal and exposure characteristics to the adjustment of adolescents following war. J Adolesc 36(1):21–30. doi:10.1016/j.adolescence.2012.09.003

Le Brocque RM, Hendrikz J, Kenardy JA (2010) The course of posttraumatic stress in children: examination of recovery trajectories following traumatic injury. J Pediatr Psychol 35(6):637–645

Liu K, Liang X, Guo L, Li Y, Li X, Xin B et al (2010) Acute stress disorder in the paediatric surgical children and adolescents injured during the Wenchuan Earthquake in China. Stress Health J Int Soc Investig Stress 26(4):262–268. doi:10.1002/smi.1288

Marsac ML, Kassam-Adams N, Delahanty DL, Widaman K, Barakat LP (2014) Posttraumatic stress following acute medical trauma in children: a proposed model of bio-psycho-social processes during the peri-trauma period. Clin Child Fam Psychol Rev 17(4):399–411. doi: 10.1007/s10567-014-0174-2

McGregor LS, Melvin GA, Newman LK (2015) Familial separations, coping styles, and PTSD symptomatology in resettled refugee youth. J Nerv Ment Dis 203(6):431–438. doi:10.1097/NMD.0000000000000312

McKinnon AC, Nixon RD, Brewer N (2008) The influence of data-driven processing on perceptions of memory quality and intrusive symptoms in children following traumatic events. Behav Res Ther 46(6):766–775. doi: 10.1016/j.brat.2008.02.008

McLaughlin KA, Koenen KC, Hill ED, Petukhova M, Sampson NA, Zaslavsky AM, Kessler RC (2013) Trauma exposure and posttraumatic stress disorder in a national sample of adolescents. J Am Acad Child Adolesc Psychiatry 52(8):815–830. e814

Meiser-Stedman R, Dalgleish T, Glucksman E, Yule W, Smith P (2009) Maladaptive cognitive appraisals mediate the evolution of posttraumatic stress reactions: a 6-month follow-up of child and adolescent assault and motor vehicle accident survivors. J Abnorm Psychol 118(4):778

Meiser-Stedman R, Smith P, Glucksman E, Yule W, Dalgleish T (2007) Parent and child agreement for acute stress disorder, post-traumatic stress disorder and other psychopathology in a prospective study of children and adolescents exposed to single-event trauma. J Abnorm Child Psychol 35(2):191–201. doi:10.1007/s10802-006-9068-1

Meiser-Stedman R, Shepperd A, Glucksman E, Dalgleish T, Yule W, Smith P (2014) Thought control strategies and rumination in youth with acute stress disorder and posttraumatic stress disorder following single-event trauma. J Child Adolesc Psychopharmacol 24(1):47–51. doi:10.1089/cap.2013.0052

Meiser-Stedman R, Smith P, Glucksman E, Yule W, Dalgleish T (2008) The posttraumatic stress disorder diagnosis in preschool-and elementary school-age children exposed to motor vehicle accidents. Am J Psychiatry 165(10):1326–1337. doi:10.1176/appi.ajp.2008.07081282

Meiser-Stedman RA, Yule W, Dalgleish T, Smith P, Glucksman E (2006) The role of the family in child and adolescent posttraumatic stress following attendance at an emergency department. J Pediatr Psychol 31(4):397–402

Meiser-Stedman R, Yule W, Smith P, Glucksman E, Dalgleish T (2005) Acute stress disorder and posttraumatic stress disorder in children and adolescents involved in assaults or motor vehicle accidents. Am J Psychiatry 162(7):1381–1383

Melhem NM, Porta G, Shamseddeen W, Payne MW, Brent DA (2011) Grief in children and adolescents bereaved by sudden parental death. Arch Gen Psychiatry 68(9):911–919

Milan S, Zona K, Acker J, Turcios-Cotto V (2013) Prospective risk factors for adolescent PTSD: sources of differential exposure and differential vulnerability. J Abnorm Child Psychol 41(2):339–353. doi:10.1007/s10802-012-9677-9

Mohler-Kuo M, Landolt MA, Maier T, Meidert U, Schönbucher V, Schnyder U (2014) Child sexual abuse revisited: a population-based cross-sectional study among swiss adolescents. J Adolesc Health 54(3):304–311. doi:10.1016/j.jadohealth.2013.08.020

Morrongiello BA, House K (2004) Measuring parent attributes and supervision behaviors relevant to child injury risk: examining the usefulness of questionnaire measures. Inj Prev 10(2):114–118. doi:10.1136/ip.2003.003459

Neuner F, Schauer E, Catani C, Ruf M, Elbert T (2006) Post-tsunami stress: a study of posttraumatic stress disorder in children living in three severely affected regions in Sri Lanka. J Trauma Stress 19(3):339–347. doi:10.1002/jts.20121

Neuner F, Schauer M, Karunakara U, Klaschik C, Robert C, Elbert T (2004) Psychological trauma and evidence for enhanced vulnerability for posttraumatic stress disorder through previous trauma among West Nile refugees. BMC Psychiatry 4(1):34

Nooner KB, Linares LO, Batinjane J, Kramer RA, Silva R, Cloitre M (2012) Factors related to posttraumatic stress disorder in adolescence. Trauma Violence Abuse 13(3):1524838012447698. doi:10.1177/1524838012447698

Nugent NR, Ostrowski S, Christopher NC, Delahanty DL (2007) Parental posttraumatic stress symptoms as a moderator of child's acute biological response and subsequent posttraumatic stress symptoms in pediatric injury patients. J Pediatr Psychol 32(3):309–318. doi:10.1093/jpepsy/jsl005

Olsson KA, Le Brocque RM, Kenardy JA, Anderson V, Spence SH (2008) The influence of pre-injury behaviour on children's type of accident, type of injury and severity of injury. Brain Inj 22(7–8):595–602. doi:10.1080/02699050802132453

Ostrowski SA, Ciesla JA, Lee TJ, Irish L, Christopher NC, Delahanty DL (2011) The impact of caregiver distress on the longitudinal development of child acute post-traumatic stress disorder symptoms in pediatric injury victims. J Pediatr Psychol 36(7):806–815

Owens JA, Fernando S, Mc Guinn M (2005) Sleep disturbance and injury risk in young children. Behav Sleep Med 3(1):18–31. doi:10.1207/s15402010bsm0301_4

Pervanidou P (2008) Biology of post-traumatic stress disorder in childhood and adolescence. J Neuroendocrinol 20(5):632–638. doi:10.1111/j.1365-2826.2008.01701.x

Pervanidou P, Kolaitis G, Charitaki S, Margeli A, Ferentinos S, Bakoula C, Lazaropoulou C, Papassotiriou I, Tsiantis J, Chrousos GP (2007) Elevated morning serum interleukin (IL)-6 or evening salivary cortisol concentrations predict posttraumatic stress disorder in children and adolescents six months after a motor vehicle accident. Psychoneuroendocrinology 32(8):991–999

Salazar AM, Keller TE, Gowen LK, Courtney ME (2013) Trauma exposure and PTSD among older adolescents in foster care. Soc Psychiatry Psychiatr Epidemiol 48(4):545–551

Salloum A, Carter P, Burch B, Garfinkel A, Overstreet S (2011) Impact of exposure to community violence, Hurricane Katrina, and Hurricane Gustav on posttraumatic stress and depressive symptoms among school age children. Anxiety Stress Coping 24(1):27–42. doi:10.1080/10615801003703193

Salmon K, Sinclair E, Bryant RA (2007) The role of maladaptive appraisals in child acute stress reactions. Br J Clin Psychol 46(2):203–210. doi:10.1348/014466506X160704

Saunders BE, Adams ZW (2014) Epidemiology of traumatic experiences in childhood. Child Adolesc Psychiatr Clin N Am 23(2):167–184. doi:10.1016/j.chc.2013.12.003

Saxe GN, Miller A, Bartholomew D, Hall E, Lopez C, Kaplow J et al (2005a) Incidence of and risk factors for acute stress disorder in children with injuries. J Trauma Inj Infect Crit Care 59(4):946–953. doi:10.1097/01.ta.0000187659.37385.16

Saxe G, Stoddard F, Chawla N, Lopez CG, Hall E, Sheridan R, King D, King L (2005b) Risk factors for acute stress disorder in children with burns. J Trauma Dissociation 6(2):37–49. doi:10.1300/J229v06n02_05

Scheeringa MS, Zeanah CH (2001) A relational perspective on PTSD in early childhood. J Trauma Stress 14(4):799–815. doi:10.1023/A:1013002507972

Scheeringa MS, Zeanah CH, Cohen JA (2011) PTSD in children and adolescents: toward an empirically based algorithm. Depress Anxiety 28:770–782

Stoddard FJ, Saxe G, Ronfeldt H, Drake JE, Burns J, Edgren C, Sheridan R (2006) Acute stress symptoms in young children with burns. J Am Acad Child Adolesc Psychiatry 45(1):87–93. doi:10.1097/01.chi.0000184934.71917.3a

Stowman S, Kearney CA, Daphtary K (2015) Mediators of initial acute and later posttraumatic stress in youths in a pediatric intensive care unit. Pediatr Crit Care Med 16(4):e113–e118. doi:10.1097/PCC.0b013e31822f1916

Thoresen S, Jensen TK, Wentzel-Larsen T, Dyb G (2014) Social support barriers and mental health in terrorist attack survivors. J Affect Disord 156:187–193. doi:10.1016/j.jad.2013.12.014

Tierens M, Bal S, Crombez G, Loeys T, Antrop I, Deboutte D (2012) Differences in posttraumatic stress reactions between witnesses and direct victims of motor vehicle accidents. J Trauma Stress 25(3):280–287. doi:10.1002/jts.21692

Trickey D, Siddaway AP, Meiser-Stedman R, Serpell L, Field AP (2012) A meta-analysis of risk factors for post-traumatic stress disorder in children and adolescents. Clin Psychol Rev 32(2):122–138. doi:10.1016/j.cpr.2011.12.001

Winston FK, Baxt C, Kassam-Adams NL, Elliott MR, Kallan MJ (2005) Acute traumatic stress symptoms in child occupants and their parent drivers after crash involvement. Arch Pediatr Adolesc Med 159(11):1074–1079. doi:10.1001/archpedi.159.11.1074

World Health Organization (2014) Main messages from the world report [Fact sheet]. Retrieved from http://www.who.int/violence_injury_prevention/child/injury/world_report/Main_messages_englis

Zona K, Milan S (2011) Gender differences in the longitudinal impact of exposure to violence on mental health in urban youth. J Youth Adolesc 40(12):1674–1690. doi:10.1007/s10964-011-9649-3

Childhood Trauma as a Public Health Issue

3

Hilary K. Lambert, Rosemary Meza, Prerna Martin, Eliot Fearey, and Katie A. McLaughlin

Trauma involves exposure to events that pose significant danger to one's safety, witnessing such an event happening to another person, or learning about a loved one experiencing such events (American Psychiatric Association 2013). Population-based data indicate that between one-third to one-half of youths in the USA have experienced sexual or physical abuse or have witnessed violence (Copeland et al. 2007; Finkelhor et al. 2005) and nearly two-thirds of children will experience some type of traumatic event by the time they reach adulthood (McLaughlin et al. 2013). The burden of trauma among children exposed to humanitarian emergencies such as war and armed conflict in low- and middle-income countries (LAMICs) is substantial (World Health Organization 2013). According to the UNICEF, in 2014 over 15 million children were exposed to violent conflicts in the Central African Republic, South Sudan, Iraq, Palestine, Syria, and Ukraine. An estimated 230 million children currently live in countries or regions impacted by armed conflicts (UNICEF 2014). Children living in areas experiencing armed conflict are at risk of internal displacement, becoming a refugee, witnessing brutal violence and death, and being orphaned, kidnapped, tortured, raped, or recruited as child soldiers (UNICEF 2009). This pervasive exposure to trauma among children worldwide is concerning from a public health perspective given that childhood exposure to trauma is associated with a range of negative outcomes across the life course, including virtually all commonly occurring forms of mental disorder, physical health problems, low academic achievement, and poor social and interpersonal functioning.

In this chapter, we first review the public health impact of childhood trauma, including consequences related to mental health, physical health, academic and socioeconomic outcomes, and interpersonal functioning. Next, we review the public health response to childhood trauma, including efforts to prevent child trauma

H.K. Lambert (✉) • R. Meza • P. Martin • E. Fearey • K.A. McLaughlin
Department of Psychology, University of Washington, Box 351525, Seattle, WA 98195, USA
e-mail: hklamb@uw.edu

exposure and prevent the mental health consequences of trauma among children and approaches to intervention and treatment delivery in low-resource settings where mental health resources are scarce. Because interpersonal violence exposure including maltreatment (i.e., physical and sexual abuse) and other forms of violence exposure (i.e., violence occurring in the home, school, or community) are more strongly associated with downstream mental health problems than non-interpersonal forms of trauma (Breslau et al. 1998; McLaughlin et al. 2013), we focus primarily on traumatic events involving interpersonal violence.

3.1 Public Health Impact of Childhood Trauma

3.1.1 Mental Health

Epidemiological studies reveal four general patterns pertaining to childhood trauma and the distribution of mental disorders in the population. First, children exposed to trauma are at markedly elevated risk for developing a mental disorder in their lifetime compared to children without exposure, and the odds of developing a lifetime mental disorder increase as trauma exposure increases (Green et al. 2010; Kessler et al. 2010; McLaughlin et al. 2010, 2012). Second, increased vulnerability for developing a mental disorder following child trauma persists across the life course. Childhood trauma is associated with elevated odds of developing a mental disorder in childhood and adolescence (McLaughlin et al. 2012) as well as in adulthood (Green et al. 2010; Kessler et al. 2010). Third, associations of childhood trauma with commonly occurring mental disorders are largely nonspecific. Children exposed to trauma are more likely to develop mood, anxiety, substance use, and disruptive behavior disorders, and there is little variation in the strength of these associations across disorder types (Green et al. 2010; Kessler et al. 2010; McLaughlin et al. 2012). Although PTSD is a common form of psychopathology among children exposed to trauma, it represents just one of the many mental disorders that occur following child trauma. Recent findings suggest that associations of child maltreatment with lifetime mental disorders operate entirely through a latent vulnerability for internalizing and externalizing psychopathology, with no direct effects on specific mental disorders that are not explained by this latent risk (Caspi et al. 2014; Keyes et al. 2012). Fourth, child trauma exposure explains a substantial proportion of mental disorder onsets in the population, both in the USA and cross-nationally (Green et al. 2010; Kessler et al. 2010; McLaughlin et al. 2012), reflecting both the high prevalence of trauma exposure in children and the strong association of child trauma with the onset of psychopathology. Together, findings from epidemiological studies show that child trauma exposure is a powerful determinant of risk for psychopathology.

PTSD is one mental health consequence of child trauma. As shown in more detail in Chap. 2 of this volume, epidemiological studies in high-income countries indicate that between 7.6 and 8.8 % of youths exposed to trauma develop PTSD at some point in the life course (Breslau et al. 2004; McLaughlin et al. 2013) and even more develop PTS symptoms (Copeland et al. 2007). The conditional probability for developing PTSD is higher following interpersonal violence than non-interpersonal forms of trauma (e.g., accidents, injuries, and natural disasters) (Breslau et al. 2004; Copeland et al. 2007; McLaughlin et al. 2013). There is considerable variation in estimates of PTSD prevalence in children in low- and middle-income countries (LAMICs). A meta-analysis of children affected by war reported PTSD prevalence rates ranging from 4.5 to 89.3 % across studies, with an overall pooled estimate of 47 % (Attanayake et al. 2009), suggesting that PTSD is particularly common in children exposed to war. Similarly high rates of PTSD have been found in children who are displaced and living as refugees (Almqvist and Brandell-Forsberg 1997; Thabet and Vostanis 1999). The burden of trauma is also remarkably high among child soldiers, who are forced to commit violence and often acts of torture. Studies of former child soldiers from Uganda and the Democratic Republic of Congo have found PTSD prevalence rates that range from 35 to 97 % across studies (Bayer et al. 2007; Derluyn et al. 2004). Among child soldiers, beatings, bombings, and torture are strongly associated with PTSD and other poor mental health outcomes (Benjet 2010).

PTSD risk in children increases with increasing exposure to trauma (Copeland et al. 2007; McLaughlin et al. 2013) and is higher among children experiencing other forms of stress and adversity (Khamis 2005). In children exposed to war, parental loss and family displacement pose a cumulative risk effect with the traumatic experience itself (Macksoud and Aber 1996; Wolff et al. 1995). PTSD rates are higher in female youth than males following virtually all forms of child trauma (McLaughlin et al. 2013), particularly interpersonal violence (Breslau et al. 2004). Children who have preexisting internalizing and externalizing psychopathology are also more likely to develop PTSD following trauma exposure (Copeland et al. 2007; McLaughlin et al. 2013).

PTSD following child trauma is often chronic. Mean recovery time in a US population sample was estimated at 14.8 months (McLaughlin et al. 2013), and a study in Germany reported that 48 % of adolescents and young adults with PTSD had not recovered after 34 to 50 months following initial assessment (Perkonig et al. 2005). Children who develop PTSD experience increased risk for developing additional internalizing and externalizing disorders (Giaconia et al. 1995; Perkonigg et al. 2000).

Considerable variability exists in the presentation of PTSD symptoms and posttraumatic psychopathology among youths in different cultural contexts (Barenbaum et al. 2004). For example, in a qualitative study on mental health problems among orphaned youth in Tanzania, authors found that the three local problems most commonly associated with trauma exposure were *unyanyasaji* (mistreated/abused), *kutopendwa* (not feeling loved), and *msongo wa mawazo* (stress/overthinking) (Dorsey et al. 2015). These problems were in turn associated with a range of symptoms including behavioral problems, sadness, grief, loneliness, losing hope, and stress that are similar to Western conceptualizations of post-trauma psychopathology. Unique symptoms such as "feeling a lack of peace" and "increased feelings of hate" that are not traditionally part of the PTSD diagnosis were also observed

(Dorsey et al. 2015). Similar findings documenting common presentations of posttraumatic psychopathology that do not map onto Western conceptualizations have been observed in other cultural contexts such as coping styles characterized by suppression of one's feelings among Khmer youth in Cambodia or symptoms described in the local language as "thinking too much" or "having an unsettled mind" among HIV-infected youth in Zambia (Kleinman and Kleinman 1991; Murray et al. 2006).

3.1.2 Physical Health

Childhood trauma is associated with increased risk for a wide range of chronic physical health conditions in adulthood (Felitti et al. 1998; Rich-Edwards et al. 2010). In a cross-national survey of adults from 14 countries, lifetime exposure to traumatic events was associated with elevated odds of developing heart disease, hypertension, asthma, chronic pain, and gastrointestinal problems, and these associations were not explained by co-occurring psychopathology (Scott et al. 2013). Child abuse predicts increased risk for poor physical health and chronic pain in adulthood (Davis et al. 2005; Widom et al. 2012) as well as specific chronic conditions such as heart disease and diabetes (Felitti et al. 1998; Rich-Edwards et al. 2010), and the effect sizes for these associations are comparable for those of the associations of child abuse with mental disorders (Wegman and Stetler 2009). Emerging evidence suggests that childhood trauma is also an important determinant of risk for chronic physical health conditions that emerge early in the life course, beginning in childhood and adolescence. Children who have experienced trauma related to interpersonal violence are more likely to experience symptoms of pain and changes in appetite or sleep (Bailey et al. 2005; Lamers-Winkelman et al. 2012; Stensland et al. 2014). Specifically, childhood trauma is associated with higher levels of somatic symptoms (Bailey et al. 2005; Lamers-Winkelman et al. 2012), including headaches (Bailey et al. 2005; Stensland et al. 2014) and stomachaches (Bailey et al. 2005), and with poor self-rated health (Annerbäck et al. 2012) in children. Clinically significant elevations in somatic symptoms have also been reported in adolescent refugees living at the Thai-Cambodian border (Mollica et al. 1997). Childhood trauma has been associated with risk for asthma in multiple studies (Cohen et al. 2008; Swahn and Bossarte 2006). A recent study utilizing a population-representative sample of US adolescents documented associations of child trauma with numerous chronic conditions, with particularly strong associations between child trauma and conditions involving pain (McLaughlin et al. in press).

PTSD symptoms may also independently contribute to physical health consequences, serve as a mediator underlying the association of child trauma and later physical health problems (Schnurr and Green 2004), or be unrelated to physical health problems. Understanding the contributions of PTSD and child trauma to poor physical health could enhance early identification and prevention of poor physical health. For example, determining which individuals are most susceptible to developing physical health problems (e.g., youth exposed to childhood trauma, youth with PTSD, or both) may inform the targeting of preventative interventions.

3 Childhood Trauma as a Public Health Issue

However, most studies do not examine childhood trauma or PTSD specifically when examining health outcomes. For example, a recent meta-analysis found that adults with PTSD exhibited worse general health, more general medical conditions, worse health-related quality of life, more pain, worse cardiorespiratory health, and poor gastrointestinal health compared to adults without PTSD, but the role of childhood trauma or early-onset PTSD was not examined (Pacella et al. 2013). Even fewer studies have examined the physical health consequences of early-onset PTSD in youth while accounting for childhood trauma. One study reported that, while controlling for childhood trauma, PTSD occurring prior to the age of 21 predicted a variety of chronic physical health conditions in adulthood including heart disease, asthma, osteoarthritis, neck or back pain, and headaches (Scott et al. 2011). Similarly, the association of child maltreatment and physical health problems like pain was mediated by current PTSD symptoms in adult women (Lang et al. 2006). In contrast, another study reported that after adjustment for childhood physical or sexual abuse, PTSD symptoms predicted only worse perceptions of overall health but not the number of medical problems in adult women (Cloitre et al. 2001). Similarly, adolescents exposed to childhood trauma reported worse physical health and more sick days per month than adolescents without trauma exposure; however, there were no differences between children with and without PTSD (Giaconia et al. 1995). Future research is needed to disentangle the complex relationships of child trauma, PTSD, and physical health consequences.

3.1.3 Academic and Socioeconomic Outcomes

Although numerous studies have observed an association between childhood trauma and poor academic functioning, some evidence suggests that this association is explained by social factors that often co-occur with trauma exposure in children, such as poverty. In some studies, childhood maltreatment is associated with low performance on standardized academic achievement tests that assess reading and math abilities (De Bellis et al. 2013), low grades (Leiter and Johnsen 1997), high rates of grade repetition (Leiter and Johnsen 1997), high eligibility for special education (Jonson-Reid 2015), and low probability of attaining a college-level education (Lansford et al. 2002). Similarly, approximately half of Iranian children living in Sweden for several years as refugees had poor academic performance, and two-thirds had difficulties speaking Swedish (Almqvist and Broberg 1999). In contrast, other studies have observed that the associations of child trauma with poor performance on standardized academic achievement tests (Eckenrode et al. 1993), low grades (Lansford et al. 2002; Eckenrode et al. 1993), high rates of grade repetition (Eckenrode et al. 1993), and low academic attainment (Boden et al. 2007) disappear with the adjustment for demographic, socioeconomic, and familial risk factors associated with child abuse. Further research is needed to disentangle whether poor academic achievement is a consequence of childhood trauma or other aspects of the early environment. Although the relationship between childhood trauma and academic achievement is uncertain, childhood trauma is more consistently associated with long-term socioeconomic outcomes in adulthood, including high unemployment (Macmillan and Hagan 2004; Zielinski 2009), low income and high odds of living below the poverty line (Macmillan 2000; Zielinski 2009), high Medicaid enrollment (Zielinski 2009), and elevated likelihood of receiving public assistance (Macmillan and Hagan 2004), even after adjustment for co-occurring risk factors in childhood. In contrast, one study reported that the association of childhood abuse and SES in adulthood did not survive after including covariates for familial and social risk in models (Mullen et al. 1996). At least some evidence suggests that child trauma influences patterns of academic achievement and socioeconomic outcomes later in life.

Scant research has investigated the academic and socioeconomic consequences of early-onset PTSD independent of childhood trauma. In one study, youth exposed to child maltreatment with and without PTSD exhibited similarly low performance on standardized academic achievement tests that assess reading and math abilities (De Bellis et al. 2013), suggesting that childhood maltreatment, but not PTSD, may be the common denominator contributing to poor academic achievement across the two groups. Similarly, adolescents exposed to childhood trauma with and without PTSD reported lower high school grades and more school suspensions and expulsions than control adolescents; however, there were no differences between the two trauma-exposed groups (Giaconia et al. 1995). Future research is needed to clarify contributions of multiple coexisting risk factors, including child trauma and PTSD, to poor socioeconomic and academic outcomes.

3.1.4 Social Functioning

Childhood trauma is associated with a range of negative long-term social and interpersonal consequences. There are numerous studies that consistently indicate a significant relationship between sexual abuse and interpersonal difficulties (Cole and Putnam 1992; DiLillo 2001; Rumstein-McKean and Hunsley 2001). Children exposed to sexual abuse are likely to be revictimized in adulthood, frequently by an intimate partner (DiLillo 2001; Follette et al. 1996; Rumstein-McKean and Hunsley 2001). Women with a history of childhood abuse also report difficulties with romantic partners, including less secure attachment (Feldman and Downey 1994), difficulty communicating about sexual arousal and comfort (Cole and Putnam 1992; DiLillo 2001), sexual dysfunction (Davis and Petretic-Jackson, 2000; DiLillo 2001; Rumstein-McKean and Hunsley 2001), and higher levels of marital separation and divorce (DiLillo, 2001; Rumstein-McKean and Hunsley 2001). Furthermore, survivors of childhood abuse experience problems in relationships with parents (e.g., feeling betrayed by a mother who did not protect them from the abuse) (Aspelmeier et al. 2007) and their children (e.g., having negative perceptions of parenting abilities) (Cole and Putnam 1992; DiLillo 2001). Finally, maltreated children exhibit numerous difficulties with peers, including fewer positive social interactions and greater peer rejection (Haskett and Kistner 1991; Kim and Cicchetti 2010). In former child soldiers in Sierra Leone, killing/harming others during war was associated with reduced pro-social behaviors (e.g., sharing with others) and higher hostility (e.g., getting into fights) (Betancourt et al. 2010a, b).

Research examining the unique impact of PTSD on social functioning in youth is scant. One study reported that adolescents exposed to childhood trauma with PTSD had worse interpersonal issues (i.e. not having other people to depend on, having communication difficulties) than both adolescents exposed to child trauma without PTSD and non-trauma-exposed adolescents (Giaconia et al. 1995), suggesting that PTSD contributes to interpersonal deficits beyond those of child trauma.

3.2 Public Health Response

Modern public health approaches consider risk factors operating at multiple levels, including macrosocial, individual, and biological, that increase the probability of a disease or disability with the ultimate goal of preventing disease onset. In the case of trauma-related problems, public health approaches to prevention and intervention consider the nature of trauma itself, the characteristics of children who are exposed to trauma, their families, and the variety of environmental factors that play a role in the likelihood of trauma exposure and trauma-related psychopathology (e.g., safety of neighborhoods) and societal factors, attitudes, and characteristics that influence trauma likelihood and intervention (e.g., societal norms regarding tolerance for interpersonal violence). This type of multilevel approach provides a public health framework for developing an array of strategies aimed at preventing the occurrence and sequelae of trauma.

Prevention aims to reduce the incidence, prevalence, duration and recurrence of mental health problems, related risks, and the impact on individuals, their families, and society (World Health Organization 2004). Different types of programs and approaches are associated with each level of prevention. Universal preventive interventions are targeted at the general population and are not based on the level of individual risk. Selective preventive interventions are targeted at individuals whose risk of developing a problem (e.g., child trauma or PTSD) is higher than average (e.g., children who live in a violent neighborhood or an area experiencing armed conflict). Indicated preventive interventions are targeted at high-risk individuals who have minimal but detectable signs or symptoms foreshadowing a problem or disorder. Finally, tertiary prevention includes both treatment and maintenance to prevent additional problems (see Fig. 3.1).

3.2.1 Preventing Trauma Exposure

From a public health perspective, preventing exposure to childhood trauma in the first place is likely to have the most meaningful population-level effect. Preventive interventions aimed at reducing childhood trauma exposure have largely focused on childhood maltreatment. Home-visiting programs that target new mothers with known risk factors for child maltreatment (e.g., poverty, maternal substance abuse),

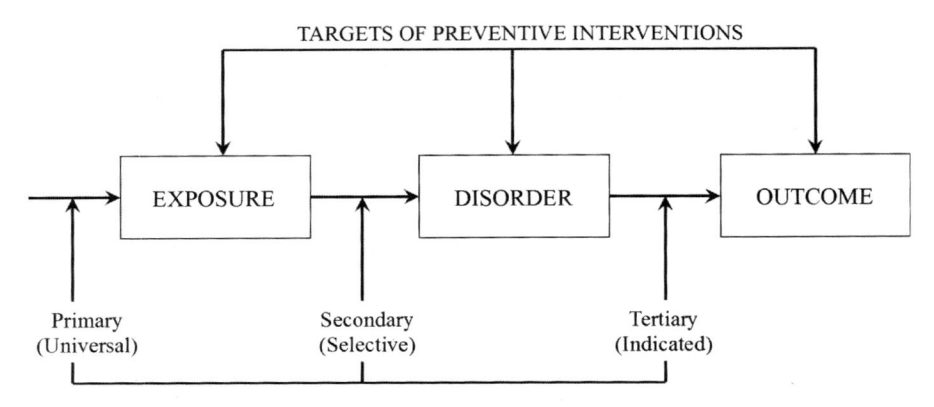

```
                    TARGETS OF PREVENTIVE INTERVENTIONS
                    ┌───────────────┬───────────────┐
                    ↓               ↓               ↓
        ┌─────────────┐    ┌─────────────┐    ┌─────────────┐
    →   │  EXPOSURE   │ →  │  DISORDER   │ →  │   OUTCOME   │
        └─────────────┘    └─────────────┘    └─────────────┘
              ↑                  ↑                  ↑
              │                  │                  │
           Primary            Secondary          Tertiary
          (Universal)         (Selective)        (Indicated)
```

Fig. 3.1 Epidemiology explicitly includes disease *prevention* as a goal. This figure depicts the targets of the three major classes of preventive interventions in epidemiology: primary, secondary, and tertiary (Adapted from Costello and Angold (1995))

such as the Nurse-Family Partnership in the USA, have been demonstrated to be effective at preventing child maltreatment and improving a wide range of child outcomes (Eckenrode et al. 2010; Miller 2015). This approach is being combined with other preventive interventions in the Durham Family Initiative (DFI) to prevent the occurrence of child maltreatment in Durham County, North Carolina. Based on evidence that risk factors for child maltreatment operate at the level of children, parents, families, neighborhood, and community levels, the DFI has created a preventive system of care that seeks to reduce risk factors at each of these levels through universal screening, early intervention for high-risk families, neighborhood- and community-level interventions, and collaboration among government agencies to provide these services (Dodge et al. 2004). For example, families may receive crisis intervention services or parent training to reduce family conflict. At the community level, organized volunteers may work to improve access to social services in high-risk neighborhoods, provide social support and respite care, and improve coordination among social service agencies. Ultimately these types of multilevel approaches are likely to be necessary to prevent the occurrence of childhood maltreatment and other forms of child trauma.

Despite the recognition of child trauma as a global phenomenon, there are strikingly few rigorous prevention studies in LAMICs. A review of child maltreatment prevention interventions revealed that 0.6 % of the studies were conducted in middle-income countries and none were conducted in low-income countries (Mikton and Butchart 2009).

3.2.2 Preventing PTSD and Trauma-Related Psychopathology

A second public health approach to childhood trauma is to prevent the onset of PTSD and other forms of trauma-related psychopathology among children exposed to trauma. Effective interventions have been developed to prevent the onset of PTSD in trauma-exposed youths in the USA that draw on techniques used in evidence-based treatments for child PTSD (e.g., trauma-focused cognitive behavior therapy). Specifically, a brief 4-session intervention that provided behavioral skills training to children who had recently experienced traumatic violence, and their parents, prevented the onset of post-traumatic stress disorder and anxiety 3 months later (Berkowitz et al. 2011). The intervention enhanced parent support by increasing communication between the child and their caregiver and provided behavioral skills to cope with post-trauma symptoms, such as deep breathing. A number of universal school-based prevention programs have been developed for trauma-exposed youth living in contexts where armed conflict and violence are common (Ager et al. 2011; Gelkopf and Berger 2009). The content of these programs vary, including techniques such as psychoeducation, skills training, resiliency strategies, and mobilization of social support. School-based interventions have resulted in improvement in PTS symptoms, anxiety, and functional impairment among children in Israel faced with ongoing terrorism (Berger et al. 2007).

A number of selective or indicated school-based interventions have been examined for youth PTSD, and the results on initial and sustained effects of the interventions have been mixed (Constandinides et al. 2011; Hasanovic et al. 2009). Other prevention efforts exist (e.g., psychological first aid—aimed at addressing mental health symptoms in the immediate aftermath of disasters, family-focused interventions that focus on keeping families together, and youth clubs that engage youth in recreational and group processing activities); however, many of these have limited evidence to support their effectiveness or have elements that have been shown to be iatrogenic with adults (e.g., psychological debriefing) (Aulagnier et al. 2004). These limitations in the child trauma prevention literature underscore the necessity for increased investment in prevention efforts and additional rigorous studies on interventions designed to prevent or decrease the impact of trauma exposure on mental health and functional outcomes among children and adolescents.

3.2.3 Trauma Treatment and the Global Mental Health Treatment Gap

Evidence-based treatments (EBTs) have been developed for children exposed to trauma, and these treatments are effective at reducing PTS symptoms and other internalizing and externalizing problems (for a review, see Dorsey et al. in press). However, most children in need of trauma treatment globally do not have access to these interventions. In LAMICs, four out of five people in need of mental health services do not receive them (World Health Organization 2010), and poor access to mental health services is especially prominent among children and adolescents (Saxena et al. 2007). Barriers to accessing and implementing EBTs in LAMICs include lack of government funds, centralization of mental health services in large cities, stigma, and the scarcity of mental health professionals (Kieling et al. 2011; Patel et al. 2011). Shortages in mental health workers significantly reduce access to mental health services, particularly for children who often comprise a large portion of the population in LAMICs.

Acceptability of EBTs across cultures is another barrier to accessing services for children in LAMICs (Patel et al. 2011). Only 10 % of randomized controlled mental health trials come from LAMICs (Kieling et al. 2011). The extent to which Western treatments for child trauma are acceptable in LAMICs is unknown. A number of culturally specific syndromes associated with child trauma have been identified in low-resource settings (e.g., Betancourt et al. 2009). Though descriptions of local syndromes are similar to Western mood, anxiety, and conduct disorders, they also consist of culturally specific symptoms that may not be addressed in Western EBTs. Moreover, contextual differences also pose a threat to acceptability and effectiveness of treatments. For instance, many EBTs for youth are designed to involve caregivers. The availability of caregivers and child-caregiver relationships may differ by culture (Murray et al. 2013), and these differences may not be reflected in Western EBTs. Other contextual factors that may impact acceptability include literacy rates among clients, language differences, religious beliefs, therapist gender, and the use of culturally specific metaphors (Kaysen et al. 2013; Patel et al. 2011).

In addition to these general treatment barriers, treating trauma-exposed youth in LAMICs comes with unique complexities. For example, displaced children living in refugee camps struggle with basic needs of food, water, and clothing, making mental health a lower priority for families. In addition, uncertainty in the child's legal status and political instability make it challenging for consistent provision of and access to mental health services. Children unaccompanied by adults are most difficult to reach as they are often victims of exploitation, abuse, forced prostitution, or child labor (Reed et al. 2012).

3.2.4 Efforts to Address Global Mental Health Barriers

To address the mass shortage of mental health professionals, many have adopted a task-sharing approach in LAMICs (Kakuma et al. 2011). Task-sharing involves the use of nonspecialists, such as lay personnel, nurses, and community health workers, in the delivery of EBTs (Patel et al. 2011). Numerous studies have demonstrated the effectiveness and feasibility of task-sharing for mental health problems such as anxiety, depression, and trauma and physical health interventions such as antiretroviral treatment and obstetric care (Dawson et al., 2013; Kakuma et al. 2011; Shumbusho et al. 2009). Though this approach has been used less frequently to treat trauma-exposed youth, studies have demonstrated that lay counselors can effectively implement child trauma treatments (Ertl et al. 2011; Murray et al. 2013).

Numerous approaches have been adopted to address the acceptability of EBTs in LAMICs such as the Design, Implementation, Monitoring, and Evaluation (DIME) process (AMHRG 2013). DIME was specifically designed for researchers and organizations implementing treatments for trauma-affected populations. The process involves (1) a qualitative assessment to identify local mental health priorities; (2) a development/adaptation and validation of culturally appropriate measures; (3) a population-based assessment to gauge the problem prevalence; (4) an intervention design of the intervention to address the problem; (5) a selection, adaptation, and implementation of interventions; and (6) an assessment of intervention impact. The DIME process has been used to develop locally relevant measures (Bolton et al. 2014), identify locally relevant mental health issues (e.g., depression-like syndrome), understand local descriptions of symptoms and causes (Murray et al. 2006), and select and adapt treatments that fit the locally identified psychosocial problems (Murray et al. 2011). Psychosocial issues that have been addressed using the DIME process include violence, HIV, and parental loss (Bolton et al. 2014; Murray et al. 2006; Murray et al. 2015). .

3.2.5 Global Intervention Efforts

Although research on the feasibility and effectiveness of child trauma treatments in LAMICs lags behind that of high-income countries, the past two decades have witnessed an increase in global efforts to study the treatment of child trauma. Child trauma treatment studies have been conducted in multiple regions in Africa (e.g., McMullen et al. 2013; Murray et al. 2015; O'Donnell et al. 2014), Asia (e.g., Zeng & Silverstein 2011), and Europe (e.g., Layne et al. 2008). Most studies have focused on children who have been impacted by war (Ertl et al. 2011; McMullen et al. 2013) and to a lesser extent orphans (Murray et al. 2013; O'Donnell et al. 2014) and refugees (Schauer et al. 2004). Despite this increase in treatment efforts, many of these studies have lacked rigorous research methods (e.g., non-randomized and pre-post designs, Jordans et al. 2009), and fewer than a dozen RCTs have been conducted on a variety of child trauma treatments in LAMICs. However, feasibility studies and RCTs have contributed to a growing literature on a number of culturally adapted treatments for childhood trauma, many of which have incorporated culturally acceptable methods in the identification of culturally relevant psychosocial problems, development of locally validated measures, and adaptation to treatments and delivery methods (Murray et al. 2015).

In particular, trauma-focused cognitive behavioral therapy (TF-CBT)—an established EBT for treatment child trauma (Cohen et al. 2006)—has been shown to be effective at reducing mental health problems with a range trauma-exposed populations including orphans (Murray et al. 2015; O'Donnell et al. 2014), former child soldiers (McMullen et al. 2013), and war-affected, sexually exploited girls (O'Callaghan et al. 2013). Notably, all of these studies included adaptations to the treatment and delivery method to fit the local context, using the DIME approach outlined above, and in some cases TF-CBT was implemented by lay counselors with local supervisors (Murray et al. 2015). While the core components of TF-CBT were maintained, major themes of adaptation included the engagement of the larger family system, incorporation of culturally appropriate stories and analogies, use of local language, and incorporation of core cultural values into treatment components. Narrative exposure therapy (NET), a short-term trauma-focused treatment developed for use in low-resource settings (Schauer et al. 2004), has also been shown to be effective in LAMICs including former child soldiers (Ertl et al. 2011), refugee children affected by the Tsunami in Sri Lanka (Catani et al. 2009), and Rwandan genocide orphans (Schaal et al. 2009). Taken together, this emerging literature points to promising new public health directions; combining approaches such as task-sharing and DIME can increase the feasibility, effectiveness, and scalability of treatments and ultimately help address the mental health treatment gap for trauma-exposed children in low-resource settings.

3.3 Conclusion and Future Directions

Findings from epidemiological studies show that the prevalence of childhood trauma worldwide is remarkably high. Childhood trauma exposure increases risk for the onset of virtually all commonly occurring forms of mental disorders and for a wide range of chronic physical health conditions across the lifespan. Childhood trauma is also consistently associated with poor long-term socioeconomic as well as social and relationship outcomes. The relationship between childhood trauma and academic achievement is uncertain, and future research is needed to disentangle whether poor academic achievement is a consequence of child trauma or social factors that often co-occur with trauma exposure in children. Furthermore, PTSD is a common mental health consequence of childhood trauma that tends to be chronic. It is unclear whether PTSD contributes to physical health, academic, socioeconomic, and interpersonal outcomes independent of childhood trauma since most studies do not account for child trauma exposure. Overall, child trauma exposure is a powerful determinant of the distribution of mental health and other poor life outcomes globally.

Developing widely applicable interventions that target these consequences is therefore of critical public health importance. Dissemination and implementation of multilevel interventions to prevent and treat childhood trauma exposure and trauma-related psychopathology and implementation adaptations to effective interventions in settings with limited access to mental health resources are critical components of a public health response to child trauma. Despite increased efforts to study the prevention and treatment of childhood trauma exposure and its sequelae, we identify several gaps in the current literature and offer recommendations for future directions. First, rigorous examinations of interventions that aim to prevent childhood trauma exposure and the onset of PTSD, which are likely to have the most widespread public health impact, are largely absent in LAMICs. Specifically, the few existing child trauma primary prevention efficacy studies, which aim to reduce the occurrence of childhood trauma, measure indirect outcomes, such as parent-child relationships, parenting skills, and conflict resolution (Khowaja et al. 2016; Oveisi et al. 2010), instead of childhood trauma exposure itself, limiting the implications of the findings. Similarly, PTSD prevention studies in low-resource settings frequently lack rigorous designs (e.g., pre-post experimental designs). Future research on childhood trauma and PTSD prevention should aim to use more rigorous experimental design, including culturally validated measurement of child trauma or mental health outcomes and the inclusion of a control group. Second, research on the efficacy and effectiveness of prevention and treatment of childhood trauma in low-resource settings still lags behind that of high-income settings. Future research should include randomized controlled trials that address a variety of common childhood traumas and measure relevant child outcomes.

Third, while evidence for the effectiveness and feasibility of child trauma treatments in low-resource settings is growing, this research has largely focused on war-affected and orphaned youth, restricting our understanding of their efficacy to specific forms of trauma. Moreover, future research is needed to develop strategies that increase accessibility and sustainability of these treatments in low-resource settings, such as the use of lay health providers in the delivery of treatment and the integration of mental health treatment into existing school and health systems. Together, these approaches will contribute to reducing the public health burden of child trauma exposure.

References

Ager A, Akesson B, Stark L, Flouri E, Okot B, McCollister F, Boothby N (2011) The impact of the school-based Psychosocial Structured Activities (PSSA) program on conflict-affected children in northern Uganda. J Child Psychol Psychiatry Allied Disciplines 52(11):1124–1133

Almqvist K, Brandell-Forsberg M (1997) Refugee children in Sweden: post-traumatic stress disorder in Iranian preschool children exposed to organized violence. Child Abuse Negl 21(4):351–366

Almqvist K, Broberg AG (1999) Mental health and social adjustment in young refugee children 3 1/2 years after their arrival in Sweden. J Am Acad Child Adolesc Psychiatry 38(6):723–730

American Psychiatric Association (2013) Diagnostic and statistical manual of mental disorders, 5th edition (DSM-5). American Psychiatric Press, Washington, DC

Annerbäck EM, Sahlqvist L, Svedin CG, Wingren G, Gustafsson PA (2012) Child physical abuse and concurrence of other types of child abuse in Sweden: associations with health and risk behaviors. Child Abuse Negl 36(7–8):585–595

Applied Mental Health Research Group (2013) Design, implementation, monitoring,and evaluation of mental health and psychosocial assistance programs for trauma survivors in low resource countries: a user's manual for researchers and program implementers. In: Module 1: qualitative assessment. United States: Johns Hopkins University Bloomberg School of Public Health

Aspelmeier JE, Elliott AN, Smith CH (2007) Childhood sexual abuse, attachment, and trauma symptoms in college females: the moderating role of attachment. Child Abuse Negl 31(5):549–566

Attanayake V, McKay R, Joffres M, Singh S, Burkle F Jr, Mills E (2009) Prevalence of mental disorders among children exposed to war: a systematic review of 7,920 children. Med Confl Surviv 25(1):4–19

Aulagnier M, Verger P, Rouillon F (2004) Efficiency of psychological debriefing in preventing post-traumatic stress disorders. Revue D'epidemiologie et de Sante Publique 52(1):67–69

Bailey BN, Delaney-Black V, Hannigan JH, Ager J, Sokol RJ, Covington CY (2005) Somatic complaints in children and community violence exposure. J Dev Behav Pediatr 26(5):341–348

Barenbaum J, Ruchkin V, Schwab-Stone M (2004) The psychosocial aspects of children exposed to war: practice and policy initiatives. J Child Psychol Psychiatry 45(1):41–62

Bayer CP, Klasen F, Adam H (2007) Association of trauma and PTSD symptoms with openness to reconciliation and feelings of revenge among former Ugandan and Congolese child soldiers. JAMA 298(5):555–559

Benjet C (2010) Childhood adversities of populations living in low-income countries: prevalence, characteristics, and mental health consequences. Curr Opin Psychiatry 23(4):356–362

Berger R, Dutton MA, Greene R (2007) School-based intervention for prevention and treatment of elementary-students' terror-related distress in Israel: a quasi-randomized controlled trial. J Trauma Stress 20(4):541–551

Berkowitz SJ, Stover CS, Marans SR (2011) The child and family traumatic stress intervention: secondary prevention for youth at risk of developing PTSD. J Child Psychol Psychiatry 52(6):676–685

Betancourt TS, Borisova II, Williams TP, Brennan RT, Whitfield TH, de la Soudiere M, Williamson J, Gilman SE (2010a) Sierra leone's former child soldiers: a follow-up study of psychosocial adjustment and community reintegration. Child Dev 81(4):1077–1095

Betancourt TS, Brennan RT, Rubin-Smith J, Fitzmaurice GM, Gilman SE (2010b) Sierra Leone's former child soldiers: a longitudinal study of risk, protective factors, and mental health. J Am Acad Child Adolesc Psychiatry 49(6):606–615

Betancourt TS, Speelman L, Onyango G, Bolton P (2009) Psychosocial problems of war-affected youth in Northern Uganda: a qualitative study. Transcult Psychiatry 46(2):238

Boden JM, Horwood LJ, Fergusson DM (2007) Exposure to childhood sexual and physical abuse and subsequent educational achievement outcomes. Child Abuse Negl 31(10):1101–1114

Bolton P, Bass JK, Zangana GAS, Kamal T, Murray SM, Kaysen D, Lejuez CW, Lindgren K, Pagoto S, Murray LK, Ahmed AMA, Amin NMM, Rosenblum M, Van Wyk SS (2014) A randomized controlled trial of mental health interventions for survivors of systematic violence in Kurdistan, Northern Iraq. BMC Psychiatry 14(1):1

Breslau N, Kessler RC, Chilcoat HD, Schultz LR, Davis GC, Andreski P (1998) Trauma and posttraumatic stress disorder in the community: the 1996 detroit area survey of trauma. Arch Gen Psychiatry 55(7):626–632

Breslau N, Wilcox HC, Storr CL, Lucia VC, Anthony JC (2004) Trauma exposure and posttraumatic stress disorder: a study of youths in Urban America. J Urban Health 81(4):530–544

Caspi A, Houts RM, Belsky DW, Goldman-Mellor SJ, Harrington H, Israel S, Meier MH, Ramrakha S, Shalev I, Poulton R, Moffitt TE (2014) The p factor: one general psychopathology factor in the structure of psychiatric disorders? Clin Psychol Sci 2(2):119–137

Catani C, Kohiladevy M, Ruf M, Schauer E, Elbert T, Neuner F (2009) Treating children traumatized by war and Tsunami: a comparison between exposure therapy and meditation-relaxation in North-East Sri Lanka. BMC Psychiatry 9:22

Cloitre M, Cohen LR, Edelman RE, Han H (2001) Posttraumatic stress disorder and extent of trauma exposure as correlates of medical problems and perceived health among women with childhood abuse. Women Health 34(3):1–17

Cohen RT, Canino GJ, Bird HR, Celedón JC (2008) Violence, abuse, and asthma in Puerto Rican children. Am J Respir Crit Care Med 178(5):453–459

Cohen JA, Mannarino AP, Deblinger E (2006) Treating trauma and traumatic grief in children and adolescents. Guilford Press, New York

Cole PM, Putnam FW (1992) Effect of incest on self and social functioning: a developmental psychopathology perspective. J Consult Clin Psychol 60(2):174–184

Constandinides D, Kamens S, Marshoud B, Flefel F (2011) Research in ongoing conflict zones: effects of a school-based intervention for Palestinian children. Peace Conflict J Peace Psychol 17(3):270–302

Copeland WE, Keeler G, Angold A, Costello EJ (2007) Traumatic events and posttraumatic stress in childhood. Arch Gen Psychiatry 64(5):577–584

Costello EJ, Angold A (1995) Developmental epidemiology. In: Cicchetti D, Cohen D (eds) Developmental psychopathology, vol 1: theory and methods. Wiley & Sons, New York

Davis DA, Luecken LJ, Zautra AJ (2005) Are reports of childhood abuse related to the experience of chronic pain in adulthood? A meta-analytic review of the literature. Clin J Pain 21(5):398–405

Davis J, Petretic-Jackson P (2000) The impact of child sexual abuse on adult interpersonal functioning: a review and synthesis of the empirical literature. Aggress Violent Behav 5(3):291–328

Dawson AJ, Buchan J, Duffield C, Homer CS, Wijewardena K (2013) Task shifting and sharing in maternal and reproductive health in low-income countries: a narrative synthesis of current evidence. Health Policy Plan 29(3):396–408

De Bellis MD, Woolley DP, Hooper SR (2013) Neuropsychological findings in pediatric maltreatment: relationship of PTSD, dissociative symptoms, and abuse/neglect indices to neurocognitive outcomes. Child Maltreat 18(3):171–183

Derluyn I, Broekaert E, Schuyten G, De Temmerman E (2004) Post-traumatic stress in former Ugandan child soldiers. Lancet 363(9412):861–863

DiLillo D (2001) Interpersonal functioning among women reporting a history of childhood sexual abuse: empirical findings and methodological issues. Clin Psychol Rev 21(4):553–576

Dodge KA, Berlin LJ, Epstein M, Spitz-Roth A, O'Donnell K, Kaufman M, Amaya-Jackson L, Rosch J, Christopoulos C (2004) The Durham family initiative: a preventive system of care. Child Welfare 83(2):109

Dorsey S, Lucid L, Murray L, Bolton P, Itemba D, Manongi R, Whetten K (2015) A qualitative study of mental health problems among orphaned children and adolescents in Tanzania. J Nerv Ment Dis 203(11):864–870

Dorsey S, McLaughlin KA, Kerns SEU, Harrison JP, Lambert HK, Briggs-King E, Cox JR, Amaya-Jackson L (2016) Evidence base update for psychosocial treatments for children and adolescents exposed to traumatic events. J Clin Child Adolesc Psychol: 1–28

Eckenrode J, Campa M, Luckey DW, Henderson CR, Cole R, Kitzman H, Anson E, Sidora-Arcoleo K, Powers J, Olds D (2010) Long-term effects of prenatal and infancy nurse home visitation on the life course of youths: 19-year follow-up of a randomized trial. Arch Pediatr Adolesc Med 164(1):9–15

Eckenrode J, Laird M, Doris J (1993) School performance and disciplinary problems among abused and neglected children. Dev Psychol 29(1):53–62

Ertl V, Pfeiffer A, Schauer E, Elbert T, Neuner F (2011) Community-implemented trauma therapy for former child soldiers in Northern Uganda: a randomized controlled trial. JAMA 306(5):503–512

Feldman S, Downey G (1994) Rejection sensitivity as a mediator of the impact of childhood exposure to family violence on adult attachment behavior. Dev Psychopathol 6:231–247

Felitti FVJ, Anda MRF, Nordenberg D, Williamson PDF, Spitz MAM, Edwards V, Koss MP, Marks JS (1998) Relationship of childhood abuse and household dysfunction to many of the leading causes of death in adults: The Adverse Childhood Experiences (ACE) Study. Am J Prev Med 14(4):245–258

Finkelhor D, Ormrod RK, Turner HA, Hamby SL (2005) The victimization of children and youth: a comprehensive, national survey. Child Maltreat 10(1):5–25

Follette VM, Polusny MA, Bechtle AE, Naugle AE (1996) Cumulative trauma: the impact of child sexual abuse, adult sexual assault, and spouse abuse. J Trauma Stress 9(1):25–35

Gelkopf M, Berger R (2009) A school-based, teacher-mediated prevention program (ERASE-Stress) for reducing terror-related traumatic reactions in Israeli youth: a quasi-randomized controlled trial. J Child Psychol Psychiatry 50(8):962–971

Giaconia RM, Reinherz HZ, Silverman AB, Pakiz B, Frost AK, Cohen E (1995) Traumas and post-traumatic stress disorder in a community population of older adolescents. J Am Acad Child Adolesc Psychiatry 34(10):1369–1380

Green JG, McLaughlin KA, Berglund PA, Gruber MJ, Sampson NA, Zaslavsky AM, Kessler RC (2010) Childhood adversities and adult psychiatric disorders in the national comorbidity survey replication I: associations with first onset of DSM-IV disorders. Arch Gen Psychiatry 67(2):113–123

Hasanovic M, Srabovic S, Rasidovic M, Sehovic M, Hasanbasic E, Husanovic J, Hodzic R (2009) Psychosocial assistance to students with posttraumatic stress disorder in primary and secondary schools in post-war Bosnia Herzegovina. Psychiatr Danub 21(4):463–473

Haskett ME, Kistner JA (1991) Social interactions and peer perceptions of young physically abused children. Child Dev 62(5):979–990

Jonson-Reid M (2015) A prospective analysis of the relationship between reported child maltreatment and special education among poor children. Child Maltreat 9(4):382–394

Jordans MJD, Tol WA, Komproe IH, De Jong JVTM (2009) Systematic review of evidence and treatment approaches: psychosocial and mental health care for children in war. Child Adolesc Mental Health 14(1):2–14

Kakuma R, Minas H, Van Ginneken N, Dal Poz MR, Desiraju K, Morris JE, Saxena S, Scheffler RM (2011) Human resources for mental health care: current situation and strategies for action. Lancet 378(9803):1654–1663

Kaysen D, Lindgren K, Zangana GAS, Murray L, Bass J, Bolton P (2013) Adaptation of cognitive processing therapy for treatment of torture victims: experience in Kurdistan, Iraq. Psychological Trauma Theory Res Practice Policy 5(2):184–192

Kessler RC, McLaughlin KA, Green JG, Gruber MJ, Sampson NA, Zaslavsky AM, Aguilar-Gaxiola S, Alhamzawi AO, Alonso J, Angermeyer M, Benjet C, Bromet E, Chatterji S, de Girolamo G, Demyttenaere K, Fayyad J, Florescu S, Gal G, Gureje O, Haro JM, Hu CY, Karam EG, Kawakami N, Lee S, Lépine JP, Ormel J, Posada-Villa J, Sagar R, Tsang A, Ustün TB, Vassilev S, Viana MC, Williams DR (2010) Childhood adversities and adult psychopathology in the WHO World Mental Health Surveys. Br J Psychiatry J Mental Sci 197(5):378–385

Keyes KM, Eaton NR, Krueger RF, McLaughlin KA, Wall MM, Grant BF, Hasin DS (2012) Childhood maltreatment and the structure of common psychiatric disorders. Br J Psychiatry J Mental Sci 200(2):107–115

Khamis V (2005) Post-traumatic stress disorder among school age Palestinian children. Child Abuse Negl 29(1):81–95

Khowaja Y, Karmaliani R, Hirani S, Khowaja AR, Rafique G, Mcfarlane J (2016) A Pilot study of a 6-week parenting program for mothers of pre-school children attending family health centers in Karachi, Pakistan. Int J Health Policy Manage 5(2):91–97

Kieling C, Baker-Henningham H, Belfer M, Conti G, Ertem I, Omigbodun O, Rohde LA, Srinath S, Ulkuer N, Rahman A (2011) Child and adolescent mental health worldwide: evidence for action. Lancet 378(9801):1515–1525

Kleinman A, Kleinman J (1991) Suffering and its professional transformation: toward an ethnography of interpersonal experience. Cult Med Psychiatry 15(3):275

Kim J, Cicchetti D (2010) Longitudinal pathways linking child maltreatment, emotion regulation, peer relations, and psychopathology. J Child Psychol Psychiatry 51(6):706–716

Lamers-Winkelman F, Schipper JCD, Oosterman M (2012) Children's physical health complaints after exposure to intimate partner violence. Br J Health Psychol 17(4):771–784

Lang AJ, Laffaye C, Satz LE, McQuaid JR, Malcarne VL, Dresselhaus TR, Stein MB (2006) Relationships among childhood maltreatment, PTSD, and health in female veterans in primary care. Child Abuse Negl 30(11):1281–1292

Lansford JE, Dodge KA, Pettit GS, Bates JE, Crozier J, Kaplow J (2002) A 12-year prospective study of the long-term effects of early child physical maltreatment on psychological, behavioral, and academic problems in adolescence. Pediatr Adolesc Med 156(8):824–830

Layne CM, Saltzman WR, Poppleton L, Burlingame GM, Pašalić A, Duraković E, Musić M, Campara N, Dapo N, Arslanagić B, Steinberg AM, Pynoos RS (2008) Effectiveness of a school-based group psychotherapy program for war-exposed adolescents: a randomized controlled trial. J Am Acad Child Adolesc Psychiatry 47(9):1048–1062

Leiter J, Johnsen MC (1997) Child maltreatment and school performance declines: an event-history analysis. Am Educ Res J 34(3):563–589

Macksoud MS, Aber JL (1996) The war experiences and psychosocial development of children in Lebanon. Child Dev 67(1):70–88

Macmillan R (2000) Adolescent victimization and income deficits in adulthood: Rethinking the costs of criminal violence from a life-course perspective. Criminol 38(2):553–588

Macmillan R, Hagan J (2004) Violence in the transition to adulthood: adolescent victimization, education, and socioeconomic attainment in later life. J Res Adolesc 14(2):127–158

McLaughlin KA, Basu A, Walsh K, Slopen N, Sumner JA, Koenen KC, Keyes KM (2016) Childhood exposure to violence and chronic physical conditions in a national sample of U.S. youth. Psychosom Med 78(9):1072–1083

McLaughlin KA, Conron KJ, Koenen KC, Gilman SE (2010) Childhood adversity, adult stressful life events, and risk of past-year psychiatric disorder: a test of the stress sensitization hypothesis in a population-based sample of adults. Psychol Med 40(10):1647–1658

McLaughlin KA, Green JG, Gruber MJ, Sampson NA, Zaslavsky AM, Kessler RC (2012) Childhood adversities and first onset of psychiatric disorders in a national sample of US adolescents. Arch Gen Psychiatry 69(11):1151–1160

McLaughlin KA, Koenen KC, Hill ED, Petukhova M, Sampson NA, Zaslavsky AM, Kessler RC (2013) Trauma exposure and posttraumatic stress disorder in a national sample of adolescents. J Am Acad Child Adolesc Psychiatry 52(8):815–830

McMullen J, O'Callaghan P, Shannon C, Black A, Eakin J (2013) Group trauma-focused cognitive-behavioural therapy with former child soldiers and other war-affected boys in the DR Congo: a randomised controlled trial. J Child Psychol Psychiatry Allied Disciplines 54(11):1231–1241

Mikton C, Butchart A (2009) Child maltreatment prevention: a systematic review of reviews. Bull World Health Organ 87(5):353–361

Miller TR (2015) Projected outcomes of nurse-family partnership home visitation during 1996–2013, USA. Prev Sci 16(6):765–777

Mollica RF, Poole C, Son L, Murray CC, Tor S (1997) Effects of war trauma on Cambodian refugee adolescents' functional health and mental health status. J Am Acad Child Adolesc Psychiatry 36(8):1098–1106

Mullen PE, Martin JL, Anderson JC, Romans SE, Herbison GP (1996) The long-term impact of the physical, emotional, and sexual abuse of children: a community study. Child Abuse Negl 20(1):7–21

Murray LK, Bass J, Chomba E, Imasiku M, Thea D, Semrau K, Cohen JA, Lam C, Bolton P (2011) Validation of the UCLA child post traumatic stress disorder-reaction index in Zambia. Int J Ment Heal Syst 5(1):24

Murray LK, Familiar I, Skavenski S, Jere E, Cohen J, Imasiku M, Mayeya J, Bass JK, Bolton P (2013) An evaluation of trauma focused cognitive behavioral therapy for children in Zambia. Child Abuse Negl 37(12):1175–1185

Murray LK, Haworth A, Semrau K, Singh M, Aldrovandi GM, Sinkala M, Thea DM, Bolton PA (2006) Violence and abuse among HIV-infected women and their children in Zambia: a qualitative study. J Nerv Mental Dis 194(8):610–615

Murray LK, Skavenski S, Kane JC, Mayeya J, Dorsey S, Cohen JA, Michalopoulos LT, Imasiku M, Bolton PA (2015) Effectiveness of trauma-focused cognitive behavioral therapy among trauma-affected children in Lusaka, Zambia : a randomized clinical trial. JAMA Pediatr 169(8):761

O'Callaghan P, McMullen J, Shannon C, Rafferty H, Black A (2013) A randomized controlled trial of trauma-focused cognitive behavioral therapy for sexually exploited, war-affected congolese girls. J Am Acad Child Adolesc Psychiatry 52(4):359–369

O'Donnell K, Dorsey S, Gong W, Ostermann J, Whetten R, Cohen JA, Itemba D, Manongi R, Whetten K (2014) Treating maladaptive grief and posttraumatic stress symptoms in orphaned children in Tanzania: group-based trauma-focused cognitive–behavioral therapy. J Trauma Stress 27(2):664–671

Oveisi S, Ardabili HE, Dadds MR, Majdzadeh R, Mohammadkhani P, Rad JA, Shahrivar Z (2010) Primary prevention of parent-child conflict and abuse in Iranian mothers: a randomized-controlled trial. Child Abuse Negl 34(3):206–213

Pacella ML, Hruska B, Delahanty DL (2013) The physical health consequences of PTSD and PTSD symptoms: a meta-analytic review. J Anxiety Disord 27(1):33–46

Patel V, Chowdhary N, Rahman A, Verdeli H (2011) Improving access to psychological treatments: lessons from developing countries. Behav Res Ther 49(9):523–528

Perkonigg A, Kessler RC, Storz S, Wittchen HU (2000) Traumatic events and post-traumatic stress disorder in the community: prevalence, risk factors and comorbidity. Acta Psychiatr Scand 101(1):46–59

Perkonigg A, Pfister H, Stein MB, Höfler M, Lieb R, Maercker A, Wittchen HU (2005) Longitudinal course of posttraumatic stress disorder and posttraumatic stress disorder symptoms in a community sample of adolescents and young adults. Am J Psychiatry 162:1320–1327

Reed RV, Fazel M, Jones L, Panter-Brick C, Stein A (2012) Mental health of displaced and refugee children resettled in low-income and middle-income countries: risk and protective factors. Lancet 379(9812):250–265

Rich-Edwards JW, Spiegelman D, Lividoti Hibert EN, Jun HJ, Todd TJ, Kawachi I, Wright RJ (2010) Abuse in childhood and adolescence as a predictor of type 2 diabetes in adult women. Am J Prev Med 39(6):529–536

Rumstein-McKean O, Hunsley J (2001) Interpersonal and family functioning of female survivors of childhood sexual abuse. Clin Psychol Rev 21(3):471–490

Saxena S, Thornicroft G, Knapp M, Whiteford H (2007) Resources for mental health: scarcity, inequity, and inefficiency. Lancet 370(9590):878–889

Schaal S, Elbert T, Neuner F (2009) Narrative exposure therapy versus interpersonal psychotherapy: a pilot randomized controlled trial with rwandan genocide orphans. Psychother Psychosom 78(5):298–306

Schauer E, Neuner F, Elbert T, Ertl V, Onyut LP, Odenwald M, Schauer M (2004) Narrative exposure therapy in children: a case study 1. Ther 2(1):18–32

Schnurr PP, Green BL (2004) Understanding relationships among trauma, post-traumatic stress disorder, and health outcomes. Adv Mind Body Med 20(1):18–29

Scott KM, Koenen KC, Aguilar-Gaxiola S, Alonso J, Angermeyer MC, Benjet C, Bruffaerts R, Caldas-de-Almeida JM, de Girolamo G, Florescu S, Iwata N, Levinson D, Lim CC, Murphy S, Ormel J, Posada-Villa J, Kessler RC (2013) Associations between lifetime traumatic events and subsequent chronic physical conditions: a cross-national, cross-sectional study. PLoS One 8(11):e80573

Scott KM, Von Korff M, Angermeyer MC, Benjet C, Bruffaerts R, de Girolamo G, Haro JM, Lépine JP, Ormel J, Posada-Villa J, Tachimori H, Kessler RC (2011) Association of childhood adversities and early-onset mental disorders with adult-onset chronic physical conditions. Arch Gen Psychiatry 68(8):838–844

Shumbusho F, van Griensven J, Lowrance D, Turate I, Weaver MA, Price J, Binagwaho A (2009) Task shifting for scale-up of HIV care: evaluation of nurse-centered antiretroviral treatment at rural health centers in Rwanda. PLoS Med 6(10):e1000163

Stensland S, Thoresen S, Wentzel-Larsen T, Zwart JA, Dyb G (2014) Recurrent headache and interpersonal violence in adolescence: the roles of psychological distress, loneliness and family cohesion: the HUNT study. J Headache Pain 15(1):35

Swahn MH, Bossarte RM (2006) The associations between victimization, feeling unsafe, and asthma episodes among US high-school students. Am J Public Health 96(5):802–804

Thabet AAM, Vostanis P (1999) Post-traumatic stress reactions in children of war. J Child Psychol Psychiatry 40(3):385–391

The United Nations Children's Emergency Fund (UNICEF), United Nations. Office of the Special Representative of the Secretary-General for Children, & Armed Conflict (2009) Machel study 10-year strategic review: children and conflict in a changing world. UNICEF, New York

The United Nations Children's Emergency Fund (UNICEF) (2014) With 15 million children caught up in major conflicts, UNICEF declares 2014 a devastating year for children [Press release]. Retrieved from http://www.unicef.org/media/media_78058.html?p=printme

Wegman HL, Stetler C (2009) A meta-analytic review of the effects of childhood abuse on medical outcomes in adulthood. Psychosom Med 71(8):805–812

Widom CS, Czaja SJ, Bentley T, Johnson MS (2012) A prospective investigation of physical health outcomes in abused and neglected children: new findings from a 30-year follow-up. Am J Public Health 102(6):1135–1144

Wolff PH, Tesfai B, Egasso H, Aradomt T (1995) The orphans of Eritrea: a comparison study. J Child Psychol Psychiatry 36(4):633–644

World Health Organization (2004) Prevention of mental disorders: effective interventions and policy options: Summary report. World Health Organization, Geneva

World Health Organization (2010) mhGAP intervention guide for mental, neurological and substance abuse disorders in non-specialized health settings. World Health Organization, Geneva

World Health Organization (2013) Mental health action plan 2013–2020. World Health Organization, Geneva

Zeng EJ, Silverstein LB (2011) China earthquake relief: participatory action work with children. Sch Psychol Int 32(5):498–511

Zielinski DS (2009) Child maltreatment and adult socioeconomic well-being. Child Abuse Negl 33(10):666–678

Applying Evidence-Based Assessment to Childhood Trauma and Bereavement: Concepts, Principles, and Practices

4

Christopher M. Layne, Julie B. Kaplow, and Eric A. Youngstrom

4.1 On the Need for Trauma- and Bereavement-Informed Assessment

Growing recognition of the high prevalence rates of trauma exposure and its severe consequences across the life span have led to international calls to action to train clinicians in essential trauma competencies (Courtois and Gold 2009; Weine et al. 2002), many of which involve assessment (Cook et al. 2014). Nevertheless, standard assessment toolkits generally fail to address this important issue. Many commonly used assessment tools do not include a *trauma* screen or measure of posttraumatic stress disorder (PTSD) symptoms (e.g., Achenbach and Rescorla 2001; Derogatis 1977; Goodman et al. (2000), creating blind spots in risk detection and case formulation that impede the ability of systems to become trauma informed

---

Author disclosures: Drs. Layne and Kaplow are lead authors of the Persistent Complex Bereavement Disorder Checklist, and are contributing authors to Trauma and Grief Component Therapy for Adolescents.

Author Disclosure and Acknowledgements: Drs. Kaplow and Layne are principal investigators of the GIFT (Grief-Informed Foundations of Treatment) Network, a practice research network established to raise the standard of care for bereaved youth and their families. The authors gratefully acknowledge the financial support of New York Life Foundation to the GIFT Network in the writing of this chapter.

C.M. Layne, PhD (✉)
UCLA/Duke University National Center for Child Traumatic Stress, and Department of Psychiatry and Biobehavioral Sciences, University of California, Los Angeles, USA
e-mail: CMLayne@mednet.ucla.edu

J.B. Kaplow, PhD, ABPP
Department of Psychiatry and Behavioral Sciences, University of Texas Health Sciences Center at Houston, Houston, USA

E.A. Youngstrom, PhD
Department of Psychology and Neuroscience, University of North Carolina at Chapel Hill, Chapel Hill, USA

© Springer International Publishing Switzerland 2017
M.A. Landolt et al. (eds.), *Evidence-Based Treatments for Trauma Related Disorders in Children and Adolescents*, DOI 10.1007/978-3-319-46138-0_4

(Ko et al. 2008). Although the accuracy with which PTSD is identified is comparatively higher than many other diagnoses (Regier et al. 2012), standard clinical interviews also yield only modestly accurate trauma-related diagnoses for both child and adult populations (Rettew et al. 2009). These findings suggest that a substantial portion of trauma-exposed youth with likely PTSD is either missed or mislabeled.

In addition, there is substantial evidence that core assessment competencies should encompass and address not only trauma but also *bereavement* in a side-by-side fashion. Childhood bereavement is one of the most frequently reported types of trauma or extreme adversity seen in clinic-referred youth (Pynoos et al. 2014) and is highly prevalent in general population samples. The worldwide lifetime prevalence of children bereaved by one or both parents was 151 million in 2011 (UNICEF 2013), not including deaths of other close loved ones such as siblings or other caregivers. Further, the death of a loved one is also identified as the most common and the most distressing type of trauma among both adults and youth (Breslau et al. 2004; Kaplow et al. 2010). In addition, grief reactions uniquely predict impaired functioning above and beyond the predictive effects of PTSD in bereaved youth (Melhem et al. 2007; Spuji et al. 2012). Such findings point to the incremental clinical utility of addressing grief above and beyond PTSD. More specifically, they underscore the need to screen for both bereavement and trauma exposure, and to assess for each outcome when primary causal risk factors are detected (grief following bereavement; PTSD following trauma exposure; both grief and PTSD following potential traumatic bereavement).

Nevertheless, few standardized assessment tools are available to measure childhood bereavement and accompanying grief reactions. Those that currently exist often do not screen for bereavement or instead lump bereavement into a generic "loss" category that also includes parental divorce and incarceration (Nader and Layne 2009). The introduction of *persistent complex bereavement disorder (PCBD)* as a proposed diagnosis in DSM-5 calls much needed attention to these important assessment issues (Kaplow et al. 2012; Kaplow, Layne, & Pynoos 2014). The inclusion of PCBD in DSM-5, as well as the proposed inclusion of *prolonged grief disorder* in ICD-11, constitute calls to action to carefully assess potentially maladaptive grief reactions and to search for causal risk, vulnerability, protective, and promotive factors that may differentially contribute to adaptive, versus maladaptive, grief reactions (Kaplow, Layne, & Pynoos 2014; Kaplow and Layne 2014; see Layne et al. 2009 for definitions and a basic conceptual framework). Thus, similar to the challenge of accurately detecting trauma and associated posttraumatic stress reactions, the lack of screening for bereavement and associated maladaptive grief reactions also creates gaps and potential blind spots in risk detection and case formulation that reduce the capacity of systems to become bereavement informed (Kaplow, Layne, & Pynoos 2014). Consequently, many traumatized and bereaved youth may remain undetected or, alternatively, may be misdiagnosed and prescribed nonoptimal or inappropriate interventions.

4.2 Strategy and Rationale for Evidence-Based Assessment

From a practical perspective, an in-depth evaluation using structured interviews and collateral informants of every potentially trauma-exposed or bereaved client is not cost-effective and may provide insufficient information to guide treatment. Indeed, universal in-depth evaluations are susceptible to high rates of false positives (overdiagnosis), especially when used in settings where trauma and bereavement have low prevalence rates (Straus et al. 2011). Ironically, too much testing can lead to less accurate assessment results, poorer treatment selection, and worse allocation of limited resources (Kraemer 1992). Thus, a potential solution to this dilemma lies in applying principles of *evidence-based assessment (EBA)*. EBA provides a rigorous yet practical way for clinicians to use assessment tools to guide clinical decision-making and treatment planning (Youngstrom 2013). EBA emphasizes the importance of selecting the best available assessment tools for the specific clinical questions at hand, gathering the best available data using those tools, and judiciously applying assessment data to make informed clinical decisions about individual patients (Hunsley 2015; Hunsley and Mash 2007).

In the remainder of this chapter, we illustrate how concepts, principles, and practices of EBA can be harnessed to enhance the capacity of health professionals to competently assess traumatized and bereaved youth. We begin with practical clinical considerations, including recommended strategies for selecting appropriate measures, enhancing assessment validity, and reasoning through differential diagnosis. We then discuss how EBA can guide not only initial assessment but also monitoring treatment response, as well as surveillance for additional major life events, across the course of treatment. We conclude with a case example illustrating the use of the CHECKS Heuristic—a clinical decision-making tool designed to help clinicians gather, organize, consolidate, integrate, and make meaning of assessment data and segue into case conceptualization and intervention planning.

4.3 Shared Clinical Wisdom: Responses to Common Questions and Concerns About Trauma- and Bereavement-Informed Assessment

Clinicians often present with similar "how to?" and "what if?" questions and concerns as they strive to apply principles of trauma- and bereavement-informed assessment to their practice with traumatized and grieving youth. In this section, we address seven frequently asked questions, framing our responses in terms of recommended competencies for applying EBA to the assessment of trauma-exposed and bereaved youth.

4.3.1 How Can I Psychologically Prepare for a Trauma- or Bereavement-Informed Assessment?

Admittedly, in most diagnostic assessments or risk screening protocols, the very act of evaluating children's symptoms, inquiring about life events or factors that may have precipitated those symptoms, and obtaining details about domain-specific functioning evokes empathy or concern in the clinician. Our experience is that assessing trauma- and bereavement-related issues can markedly intensify a clinician's personal reactions—particularly if the young patient is willing and able to share specific details, thoughts, and feelings about the traumatic event or the loss. As such, *vicarious traumatization* (disturbances in the therapist's cognitive frame of reference including world view and identity; Palm et al. 2004) and *secondary traumatic stress* (emotional distress experienced by an individual having close contact with a trauma survivor; Figley and Kleber 1995) become even more important considerations. These adverse reactions commonly arise when clinicians feel unprepared for what is being shared or become reminded of their own trauma or loss histories. Clinicians thus need to be self-reflective prior to initiating assessments of traumatized or bereaved youth by taking note of their own capacity to listen and be fully present when faced with distressing or provocative content.

Regardless of their own life experiences, clinicians often feel uncomfortable and unsure regarding how to respond (What should I say? What shouldn't I say? What if I start to cry?) when youth reveals disturbing or distressing information during an assessment. It is important to remember that sympathetic listening and bearing witness can be the single most therapeutic aspect of the assessment process, especially if this is the first time the child has shared his/her trauma or loss history. It is often comforting for clinicians to recognize that their ability to express warmth and empathy through body language, not necessarily through words, can play an instrumental role in facilitating the assessment process and establishing a strong rapport with the child. Our studies have found that these unspoken features of quality adult-child communication (maintaining good eye contact, appearing engaged and interested, conveying warmth, smiling as appropriate, etc.) can effectively facilitate children's adaptive psychological functioning following a trauma or a loss (Howell et al. in press; Shapiro et al. 2014).

4.3.2 How Can I Find Measures of PTSD and Maladaptive Grief?

One strategy for locating specialized measures for traumatized or bereaved youth is to review the *Measures Review Database* compiled by the National Child Traumatic Stress Network. This no-cost service (http://www.nctsn.org/resources/online-research/measures-review) describes measures of traumatic events, posttraumatic stress reactions, grief, and associated reactions; summarizes test reliability and validity data; and includes details for obtaining the measure. This database allows clinicians to quickly and efficiently access, evaluate, and compare (when available) information about different measures. The website includes a search function that allows users to identify specific measures by title, author, specific symptom domains assessed, and specific populations.

As a second search strategy, Table 4.1 summarizes selected instruments for assessing DSM-5 ASD, PTSD, and maladaptive grief reactions in preschoolers, school-aged children, and adolescents. Although a comprehensive summary of all measures available is beyond the scope of this chapter, these measures generally reflect those that have seen most widespread use across diverse populations in the childhood traumatic stress field.

Table 4.1 Recommended child and adolescent measures of acute stress, posttraumatic stress, and grief reactions

Construct	Name of measure	Type of measure	Number items	Psychometric data	Reference
Trauma exposure, including complex trauma exposure	Traumatic Experiences Screening Instrument (TESI)	Computer-assisted self-report questionnaire 10–12 min to complete 5th grade reading level	8 types of nonvictimization adversity (including loss) 13 types of interpersonal victimization including emotional abuse and neglect	Test-retest reliability Criterion-referenced validity Predictive validity	Ford, J.D., Grasso, D.J., Hawke, J., & Chapman, J. F. (2013). Poly-victimization among juvenile justice-involved youths. Child Abuse & Neglect, 37, 788–800. Inquiries: Julian Ford jford@uchc.edu
25 adverse childhood experiences and potentially traumatic events, including complex trauma exposure (Also assesses four DSM-5 PTSD symptom clusters, dissociative symptoms, trauma-related functional impairment)	Structured Trauma-Related Experiences and Symptoms Screener (STRESS)	Self-report (optionally computer-administered) instrument for youth ages 7–18	Age at occurrence of 18 DSM-5 traumatic events (noninterpersonal, interpersonal victimization, sexual victimization) and neglect 21 items measure distress	Internal consistency Criterion-referenced validity Convergent validity	Grasso, D. J., Felton, J.W., & Reid-Quinones, K. (2015) The Structured Trauma-Related Experiences and Symptoms Screener (STRESS): Development and preliminary psychometrics. Child Maltreatment, 20, 214–220. Inquires: Damion Grasso dgrasso@uchc.edu

(continued)

Table 4.1 (continued)

Construct	Name of measure	Type of measure	Number items	Psychometric data	Reference
DSM-IV criteria for Acute Stress Disorder (four associated features including subjective life threat, family context, coping)	Acute Stress Checklist for Children (ASC-Kids)	Child/adolescent self-report measure for youth (ages 8–17)	29 items rated on 3-point Likert scale	Test-retest reliability within 1 week = .76 Internal consistency = .86 Convergent validity with PTSD symptom scale r = .77 Being validated for DSM-5 Short forms in English, Spanish underway	Kassam-Adams, N. (2006). The acute stress checklist for children (ASC-Kids): Development of a child self-report measure. Journal of Traumatic Stress, 19(1), 129–139. Kassam-Adams, N, Gold, J, Montaño, Z, Kohser, K, Cuadra, A, Muñoz, C, Armstrong, FD. (2013). Development and psychometric evaluation of child acute stress measures in Spanish and English. Journal of Traumatic Stress, 26(1):19–27. doi: 10.1002/jts.21782
DSM-5 criteria for PTSD Trauma History Profile obtains comprehensive trauma history, including ages of exposure and trauma-specific details	UCLA DSM-5 PTSD Reaction Index for Children and Adolescents	Child/adolescent self-report measure (ages 7–18) Caregiver-report version (ages 7–18)	23 item Trauma History Screen 23 item trauma and loss-specific details 32 item DSM-5 PTSD symptoms plus Dissociative subtype Functional impairment Rated on 5-point Likert scale	Being validated for DSM-5	Pynoos R.S. & Steinberg, A.M. © 2014; The UCLA PTSD Reaction Index for Children and Adolescents, University of California, Los Angeles. Pynoos R.S. & Steinberg, A.M. © 2014; The UCLA PTSD Reaction Index for Children and Adolescents – Parent/Caregiver Version, University of California, Los Angeles. Licensing available from Behavioral Health Innovations at reactionindex.com Inquiries: Preston Finley HFinley@mednet.ucla.edu

Modified DSM-5 criteria for PTSD in young children Trauma History Profile obtains comprehensive trauma history, including ages of exposure and trauma-specific details	UCLA DSM-5 PTSD Reaction Index for Young Children (Parent/Caregiver Version)	Parent/adult caregiver of children (aged 6 and under)	22 item Trauma History Screen 22 item trauma and loss-specific details 19 item DSM-5 PTSD symptoms 48 functional impairment items Rated on 5-point Likert scale	Being validated for DSM-5	Steinberg A, Pynoos R, Lieberman A, Osofsky J, & Vivrette R (in preparation). UCLA DSM-5 PTSD Reaction Index for Young Children (Parent/Caregiver Version). Inquiries: Preston Finley HFinley@mednet.ucla.edu
DSM-5 criteria for PTSD; includes screen for trauma exposure Provides "probable" diagnostic cut-off score	Young Child PTSD Checklist (YCPC)	Caregiver report for youth ages 1–6	42 total items 13 items evaluate event occurrence, age, number of times. 29 symptom items rated on 5-point Likert scale	Being validated for DSM-5	Scheeringa, M.S. (2010). Young Child PTSD Checklist. Tulane University School of Medicine. http://tulane.edu/som/departments/psychiatry/ScheeringaLab/manuals-training.cfm
DSM-5 criteria for PTSD (PTSD Criterion B, Criterion C, Criterion D, Criterion E; also provides dissociative subtype symptom cluster score)	CAPS-CA-5 (Clinician-Administered PTSD Scale for DSM-5- Child/Adolescent Version)	Semi-structured interview for children, adolescents (ages 7 and above)	30 items Items rated with single severity score from 0 (absent) to 4 (Extreme/Incapacitating)	Being validated for DSM-5	Pynoos, R. S., Weathers, F. W., Steinberg, A. M., Marx, B. P., Layne, C. M., Kaloupek, D. G., Schnurr, P. P., Keane, T. M., Blake, D. D., Newman, E., Nader, K. O., & Kriegler, J. A. (2015).Clinician-Administered PTSD Scale for DSM-5 – Child/Adolescent Version. www.ptsd.va.gov

(continued)

Table 4.1 (continued)

Construct	Name of measure	Type of measure	Number items	Psychometric data	Reference
DSM-5 criteria for PTSD PTSD diagnosis, plus alternative empirically validated procedure for young children (PTSD-AA) requiring only 1 of 7 Criterion C symptoms (avoidance and numbing) instead of 3	Diagnostic Infant Preschool Assessment (DIPA) PTSD Module	Caregiver report semi-structured clinical interview (ages 1–6)	Responses coded for frequency, duration, onset, functional impairment	Test-retest reliability (18 day average) ICC = .87 Concurrent criterion validity (referenced to Child Behavior Checklist PTSD scale) ranged from kappa = .17 (DSM-IV criteria) to .48 (PTSD-AA)	Scheeringa, M.S., & Haslett, N. (2010). The reliability and criterion validity of the Diagnostic Infant and Preschool Assessment: A new diagnostic instrument for young children. Child Psychiatry & Human Development, 41, 3, 299–312 http://tulane.edu/som/departments/psychiatry/ScheeringaLab/manuals-training.cfm
DSM-5 proposed criteria for PCBD (additional items assess proposed Traumatic Bereavement Specifier)	Persistent Complex Bereavement Disorder (PCBD) Checklist	Child/adolescent self-report measure for bereaved youth ages 8–18	39 items rated on a 5-point Likert scale	Good content validity, criterion-referenced and incremental validity Additional psychometric analyses underway	Layne, C.M., Kaplow, J.B., & Pynoos, R.S. (2014). Persistent Complex Bereavement Disorder (PCBD) Checklist and Test Administration Manual– Youth Version 1.0. University of California, Los Angeles. Kaplow JB, Layne CM, Oosterhoff B et al. (under review). Test validation of the Persistent Complex Bereavement Disorder (PCBD) Checklist: A developmentally-informed assessment tool for bereaved youth. Licensing: http://oip.ucla.edu/pcbd-checklist-test-license Inquiries: Christopher Layne cmlayne@mednet.ucla.edu

4.3.3 What Should I Consider When Searching for the Most Appropriate Trauma- and Bereavement-Informed Assessment Tools for Youth?

A crucial step in validly assessing children's responses to trauma and bereavement involves selecting measures that are sensitive to developmental factors and age-relevant norms. Unfortunately, many measures used with children and adolescents are simply downwardly extended adaptations of measures originally developed for adults (Hunsley and Mash 2007). Although such adapted measures carry the apparent convenience of generalizing to adult populations, there is substantial evidence that childhood PTSD and grief may manifest differently than adult PTSD and grief (Kaplow et al. 2012; see Chaps. 1 and 5 this volume) and indeed may be influenced by different configurations of risk, vulnerability, and protective factors (Kaplow, Howell et al. 2014; Layne et al. 2009). In our experience, commencing test construction with a developmentally informed theory, a youth (as opposed to adult) sample, and a child-friendly test item pool can produce a final test that differs markedly from a downwardly adapted adult test (Kaplow, Layne, & Pynoos 2014).

4.3.4 How Can I Assess a Child Who Is Very Avoidant?

Avoidance can manifest in various ways when assessing bereaved children and adolescents. The most common form of avoidance is simply hesitancy to talk; however, avoidance can also be expressed through fidgetiness, repeatedly changing the subject, or replying with "I don't know" to most questions. Although clinicians can find it frustrating to interview youth who do not want to talk about "bad things" that may have happened to them, avoidance or hesitancy is often the norm. Using standardized, developmentally appropriate assessment tools to assess posttraumatic stress and grief reactions using language that children can readily relate to can be very helpful in this regard (see Table 4.1). Traumatized or bereaved children often feel strange, different, abnormal, or socially alienated due to what they have endured—a state that can intensify their hesitancy to talk openly about the event. Nevertheless, these same children often feel validated when they hear or see items on a standardized questionnaire that resemble their personal experiences, often responding with statements such as "I thought that was just me" or "Maybe I'm not so crazy" to items that resonate with them. To address the needs of more avoidant youth, standardized questionnaires can be administered in a variety of ways, including ways that do not require in-depth conversation. For example, the clinician can read questions and invite the child to circle his/her responses without saying a word. This can reduce the pressure children feel to verbalize their most personal thoughts and feelings during an initial encounter with a new adult. Standardized questionnaires also provide structure to the assessment process itself, serving as a guide for novice clinicians so they are not left wondering "What should I ask next?"—a dilemma that often arises with reserved and reluctant youth.

Beyond standardized questionnaires, other techniques are also useful for engaging avoidant youth. For youth who fidget during the assessment, it can be helpful to have toys available that they can hold and manipulate. Younger children who have difficulty with verbally responding to assessment questions often respond more readily when the clinician creates a game by writing response options on sheets of paper (e.g., *Not At All* on Page 1; *A Little Bit* on Page 2, etc.), arranging the sheets in a row on the floor, and asking the child to jump from answer to answer. For youth who repeatedly respond "I don't know," it can be useful to distinguish between "I don't know" versus "I don't want to talk about it." This empowers the youth to tell the clinician if something is too hard to discuss at the time while providing useful information about topics that evoke distress. More generally, it is important to recognize that avoidance itself is a critical aspect of the assessment. By paying close attention to specific words or topics the child wishes to avoid, the clinician can form hypotheses about which aspects of the trauma or death are most difficult to process (and thus require more attention in treatment).

4.3.5 Why Is It So Easy to Misdiagnose PTSD or Maladaptive Grief?

PTSD and maladaptive grief can often be masked by other psychological or behavioral difficulties. Although PTSD can appear as a comorbid condition with ADHD (Cuffe et al. 1994; Weinstein et al. 2000) and PTSD and dissociative symptoms both predict future attention problems in children (Kaplow et al. 2008), children with PTSD can also be misdiagnosed as having ADHD. In our experience, this may be due to the inherent difficulty in distinguishing between behavioral manifestations of (a) hyperactivity versus hyperarousal, (b) inattention versus avoidance or dissociation, and (c) fidgetiness versus reexperiencing symptoms. The close overlap between these symptom pairings (the first reflecting ADHD, the second PTSD) underscores the need to carefully assess whether the onset of possible ADHD symptoms temporally corresponds with the occurrence of potentially traumatic events. In such cases, the trio of hypotheses that (1) ADHD is present and PTSD is not, (2) ADHD is comorbid with and potentially masking underlying PTSD, or, alternatively, (3) ADHD-like symptoms actually reflect the presence of PTSD and are not actually ADHD, should each be evaluated.

Bereaved youth are also sometimes referred for services on the basis of suicidal ideation. However, it is quite common for youth to express a wish to die following the death of a loved one given that their intense separation distress can evoke reunification fantasies about being with the person again in an afterlife, depending on their spiritual or religious beliefs. Further, youths' existential/identity distress may also reflect the perceptions that life feels empty, joyless, and meaningless without the deceased's physical presence (Kaplow et al. 2013). Although the presence of these grief reactions does not necessarily diminish a bereaved child's risk for suicide, the capacity to understand and compassionately label the motivation behind the apparent suicidal ideation can be essential for engagement, case conceptualization, and treatment planning. Indeed, suicidal thoughts stemming from a major depressive episode call for a different treatment approach than suicidal thoughts stemming from a strong wish to, for example, be reunited with the deceased in an afterlife. Clinicians' ability to accurately assess and discriminate between children's intense grief reactions (Kaplow, Layne, & Pynoos 2014) versus suicidal ideation (King et al. 2013) can provide opportunities to sympathetically validate a child's underlying grief ("This helps me understand how much you really miss him"). Exercising the same bereavement competencies can also prevent instances in which the clinician inadvertently overpathologizes and invalidates a child's grief reactions (e.g., immediately launching into safety planning after hearing a child disclose a wishful reunification fantasy).

4.3.6 Why Do We Need to Determine Whether It's a Traumatic Stress Reaction Versus a Grief Reaction? Does Making a Distinction Make a Difference?

Posttraumatic stress and grief reactions often do *co-occur* following a death—especially if the death occurred under traumatic circumstances. The resulting interplay between posttraumatic stress and grief reactions can powerfully influence the nature and course of children's adjustment (Kaplow et al. 2012, 2013; Layne et al. 2001, 2008; Pynoos 1992). In particular, the co-occurring presence of both posttraumatic stress and grief reactions predicts the prolonged course of both sets of reactions (Nader et al. 1990).

Nevertheless, the child bereavement literature has at times shown a tendency to conflate posttraumatic stress and grief reactions to the extent that these constructs are conceptually bundled together, taught, and treated as essentially the same entity. For example, childhood traumatic grief is defined as a special case of PTSD in which PTSD symptoms evoked by the circumstances of the death encroach upon and interfere with the child's ability to engage in essential grief-related tasks—thereby calling for primarily trauma-focused treatment components to assist bereaved children (e.g., Cohen et al. 2002; Mannarino and Cohen 2011).

Although we agree that PTSD reactions can reduce or inhibit children's ability to manage their grief (and, conversely, that grief reactions can reduce or inhibit children's ability to manage their posttraumatic stress reactions), our experience as test developers, researchers, and trained clinicians leads us to conclude that defining maladaptive grief as a special-case variant of PTSD blurs the boundaries between the two constructs, introduces confusion, and raises questions regarding whether maladaptive grief reactions consist of anything other than a variant of PTSD symptoms. We thus advocate that PTSD and grief be conceptualized and assessed as distinct but related constructs—constructs that can jointly arise from exposure to the same death (e.g., *traumatic bereavement*, in which the circumstances of the death contain traumatogenic elements; Kaplow, Howell et al. 2014)—but can also arise from exposure to distinctly different events (e.g., trauma, *and* bereavement under peaceful circumstances) (Pynoos 1992).

The overlapping subfields of childhood trauma and childhood bereavement clearly have more work to do to delineate—both conceptually and empirically—the boundaries between PTSD and grief and the diverse ways in which PTSD symptoms and grief reactions can intersect to produce impairment in children and teens. Nevertheless, although in its early stages, the current literature points to the importance of distinguishing between PTSD symptoms and grief reactions, given that the two constructs may have different configurations of causal risk factors, vulnerability factors, protective factors, and outcomes, and thus call for different treatment components given evidence of their different treatment response trajectories (Grassetti et al. 2015). Clinicians' ability to formulate an effective treatment plan for traumatized and bereaved youth may thus depend on their ability to accurately assess and discriminate between PTSD symptoms versus grief reactions.

4.3.7 Can We (as Clinicians) Assume That Exposure to Objectively Traumatic Circumstances of a Death Will Probably Result in a Traumatic Stress Response (i.e., PTSD)?

The short answer is no. Our research and clinical work have taught us that the specific manner of death (e.g., progressive deteriorating death due to cancer, sudden death due to heart attack, suicide) may be differentially linked to posttraumatic stress and grief reactions but perhaps in counterintuitive ways. As described earlier, children whose parent died after a prolonged wasting illness exhibited higher posttraumatic stress and maladaptive grief reactions than children whose parent died due to seemingly more traumatic causes, including sudden heart attack or stroke (Kaplow, Howell et al. 2014). The complexity of the circumstances surrounding the deaths of loved ones, as well as the often dramatic variability in how different children grieve, underscores the need to assess the broader socioenvironmental context that surrounds each death. This includes potentially traumatogenic elements of the death itself (e.g., intense suffering, physical deterioration, ineffectual attempts to resuscitate the person), as well as potential trauma reminders (e.g., people crying, hospitals, ambulances) and loss reminders (e.g., the deceased's name, photos, belongings) (Kaplow and Layne 2014; Layne et al. 2006).

As a case example, prior to evaluating a 9-year-old girl who was in a car crash in which her mother was killed, one of the authors (J.K.) hypothesized that the girl would likely exhibit elevated levels of posttraumatic stress reactions given that she had directly witnessed the gruesome death of her mother from the backseat. Instead, the assessment revealed that the girl's primary presenting issue was maladaptive grief marked by intense separation distress (unrelenting yearning and longing for her mother) as the most prominent domain. The girl presented as extremely tearful and sorrowful throughout the assessment, stating "My mom was my best friend. I just want her back. I just need to see her again." Her extreme sadness and despair were palpable, yet she showed no trace of PTSD. These assessment data led to an effective treatment plan focused on helping her strengthen and maintain a strong and healthy connection to her deceased mother while changing the relationship to one based in memory and spiritual connection in accordance with the child's own belief system. In contrast, it was evident that conducting a trauma narrative focusing on the circumstances of her mother's death (i.e., describing the accident in explicit detail) would not be helpful but would instead fail to validate the child's reactions and potentially evoke greater distress. Nevertheless, the therapist remained open to the possibility that PTSD symptoms could arise or become more prominent at a later point in time and incorporated this into a plan for ongoing monitoring.

As a contrasting example, the same author evaluated a 12-year-old boy who experienced the death of his mother to cancer after she had endured invasive treatments for 3 years. When asked what the hardest part of this experience was, the boy reported that it was neither the death itself nor witnessing the ongoing treatment that was the most difficult. Instead, it was listening to his parents crying together in their bedroom late at night and overhearing his mother sobbing, "I know the treatment isn't working. But I'm not ready to say goodbye." The boy reported extremely high levels of posttraumatic stress, including reexperiencing symptoms of the night he overheard his parents' agonized cries. An assessment of the boy's grief reactions revealed a typical grief response that did not reflect clinical impairment.

In summary, these case examples illustrate the importance of conducting a thorough trauma- and bereavement-informed assessment while avoiding the presumption that "unnatural" (sudden and/or violent) deaths will necessarily lead to PTSD or that "natural" (anticipated and nonviolent) deaths pose a low risk for PTSD or other adverse psychological consequences given that they presumably help the child prepare for the impending loss. Similarly, it is important to recognize that children exposed to the death of a loved one can develop both PTSD and maladaptive grief and that the presence of each set of reactions can prolong and intensify the course of the other (Pynoos 1992). Trauma- and bereavement-informed assessment tools can be valuable guides to treatment planning by clarifying whether one set of reactions is more prominent than the other, thereby identifying the most useful starting point for intervention.

4.4 How Can EBA Facilitate the Competent Use of Tests?

In the following section, we illustrate how EBA concepts, principles, and practices can improve both efficiency (not assessing at points where it is not informative) and effectiveness (using appropriately designed tools to inform and guide specific clinical decisions as they arise) when applied to settings that serve traumatized and bereaved youth (Youngstrom 2013). We divide the EBA process into four main stages that should be viewed as fluid (adaptable to individual cases, iterating steps multiple times as needed) rather than strictly sequential. Stages include (1) preparations prior to meeting the client, (2) routine evaluation, (3) in-depth assessment, and (4) assessment during active treatment and follow-up.

4.4.1 Stage 1: Preparation (Adopting EBA in a Trauma- and Bereavement-Informed Clinic)

Careful preparation is needed to optimize the quality and effectiveness of EBA in a given clinical setting. Although requiring a few hours or days to incorporate, these preparations can pay dividends many times over in time saved and improved results. A first step is to identify the most common referral questions and diagnostic issues encountered in a given practice setting. In most trauma clinics, referral questions typically center on whether a child/adolescent has been exposed to a certain form of trauma or loss and how he/she is reacting to that event. In many cases, however, a history of trauma may be suspected, but primary presenting issues revolve around behavioral problems (e.g., risky behaviors, oppositional behaviors, substance use). Informally, this review of common referring problems and diagnostic issues can take the form of jotting down a list from memory or pulling a sample of files and tallying the results. Calculating summary statistics from electronic records often yields more detailed and precise estimates.

A second step is to compare and benchmark these locally observed base rates against the rates reported by similar practice settings (Rettew et al. 2009; Youngstrom et al. 2014). Are local base rates similar to, lower than (pointing to the possibility of under-detection/false negatives), or higher than (pointing to the possibility of over-detection/false positives) credible external benchmarks? Conducting this step helps to evaluate whether the base rates observed in the clinician's practice setting appear to be reasonable when compared to similar practice settings. As an example, are rates of exposure to trauma and bereavement observed in a given school-based clinic consistent with those reported in epidemiologic studies of similar populations? Comparing local base rates to external benchmarks may reveal actual population-based differences or, alternatively, coverage gaps in the risk screening and evaluation process or differences in referral procedures. Given base rates of trauma and bereavement (and associated posttraumatic stress and grief reactions) reported in diverse populations, trauma and bereavement issues are commonplace in many practice settings and call for systematic risk screening (Breslau et al. 2004; Courtois and Gold 2009; Kaplow et al. 2010).

Last, we need to review our assessment tools and protocols to ensure we have useful and valid tools available to assess the most prevalent exposures and common conditions in our setting (see Sect. 4.2 for information regarding how to identify and select these measures). Keeping a list of the most common conditions also reminds us to consider common differential diagnoses or potential comorbid diagnoses as an integral part of clinical assessment. Without such reminders and/or a structured interview, clinicians tend to miss at least one diagnosis per case on average and consequently underestimate comorbidity (Jensen-Doss et al. 2014; Rettew et al. 2009).

4.4.2 Stage 2: Routine Evaluation of Trauma and Bereavement and Associated Distress

Gathering data regarding the most commonly presenting clinical problems also helps to reengineer routine evaluation procedures. For example, if common reasons for referral are suspected to reflect posttraumatic stress *and* grief reactions, then a reasonable policy is to require presenting clients to complete measures with broad coverage of both constructs (e.g., trauma exposure and PTSD—see Elhai et al. 2013; Foa et al. 2001; bereavement and PCBD-see Layne, Kaplow, & Pynoos 2014).

Because (as noted earlier) most commonly used measures do not screen for trauma or bereavement, it is advisable to identify those that do include a systematic evaluation of these risk factors. Options range from a standardized checklist of verbal questions that include whether clients have lost someone close to them or were exposed to a traumatic event (Gawande 2010) to systematic screening tools that cover a broad range of types of traumatic events and losses (e.g., Pynoos et al. 2014; see Table 4.1). Broad range trauma- and bereavement-informed screening tools can help clinicians identify, visually depict, and address *risk factor caravans*—clusters of co-occurring traumatic events and losses that accumulate in number, accrue in their adverse effects, and cascade forward across development (Layne, Briggs-King et al. 2014). For example, using the Trauma History Profile in a large clinic-referred US sample, Pynoos et al. (2014) identified five mutually exclusive risk factor caravans that differed in their compositions of risk factors, age of onset, and patterns of occurrence and recurrence across childhood and adolescence. Identifying which risk factors cluster together helps clinicians to become more aware of an increased likelihood of other types of trauma. The first caravan—comprised of neglect, emotional abuse, impaired caregiver, domestic violence, and physical abuse—tended to co-occur and have its onset early in development (0–5 years). In contrast, the fourth risk factor caravan is comprised of sexual abuse, sexual assault/rape, and physical assault, which tend to occur at a later developmental stage (primarily 6–12 years).

Such knowledge of the developmental epidemiology of the prevalence rates and initial onset of many different types of childhood trauma and loss promotes trauma- and bereavement-informed assessment in at least three ways. First, knowing which types of trauma and loss exposures are most prevalent across different developmental periods informs risk screening by identifying which types of events clinicians should be most vigilant for when assessing youths of different ages. Second, knowing which types of traumata tend to co-occur in clusters assists in risk screening because each type of trauma acts as a *risk marker* by signaling an increased risk for the presence of (either temporally prior, concurrent, or subsequent to) its co-occurring caravan companions (Layne et al. 2009). Risk markers promote risk screening by underscoring the need for careful assessment of the entire cluster of risk factors when at least one risk factor is detected. Third, knowledge of the average age of onset for specific types of trauma and loss helps to sequence the order in which different risk factors tend to occur, co-occur, and cascade forward across development. For example, in the fourth risk factor caravan, sexual abuse tends to precede sexual assault/rape and physical assault in onset, highlighting a window of opportunity for early intervention to prevent sexual abuse from cascading into subsequent risk factors.

4.4.3 Stage 3: In-Depth Focus on the Individual in the Context of Trauma and Bereavement

After evaluating exposure to risk factors such as trauma and bereavement, as well as commonly observed reactions to these events, clinicians can move toward a systematic in-depth assessment for trauma- or bereavement-related clinical impairment. The fact that, by definition, trauma- and stressor-related disorders such as PTSD and PCBD have their primary etiologic (causal) origins (trauma and bereavement, respectively) located outside the individual—within the surrounding physical and social ecology—sets these disorders apart from heavily biologically determined psychiatric disorders (bipolar disorder, schizophrenia, etc.). This distinction regarding the primary locus of causation of environmentally caused disorders underscores the need for a thorough ecological assessment that searches for factors that play influential roles in causing, maintaining, worsening, or mitigating clinically significant distress and impairment.

An ecologically informed assessment should involve a systematic search for a variety of potential contributing factors (Layne et al. 2009, Layne, Steinberg et al. 2014). These factors include theorized:

(a) Direct-effect causal contributors to adjustment, including *causal risk factors* (e.g., sexual abuse, physical abuse, bereavement) and *promotive factors* (healthy attachment relationships)
(b) Interactive-effect moderator variables. Moderator variables include *vulnerability factors* and *protective factors* (use the Double Check Heuristic, described below, as a visual aid).
- Vulnerability factors interact with the causal risk factor to *exacerbate* its harmful effects on a negative outcome. For example, poor familial support (vulnerability factor) after a rape (risk factor) can worsen PTSD symptoms (negative or undesirable outcome).
- Vulnerability factors can also interact with the causal risk factor to *intensify* its negative effects on a positive outcome. For example, peer rejection (vulnerability factor) following a rape (risk factor) can further diminish self-esteem (positive or desirable outcome).
- Protective factors interact with the causal risk factor to *buffer* or mitigate its effects on a negative outcome. For example, peer social support (protective factor) after a car accident (risk factor) can lessen PTSD symptoms (negative outcome).
- Protective factors also interact with the causal risk factor to *diminish* its harmful effects on a positive outcome—for example, positive parent-child communication (protective factor) about a difficult death (risk factor) can preserve a child's ability to grieve in adaptive ways (positive outcome).

(c) *Mediator variables* (e.g., trauma reminders, loss reminders, secondary adversities) that convey the prior effects of causal risk factors (trauma, bereavement) to subsequent outcomes (PTSD, PCBD) and thus help to maintain or worsen distress over time (Kaplow et al. 2012; Kaplow and Layne 2014; Layne et al. 2006)

Mediator variables can also consist of risky behavior and functional impairment resulting from developmentally prior causal risk factors (e.g., physical and emotional abuse in childhood), that then co-occur and accumulate within a given developmental period (substance abuse in early adolescence), and cascade forward into a subsequent developmental period where they carry their own risks in a chain reaction snowballing effect (addiction and reckless driving in late adolescence) (Layne, Greeson et al. 2014; Oosterhoff, Kaplow, and Layne, in press). These findings underscore the need for risk screening for both trauma exposure and co-occurring risky behavior to create opportunities for early intervention (Layne, Greeson et al. 2014).

The need for conceptual clarity and measurement precision when evaluating the ecologies that surround traumatized and bereaved youth is illustrated by evidence of differential relations between theorized causal risk factors and their consequences. For example, a recent study found that children bereaved by deaths after a prolonged illness report higher rates of posttraumatic stress and maladaptive grief than children bereaved by sudden deaths (Kaplow, Howell et al. 2014). Further, a study of war-exposed youth revealed that different types of war exposure (e.g., life threat, physical harm, traumatic bereavement, material loss) differentially contributed to PTSD and depression symptoms reported 4 years after the war and were mediated by different pathways of influence, including trauma reminders, interpersonal adversities, and existential adversities (Layne et al. 2010). Such findings point to the conclusion that childhood causal risk factors are not functionally interchangeable. Rather, simple summative scoring (creating a simple sum of different types of adverse childhood events, where a higher total score denotes greater risk) loses theoretically informative and clinically actionable information—including identifying which mediated pathways (e.g., parent-adolescent conflict, trauma reminders) are the most promising sites for intervention (Layne, Briggs-King et al. 2014).

Stage 3 uses more rigorous tools, including semi-structured or structured diagnostic interviews that focus on PTSD, related conditions, and environmental vulnerability and protective factors (Sheehan et al. 1998). The reliability of these methods is substantially higher than unstructured interviews (Garb 1998), increasing the accuracy of both diagnosis and ensuing treatment choices. In our experience, some clinicians may shy away from structured interviews due in part to the assumption that they might damage therapeutic rapport. However, such assumptions appear to be unfounded: Patients often prefer structured approaches and perceive the clinician as having a more comprehensive understanding of them and their situation (Bruchmuller et al. 2011; Suppiger et al. 2009). Semi-structured interviews carry the added advantage of offering the clinician greater flexibility in addressing developmental (Kaplow et al. 2012; Kaplow and Layne 2014) and cultural factors (Contractor et al. 2015) that may modify the clinical manifestations of posttraumatic stress or grief reactions. In this stage of evaluation, diagnostic interviews and self-report checklists complement one another in guiding and informing clinical diagnosis and treatment goal setting.

Consistent with basic tenets of EBA, an additional component of treatment planning involves integrating clients' values and informed wishes. Incorporating clients' values and informed wishes is consistent with recent calls for EBA to integrate *idiographic* (client-centered or client-nominated) information, such as asking clients to identify their highest priority or "top" problems, with *nomothetic* (norm-referenced) information as gathered using standardized tests. This integrative approach captures the complementary strengths of both methods, including client engagement and making treatment outcomes transparently relevant to clients (Weisz et al. 2011). Being sensitive to clients' values is especially relevant to the assessment of trauma-exposed and bereaved youth for whom developmental factors, culture, and personal life experiences may markedly influence how distress, impairment, and/or adaptation are exhibited (Kaplow et al. 2012). Clients' beliefs about the causes of their distress reactions, as well as how to best address them, also vary widely and can influence their willingness to engage in assessment and treatment. When patient beliefs align with clinicians' line of questioning and use of assessment tools, the chances of rapport building, treatment adherence, and treatment success markedly improve (Yeh et al. 2005). For example, many traumatized or bereaved families turn to their religious and/or spiritual beliefs to make meaning of their adverse experiences. In our experience, using assessment questions and tools that invite family members to share their individual spiritual beliefs can convey a sense of sympathetic validation and support that helps to strengthen the therapeutic alliance (Howell et al. 2015).

4.4.4 Stage 4: Assessment During Active Treatment and Follow-Up

If the in-depth assessment finds that trauma- or bereavement-related clinical impairment is probably present and a major focus of treatment, then the goal of assessment shifts to measuring therapeutic process and progress (Youngstrom and Frazier 2013). Process measures can include tracking whether the patient completes homework assignments, such as keeping track of trauma reminders and associated reactions. Technology now makes it possible to automatically schedule client reminders for activities and to track completion rates. A variety of progress measures are available that are brief and sensitive to change, allowing clinicians to monitor therapeutic progress (e.g., Wells et al. 1996; see Beidas et al. 2015, for a review of no-cost measures). Longer measures can be burdensome if used every session but can be repeated periodically to evaluate whether significant change has occurred. Session-by-session progress measures, even though brief, can significantly improve outcomes and provide a valuable cue to revisit diagnosis or treatment planning if the client is not making expected gains. Once clients have reached their goals, termination planning can incorporate monitoring strategies that can trigger a booster session or return to treatment. Identifying bereavement-related anniversaries, developmental milestones, or other reminder-laden situations ahead of time, and explicitly planning how to manage them, improves the prospect for maintaining treatment gains (Lambert 2010).

4.5 Making Sense of Assessment Data Using the *Double Checks Heuristic*

Clinical training approaches that emphasize EBA competencies encourage the use of several clinical reasoning strategies when conducting in-depth clinical evaluations (e.g., Hoge et al. 2003). A first strategy is to consider more than one clinical hypothesis or explanation. This strategy acts as a check against the biasing tendency to preferentially search for and weight confirming evidence over disconfirming evidence. This strategy is especially useful in clinical settings where comorbidity is common, and "all of the above" (e.g., the client has PTSD *and* depression *and* anxiety) may be a legitimate clinical decision for some clients.

A second, recently proposed strategy is the *Double Checks Heuristic* (Layne, Steinberg et al. 2014), a clinical reasoning and conceptual tool for organizing assessment data, case formulation, and treatment planning. The heuristic is designed to complement recent efforts to develop science-informed case formulation procedures (Christon et al. 2015) by guiding clinicians in assigning assessment data to different hypothesized roles in the working clinical theory. Each role in the model (e.g., protective factors, vulnerability factors, negative outcomes such as PTSD) is represented by a conceptual bin into which relevant evidence is sorted. Applying the heuristic involves systematically conceptualizing clients within the context of their surrounding ecology and sorting pieces of evidence into the conceptual bin to which they are hypothesized to belong in the model. The heuristic initially focuses on collecting data and formulating a working clinical theory, which logically segues into formulating an intervention plan by identifying intervention objectives associated with each conceptual bin (Fig. 4.1).

The Double Checks Heuristic carries five primary strengths that promote EBA. First, it helps clinicians manage complex assessment data by systematically unpacking, organizing, and making sense of complex ecologies comprised of many different factors. Second, it is compatible with positive youth development and positive psychology principles in its balanced focus on checking for bad things (causal risk factors, vulnerability factors, negative outcomes, inhibitory factors/barriers) with an equal strength-based emphasis on checking for good things (promotive factors, facilitative/catalytic factors, positive outcomes, protective factors) that can be therapeutically harnessed or evaluated as outcomes (Layne et al. 2009). Third, it strengthens clinical reasoning skills by facilitating deep-level cognitive processing including understanding (distinguishing between risk factors vs. vulnerability factors), analysis (sorting data into different conceptual bins), synthesis (integrating the conceptual bins to generate a working clinical theory, hypotheses, and treatment plan), and evaluation (weighing the evidence to test a hypothesis) (Anderson et al. 2001). Fourth, it helps to translate case conceptualization into treatment planning by helping clinicians to consider what they wish to achieve in relation to each conceptual bin. In particular, the heuristic facilitates intervention planning by aligning *intervention foci* (the conceptual bin where you wish to intervene, e.g., protective factors), *intervention objectives* (what you wish to achieve, e.g., mobilize social support to reduce distress evoked by trauma reminders), and *practice elements* (how you will achieve it, e.g., teach clients social support recruitment skills) (e.g., Saltzman et al. in press). Last, the heuristic helps clinicians to think integratively by strategizing

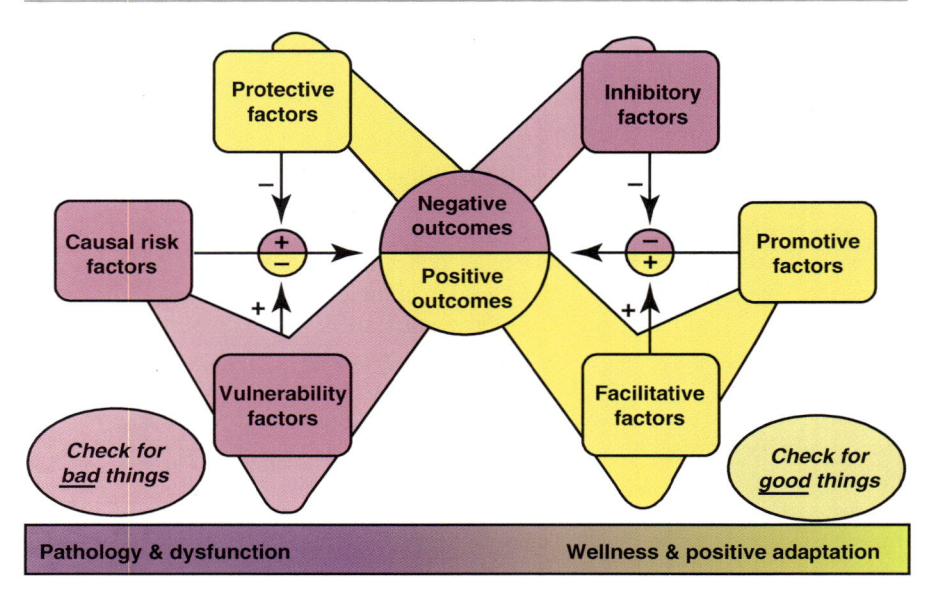

Fig. 4.1 The Double Checks Heuristic (Adapted from Layne, Steinberg et al. 2014). The valence (+ or −) of the direct effects of the causal risk factors and promotive factors on the outcome varies as a function of the valence (positive versus negative) of the outcome. In contrast, protective and inhibitory factors are always associated with a reduction of those direct effects, and vulnerability and facilitative factors are always associated with an intensification of those direct effects

Fig. 4.2 The CHECKS Heuristic

how to harness different elements of the model in synergistic ways. For example, youths can derive more benefit from a strong social network (a promotive factor) when given ready access to in-person visits or phone calls (a facilitative factor).

Newer clinicians and teams of clinicians in group supervision settings (where time for in-depth case discussion is more limited) can benefit from a simplified version of the Double Checks Heuristic called the CHECKS Heuristic (Fig. 4.2). The acronym CHECKS is comprised of C (*what caused the problem?* (causal risk factor)), H (*what might help the problem to get better?* (protective factor)), E (*what might exacerbate the problem?* (vulnerability factor)), C (*what is the most pressing consequence?* (negative outcome)), K (*what are the key intervention objectives?* (highest treatment priorities)), and S (*how do we know whether treatment is successful?* (monitoring treatment progress)). In the next section, we demonstrate how the CHECKS Heuristic can be used throughout the assessment process, beginning with case formulation but extending into ongoing monitoring and surveillance efforts as new causal risk factors, protective factors, or vulnerability factors are identified over time.

In summary, EBA helps to make clinical reasoning a more explicit, balanced, systematic, and quantifiable process. The heuristics and skills described earlier help clinicians to organize and formulate assessment data into a working clinical theory that systematically considers and evaluates competing possibilities.

4.6 Case Example: Conducting a Trauma-Informed Assessment Using EBA Principles

Melinda ("Mindy"), a 15-year-old Caucasian female, was referred to an outpatient mental health clinic by her school counselor who reported that, during the last 2 months, Mindy's grades have dropped substantially, she has been skipping school, and she has not completed any of her homework assignments. In her second meeting with the school counselor, Mindy disclosed that she had been raped by her best friend's brother 2 months before and has had difficulty focusing on school ever since then. The school counselor quickly initiated contact with Child Protective Services, and an investigation is ongoing. The school counselor reported that Mindy informed her parents (who are divorced) about the rape the day after it happened. When asked by the school counselor about her parents' reaction, Mindy stated, "My dad [Craig] was furious and said he wouldn't rest until this guy was in jail. He also told me he loves me and he wouldn't let anything like this happen again. But my mom got really mad at me and said I probably did something to provoke him. Like I shouldn't have been wearing such a tight-fitting t-shirt."

In an initial evaluation, the clinician, Ms. Morgan (M.S.W.), met with Mindy's mother, Janice, to review limits of confidentiality, obtain a developmental and psychosocial history, and gain a better understanding of Janice's perspective on the presenting issues. Janice stated that she was "fed up with Mindy's attitude about school" and that she "doesn't know what to do with her anymore." She also reported that although she was very upset that Mindy was raped, she thinks Mindy "also learned an important lesson about flirting with older boys." Janice stated, "I know she says she was trying to fight him off, but Mindy is always looking for attention, so I'm not sure I fully believe that." When asked specifically about the timing of when the school problems began, Janice noted that they actually began about 8 months ago, right around the time that Janice's mother died, but that things have gotten progressively worse since the rape. Janice stated, "My mom's death was hard on all of us. She started living with Mindy and me when Craig and I got divorced, which was about 4 years ago. She was like a second mother to Mindy. Mindy always seemed much more comfortable talking to her grandmother than to me." Janice said tearfully, "Mindy screamed at me just last week that she wishes it was me who died and not her grandmother." At the end of their meeting, Ms. Morgan asked Janice to complete several measures in the waiting area including a measure of her own grief reactions relating to the death of mother, as well as a measure of Mindy's psychosocial functioning in various developmental domains (the Strengths and Difficulties Questionnaire).

After meeting with Mindy's mother, Ms. Morgan met with Mindy alone. Mindy appeared anxious and fidgety but also polite and somewhat withdrawn. When asked whether she knew why she had been referred to the clinic, Mindy said, "I guess it's because I'm failing my classes." The clinician explained that although she wanted to better understand why Mindy was having school difficulties, her job was to listen to what was bothering her and to get to know her better. Ms. Morgan also explained that she helps teens talk about bad things that happened to them and helps them cope with the many different types of reactions that kids can have after a scary or upsetting event. After this initial conversation, Mindy began to look somewhat relieved and a bit more relaxed.

Ms. Morgan started the evaluation by reviewing limits of confidentiality. After stating that she would need to let her parents or the authorities know if Mindy were being hurt, Mindy quickly said, "You don't need to worry about that—everyone already knows what happened to me. And I know my school counselor already told you, too." The clinician told Mindy that she was hoping to hear about what happened in Mindy's own words so she could better understand her experience. Mindy hesitated and then briefly stated, "I was raped. But I don't want to talk about it. There is a court date coming up and they think I'll have to testify. I just wish I could forget about it and push it out of my mind." Ms. Morgan validated Mindy's strong desire to avoid thinking or talking about the event and told her that she didn't need to share more details unless she wanted to. Ms. Morgan also reassured Mindy that kids often feel better after talking through upsetting experiences, and there would be more time for that later if she felt comfortable.

Ms. Morgan then conducted a brief clinical interview with Mindy in which she reviewed her developmental and psychosocial history. Mindy reported that her parents divorced several years ago and that, although she has a good relationship with her father, she doesn't see him very frequently because he moved out of state. She indicated that she lives with her mother and her younger sister, who is 10 years old. Mindy said, "My sister and I are really close. I think it's hard for her to see me so upset all the time. She looks up to me and wants to do everything I do. But now she sees how kids make fun of me and bully me on Facebook and she can't understand why they do that." Mindy indicated that since the rape, her former best friend (Sara) and other girls at school have been calling her names when she walks by (e.g., "slut"), posting mean and accusatory statements on Facebook (e.g., "Don't pretend like you didn't want it"), and taping derogatory comments on her locker. When Ms. Morgan empathically commented on how hard that must be for her, Mindy stated, "It's almost worse than what Jake did to me. Every time they make fun of me, it just reminds me again about what happened, and I start to have that sick feeling in my stomach. It's like I feel trapped no matter where I go, and I just wish I could turn my brain off. I used to like going to school, but now I hate it and can't wait to go home."

The clinician then administered the Trauma History section of the UCLA PTSD Reaction Index. When asked about other scary or very upsetting events that may have happened to her, Mindy reported that her grandmother died suddenly of a heart attack about 8 months ago. When Ms. Morgan asked if she could tell her more about that, Mindy described missing her grandmother even more since the rape took place, stating "I know my grandma would have been much more understanding than my mom. She would have never made me feel like it was my fault." As directed by the PTSD RI, Ms. Morgan then asked Mindy to identify the one event that bothers her the most now. Mindy said, "I'm always missing my grandma, but I can't stop thinking about what Jake did to me no matter how hard I try to get it out of my mind. So I guess it's that" (the rape). During the remaining test administration, Mindy endorsed a number of PTSD symptoms as happening much or most of the time, including "I try to stay away from people, places or things that remind me about what happened," "I have thoughts like I will never be able to trust other people," "I have upsetting thoughts, pictures or sounds of what happened come into my mind when I don't want them to," and "I feel ashamed or guilty about what happened."

Next, Ms. Morgan asked whether Mindy felt comfortable sharing more about what happened. Mindy then explained that she had been best friends with Sara since the sixth grade and had slept over at her house many times in the past. She said that this time was different because Sara's older brother, Jake, whom Mindy had only met a couple of times before, was home from college and came back to the house around 1:00 am after going to a party with some friends. When he came back to the house, Sara was asleep and Mindy was half asleep in the bottom bunk of Sara's bunk bed. Jake came into Sara's bedroom, nudged Mindy, and asked whether she wanted to "hang out." When Mindy said she was too tired, Jake sat down on the bed next to her and told her to move over. She could smell alcohol on his breath, and he was slurring his words. When Mindy refused to move over, Jake said, "You're being a bad girl – just relax" and started taking off his clothes. He then climbed on top of her, covered her mouth with his hand, and raped her. Mindy stated that she tried to fight him off, but he was too strong. She also said, "I kept thinking that I might suffocate or die – his hands were covering my nose and my mouth and I could barely breathe." Mindy said she was certain that Sara woke up and knew what was happening. She said, "I can't believe she didn't stop him. There's no way she could have thought I actually wanted him to do that – she knew I was a virgin and was waiting until I had a real boyfriend. After he finally stopped and left the room, I cried for hours, and she just pretended to be asleep. I guess maybe she doesn't want to know the truth."

When they awoke the next morning, Sara acted as though nothing had happened. When Mindy confronted her and told her that Jake made her have sex, Sara said, "My brother wouldn't do that. Come on, Mindy, you said you had a crush on him." Mindy called her mother to come get her from Sara's house and has not talked to Sara since their confrontation. Mindy stated,

> It just hurts so much that someone you trust can turn on you like that – I thought I could always count on her, and now she's my enemy. I know she doesn't want her brother to go to jail, but it's like she's out to prove that this was all my fault. I think she wants me to be too scared to testify by constantly bullying me. But I honestly don't think it can get any worse.

When Ms. Morgan asked Mindy about specific people, places, or things that she tries to avoid now, she said she feels "panicky" when she sees her former best friend at school because just seeing her from a distance reminds Mindy of the rape. She also said that hearing rude and derogatory remarks from other kids at school also brings up bad memories of that night. Finally, Mindy described a relaxation exercise in her physical education class. The minute her teacher said "relax," she was flooded with memories of the rape because it brought to mind Jake telling her over and over again to "just relax."

Given Mindy's recent history of losing her grandmother, Ms. Morgan also administered the Persistent Complex Bereavement Disorder (PCBD) Checklist. Notable during the administration was Mindy's disclosure that she felt responsible for her grandmother's death: "If I hadn't been fighting with my mom so much, my grandma wouldn't have been so stressed and probably wouldn't have had a heart attack." Ms. Morgan also administered the Short Mood and Feelings Questionnaire to evaluate potential depressive symptoms. Mindy endorsed three items as true (i.e., most of the time): "I felt I was no good anymore," "I found it hard to think properly or concentrate," and "I felt lonely." Last, given Mindy's trauma and loss history, perceived lack of support from her mother and friends, and endorsement of multiple PTSD symptoms and depressive symptoms, Ms. Morgan administered the Suicidal Ideation Questionnaire. Mindy endorsed none of the items, stating "I know things are bad right now but I would never kill myself. I would never leave my sister–she needs me even more now that Grandma is gone."

At the conclusion of the evaluation, Ms. Morgan explained that she would be reviewing the measures and would come up with a plan for how best to help Mindy based on the results. Ms. Morgan praised Mindy for sharing her very personal story, including her own thoughts and feelings, and asked Mindy if she had any questions. Mindy replied, "Does this kind of stuff really happen to other kids? I feel like I'm jinxed or weird or something." Ms. Morgan reassured Mindy that feeling jinxed or different from other kids are common reactions to being raped but that she has helped many other teens who've been through similar experiences and feels confident that she can help Mindy, too.

4.6.1 Conceptualizing Mindy's Case Using the CHECKS Heuristic

1. **What *caused* the problem?** *Goal: Identify causal risk factor(s).*
    Ms. Morgan utilized parent and child clinical interviews as well as the Self-Report Trauma History portion of the UCLA PTSD RI to determine that Mindy had experienced two potentially traumatic events—the rape and the sudden death of her grandmother. This allowed Ms. Morgan to identify the most common or likely outcomes of these events (i.e., PTSD and PCBD) and ensure that she had the appropriate assessment tools to measure those primary outcomes.
2. **What are the primary *consequences*?** *Goal: Identify the primary causal consequence(s) of exposure to the primary causal risk factor(s).*
    Results of Mindy's PTSD RI reveal that she meets criteria for PTSD. Although she does not meet full criteria for PCBD, Mindy highly endorsed a number of items on the PCBD Checklist reflecting separation distress (e.g., missing her grandmother so much that her heart aches) as well as circumstance-related

distress (e.g., feeling responsible for the death and thinking about ways in which the death could have been prevented) (Kaplow et al. 2013). According to the Short Mood and Feelings Questionnaire, Mindy does not appear to be at significant risk for clinical depression. Other presenting issues based on clinical interviews and the parent-report version of the Strengths and Difficulties Questionnaire (SDQ) include inattention, social withdrawal, and being bullied or picked on by others. Identified strengths on the SDQ include being considerate of others' feelings and being kind to younger children. Given that Mindy meets full criteria for PTSD, the clinician's case conceptualization focuses on PTSD as the primary presenting issue.

3. **What resources (both internal and external) may _help_ the problem?** *Goal: Identify potential protective factors (things in the ecology that lessen the effects of the causal risk factor).*

    Mindy's relationship with her sister appears to be protective in that she does not allow herself to think of suicide given how devastating it would be for her sister. Because she feels comfortable talking to her father about what happened, he may be able to serve as an important source of support if they can connect regularly. Mindy's willingness to talk openly with the therapist about her assault may be indicative of a more emotionally expressive form of coping, which can assist in reducing PTSD symptoms. During the clinical interview, Mindy also revealed that she enjoys painting, hopes to be an artist one day, and already sold a couple of her pieces to a local art dealer. Mindy's artistic abilities may help her by allowing for a more creative outlet to express her distress and grief.

4. **What factors (both internal and external) may _exacerbate_ the problem?** *Goal: Identify potential vulnerability factors (things in the ecology that intensify the effects of the causal risk factor).*

    Ms. Morgan's evaluation identified a number of potential vulnerability factors (both intrinsic and extrinsic to Mindy) that may exacerbate her PTSD symptoms. With respect to her (*extrinsic*) social ecology, theorized vulnerability factors include her perception of her mother as being nonsupportive, the death of her grandmother (who served as a primary source of emotional support, especially after her parents divorced), being bullied in school, and the loss of her best friend with whom she became estranged when she sided with her brother after the assault. The mother's own self-reported maladaptive grief reactions also appear to be elevated; thus, the mother's grief may be contributing to her difficulties in providing support to Mindy. Additional vulnerability factors within the social ecology include frequent exposure to trauma reminders including seeing her best friend in school, and hearing and seeing derogatory comments made by other youth at school and on Facebook. Mindy's theorized intrinsic vulnerability factors include maladaptive cognitions focusing on self-blame and feeling as if she is "jinxed" as a result of the rape.

5. **What are _key_ intervention objectives?** *Goal: Begin case conceptualization and treatment planning based on the integrated assessment data.*

    Based on the evaluation results, the clinician identifies several primary *intervention objectives* that address the effects of trauma, bereavement, and their interplay during adolescence (e.g., Saltzman et al. in press). These include (1) reducing PTSD symptoms; (2) reducing maladaptive grief reactions, particularly separation distress and circumstance-related distress (Kaplow et al. 2013); and (3) increasing adaptive school-related behaviors (e.g., attending class, completing homework assignments).

Ms. Morgan also identifies specific *practice elements* intended to reduce therapeutically modifiable vulnerability factors (things that can be changed) and to harness protective factors. These factors include:

1. Facilitate more adaptive and supportive parent-child interactions between Mindy and her mother that will help her deal with her daily trauma reminders, distress symptoms, and social adversities and provide the support she needs to perform well at school.
2. Help Mindy harness her capacity for expressive coping, particularly through her artistic abilities, to help her manage her posttraumatic stress reactions, grief reactions, and social adversities.
3. Inform Janice, the school counselor, and school teachers of Mindy's potential trauma reminders in order to reduce preventable exposures and help Mindy improve her school behavior and performance.
4. Use cognitive-behavioral strategies to reduce Mindy's maladaptive thoughts regarding self-blame and derogatory self-statements.
5. Harness Mindy's supportive relationship with her father to furnish another safe person with whom she can talk about the assault and about distressing reminders as needed. Mindy's father is skilled in computers and can also teach her how to better protect herself online (e.g., security settings, reporting abuse).
6. Find healthy ways in which Mindy can feel a sense of ongoing connection to her deceased grandmother and continue to draw strength from that unique and important relationship.

6. **Is treatment *successful*? Why or why not?** *Goal: Monitor treatment progress and identify theorized mechanisms of therapeutic change (active ingredients of treatment).*

Ms. Morgan plans to readminister the test battery at regular intervals throughout treatment to monitor therapeutic progress and make adjustments as needed. She will also continue to monitor vulnerability and protective factors she has targeted in her treatment plan, both to evaluate their theorized role as mechanisms of therapeutic change, as well as to ensure that she is effectively addressing her intervention foci. She will take timely course correction steps as needed if her monitoring procedure reveals a lack of adequate therapeutic progress to increase the chance of a successful treatment outcome (Lambert 2010), including a return to the CHECKS Heuristic to troubleshoot additional targets for intervention (e.g., vulnerability factors). Finally, the clinician will incorporate surveillance in her ongoing assessment activities by continuing to look for other potential adversities or sources of distress that may arise during the course of treatment. If detected, she will also adjust her treatment plan accordingly.

Conclusion

In this chapter, we advocated for the need for both trauma-informed and bereavement-informed EBA in recognition of the frequent co-occurrence of trauma and bereavement and the fact that each may carry different constellations of causal risk factors, vulnerability factors, protective factors, and outcomes. We also emphasized the value that EBA principles and methods can add to furnishing clinicians with best-practice tools for assessing traumatized and bereaved youth. We proposed that EBA holds great promise for raising the standard of care for traumatized and bereaved youth, including promoting the competent use of tests in ways that maximize both efficiency and effectiveness and raise the standard of care. We illustrated this promise by describing how EBA can guide and inform the entire arc of therapy, ranging from risk screening through clinical assessment, case conceptualization, treatment planning, monitoring treatment response, evaluating treatment outcomes, surveillance for new stressors, and monitoring posttreatment adjustment (e.g., key developmental milestones and transitions). We introduced a heuristic for organizing different types of assessment data and demonstrated how it can be used to facilitate case conceptualization, treatment planning, monitoring therapeutic progress, and treatment outcome evaluation. We concluded with a case study that demonstrated how these EBA principles and tools can be used in concert to evaluate and treat a traumatized and bereaved child.

References

Achenbach TM, Rescorla LA (2001) Manual for the ASEBA School-Age Forms & Profiles. University of Vermont, Burlington

Anderson LW, Krathwohl D, Airasian P, Cruikshank KA, Mayer RE, Pintrich P, Rathers J, Wittrock C (2001) A taxonomy for learning, teaching, and assessing: a revision of bloom's taxonomy of educational objectives, Complete edn. Longman, New York

Beidas RS, Stewart RE, Walsh L, Lucas S, Downey MM, Jackson K, Mandell DS (2015) Free, brief, and validated: standardized instruments for low-resource mental health settings. Cogn Behav Pract 22:5–19

Breslau N, Peterson EL, Poisson LM, Schultz LR, Lucia VC (2004) Estimating posttraumatic stress disorder in the community: lifetime perspective and the impact of typical traumatic events. Psychol Med 34:889–898

Bruchmuller K, Margraf J, Suppiger A, Schneider S (2011) Popular or unpopular? Therapists' use of structured interviews and their estimation of patient acceptance. Behav Ther 42(4):634–643

Christon LM, McLeod BD, Jensen-Doss A (2015) Evidence-based assessment meets evidence-based treatment: an approach to science-informed case conceptualization. Cogn Behav Pract 22:36–48

Cohen JA, Mannarino AP, Greenberg T, Padlo S, Shipley C (2002) Trauma. Violence Abuse 3(4):307–328

Contractor AA, Claycomb MA, Byllesby BM, Layne CM, Kaplow JB, Steinberg AM, Elhai J (2015) Hispanic ethnicity and Caucasian race: relations with posttraumatic stress disorder's factor structure in clinic-referred youth. Psychol Trauma 7(5):456–464

Cook JM, Newman E, The New Haven Trauma Competency Group (2014) A consensus statement on trauma mental health: the new haven competency conference process and major findings. Psychol Trauma Theor Res Pract Policy 6:300–307

Courtois CA, Gold SN (2009) The need for inclusion of psychological trauma in the professional curriculum: a call to action. Psychol Trauma Theory Res Pract Policy 1:3–23

Cuffe SP, McCullough EL, Pumariega AJ (1994) Comorbidity of attention deficit hyperactivity disorder and posttraumatic stress disorder. J Child Family Stud 3(3):327–336

Derogatis L (1977) SCL-90: administration, scoring, and procedures manual for the revised version. Johns Hopkins University School of Medicine, Baltimore

Elhai JD, Layne CM, Steinberg AM, Brymer MJ, Briggs EC, Ostrowski SA, Pynoos RS (2013) Psychometric properties of the UCLA PTSD Reaction Index Part II: Investigating factor structure findings in a national clinic-referred youth sample. J Trauma Stress 26:10–18

Figley CR, Kleber RJ (1995) Beyond the "victim": secondary traumatic stress. In: Kleber RJ, Figley CR, Gersons BPR (eds) Beyond trauma: cultural and societal dynamics. Plenum, New York, pp. 75–98

Foa EB, Johnson KM, Feeny NC, Treadwell KR (2001) The child PTSD Symptom Scale: a preliminary examination of its psychometric properties. J Clin Child Psychol 30:376–384

Garb HN (1998) Studying the clinician: judgment research and psychological assessment. American Psychological Association, Washington, DC

Gawande A (2010) The checklist manifesto. Penguin, New York

Goodman R, Ford T, Simmons H, Gatward R, Meltzer H (2000) Using the Strengths and Difficulties Questionnaire (SDQ) to screen for child psychiatric disorders in a community sample. Br J Psychiatry 177:534–539

Grassetti SN, Herres J, Williamson AA, Yarger HA, Layne CM, Kobak R (2015) Narrative focus predicts symptom change trajectories in group treatment for traumatized and bereaved adolescents. J Clin Child Adolesc Psychol 44:933–941

Hoge MA, Tondora J, Stuart GW (2003) Training in evidence-based practice. Psychiatr Clin North Am 26:851–865

Howell KH, Barrett-Becker EP, Burnside AN, Wamser-Nanney R, Layne CM, Kaplow JB (2016) Children facing parental cancer versus parental death: the buffering effects of positive parenting and emotional expression. J Child Family Stud 25;152–164

Howell KH, Shapiro DN, Layne CM, Kaplow JB (2015) Individual and psychosocial mechanisms of adaptive functioning in parentally bereaved children. Death Stud 39:296–306

Hunsley J (2015) Translating evidence-based assessment principles and components into clinical practice settings. Cogn Behav Pract 22:101–109

Hunsley J, Mash EJ (2007) Evidence-based assessment. Annu Rev Clin Psychol 3:29–51

Jensen-Doss A, Youngstrom EA, Youngstrom JK, Feeny NC, Findling RL (2014) Predictors and moderators of agreement between clinical and research diagnoses for children and adolescents. J Consult Clin Psychol 82:1151–1162

Kaplow J, Hall E, Koenen K, Dodge K, Amaya-Jackson L (2008) Dissociation predicts later attention problems in sexually abused children. Child Abuse Negl 32:261–275

Kaplow JB, Howell KH, Layne CM (2014) Do circumstances of the death matter? Identifying socioenvironmental risks for grief-related psychopathology in bereaved youth. J Trauma Stress 27(1):42–49

Kaplow JB, Layne CM (2014) Sudden loss and psychiatric disorders across the life course: Toward a developmental lifespan theory of bereavement-related risk and resilience. Am J Psychiatry 171(8):807–810

Kaplow JB, Layne CM, Pynoos RS (2014) Persistent Complex Bereavement Disorder as a call to action: using a proposed DSM-5 diagnosis to advance the field of childhood grief. Trauma Stress Points 28(1) http://sherwood-istss.informz.net/admin31/content/template.asp?sid=35889&ptid=1686&brandid=4463&uid=0&mi=3773102&ps=35889

Kaplow JB, Layne CM, Pynoos RS, Cohen JA, Lieberman A (2012) DSM-V diagnostic criteria for bereavement-related disorders in children and adolescents: developmental considerations. Psychiatry 75(3):243–266

Kaplow JB, Layne CM, Saltzman WR, Cozza SJ, Pynoos RS (2013) Using multidimensional grief theory to explore effects of deployment, reintegration, and death on military youth and families. Clin Child Fam Psychol Rev 16:322–340

Kaplow JB, Saunders J, Angold A, Costello EJ (2010) Psychiatric symptoms in bereaved versus non-bereaved youth and young adults: a longitudinal, epidemiological study. J Am Acad Child Adolesc Psychiatry 49:1145–1154

King CA, Ewell Foster C, Rogalski K (2013) Teen suicide risk: a practitioner guide to screening, assessment, and care management. Guilford, New York

Ko SJ, Ford JD, Kassam-Adams N, Berkowitz SJ, Wilson C, Wong M, Brymer MJ, Layne CM (2008) Creating trauma-informed systems: child welfare, education, first responders, health care, juvenile justice. Prof Psychol Res Pract 39:396–404

Kraemer HC (1992) Evaluating medical tests: Objective and quantitative guidelines. Sage, Newbury Park

Lambert MJ (2010) Prevention of treatment failure: the use of measuring, monitoring, and feedback in clinical practice. American Psychological Association, Washington, DC

Layne CM, Beck CJ, Rimmasch H, Southwick JS, Moreno MA, Hobfoll SE (2009) Promoting "resilient" posttraumatic adjustment in childhood and beyond: "unpacking" life events, adjustment trajectories, resources, and interventions. In: Brom D, Pat-Horenczyk R, Ford J (eds) Treating traumatized children: risk, resilience, and recovery. Routledge, New York, pp. 13–47

Layne CM, Briggs-King E, Courtois C (2014) Introduction to the Special Section: Unpacking risk factor caravans across development: Findings from the NCTSN Core Data Set. Psychol Trauma Theory Res Pract Policy 6(Suppl 1):S1–S8

Layne CM, Greeson JKP, Kim S, Ostrowski SA, Reading S, Vivrette RL, Briggs EC, Fairbank JA, Pynoos RS (2014) Links between trauma exposure and adolescent high-risk health behaviors: findings from the NCTSN Core Data Set. Psychol Trauma Theory Res Pract Policy 6(Suppl 1):S40–S49

Layne CM, Kaplow JB, Pynoos RS (2014) Persistent Complex Bereavement Disorder (PCBD) checklist – youth version 1.0. University of California, Los Angeles

Layne CM, Olsen JA, Baker A, Legerski JP, Isakson PA, Duraković-Belko E, Dapo N, Campara N, Arslanagić B, Saltzman WR, Pynoos RS (2010) Unpacking trauma exposure risk factors and differential pathways of influence: predicting post-war mental distress in bosnian adolescents. Child Dev 81:1053–1076

Layne CM, Pynoos RS, Saltzman WR, Arslanagić B, Black M, Savjak N, Popovi T, Durakovi E, Mu M, Campara. N, Djapo. N, Houston R (2001) Trauma/grief-focused group psychotherapy: school-based postwar intervention with traumatized Bosnian adolescents. Group Dyn Theory Res Pract 5:277

Layne CM, Saltzman WR, Poppleton L, Burlingame GM, Pašalić A, Duraković E, Musić M, Campara N, Dapo N, Arslanagić B, Steinberg AM, Pynoos RS (2008) Effectiveness of a school-based group psychotherapy program for war-exposed adolescents: a randomized controlled trial. J Am Acad Child Adolesc Psychiatry Child Adolesc Psychiatry 47:1048–1062

Layne CM, Steinberg JR, Steinberg AM (2014) Causal reasoning skills training for mental health practitioners: promoting sound clinical judgment in evidence-based practice. Train Educ Prof Psychol 8:292–302

Layne CM, Warren JS, Saltzman WR, Fulton J, Steinberg AM, Pynoos RS (2006) Contextual influences on post-traumatic adjustment: retraumatization and the roles of distressing reminders, secondary adversities, and revictimization. In: Schein LA, Spitz HI, Burlingame GM, Muskin PR (eds) Group approaches for the psychological effects of terrorist disasters. Haworth, New York, pp. 235–286

Mannarino AP, Cohen JA (2011) Traumatic loss in children and adolescents. J Child Adolesc Trauma 4:22–33

Melhem NM, Moritz G, Walker M, Shear MK, Brent D (2007) Phenomenology and correlates of complicated grief in children and adolescents. J Am Acad Child Adolesc Psychiatry 46(4):493–499

Nader KO, Layne CM (2009, September) Maladaptive grieving in children and adolescents: discovering developmentally-linked differences in the manifestation of grief. Trauma Stress Points 23(5):12–16

Nader K, Pynoos R, Fairbanks L, Calvin F (1990) Children's PTSD reactions one year after a sniper attack at their school. Am J Psychiatry 147:1526–1530

Oosterhoff B, Kaplow JB, Layne CM (in press). Trajectories of adolescent binge drinking in trauma-exposed youth differentially predict subsequent adjustment in emerging adulthood. *Translational issues in psychological science*

Palm KM, Polusny MA, Follette VM (2004) Vicarious traumatization: potential hazards and interventions for disaster and trauma workers. Prehosp Disaster Med 19:73–78

Pynoos RS (1992) Grief and trauma in children and adolescents. Bereavement Care 11:2–10

Pynoos RS, Steinberg AM, Layne CM, Liang LJ, Vivrette RL, Briggs EC, Kisiel CL, Habib M, Belin TR, Fairbank J (2014) Modeling constellations of trauma exposure in the National Child Traumatic Stress Network Core Data Set. Psychol Trauma Theory Res Pract Policy 6(Suppl 1):S9–S17

Regier DA, Narrow WE, Clarke DE, Kraemer HC, Kuramoto SJ, Kuhl EA, Kupfer DJ (2012) DSM-5 field trials in the United States and Canada, part II: test-retest reliability of selected categorical diagnoses. Am J Psychiatry 170:59–70

Rettew DC, Lynch AD, Achenbach TM, Dumenci L, Ivanova MY (2009) Meta-analyses of agreement between diagnoses made from clinical evaluations and standardized diagnostic interviews. Int J Methods Psychiatr Res 18:169–184

Saltzman WR, Layne CM, Pynoos RS, Olafson E, Kaplow JB, Boat B (in press) Trauma and Grief Component Therapy for Adolescents: A Modular Approach to Treating Traumatized and Bereaved Youth. Cambridge University Press

Shapiro D, Howell K, Kaplow J (2014) Associations among mother-child communication quality, childhood maladaptive grief, and depressive symptoms. Death Stud 38:172–178

Sheehan DV, Lecrubier Y, Sheehan KH, Amorim P, Janavs J, Weiller E, Hergueta T, Baker R, Dunbar GC (1998) The Mini-International Neuropsychiatric Interview (M.I.N.I.): the development and validation of a structured diagnostic psychiatric interview for DSM-IV and ICD-10. J Clin Psychiatry 59:22–33

Spuji M, Prinzie P, Zijderlaan J, Stikkelbroe Y, Dillen L, de Roos C, Boelen PA (2012) Psychometric properties of the Dutch inventories of prolonged grief for children and adolescents. Clin Psychol Psychother 19:540–551

Straus SE, Glasziou P, Richardson WS, Haynes RB (2011) Evidence-based medicine: how to practice and teach EBM, 4 edn. Churchill Livingstone, New York

Suppiger A, In-Albon T, Hendriksen S, Hermann E, Margraf J, Schneider S (2009) Acceptance of structured diagnostic interviews for mental disorders in clinical practice and research settings. Behav Ther 40(3):272–279

UNICEF (2013) Statistics by area/HIV/AIDS: orphan estimates.. http://www.childinfo.org/hiv_aids_orphanestimates.php

Weine S, Danieli Y, Silove D, Van Ommeren M, Fairbank JA, Saul J (2002) Guidelines for international training in mental health and psychosocial interventions for trauma exposed populations in clinical and community settings. Psychiatry 65:156–164

Weinstein D, Staffelbach D, Biaggio M (2000) Attention-deficit hyperactivity disorder disorder and posttraumatic stress disorder: differential diagnosis in childhood sexual abuse. Clin Psychol Rev 20(3):359–378

Weisz JR, Chorpita BF, Frye A, Ng MY, Lau N, Bearman SK, Hoagwood KE (2011) Youth top problems: using idiographic consumer-guided assessment to identify treatment needs and to track change during psychotherapy. J Consult Clin Psychol 79:369–380

Wells GM, Burlingame GM, Lambert MJ, Hoag MJ, Hope CA (1996) Conceptualization and measurement of patient change during psychotherapy: development of the outcome questionnaire and youth outcome questionnaire. Psychother Theory Res Pract Train 33:275–283

Yeh M, Hough RL, Fakhry F, McCabe KM, Lau AS, Garland AF (2005) Why bother with beliefs? Examining relationships between race/ethnicity, parental beliefs about causes of child problems, and mental health service use. J Consult Clin Psychol 73(5):800–807

Youngstrom EA (2013) Future directions in psychological assessment: combining evidence-based medicine innovations with psychology's historical strengths to enhance utility. J Clin Child Adolesc Psychol 42(1):139–159

Youngstrom EA, Choukas-Bradley S, Calhoun CD, Jensen-Doss A (2014) Clinical guide to the evidence-based assessment approach to diagnosis and treatment. Cogn Behav Pract 22:20–35

Youngstrom EA, Frazier TW (2013) Evidence-based strategies for the assessment of children and adolescents: measuring prediction, prescription, and process. In: Miklowitz DJ, Craighead WE, Craighead L (eds) Developmental psychopathology, 2 edn. Wiley, New York, pp. 36–79

Psychological and Biological Theories of Child and Adolescent Traumatic Stress Disorders

Julian D. Ford and Carolyn A. Greene

5.1 Introduction

In order to assess and treat child and adolescent traumatic stress disorders, clinicians need a guiding theoretical framework for conceptualizing the origins, course, and contributing (risk and protective) factors for these disorders. The current chapter therefore provides an overview of the leading psychobiological theories of childhood traumatic stress disorders. The chapter begins with a brief historical chronology of the dominant theories, followed by a summary of the scientific research that has informed theory development in the traumatic stress field. Then the major current theories of child and adolescent traumatic stress disorders are described, including learning/conditioning, cognitive/information processing, interpersonal/resources, developmental, and intergenerational theories. The chapter concludes with a discussion of the implications of these theories for clinical assessment and treatment of childhood traumatic stress disorders.

5.2 A Brief History of the Emergence of Theoretical Models of Traumatic Stress Disorders

The earliest theories of traumatic stress disorders were formulated more than 150 years ago in order to provide a biomedical explanation for mental breakdowns observed in soldiers (e.g., soldier's heart) following combat and in railway personnel (e.g., railway spine syndrome). Next, *psychodynamic* theories emerged with the

---

J.D. Ford, PhD, ABPP (✉)
University of Connecticut Schools of Medicine and Law,
263 Farmington Avenue MC1410 L4055, Farmington, CT 06030-1410, USA
e-mail: jford@uchc.edu

C.A. Greene, PhD
University of Connecticut Health Center, 65 Kane Street, West Hartford, CT 06119, USA
e-mail: cgreene@uchc.edu

© Springer International Publishing Switzerland 2017
M.A. Landolt et al. (eds.), *Evidence-Based Treatments for Trauma Related Disorders in Children and Adolescents*, DOI 10.1007/978-3-319-46138-0_5

advent of psychoanalysis, focusing initially on emotional conflicts caused by childhood sexual abuse and subsequently on personality and a putative psychological vulnerability to emotional distress. As behaviorism began to hold sway in the early to middle twentieth century, *learning* theories based on the principles of classical and operant conditioning were developed, with the application of research on fear to conceptualizations of traumatic stress disorders in ascendance concurrently with the first formal codification of posttraumatic stress disorder (PTSD) in 1980.

Cognitive behavioral theories of anxiety and affective disorders developed in the middle twentieth century and rapidly were adapted to complement and extend learning theory models of traumatic stress disorders in *cognitive* theories that invoked cognitive appraisals and errors as a pathway paralleling the behavioral conditioning processes in the origins and persistence of these disorders. Advances in information processing science led to the elaboration of learning and cognitive theories with conceptual models that identified potential mechanisms of altered *information processing* in the traumatic stress disorders (e.g., sensory/perceptual and verbal processing; working, procedural, and episodic/narrative memory). Advances in research since the 1980s have resulted in key insights in three areas relevant to theory: (1) potential changes in brain structure and functioning associated with altered information processing in traumatic stress disorders; (2) neurochemistry of the brain and body associated with anxiety, fear, depression, and aggression; and (3) genetic risk and protective factors for traumatic stress disorders and stress-related epigenetic alterations in genes that may occur as both a cause and effect of traumatic stress disorders. As a result, *biological* theories of trauma-altered information processing emerged in the 1990s and are constantly being refined by new research.

In addition, over the past 50 years, research on the social determinants of physical and psychological health has informed the development of socioecological theories of traumatic stress disorders. This has spurred the transformation of psychodynamic and family systems theories into *interpersonal* theories of psychopathology and childhood traumatic stress disorders, Related research on social support and socioeconomic assets and stressors by social and community psychologists and public health scientists has resulted in a parallel social determinants model of traumatic stress disorders, *conservation of resources* theory.

No single theory alone can fully account for the origins and persistence of childhood traumatic stress disorders. However, taken together, the existing portfolio of theoretical models provides clinicians with a powerful set of concepts and tools for understanding the processes that must be assessed and targeted for treatment in order to enable children and adolescents (and their families and social support networks) to recover from traumatic stress disorders.

5.3 Scientific Research Informing the Development of Child Traumatic Stress Theory

Child and adolescent traumatic stress disorders by definition are the psychopathological sequelae of exposure to traumatic stressors. Scientific research has shown that the origins and course of children's traumatic stress disorders involve a complex set of biopsychosocial factors that must be taken into account in order for traumatic stress theories to be empirically grounded.

In the first place, there are many sequelae of exposure to traumatic stressors that occur in a multiplicity of combinations. PTSD includes diverse symptoms of intrusive reexperiencing, avoidance, altered cognition/emotion, hyperarousal (including problems with sleep, aggression, self-harm, and reckless behavior), and dissociation. Further complexity is added by the finding that children exposed to traumatic stressors also are at risk for developing serious problems with anxiety, phobias, depression, disruptive behavior (including attention deficits, impulsivity, oppositional-defiance, and delinquency), learning, eating/weight, sexual behavior, addictions, psychosis, mania, and suicidality (see Chap. 1). Traumatic stress disorder theories must be able to account for the multifaceted clinical sequelae of exposure to traumatic stressors in children and adolescents, including the emergence or exacerbation of disorders that overlap with, but may extend well beyond, PTSD.

PTSD also has a highly variable course, often not emerging as a full-blown disorder for months or years after exposure to traumatic stressors, with symptoms that wax and wane in intensity and frequency over time (Andrews et al. 2007). Many trauma-exposed children never experience sufficient symptoms and impairment to be diagnosed with PTSD, or have episodes of PTSD that appear to improve or even disappear without any treatment. Others develop chronic and severe PTSD, but even they may have periods of relative remission as well as worsening of the symptoms. Theory thus must account for not only the origins of PTSD but also for the often fluctuating course of child and adolescent traumatic stress disorders (including but not limited to PTSD), and they must explain why these disorders are chronic in some cases and transient in others (Schnurr et al. 2004).

Third, many children and adolescents who are exposed to traumatic stressors never develop PTSD or other trauma-related disorders but instead appear asymptomatic or unimpaired and resistant to psychopathology—and those who do develop a trauma-related disorder may be resilient and later fully recover without subsequent recurrences (Layne et al. 2008). Several risk and protective factors for PTSD have been empirically identified (see Chap. 2). These do not *cause* traumatic stress disorders but instead influence the likelihood that a disorder will emerge after exposure to traumatic stressors. Theories must account for the operation of risk and protective factors as moderators or mediators of the relationship between children's exposure to traumatic stressors and the development or persistence of (and recovery from) traumatic stress disorders.

Fourth, the nature of the child's acute (peritraumatic, i.e., during or within hours or a few days later) reactions to traumatic stressors have been found to be predictive of the risk of posttraumatic stress symptoms (Birmes et al. 2003; Kumpula et al. 2011) and persistent PTSD (Miron et al. 2014).

Finally, child and adolescent traumatic stress disorders have been shown in numerous scientific studies to be predicted by and associated with the intensity or "dose" of exposure to traumatic stressors and related forms of childhood adversity (e.g., parental mental health or substance abuse problems) (Cloitre et al. 2009; D'Andrea et al. 2012). Several features of traumatic stressors have been shown to be

Table 5.1 Stressor features that increase risk of developing a traumatic stress disorder

Intentional physical or sexual violence perpetrated by another person or group (such as domestic, war, or community violence, terrorist attacks, or torture)
Betrayal by a person or organization responsible for protecting the safety and rights of vulnerable individuals (such as physical or sexual abuse by a caregiver or priest)
Violation of victims' bodies or selves or homes by extreme violence or destruction (such as war atrocities, rape, or destruction of home and community in a disaster)
Coercion used to destroy people's self-respect and will to resist (such as combined physical and emotional abuse, domestic violence, or torture)
Prolonged complete isolation from human contact and social interaction (such as solitary confinement of prisoners of war, kidnapping victims, or abused children)
Lengthy duration or numerous repetitions of exposure to traumatic stressors or of uncertainty in the face of imminent exposure (such as chronic abuse, violence, or premature deaths, or living in a violent family, war zone, or disaster-prone area)
Multiple concurrent or sequential types of traumatic stressors (poly-victimization)

associated with most severe immediate stress reactions and an elevated likelihood of developing traumatic stress disorders (Table 5.1).

Despite their many differences, these highly traumagenic stressors share several common features. They involve *confrontation with actual or imminent death, severe physical injury, or violation of the body's privacy and integrity* (e.g., sexual assault, torture) that constitutes a direct or vicarious threat to the person's survival and evoke an array of biological adaptations that may be the biological basis for a wide range of traumatic stress disorders (De Bellis and Zisk 2014; McLaughlin et al. 2015; Suzuki et al. 2014; Teicher and Samson 2016; Van Dam et al. 2014). A second common denominator is *unpredictability and uncontrollability* and a resultant sense of helplessness (Pivovarova et al. 2016), even for individuals who are prepared by training or forewarning (e.g., emergency first responders, military personnel) or by either past or current experience (e.g., victims of repeated episodes of abuse or domestic or community violence) (Foa et al. 1992). Third, exposure to stressors that involve multiple types of danger, harm, and victimization tends to increase the likelihood and severity of traumatic stress disorders—among children and adolescents this has been referred to as *poly-victimization* (Turner et al. 2016). Fourth, stressors that are the result of *intentional actions by other human beings*, especially when those persons occupy a position of responsibility and authority (e.g., adult family members, caregivers, faith leaders, educators, coaches), evoke not only fear but also a sense of betrayal and distrust that has been shown to undermine the child's capacities for emotion regulation (Bradley et al. 2011; Dvir et al. 2014; Valdez et al. 2014) and security in primary attachment relationships (Feldman and Vengrober 2011; Kim et al. 2011; Levendosky et al. 2011). In adults as well, stressors are most likely to lead to traumatic stress disorders when they involve a fundamental betrayal of trust due to breaches in the social contract (e.g., genocide, war atrocities, torture, intimate partner violence, sexual assault, institutional violence, or exploitation) (Smith and Freyd 2014).

5 Psychological and Biological Theories of Child and Adolescent

To further complicate matters, research suggests that children (Copeland et al. 2010; Verlinden et al. 2013) can develop the symptoms of traumatic stress disorders after experiencing relatively normative stressors that do not involve exposure to severe or life-threatening violence, injury, violation, exploitation, or loss. Therefore, traumatic stress disorder theory must account for how stressors that do not constitute a survival threat may nevertheless lead to profound psychobiological shifts in how children experience themselves (i.e., as victimized, powerless, and unprotected) and other persons and the world (i.e., as untrustworthy at best, and at worst as posing a threat that cannot be more than partially anticipated, prevented, or coped with).

To summarize briefly, research has demonstrated that traumatic stressors may take many forms and may lead to an equally wide spectrum of traumatic stress disorders depending upon not only the nature of the traumatic stressor(s) but also risk and protective factors that amplify or mitigate the adverse effects of experiencing helplessness or betrayal when confronted with a fundamental threat to survival. A variety of theories have been formulated to explain how traumatic stressors may lead to a plethora of life-altering biopsychosocial changes.

5.4 Fear Conditioning and Learning Theories

Behaviorist theories of traumatic stress disorders propose that they are the result of persistent fear reactions that are the product of two forms of learning: classical (respondent) and operant (instrumental) conditioning (Foa et al. 1989). Classical conditioning of fear involves the pairing of neutral stimuli with highly aversive stimuli. When a child experiences a traumatic event, there are many aversive aspects of the event that threaten the child's sense of safety and survival (e.g., verbal and nonverbal behavior that is terrifying and confusing for the child, the physical shock and pain of severe injury or assault). When a traumatized child encounters similar behavioral or physical cues subsequently, this can elicit similar fear reactions even if there is no objective danger or harm. Moreover, traumatic events involve many contextual stimuli that are not directly harmful but that become infused with a sense of threat or danger as a result of their co-occurrence with the traumatically harmful aspects of the event. Thus, apparently neutral or even positive stimuli such as innocuous or pleasant sounds, sights, smells, tastes, times of day, places, or behavior by other persons may come to elicit fear reactions that are disproportionate to the child's current circumstances but directly proportional to the survival threat or harm experienced in a traumatic event. Childhood PTSD thus can be understood as the result of apparently irrational fear that is a conditioned response triggered by previously neutral stimuli which have become conditioned stimuli as a result of their association with the experience of traumatic survival threats (i.e., unconditioned aversive stimuli that elicit an unconditioned [automatic, unlearned] reaction of fear). Classically conditioned fear thus potentially can account for PTSD's intrusive reexperiencing and hyperarousal symptoms.

The second factor in this two-factor behavioral theory of PTSD is operant conditioning. In contrast to the direct stimulus-response (S-R) mechanisms postulated in classical conditioning, operant conditioning involves an increase in the likelihood or frequency of behavior as a result of the consequences that follow the behavior (i.e., S-R-C). Behavior is learned or modified in order to either acquire desired outcomes ("reinforcers," e.g., approval or support from family or peers; feelings of pleasure, security, or accomplishment), or to avoid aversive outcomes (e.g., criticism, rejection, deprivation, helplessness, physical pain, or potentially traumatic threats or harm). A child who has experienced sexual abuse may not only feel an aversion to physical or emotional contact and intimacy as a result of classical conditioning but as a result of operant conditioning may also learn to avoid people, places, situations, and even thoughts or feelings that could lead to sexual contact specifically and to physical or emotional contact or intimacy more generally. Therefore, operant conditioning can potentially account for additional PTSD symptoms related to avoidance of reminders of traumatic events and social detachment and emotional numbing.

However, S-R and S-R-C fear conditioning and avoidance learning theories cannot fully account for PTSD's symptoms. In the *DSM-III* and *DSM-IV* formulations of PTSD, symptoms of anhedonia, anger, psychogenic amnesia, and flashbacks appeared to involve profound changes in not only conditioned reactions but also cognitive processing (e.g., the individual's core beliefs and ability to consciously process information). As a result, theory that accounts for changes in beliefs that reflect a person's basic sense of meaning was called for (Foa et al. 1989). The expanded set of symptoms proposed for PTSD in the *DSM*-5 increased the relevance of this proposed expansion beyond fear conditioning theories, by explicitly identifying problems with core beliefs, dysregulation as well as distress in a wide range of emotions (not only fear), blame of self and others, and self-harming, reckless, or aggressive behavior. Therefore, cognitive theories of PTSD have been developed to fill the gaps left by behavioral conditioning theories.

5.5 Cognitive and Information Processing Theories

Cognitive theories of childhood traumatic stress disorders hypothesize that exposure to traumatic stressors may alter fundamental beliefs or schemas (e.g., mental representations of the world as a dangerous place, people as harmful and untrustworthy, and oneself as powerless and damaged) and also the underlying cognitive processes (e.g., memory, planning, problem solving) that are the basis for these fundamental beliefs (Brewin and Holmes 2003). Schemas are filters or "blueprints" (Dalgleish 2004) that people use to match what they experience on a sensory, perceptual, emotional, and ultimately cognitive level with what they know from prior experience. The experience of exposure to a traumatic stressor tends to contradict the most commonly held schemas (such as safety, trust, and self-confidence), potentially leading to radical shifts in basic assumptions about self, relationships, and the world. However, schemas are relatively resistant to change, so it has been hypothesized that the contradictory information provided by psychological trauma may be sequestered separately from existing schemas in what has been described as "active memory" (Horowitz 1997). The contradiction between pre-trauma schemas and trauma-related beliefs is evident in many PTSD symptoms. Intrusive reexperiencing of trauma memories or in reaction to reminders of traumatic events is distressing due to the contrast between the trauma-related knowledge of danger, betrayal, powerlessness, and unpreparedness versus schemas based upon safety, trust, and self-efficacy. Avoidance symptoms constitute a cognitive as well as behavioral attempt to keep trauma-related knowledge out of consciousness so that it will not intrude on "active memory." Hyperarousal and hypervigilance are the bodily and mental manifestations of cognitive attempts to anticipate and prepare for further traumatic exposure. Finally, the recently added PTSD symptoms of altered cognitions and emotions are a direct expression of changes in core schemas and related emotions following traumatic exposure.

Beliefs and schemas do not occur in isolation, like separate islands of cognition, however. Instead, they form an "associative network" of interconnected ("associated") perceptions, emotions, and thoughts that each person develops based on life experiences. An extension of cognitive schema theory incorporating the concept of associative networks was developed in order to explain how traumatic stress disorders involve an organized network of distressing (principally either anxiety or anger) or absent (numbed) emotions and corresponding trauma-infused schemas (or appraisals) that are organized around core guiding beliefs that people and the world are dangerous and the self is powerless or ineffective (Tryon 1998). One cognitive theory specifically describes PTSD as involving an associative network of fear-based appraisals (Ehlers and Clark 2000). This fear network cognitive theory identifies autobiographical memory as a key cognitive feature of PTSD in addition to altered schemas involving negative appraisals.

Subsequent cognitive theories have elaborated these concepts by considering how PTSD may involve fundamental changes not only in cognitions per se but also trauma survivors' cognitive *information processing*. A dual process theory of traumatic stress disorders postulates two modes of information processing relevant to PTSD (Brewin 2014). The first information processing mode is episodic (i.e., narrative, autobiographical) and is primarily verbally mediated. The second form of information processing is perceptual, a largely automatic nonconscious intake, storage, and retrieval of memories in the form of sensory and bodily reactions to experiences. Episodic and perceptual information processing are unique and complementary, together providing complete and meaningful memories in every life experience. Dual process theory hypothesizes that traumatic stressors lead to an imbalance in which the perceptual mode dominates and episodic processing becomes impoverished. A further elaboration of cognitive theory integrates these cognitive theories of PTSD in a "SPAARS" theoretical framework (Dalgleish 2004). PTSD is theorized to involve alterations in *verbal* information processing (Brewin's episodic processing), including schemas (S), propositions (i.e., basic beliefs or appraisals, P), and *nonverbal* information processing (i.e., sensory-perceptual knowledge, A, which is similar to Brewin's perceptual processing). When these three information processing modalities are altered by exposure to traumatic stressors, this is hypothesized to correspondingly change an individual's associative representational systems (ARS).

Social learning theory was formulated more than 50 years ago in order to integrate behavioral conditioning and cognitive theories of human behavior. Social cognitive theory is an extension of social learning theory that emphasizes the role that self-related schemas—and self-efficacy, the belief in one's ability to "organize and execute courses of action to generate desired outcomes" (Waldrep and Benight 2008, p. 604)—play in moderating the effects of environmental demands on behavior, cognition, and emotion. A particular form of self-efficacy—"coping self-efficacy," the belief in one's ability to effectively cope with stressors—has been postulated (and shown empirically (Cieslak et al. 2008)) to provide a connection between negative appraisals and PTSD symptoms. Persons viewing themselves as ineffective copers had more severe PTSD symptoms when they also had trauma-altered cognitive schemas than persons who were more confident in their ability to cope with stressors (i.e., high coping self-efficacy). Thus, core beliefs about self-efficacy specifically related to coping may be a key factor to assess and treat in PTSD.

A related line of theory is based on the fact that traumatic stress disorders in childhood involve problems with attention or concentration and cognitive avoidance (i.e., avoiding thoughts that are reminders of traumatic events) as well as alterations in memory and schemas. Research on anxiety disorders has identified *attention bias to threat* as a potential cognitive mechanism contributing to PTSD (Iacoviello et al. 2014). Attention bias to threat refers to a tendency to allocate attention to either recognizing or avoiding awareness of potential threats or avoiding awareness of threat (Pine 2007). These two forms of attention bias are consistent with the PTSD symptoms of hypervigilance (i.e., bias toward paying attention to threats) and avoidance (i.e., bias toward avoiding awareness of threats). A study with highly traumatized adolescents and adults found that those with PTSD were more prone to shift their attention toward stimuli associated with threats and that attention bias toward threat was associated with intense physical arousal (startle responses) in laboratory activities involving learning and unlearning of fear cues (Fani et al. 2012b). The adults in that study who had PTSD and showed attention bias to threat also had a unique pattern of brain activity (Fani et al. 2012a). This included higher levels of activation of the "executive" area of the brain (the dorsolateral prefrontal cortex), which suggests that they were making a conscious effort to focus their attention (similar to what would be expected if an individual is hypervigilant). In addition, when they avoided paying attention to threats, the adults with PTSD had higher levels of activation in the "emotion processing" areas of the brain, the ventromedial prefrontal cortex and the anterior cingulate.

5.6 Biological and Genetic Theories

The trauma-related alterations in information processing, associative networks, and schemas postulated by cognitive theories of PTSD raise the question of how biological changes in brain structure and function contribute to PTSD. Findings from neuroimaging studies of childhood PTSD (De Bellis and Zisk 2014; Morey et al.

2016) and survivors of childhood maltreatment and family violence (Teicher and Samson 2016) point to alterations in children's brain structure and function that differ from those for adults with PTSD in ways that are consistent with what is known about brain development in childhood generally and mirror the cognitive and behavioral differences between children and adults (e.g., immature attentional, impulse control, and executive functions in children).

Despite differences in findings concerning the structural integrity, size, and patterns of neural activation in traumatized children's brains, neuroimaging research supports a theoretical model of childhood PTSD as resulting from impaired activation in and between three key brain areas: (1) emotion regulation and executive function (e.g., medial and dorsolateral prefrontal cortices), (2) stress reactivity and emotional distress (e.g., the amygdala or insula), and (3) screening and organizing perceptual and cognitive information (e.g., the thalamus, striatum, and hippocampus). Research on the neurobiology of PTSD provides evidence of alterations in brain chemistry (i.e., neurotransmitters, e.g., serotonin and catecholamines; neuropeptides, e.g., neuropeptide Y) and has shown that alterations in the chemistry of the brain's internal communication and self-regulation systems play a role in altered brain structure and activation in PTSD, particularly when trauma was experienced in childhood (Opmeer et al. 2014; Southwick et al. 1999). Biological theories of PTSD therefore postulate that the disorder results when exposure to traumatic stressors leads to a sensitization of the brain's neural (electrical and chemical) connections responsible for self- protection and mobilization (i.e., stress reactivity and mood management), such that the child's "learning brain" shifts to become a "survival brain" (Ford 2009, p. 35) concerned primarily with vigilance to and avoidance of threats or reminders of past experiences in which harm occurred.

Neuroimaging and neurobiological research on PTSD also points to a key role for genetics. For example, a genotype involved in the production of neuropeptide Y (NPY), a brain chemical that is active in the amygdala and involved in stress reactivity, has been shown to be associated with heightened activation of the amygdala (the brain's alarm center) and downregulation of the cingulate cortex (part of the brain that adjusts the brain's stress reactivity)—but only for people who had a history of childhood emotional maltreatment (Opmeer et al. 2014). Thus, a person's genetic inheritance may lead to proneness to increased stress reactivity (and potentially to PTSD) if that individual is exposed to traumatic stressors in childhood. Family and twin studies suggest that PTSD may be "heritable" (that is, inborn genetic differences may predispose people to develop PTSD) (Guffanti et al. 2013; Liberzon et al. 2014; Sumner et al. 2014; White et al. 2013; Wolf et al. 2014). The potential heritability of PTSD does not mean that people who share the same or similar genetic inheritance automatically or inevitably will develop PTSD—only that when one of two twins or family members who share some or all of the same genes develops PTSD, it is more likely that the other twin or family member also has had or will have PTSD than if neither of them develop PTSD. Whether this is actually the result of genetic inheritance or other related factors (such as a shared family environment) has not been definitively established, and a wide range of genetic variations (polymorphisms) potentially related to PTSD have been identified, but genome-wide studies are needed in order to avoid chance findings with single-candidate gene polymorphisms (Koenen et al. 2013). Nevertheless, it appears that genetic vulnerability to the adverse effects of childhood trauma exposure may take several forms, including increased risk of (1) further exposure to traumatic stressors, (2) PTSD, (3) other psychopathology (e.g., depression, suicidality) (Enoch et al. 2013; Kohrt et al. 2015), and (4) alterations in the expression of genes as a result of life experiences (epigenetics), which may account for the adverse effects of traumatic experiences across the life span (Nusslock and Miller 2016) and across generations (Bowers and Yehuda 2016).

Although genes associated with a variety of psychological processes (e.g., memory, mood, addiction) have been tentatively linked to PTSD, the most consistent evidence links PTSD with variants of genes involved in the body's peripheral stress response systems—the hypothalamic-pituitary-adrenal axis that produces "stress" chemicals (e.g., adrenaline, cortisol) and the autonomic nervous system that regulates physical arousal (e.g., heart rate, blood pressure, muscle tension) (Koenen et al. 2013). Psychophysiological research has identified extremes of both low and high levels of physical arousal in PTSD (Bauer et al. 2013; Marinova and Maercker 2015). A theory of "fear load" as the basis for PTSD has been postulated based on these converging lines of psychophysiology, neurobiology, and genetics research (Norrholm et al. 2015). Fear load is the individual's tendency to react biologically to stressors with fear, which would be consistent with learning theories (i.e., a heightened likelihood of classical conditioning and social learning of chronic fearfulness following traumatic exposure) and cognitive theories (i.e., biased attention and information processing resulting in recurrent intrusive memories and hypervigilance).

5.7 Interpersonal/Resources Theories

Traumatic stressors may disrupt, compromise, or even destroy the resources that children and their families depend upon for safety, health, and well-being. Those resources (i.e., "objects, personal characteristics, conditions or energies that are valued by individuals or serve as a means to acquire other resources," Walter et al. 2008, p. 157) also serve as crucial buffers that can prevent or mitigate against the adverse psychosocial and physical impacts of traumatic stressors. Object resources include housing, food, vehicles, clothing, and technology. Personal resources include self-esteem, self-efficacy, and physical and psychological hardiness. Condition resources include relationships, social networks, ethnocultural group memberships, and socioeconomic status. Energy resources include time, electricity, fuel, and money. Conservation of resources theory postulates that the loss of resources is more salient than resource gains, hence the potentially powerful and long-lasting impact of traumatic stressors that diminish people's access to resources (e.g., disasters that destroy homes and communities, abuse that results in a fundamental loss of trust in and separation from home or caregivers). The theory postulates preventing and recovering from exposure to traumatic adversity requires increased levels of or access to resources, at the very time when key resources may be depleted or inaccessible. Thus, PTSD can be understood as a drastic reduction in resources that results in a vicious cycle of progressively more depleted or inaccessible resources and escalating rather than diminishing distress and suffering. When a child is traumatized by domestic or community violence or bullying in the school or peer group, resources from all domains are likely to be less available in the aftermath than previously. Home or school may no longer be a safe place, leading not only to fear and sadness but also potentially to hunger, vulnerability to illness, and sleep problems. Self-esteem, self-efficacy, and the ability to trust and cooperate may be diminished as result of the emotional injury sustained. The child's security as a valued member of the family, school, and community may be severely compromised. Additionally, time and physical energy that had been available to enjoy life, learn and achieve, and grow and mature may be taken away by the demands of coping with fear or participating in therapeutic or rehabilitative services. Thus, PTSD involves not only threat and fear but the loss of vital resources when they are most needed in order to be able to regain safety and recover from danger and injury.

Social support is a key resource that often is disrupted or diminished when children experience traumatic stressors. Social support may take the form of emotional, informational, or tangible support and may be linked to specific sources, such as kin relations (spouse, family, relatives), non-kin informal networks (friends, neighbors, coworkers), and people outside the immediate support circles (charitable organizations, professional service providers). Most often, social support is measured by the individual's subjective appraisal that adequate support is available and helpful if needed. Social support also may be measured more objectively in terms of the actual help that a person receives from others (received social support) or of the closeness and position of the person in relationship to a network of potential sources of social support (social embeddedness). Self-efficacy and social support are closely linked: people with more confidence in themselves are more likely to seek and receive social support, and people with strong social support networks are more likely to feel and be effective in coping with stressors.

5.8 Developmental Trauma Theories

The impact of exposure to traumatic stressors is inextricably interwoven with—and potentially highly disruptive to—the inherently immature child's biological and psychosocial development. Children exposed to traumatic stressors thus may experience profound alterations in the development of their bodies, minds, and relationships which can lead not only to PTSD or related symptoms but also to lifelong gaps, deficits, or limitations in their mental and physical health. The adverse impact of exposure to traumatic stressors on childhood development has been well documented in several key biopsychosocial domains including (a) emotion regulation, (b) executive functions (i.e., attention, learning, problem solving, and working (short-term), declarative (verbal), and narrative (autobiographical) memory), (c) personality formation and integration, and (d) relationships (attachment). Emotion dysregulation has been identified as a core developmental impairment associated with childhood exposure to traumatic stressors (D'Andrea et al. 2012). Emotion regulation involves monitoring and maintaining the integrity of the body and self either automatically or self-reflectively (i.e., cognitively).

Emotion regulation begins in infancy, initially with relatively automatic reactions to distress (crying) and pleasure (visual attention, smiling) (Perry et al. 2016). If the infant has repeated success in coping with mild brief episodes of fear, self-regulation is enhanced. The calming presence of a caregiver who helps the infant to titrate the extent of exposure to frightening stimuli and contexts is a crucial source of attachment security that enables the infant to learn self-regulation by experiencing co-regulation (Evans and Porter 2009). Traumatic stressors, especially when they disrupt or compromise the secure infant-caregiver attachment bond, can result in lasting impairments when they prevent the infant from achieving the crucial developmental milestone of learning how to regulate the body when experiencing fear or associated distress (Moutsiana et al. 2014).

In the second and third years of life, continued rapid growth in the brain infrastructure enables the child to develop awareness of self and others as separate individuals with distinct goals, expectations, and emotions. When traumatic events occur, especially if they compromise caregiving, the toddler's neural and neurochemical circuits are likely to become organized by stress reactivity, leading to persistent states of extreme emotional distress (e.g., paralyzing shame, absence of empathy, anger expressed in aggressive behavior) and impairment in the ability to express or modulate these internalized or externalized emotion states and to inhibit impulses, think clearly, set and achieve goals, and trust and cooperate in relationships (Dackis et al. 2015; Kim-Spoon et al. 2013).

In middle childhood and preadolescence, posttraumatically dysregulated affect and impulses can cause or exacerbate a wide range of internalizing (e.g., depression, agoraphobia, panic, obsessive-compulsive, social anxiety, phobias, dissociative disorders), externalizing (e.g., oppositional defiant or conduct disorder, attentional or impulse control disorders, mania/bipolar disorder), and psychosomatic (e.g., eating disorders, sexual, and sleep disorders) problems. These problems in turn compromise successful development and performance in school and activities and with peers and family. Impaired emotion regulation in adolescence can become even more complex, including substance use or personality disorders and serious problems in the legal, school, family, and community domains (e.g., incarceration, truancy, teen pregnancy, gang involvement, suicidality). Traumatic stress disorders thus can not only cause severe immediate symptoms but moreover can alter a child's entire life course by undermining the development of foundational capacities such as emotion regulation (Nusslock and Miller 2016).

5.9 Intergenerational Transmission Theories

The powerful influence of family relationships on child and adolescent development and the empirical finding that parental PTSD severity is associated with children's posttraumatic distress (Lambert et al. 2010) suggest that theories of child traumatic stress disorders would be incomplete unless they address the role of family and intergenerational processes. Experiencing sexual, physical, and/or emotional abuse in childhood has been linked with an increased risk of adult interpersonal revictimization (Classen et al. 2005; Messman and Long 1996) and intimate partner violence (Barrett 2010; Lilly et al. 2014; Widom et al. 2014). It is not surprising, therefore, that the offspring of parents who have been maltreated as children are at increased risk of exposure to violence and other negative life events in their family environment (Collishaw et al. 2007). There also is evidence of elevated risk of child maltreatment perpetration by child abuse victims (Thornberry et al. 2013) and when intimate partner violence occurs (Bidarra et al. 2016; Jouriles et al. 2008). Thus, children of parents who experienced abuse or violence in their own lives are more likely to be exposed to potentially traumatic events and to develop traumatic stress disorders if they (the children) are exposed to traumatic stressors. In fact, the influence of parental PTSD is so salient that children with parents who are experiencing PTSD symptoms have been found to be at greater risk for emotion regulation difficulties, anxiety and depression, and general behavioral problems even when the children have not been exposed to trauma (Enlow et al. 2011; Leen-Feldner et al. 2013). When children of adults with PTSD are exposed to trauma, they are also more likely to develop posttraumatic stress reactions themselves (Chemtob et al. 2010; Leen-Feldner et al. 2013). Further, parental PTSD severity is associated with children's posttraumatic distress and reactivity (Lambert et al. 2014; Morris et al. 2012).

Parents' emotion regulation (or dysregulation) has been conceptualized as a mediator of the intergenerational transmission of traumatic stress disorders. Parents who are able to regulate their own emotion states are better able to serve as role models of the adaptive expression and management of emotional experiences (Bariola et al. 2011) and more prepared to assist their child in using adaptive emotion regulation skills when distressed (Morris et al. 2007). Conversely, emotionally dysregulated parents tend to be unavailable or unable to provide their traumatized child with the supportive, instructional, and empathic responses to their emotional distress that is necessary for the child to recover from trauma-related distress (Kim and Cicchetti 2010), and they are apt to inadvertently model reactive emotional responses (Compas et al. 2001; Pears and Fisher 2005; Shipman et al. 2007; Valiente et al. 2007) that are likely to increase the child's distress and emotion dysregulation.

One potential pathway for the intergenerational familial transmission of PTSD is parents' discipline style and parenting behaviors. While there is mixed support for an intergenerational cycle of abuse in which parents who have experienced maltreatment in childhood are more likely to become physically abusive parents (Thornberry et al. 2012), the majority of parents who have experienced childhood maltreatment do not engage in abusive practices (Berlin et al. 2011). Nevertheless, offspring of maltreated children are at greater risk of poor mental health outcomes, and numerous studies have explored other parenting practices that might explain this association (Bailey et al. 2012; Chemtob and Carlson 2004; Ehrensaft et al. 2015; Rijlaarsdam et al. 2014; Ruscio 2001). Childhood sexual abuse has been associated with greater use of permissive and decreased use of authoritarian, parenting practices, suggesting difficulty providing structure, guidance, and consistent discipline (DiLillo and Damashek 2003; Ruscio 2001). Maternal history of emotional and physical abuse has been associated with greater use of psychological control with one's offspring (Zalewski et al. 2013). Other potential intergenerational links between parent and child PTSD include parenting stress (Barrett 2009; Pereira et al. 2012; Steele et al. 2016), lower parenting self-competence (Bailey et al. 2012; Cole et al. 1992; Ehrensaft et al. 2015), lower parental warmth (Barrett 2009) and higher levels of disengagement, intrusiveness, or an unpredictable alternation of both extremes (Driscoll and Easterbrooks 2007; Moehler et al. 2007).

In addition, the nature of the attachment system may be an important factor in the outcomes associated with childhood trauma, as adult survivors of childhood abuse are at risk of developing disorganized attachments with their children (Berthelot et al. 2015; Lyons-Ruth and Block 1996). Likewise, maltreated children are more likely to have insecure and atypical attachments with their caregivers than non-maltreated children (Cicchetti and Toth 1995; Cook et al. 2005). These inadequate bonds may place children in families affected by trauma at greater risk of psychological distress (Shapiro and Levendosky 1999). Conversely, a secure attachment can be a protective factor that helps to promote resiliency in the face of traumatic experiences (Shapiro and Levendosky 1999). In a study of maltreated and non-maltreated children, Alink, Cicchetti, Kim, and Rogosch (Alink et al. 2009) found that, while maltreated children scored lower on a measure of emotion regulation than non-maltreated children, this was true only for children with an insecure attachment style. For securely attached children, maltreatment was unrelated to emotion regulation. A secure parent-child attachment bond thus may provide sufficient safety and security to sustain—or restore—the child's emotion regulation in the face of maltreatment.

A family environment characterized by chronic stress, aggression, or chaotic patterns of interaction (Morris et al. 2007; Repetti et al. 2002) may also impede a caregiver's ability to respond supportively following trauma (Nelson et al. 2009) and erode family processes that support children's recovery from trauma, such as routines, relationships, and family coping resources (Kiser and Black 2005), and are a risk factor for traumatic stress disorders in children and adolescents (Trickey et al. 2012). A study of traumatized urban youth found that high levels of reexperiencing and avoidance symptoms were associated with a lower value placed on family routines, while lower levels of emotional and behavioral problems were associated with higher levels of family structure, emotional support, and family organization (Kiser et al. 2010).

Finally, a discussion of intergenerational transmission theories would not be complete without recognition of the protective role that supportive relationships and effective parenting can have in fostering resilient outcomes for children who have experienced trauma (Howell 2011). As noted above, a secure parent-child attachment can buffer the effects of trauma (Alink et al. 2009; Shapiro and Levendosky 1999). Relatedly, a mother's ability to sensitively contain her child's distress, respond with appropriate affect, and maintain a supportive, calming presence is associated with resilient outcomes in young children (Feldman and Vengrober 2011). Among adolescents, family support has been found to buffer the psychological effects of violence exposure (Kliewer et al. 2001).

> **Conclusions**
>
> Theories of traumatic stress disorders represent a translation of scientific and clinical knowledge into an account of how people adapt following exposure to traumatic stressors. Posttraumatic adaptations include survival-based forms of *learning* (e.g., classically conditioned fear or anxiety), *cognition* (e.g., hypervigilance, perceived helplessness), *memory* (e.g., intrusive reexperiencing), and *behavioral coping* (e.g., avoidance, reactive aggression). Theories also have been formulated to account for the altered *physiological states* (e.g., hyperarousal, dissociation) and changes in *personal relationships/resources* (e.g., detachment, diminished social support) that occur as a byproduct of—but also may amplify and increase the chronicity of —traumatic stress disorders. Theories of *developmental trauma* additionally have been developed to explain the impact of traumatic stressors occurring during childhood (particularly those involving abuse or other forms of victimization) on the child's development of cognition, behavior, physiology, and relationships. Theories of *intergenerational transmission* of child traumatic stress disorders describe how parents' own traumatic stress difficulties and emotion dysregulation can adversely affect their children's development and increase the risk of child traumatic stress disorders.
>
> These theories of childhood traumatic stress disorders have played a critical role in the development of the treatment interventions for traumatized children presented in this book. Behavioral therapies translate learning theories into interventions designed to enable traumatized children to learn ways to respond to memories and reminders of past traumas that reduce fear and anxiety and restore confidence and hope (e.g., trauma memory exposure). Cognitive therapies provide traumatized children with new ways of thinking that enable them to overcome trauma-related beliefs and transform trauma memories into coherent personal narratives. Interpersonal therapies help traumatized children and their families to develop supportive relationships that can counteract trauma-related emotional and spiritual detachment and prevent further traumatization. Finally, developmental trauma therapies (e.g., ARC [see Chap. 14], SPARCS, STAIR-NST, TARGET (see Chap. 21), or TST [see Chap. 17]) assist traumatized children in developing or restoring biopsychosocial self-regulation capacities (especially emotion regulation) for parents/caregivers as well as traumatized children in order to restore healthy intergenerational relationships and child/adolescent development (Ford et al. 2013). Theory thus can fundamentally inform and guide the essential undertaking of creating, refining, and delivering the empirically supported therapies for children with traumatic stress disorders that are described in the subsequent chapters in this book.

References

Alink LRA, Cicchetti D, Kim J, Rogosch FA (2009) Mediating and moderating processes in the relation between maltreatment and psychopathology: mother-child relationship quality and emotion regulation. J Abnorm Child Psychol 37:831–843

Andrews B, Brewin CR, Philpott R, Stewart L (2007) Delayed-onset posttraumatic stress disorder: a systematic review of the evidence. [Electronic Electronic; Print]. Am J Psychiatry 164(9):1319–1326

Bailey HN, DeOliveira CA, Wolfe VV, Evans EM, Hartwick C (2012) The impact of childhood maltreatment history on parenting: a comparison of maltreatment types and assessment methods. Child Abuse Negl 36:236–246. doi:10.1016/j.chiabu.2011.11.005

Bariola E, Gullone E, Hughes EK (2011) Child and adolescent emotion regulation: the role of parental emotion regulation and expression. [Research Support, Non-U.S. Gov't Review]. Clin Child Fam Psychol Rev 14(2):198–212. doi:10.1007/s10567-011-0092-5

Barrett B (2009) The impact of childhood sexual abuse and other forms of childhood adversity on adulthood parenting. J Child Sex Abus 18:489–512. doi:10.1080/10538710903182628

Barrett B (2010) Childhood sexual abuse and adulthood parenting: the mediating role of intimate partner violence. J Aggress Maltreat Trauma 19(3):323–346. doi:10.1080/10926771003705205

Bauer MR, Ruef AM, Pineles SL, Japuntich SJ, Macklin ML, Lasko NB, Orr SP (2013) Psychophysiological assessment of PTSD: a potential research domain criteria construct. Psychol Assess 25(3):1037–1043. doi:10.1037/a0033432

Berlin LJ, Appleyard K, Dodge KA (2011) Intergenerational continuity in child maltreatment: mediating mechanisms and implications for prevention. Child Dev 82(1):162–176

Berthelot N, Ensink K, Bernazzani O, Normandin L, Luyten P, Fonagy P (2015) Intergenerational transmission of attachment in abused and neglected mothers: the role of trauma-specific reflective functioning. Infant Ment Health J 36(2):200–212. doi:10.1002/imhj.21499

Bidarra ZS, Lessard G, Dumont A (2016) Co-occurrence of intimate partner violence and child sexual abuse: prevalence, risk factors, and related issues. Child Abuse Negl 55:10–21. doi:10.1016/j.chiabu.2016.03.007

Birmes P, Brunet A, Carreras D, Ducasse JL, Charlet JP, Lauque D et al (2003) The predictive power of peritraumatic dissociation and acute stress symptoms for posttraumatic stress symptoms: a three-month prospective study. Am J Psychiatry 160(7):1337–1339. doi:10.1176/appi.ajp.160.7.1337

Bowers ME, Yehuda R (2016) Intergenerational transmission of stress in humans. Neuropsychopharmacology 41(1):232–244. doi: 10.1038/npp.2015.247

Bradley B, DeFife JA, Guarnaccia C, Phifer J, Fani N, Ressler KJ, Westen D (2011) Emotion dysregulation and negative affect: association with psychiatric symptoms. J Clin Psychiatry 72(5):685–691. doi:10.4088/JCP.10m06409blu

Brewin CR, Holmes EA (2003) Psychological theories of posttraumatic stress disorder. Clin Psychol Rev 23(3):339–376

Brewin CR (2014) Episodic memory, perceptual memory, and their interaction: foundations for a theory of posttraumatic stress disorder. Psychol Bull 140(1):69–97. doi: 10.1037/a0033722

Chemtob CM, Carlson JG (2004) Psychological effects of domestic violence on children and their mothers. Int J Stress Manag 11(3):209–226. doi:10.1037/1072-5245.11.3.209

Chemtob CM, Nomura Y, Rajendran K, Yehuda R, Schwartz D, Abramovitz R (2010) Impact of maternal posttraumatic stress disorder and depression following exposure to the September 11 attacks on preschool children's behavior. Child Dev 81(4):1129–1141

Cicchetti D, Toth SL (1995) A developmental psychopathology perspective on child abuse and neglect. J Am Acad Child Adolesc Psychiatry 34(5):541–565

Cieslak R, Benight CC, Caden Lehman V (2008) Coping self-efficacy mediates the effects of negative cognitions on posttraumatic distress. Behav Res Ther 46(7):788–798. S0005-7967(08)00069-7 [pii] 10.1016/j.brat.2008.03.007

Classen CC, Palesh OG, Aggarwal R (2005) Sexual revictimization: a review of the empirical literature. Trauma Violence Abuse 6(2):103–129. doi:10.1177/152483005275087

Cloitre M, Stolbach BC, Herman JL, van der Kolk B, Pynoos R, Wang J, Petkova E (2009) A developmental approach to complex PTSD: childhood and adult cumulative trauma as predictors of symptom complexity. J Trauma Stress 22(5):399–408. doi:10.1002/jts.20444

Cole PM, Woolger C, Power TG, Smith KD (1992) Parenting difficulties among adult survivors of father-daughter incest. Child Abuse Negl 16:239–249

Collishaw S, Dunn J, O'Connor TG, Golding J, Avon Longitudinal Study of Parents and Children Study Team (2007) Maternal childhood abuse and offspring adjustment over time. Dev Psychopathol 19:367–383

Compas BE, Connor-Smith JK, Saltzman H, Thomsen AH, Wadsworth ME (2001) Coping with stress during childhood and adolescence: problems, progress, and potential in theory and research. Psychol Bull 127(1):87–127

Cook A, Spinazzola J, Ford J, Lanktree C, Blaustein M, Cloitre M et al (2005) Complex trauma in children and adolescents. Psychiatr Ann 35(5):390–398

Copeland WE, Keeler G, Angold A, Costello EJ (2010) Posttraumatic stress without trauma in children. Am J Psychiatry 167(9):1059–1065. doi:10.1176/appi.ajp.2010.09020178

Dackis MN, Rogosch FA, Cicchetti D (2015) Child maltreatment, callous-unemotional traits, and defensive responding in high-risk children: an investigation of emotion-modulated startle response. Dev Psychopathol 27(4 Pt 2):1527–1545. doi:10.1017/S0954579415000929

Dalgleish T (2004) Cognitive approaches to posttraumatic stress disorder: the evolution of multirepresentational theorizing. [Review]. Psychol Bull 130(2):228–260. doi:10.1037/0033-2909.130.2.228

D'Andrea W, Ford JD, Stolbach B, Spinazzola J, van der Kolk BA (2012) Understanding interpersonal trauma in children: why we need a developmentally appropriate trauma diagnosis. Am J Orthopsychiatry 82(2):187–200. doi:10.1111/j.1939-0025.2012.01154.x

De Bellis MD., Zisk A (2014) The biological effects of childhood trauma. Child Adolesc Psychiatr Clin N Am 23(2):185–222, vii. doi: 10.1016/j.chc.2014.01.002

DiLillo D, Damashek A (2003) Parenting characteristics of women reporting a history of childhood sexual abuse. Child Maltreat 8(4):319–333. doi:10.1177/1077559503257104

Driscoll JR, Easterbrooks MA (2007) Young mothers' play with their toddlers: individual variability as a function of psychosocial factors. Infant Child Dev 16:649–670. doi:10.1002/icd.515

Dvir Y, Ford JD, Hill M, Frazier JA (2014) Childhood maltreatment, emotional dysregulation, and psychiatric comorbidities. Harv Rev Psychiatry 22(3):149–161. doi:10.1097/HRP.0000000000000014

Ehlers A, Clark DM (2000) A cognitive model of posttraumatic stress disorder. Behav Res Ther 38(4):319–345

Ehrensaft MK, Knous-Westfall HM, Cohen P, Chen H (2015) How does child abuse history influence parenting of the next generation. Psychol Viol 5(1):16–25

Enlow MB, Kitts RL, Blood E, Bizarro A, Hofmeister M, Wright RJ (2011) Maternal posttraumatic stress symptoms and infant emotional reactivity and emotion regulation. Infant Behav Dev 34(4):487–503

Enoch MA, Hodgkinson CA, Gorodetsky E, Goldman D, Roy A (2013) Independent effects of 5′ and 3′ functional variants in the serotonin transporter gene on suicidal behavior in the context of childhood trauma. J Psychiatr Res 47(7):900–907. doi:10.1016/j.jpsychires.2013.03.007

Evans CA, Porter CL (2009) The emergence of mother-infant co-regulation during the first year: links to infants' developmental status and attachment. Infant Behav Dev 32(2):147–158. doi:10.1016/j.infbeh.2008.12.005

Fani N, Jovanovic T, Ely TD, Bradley B, Gutman D, Tone EB, Ressler KJ (2012a) Neural correlates of attention bias to threat in post-traumatic stress disorder. Biol Psychol 90(2):134–142. doi:10.1016/j.biopsycho.2012.03.001

Fani N, Tone EB, Phifer J, Norrholm SD, Bradley B, Ressler KJ et al (2012b) Attention bias toward threat is associated with exaggerated fear expression and impaired extinction in PTSD. Psychol Med 42(3):533–543. doi:10.1017/S0033291711001565

Feldman R, Vengrober A (2011) Posttraumatic stress disorder in infants and young children exposed to war-related trauma. J Am Acad Child Adolesc Psychiatry 50(7):645–658. doi:10.1016/j.jaac.2011.03.001

Foa EB, Steketee G, Rothbaum BO (1989) Behavioral/cognitive conceptualizations of post-traumatic stress disorder. Behav Ther 20(2):155–176

Foa EB, Zinbarg RE, Rothbaum BO (1992) Uncontrollability and unpredictability in post-traumatic stress disorder: an animal model. Psychol Bull 112(2):218–238

Ford JD (2009) Neurobiological and developmental research: clinical implications. In: Courtois CA, Ford JD (eds) Treating complex traumatic stress disorders: an evidence-based guide. Guilford Press, New York

Ford JD, Blaustein M, Habib M, Kagan R (2013) Developmental trauma-focused treatment models. In: Ford JD, Courtois CA (Eds.), Treating complex traumatic stress disorders in children and adolescents: Scientific foundations and therapeutic models. Guilford Press, New York:261–276

Guffanti G, Galea S, Yan L, Roberts AL, Solovieff N, Aiello AE et al (2013) Genome-wide association study implicates a novel RNA gene, the lincRNA AC068718.1, as a risk factor for post-traumatic stress disorder in women. Psychoneuroendocrinology 38(12):3029–3038. doi:10.1016/j.psyneuen.2013.08.014

Horowitz MJ (1997) Stress response syndromes: PTSD, grief, and adjustment disorders, 3 edn. Jason Aronson, Lanham

Howell KH (2011) Resilience and psychopathology in children exposed to family violence. Aggress Violent Behav 16:562–569

Iacoviello BM, Wu G, Abend R, Murrough JW, Feder A, Fruchter E et al (2014) Attention bias variability and symptoms of posttraumatic stress disorder. J Trauma Stress 27(2):232–239. doi:10.1002/jts.21899

Jouriles EN, McDonald R, Slep AMS, Heyman RE, Garrido E (2008) Child abuse in the context of domestic violence: prevalence, explanations, and practice implications. Violence Vict 23(2):221–235

Kim J, Cicchetti D (2010) Longitudinal pathways linking child maltreatment, emotion regulation, peer relations, and psychopathology. J Child Psychol Psychiatry 51(6):706–716

Kim K, Trickett PK, Putnam FW (2011) Attachment representations and anxiety: differential relationships among mothers of sexually abused and comparison girls. J Interpers Violence 26(3):498–521. doi:10.1177/0886260510363416

Kim-Spoon J, Cicchetti D, Rogosch FA (2013) A longitudinal study of emotion regulation, emotion lability-negativity, and internalizing symptomatology in maltreated and nonmaltreated children. Child Dev 84(2):512–527. doi:10.1111/j.1467-8624.2012.01857.x

Kiser LJ, Black MM (2005) Family processes in the midst of urban poverty: what does the trauma ltierature tell us? Aggress Violent Behav 10:715–750. doi:10.1016/j.avb.2005.02.003

Kiser LJ, Medoff DR, Black MM (2010) The role of family processes in childhood traumatic stress reactions for youths living in urban poverty. Traumatology (Tallahass Fla) 16(2):33–42. doi:10.1177/1534765609358466

Kliewer W, Murrell L, Mejia R, de Torres Y, Angold A (2001) Exposure to violence against a family member and internalizing symptoms in Colombian adolescents: the protective effects of family support. J Consult Clin Psychol 69(6):971–982. doi:10.1037/AW22-006X.69.6.971

Koenen KC, Duncan LE, Liberzon I, Ressler KJ (2013) From candidate genes to genome-wide association: the challenges and promise of posttraumatic stress disorder genetic studies. Biol Psychiatry 74(9):634–636. doi:10.1016/j.biopsych.2013.08.022

Kohrt BA, Worthman CM, Ressler KJ, Mercer KB, Upadhaya N, Koirala S et al (2015) Cross-cultural gene- environment interactions in depression, post-traumatic stress disorder, and the cortisol awakening response: FKBP5 polymorphisms and childhood trauma in South Asia GxE interactions in South Asia. Int Rev Psychiatry 27(3):180–196. doi:10.3109/09540261.2015.1020052

Kumpula MJ, Orcutt HK, Bardeen JR, Varkovitzky RL (2011) Peritraumatic dissociation and experiential avoidance as prospective predictors of posttraumatic stress symptoms. J Abnorm Psychol 120(3):617–627. doi:10.1037/a0023927

Lambert SF, Nylund-Gibson K, Copeland-Linder N, Ialongo NS (2010) Patterns of community violence exposure during adolescence. Am J Commun Psychol, 46(3–4):289–302. doi:10.1007/s10464-010-9344-7

Lambert JE, Holzer J, Hasbun A (2014) Association between parents' PTSD severity and children's psychological distress: a meta-analysis. J Trauma Stress 27(1):9–17. doi:10.1002/jts.21891

Layne C, Beck C, Rimmasch H, Southwick J, Moreno M, Hobfoll S (2008) Promoting 'resilient' posttraumatic adjustment in childhood and beyond. In: Brom D, Pat-Horenczyk R, Ford JD (eds) Treating traumatized children : risk, resilience, and recovery. Routledge, London

Leen-Feldner EW, Feldner MT, Knapp A, Bunaciu L, Blumenthal M, Amstadter AB (2013) Offspring psychological and biological correlates of parental posttraumatic stress: review of the literature and research agenda. Clin Psychol Rev 33:1106–1133

Levendosky AA, Bogat GA, Huth-Bocks AC, Rosenblum K, von Eye A (2011) The effects of domestic violence on the stability of attachment from infancy to preschool. J Clin Child Adolesc Psychol 40(3):398–410. doi:10.1080/15374416.2011.563460

Liberzon I, King AP, Ressler KJ, Almli LM, Zhang P, Ma ST et al (2014) Interaction of the ADRB2 gene polymorphism with childhood trauma in predicting adult symptoms of posttraumatic stress disorder. JAMA Psychiat 71(10):1174–1182. doi:10.1001/jamapsychiatry.2014.999

Lilly MM, London MJ, Bridgett DJ (2014) Using SEM to examine emotion regulation and revictimization in predicting PTSD symptoms among childhood abuse survivors. Psychol Trauma Theory Res Pract Policy 6(6):644–651

Lyons-Ruth K, Block D (1996) The disturbed caregiving system: relations among childhood trauma, maternal caregiving, and infant affect and attachment. Infant Ment Health J 17(3):257–275

Marinova Z, Maercker A (2015) Biological correlates of complex posttraumatic stress disorder: state of research and future directions. Eur J Psychotraumatol 6:25913. doi: http://dx.doi.org/10.3402/ejpt.v6.25913

McLaughlin KA, Peverill M, Gold AL, Alves S, Sheridan MA (2015) Child maltreatment and neural systems underlying emotion regulation. J Am Acad Child Adolesc Psychiatry 54(9):753–762. doi:10.1016/j.jaac.2015.06.010

Messman TL, Long PJ (1996) Child sexual abuse and its relationship to revictimization in adult women: a review. Clin Psychol Rev 16(5):397–420

Miron LR, Orcutt HK, Kumpula MJ (2014) Differential predictors of transient stress versus posttraumatic stress disorder: evaluating risk following targeted mass violence. Behav Ther 45(6):791–805. doi:10.1016/j.beth.2014.07.005

Moehler E, Biringen Z, Poustka L (2007) Emotional availability in a sample of mothers with a history of abuse. Am J Orthopsychiatry 77(4):624–628. doi:10.1037/0002-9432.77.4.624

Morey RA, Haswell CC, Hooper SR, De Bellis MD (2016) Amygdala, hippocampus, and ventral medial prefronta cortex volumes differ in maltreated youth with and without chronic posttraumatic stress disorder. Neuropsychopharmacology 41(3):791–801. doi:10.1038/npp.2015.205

Morris AS, Silk JS, Steinberg L, Myers SS, Robinson LR (2007) The role of the family context in the development of emotion regulation. Soc Dev 16(2):361–388. doi:10.1111/j.1467-9507.2007.00389.x

Morris AS, Gabert-Quillen C, Delahanty D (2012) The association between parent PTSD/Depression symptoms and child PTSD symptoms: a meta-analysis. J Pediatr Psychol 37:1076–1088

Moutsiana C, Fearon P, Murray L, Cooper P, Goodyer I, Johnstone T, Halligan S (2014) Making an effort to feel positive: insecure attachment in infancy predicts the neural underpinnings of emotion regulation in adulthood. J Child Psychol Psychiatry 55(9):999–1008. doi:10.1111/jcpp.12198

Nelson JA, O'Brien M, Blankson AN, Calkins SD, Keane SP (2009) Family stress and parental responses to children's negative emotions: tests of the spillover, crossover, and compensatory hypotheses. [Research Support, N.I.H., Extramural]. J Fam Psychol 23(5):671–679. doi:10.1037/a0015977

Norrholm SD, Glover EM, Stevens JS, Fani N, Galatzer-Levy IR, Bradley B et al (2015) Fear load: The psychophysiological over-expression of fear as an intermediate phenotype associated with trauma reactions. Int J Psychophysiol 98(2 Pt 2):270–275. doi:10.1016/j.ijpsycho.2014.11.005

Nusslock R, Miller GE (2016) Early-Life adversity and physical and emotional health across the lifespan: A neuroimmune network hypothesis. Bio Psychiat 80:3–32. doi: 10.1016/j.biopsych.2015.05.017

Opmeer EM, Kortekaas R, van Tol MJ, van der Wee NJ, Woudstra S, van Buchem MA et al (2014) Interaction of neuropeptide Y genotype and childhood emotional maltreatment on brain activity during emotional processing. Soc Cogn Affect Neurosci 9(5):601–609. doi:10.1093/scan/nst025

Pears KC, Fisher PA (2005) Emotion understanding and theory of mind among maltreated children in foster care: evidence of deficits. Dev Psychopathol 17(1):47–65

Pereira J, Vickers K, Atkinson L, Gonzalez A, Wekerle C, Levitan R (2012) Parenting stress mediates between maternal maltreatment history and maternal sensitivity in a community sample. Child Abuse Negl 36:433–437. doi:10.1016/j.chiabu.2012.01.006

Perry NB, Swingler MM, Calkins SD, Bell MA (2016) Neurophysiological correlates of attention behavior in early infancy: implications for emotion regulation during early childhood. J Exp Child Psychol 142:245–261. doi:10.1016/j.jecp.2015.08.007

Pine DS (2007) Research Review: A neuroscience framework for pediatric anxiety disorders. J Child Psychol Psychiat 48(7):631–648

Pivovarova E, Tanaka G, Tang M, Bursztajn HJ, First MB (2016) Is helplessness still helpful in diagnosing posttraumatic stress disorder? J Nerv Ment Dis 204(1):3–8. doi:10.1097/NMD.0000000000000416

Repetti RL, Taylor SE, Seemant TE (2002) Risky families: family social environment and the mental and physical health of offspring. Psychol Bull 128:330–366

Rijlaarsdam J, Stevens GW, Jansen PW, Ringoot AP, Jaddoe VWV, Hofman A et al (2014) Maternal childhood maltreatment and offspring emotional and behavioral problems: maternal and paternal mechanisms of risk transmission. Child Maltreat 19(2):67–78

Ruscio AM (2001) Predicting the child-rearing practices of mothers sexually abused in childhood. Child Abuse Negl 25:369–387

Schnurr PP, Lunney CA, Sengupta A (2004) Risk factors for the development versus maintenance of posttraumatic stress disorder. J Trauma Stress 17(2):85–95. doi:10.1023/B:JOTS.0000022614.21794.f4

Shapiro D, Levendosky A (1999) Adolescent survivors of childhood sexual abuse: the mediating role of attachment style and coping in psychological and interpersonal functioning. Child Abuse Negl 23(11):1175–1191

Shipman KL, Schneider R, Fitzgerald MM, Sims C, Swisher L, Edwards A (2007) Maternal emotion socialization in maltreating and non-maltreating families: implications for children's emotion regulation. Soc Dev 16(2):268–285. doi:10.1111/j.1467-9507.2007.00384.x

Smith CP, Freyd JJ (2014) The courage to study what we wish did not exist. J Trsauma Dissociation 15(5):521–526. doi:10.1080/15299732.2014.947910

Southwick SM, Paige S, Morgan CA 3rd, Bremner JD, Krystal JH, Charney DS (1999) Neurotransmitter alterations in PTSD: catecholamines and serotonin. [Review]. Semin Clin Neuropsychiatry 4(4):242–248. doi:10.153/SCNP00400242

Steele H, Bate J, Steele M, Dube SR, Danskin K, Knafo H et al (2016) Adverse childhood experiences, poverty, and parenting stress. Can J Behav Sci 48(1):32–38. doi:10.1037/cbs0000034

Sumner JA, Pietrzak RH, Aiello AE, Uddin M, Wildman DE, Galea S, Koenen KC (2014) Further support for an association between the memory-related gene WWC1 and posttraumatic stress disorder: results from the Detroit Neighborhood Health Study. Biol Psychiatry 76(11):e25–e26. doi:10.1016/j.biopsych.2014.03.033

Suzuki A, Poon L, Papadopoulos AS, Kumari V, Cleare AJ (2014) Long term effects of childhood trauma on cortisol stress reactivity in adulthood and relationship to the occurrence of depression. Psychoneuroendocrinology 50:289–299. doi:10.1016/j.psyneuen.2014.09.007

Teicher MH, Samson JA (2016) Annual research review: enduring neurobiological effects of childhood abuse and neglect. J Child Psychol Psychiatry 57(3):241–266. doi:10.1111/jcpp.12507

Thornberry TP, Knight KE, Lovegrove PJ (2012) Does maltreatment beget maltreatment? A systematic review of the intergenerational literature. Trauma Violence Abuse 13(3):135–152

Thornberry TP, Henry KL, Smith CA, Ireland TO, Greenman SJ, Lee RD (2013) Breaking the cycle of maltreatment: the role of safe, stable, and nurturing relationships. J Adolesc Health 53(4 Suppl):S25–S31

Trickey D, Siddaway AP, Meiser-Stedman R, Serpell L, Field AP (2012) A meta-analysis of risk factors for post-traumatic stress disorder in children and adolescents. Clin Psychol Rev 32:122–138

Tryon WW (1998) A neural network explanation of posttraumatic stress disorder. J Anxiety Disord 12(4):373–385

Turner HA, Shattuck A, Finkelhor D, Hamby S (2016) Polyvictimization and youth violence exposure across contexts. J Adolesc Health 58(2):208–214. doi:10.1016/j.jadohealth.2015.09.021

Valdez CE, Bailey BE, Santuzzi AM, Lilly MM (2014) Trajectories of depressive symptoms in foster youth transitioning into adulthood: the roles of emotion dysregulation and PTSD. Child Maltreat 19(3–4):209–218. doi:10.1177/1077559514551945

Valiente C, Lemery-Chalfant K, Reiser M (2007) Pathways to problem behaviors: chaotic homes, parent and child effortful control, and parenting. Soc Dev 16(2):249–267. doi:10.1111/j.1467-9507.2007.00383.x

Van Dam NT, Rando K, Potenza MN, Tuit K, Sinha R (2014) Childhood maltreatment, altered limbic neurobiology, and substance use relapse severity via trauma-specific reductions in limbic gray matter volume. JAMA Psychiat 71(8):917–925. doi:10.1001/jamapsychiatry.2014.680

Verlinden E, Schippers M, Van Meijel EP, Beer R, Opmeer BC, Olff M et al (2013) What makes a life event traumatic for a child? The predictive values of DSM-Criteria A1 and A2. Eur J Psychotraumatol 4. doi:10.3402/ejpt.v4i0.20436

Waldrep E, Benight CC (2008). Social cognitive theory. In Reyes G, Elhai JD, Ford JD (Eds.), Encyclopedia of psychological trauma. John Wiley & Sons, Hoboken, New Jersey:604-606

Walter K, Hall B, Hobfoll S (2008) Conservation of resources theory. In G Reyes JD.Elhai JD Ford (Eds.), Encyclopedia of psychological trauma. John Wiley & Sons, Hoboken, New Jersey:157–159

White S, Acierno R, Ruggiero KJ, Koenen KC, Kilpatrick DG, Galea S et al (2013) Association of CRHR1 variants and posttraumatic stress symptoms in hurricane exposed adults. J Anxiety Disord 27(7):678–683. doi:10.1016/j.janxdis.2013.08.003

Widom CS, Czaja SJ, Dutton MA (2014) Child abuse and neglect and intimate partner violence victimization and perpetration: a prospective investigation. Child Abuse Negl 38:650–663. doi:10.1016/j.chiabu.2013.11.004

Wolf EJ, Mitchell KS, Logue MW, Baldwin CT, Reardon AF, Aiello A et al (2014) The dopamine D3 receptor gene and posttraumatic stress disorder. J Trauma Stress 27(4):379–387. doi:10.1002/jts.21937

Zalewski M, Cyranowski JM, Cheng Y, Swartz HA (2013) Role of maternal childhood trauma on parenting among depressed mothers of psychiatrically ill children. Depress Anxiety 30(9):792–799

Part II

Interventions

Preventative Early Intervention for Children and Adolescents Exposed to Trauma

Alexandra C. De Young and Justin A. Kenardy

6.1 Introduction

Prevention of psychological disorders, especially those that first emerge during childhood, has the potential to minimise human suffering and societal costs across the lifespan. There are three categories of prevention interventions: primary (i.e. aims to prevent the occurrence of a disease/injury), secondary (i.e. aims to reduce the impact of a disease/injury early on) and tertiary (i.e. aims to minimise the impact of an ongoing disease/injury). Preventative early interventions (which will be a term used throughout this chapter) are a type of secondary intervention that aims to prevent or reduce risk for the development of the disorder becoming chronic and to return individuals to their original level of functioning as soon as possible.

Posttraumatic stress disorder (PTSD), unlike many other disorders, usually has a clear aetiology as well as a therapeutic window of opportunity (approximately 3 months) to intervene before symptoms become chronic. Therefore PTSD is a particularly good target for preventive early intervention programs. In addition, during childhood, exposure to potentially traumatic events (PTEs) is particularly common, with approximately half to two-third of children experiencing at least one trauma (such as abuse, witnessing domestic violence, serious illness or injury, natural disaster or terrorism) by the time they turn 16 (Copeland et al. 2007; Landolt et al. 2013). Although the majority of children are resilient or will recover relatively quickly from initial high levels of distress, a clinically

---

A.C. De Young (✉)
Centre for Children's Burns and Trauma Research, Centre for Child Health Research, University of Queensland, Brisbane, QLD, Australia
e-mail: adeyoung@uq.edu.au

J.A. Kenardy
School of Psychology and Recover Injury Research Centre, University of Queensland, Brisbane, QLD, Australia
e-mail: j.kenardy@uq.edu.au

meaningful number, approximately 15.9 %, will go on to develop PTSD (Alisic et al. 2014). Even when a child does not meet full diagnostic criteria, symptoms can still be very distressing and lead to functional impairment on a day-to-day basis (Carrion et al. 2002). Research has shown that if left untreated, PTSD symptoms (PTSS) can follow a chronic and debilitating course that can significantly derail a child from their normal developmental trajectory and have a measurable impact on physical health outcomes (Le Brocque et al. 2010; Nugent et al. 2015). Comorbidity with PTSD is the rule rather than the exception (e.g. separation anxiety, oppositional defiant behaviour and phobias in younger children and depression, substance abuse and anxiety in older children), and PTSS are often present before new-onset disorders emerge after a trauma (Davis and Siegel 2000; De Young et al. 2012). These other disorders may mistakenly become the focus of treatment.

Despite a strong evidence base for the efficacy of trauma-focused cognitive behavioural therapy (TF-CBT) in treating childhood PTSD, for a myriad of reasons, very few children and adolescents who develop PTSD receive access to appropriate psychosocial services. Even when offered or directly referred to intervention programmes, uptake and engagement are typically poor with high rates of early treatment termination (Australian Centre for Posttraumatic Mental Health 2013). Taken together, it is clear that early identification and interventions for preventing the development of persistent PTSS after childhood trauma are of considerable public health significance. This chapter will (1) discuss the key theoretical and conceptual models for PTSD that help guide what should be considered for the identification of at risk children and inform timing and content of preventative early intervention programmes, (2) provide an overview of existing preventative early interventions, (3) discuss special considerations and challenges of providing early intervention in this population and (4) review the empirical evidence base for preventative early interventions following single-event traumas.

Definitions for prevention and early intervention vary in the trauma literature. For the purposes of this chapter, the authors define 'preventative early intervention' as an intervention that is conducted within the first 4 weeks of exposure to a PTE and aims to (1) prevent a PTE becoming a traumatic event/s or preventing exposure to other secondary PTEs (e.g. during medical care after injury) and (2) prevent the development and escalation of acute and persistent PTSS and other negative psychological reactions. Typology of preventative interventions includes universal, selective or indicated approaches. In the paediatric trauma literature, *universal interventions* would be those aimed at all children following exposure to a PTE. *Selective interventions* are designed for children experiencing elevated PTSS but not presenting with any other risk factors (e.g. pre-existing psychopathology, trauma history, poor social support, parent distress), and *indicated interventions* are targeted towards children presenting with marked distress and have additional risk factors for poor long-term outcomes.

Due to the complexities associated with identifying and treating children who have experienced interpersonal or chronic trauma (i.e. sexual and physical abuse, domestic violence, war) and that often problems are not identified until they become chronic, this chapter will only be discussing early interventions provided after single-event traumas, such as serious illness and injury, natural disasters and single assaults or terrorist attacks.

6.2 Theoretical Underpinnings and Conceptual Models for Early Intervention

This section will review the key evidence-based conceptual models that can be used to aid the early identification of children and family members who are at risk of poor outcomes. These models also assist in determining timing and targets for preventative early interventions within the acute period following medical trauma, disasters and terrorism.

6.2.1 Pediatric Psychosocial Preventative Health Model (PPPHM)

The PPPMH model (Kazak 2006) is guided by social ecological perspectives and incorporates a biopsychosocial framework designed to guide decisions on the type and level of preventative care needed for children and families in healthcare settings. Kazak (2006) proposes an important shift from a deficit-based approach towards a competence-based framework. The model is based on the assumption that the majority of children and families who experience an injury or serious illness are competent and will most likely cope and adjust well to the acute medical event and treatment that follows. Further, it is considered normal, and even adaptive at times, to experience some stress symptoms during the acute period (Kazak 2006). However, a smaller number of children and/or family members are vulnerable and may have risk factors present that predispose them to or exacerbate clinically significant levels of distress. The PPPMH model therefore incorporated and adapted the public health prevention framework of universal, selective and indicated to take into account the natural variability in human responses and to help match assessment and intervention to level of need.

In this model (see Fig. 6.1), *universal* represents the majority of families who present to healthcare settings and appear to be resilient or experiencing distress but coping well. It is recommended that families are provided with general support and information to support their competence and all children and parents are screened for the presence of risk factors or signs of acute distress. *Targeted* (or selective) interventions are aimed at families where signs of acute distress and/or risk factors are evident. It is suggested that early interventions should be aimed at reducing specific symptoms and monitoring distress over time (e.g. through rescreening at key transition times). The minority of families at the top of this model, *clinical/treatment*, are those experiencing clinically significant, persistent and/or escalating levels of distress and are in need of specialist psychological intervention and support.

Pediatric Psychosocial Preventive Health Model

ADDRESSING TRAUMATIC STRESS IN THE PEDIATRIC HEALTHCARE SETTING

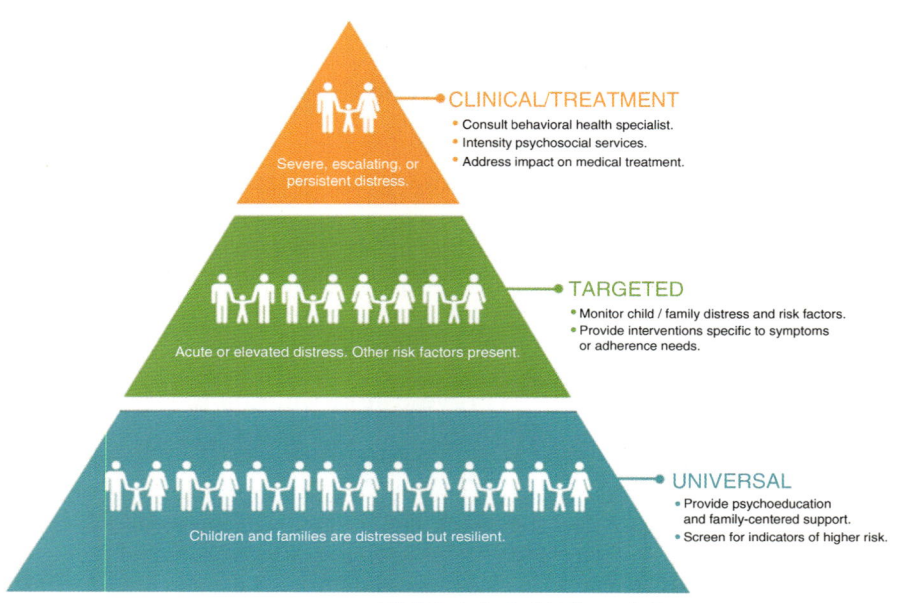

[Pyramid diagram with three tiers:

- **CLINICAL/TREATMENT** (top, orange): Severe, escalating, or persistent distress.
  - Consult behavioral health specialist.
  - Intensity psychosocial services.
  - Address impact on medical treatment.

- **TARGETED** (middle, green): Acute or elevated distress. Other risk factors present.
  - Monitor child / family distress and risk factors.
  - Provide interventions specific to symptoms or adherence needs.

- **UNIVERSAL** (bottom, teal): Children and families are distressed but resilient.
  - Provide psychoeducation and family-centered support.
  - Screen for indicators of higher risk.

©2011 Center for Pediatric Traumatic Stress]

Fig. 6.1 Pediatric Psychosocial Preventative Health Model (Reproduced with permission from the Center for Pediatric Traumatic Stress (CPTS) at Nemours Children's Health System © 2011. All rights reserved. The PPPHM may not be reproduced in any form for any purpose without the express written permission of CPTS. To obtain permission to use reproduce the PPPHM, contact Anne Kazak, PhD ABPP at anne.kazak@nemours.org)

6.2.2 Integrative Model of Paediatric Medical Traumatic Stress (PMTS)

The PMTS model is another useful framework to understand both the normative and problematic child and family responses throughout the injury or illness and treatment journey (Kazak et al. 2006). PMTS is defined as "a set of psychological and physiological responses of children and their families to pain, injury, medical procedures, and invasive or frightening treatment experiences" (Health Care Toolbox: Basics of trauma-informed care 2013). The PMTS model provides an excellent guide for assessment and treatment tailored to three key stages of recovery following medical trauma. This model has recently been re-evaluated and updated based on the significant growth in research in the area over the past 10 years and is now referred to as the *Integrative Trajectory Model of Pediatric Medical Traumatic Stress* (Price et al. 2015). This model describes child and family adjustment across the following three phases: Phase I (peri-trauma), Phase II (acute medical care (was early, ongoing, evolving)) and Phase III (ongoing care or discharge from care (was longer term)).

During Phase I, the goal is to modify the subjective experience of PTEs by providing trauma-informed care and to screen for risk. During Phase II, the goal is to screen for risk and to prevent or reduce traumatic stress. Finally, the goal of intervention during Phase III is to screen and treat significant traumatic stress. The revised model reinforces the important role that subjective appraisals (e.g. perceived life threat) play in predicting PMTS. Importantly, the revised model now incorporates four recovery trajectories, resilient, recovery, chronic and escalating PMTS, to account for the different psychological response patterns that can occur over time. It also places more emphasis on the need to consider child outcomes within the context of how their family members are also responding and coping.

6.2.3 Biopsychosocial Model of PTSD

Recently, Marsac et al. (2014) proposed a new biopsychosocial model focusing on processes that occur during the peri-trauma period after acute medical events that are hypothesised to contribute specifically to the development and maintenance of persistent PTSS. This model aims to inform the early identification of at-risk children, preventative interventions and clinical care. The authors have integrated biological, psychological and social/environmental theories and other risk factors identified by the empirical evidence base into this model. Pre-trauma represents the first phase of this model, and the key biological (i.e. child genetic predisposition, sex, age), psychological (i.e. child pre-event emotional functioning) and social/environmental (i.e. child trauma history, family functioning, community support and culture) factors are presented to indicate which children may be at greater risk of PTSD and may need additional monitoring or support. The peri-trauma phase is the focus of this model, and the possible intra- and interrelationships amongst the variables to consider for risk assessment and targets of intervention include biological (i.e. initial memory formation, hormone response, cardiovascular reactions), psychological (i.e. early child PTSS, cognitive appraisals, coping) and social/environmental (i.e. trauma severity, medical team support, community support, parent PTSS, parent appraisals, parent coping assistance) processes. Finally, the variables proposed to contribute to PTSS during the post-trauma period include physical injury recovery (i.e. biological), non-PTSS emotional reactions (i.e. psychological) and parent coping assistance and community support (i.e. social). This model is still in its infancy and requires validation, but it is based on a solid empirical and clinical evidence base and provides good directions for future research.

6.2.4 Conceptual Models for Natural Disasters

La Greca, Vernberg and colleagues (La Greca et al. 1996; Vernberg et al. 1996) have developed an integrative conceptual model for predicting children's reactions to natural disasters. This model was based on existing theories, research and the author's clinical experiences and has received some empirical support. It includes the following four factors that may either increase or decrease a child's likelihood of developing PTSD: (1) exposure to traumatic event (i.e. perceived and actual life threat, losses and disruptions), (2) individual child characteristics (i.e. gender, age and ethnicity), (3) characteristics of the post-disaster recovery environment (i.e. presence of major life events and access to social support) and (4) coping skills (i.e. positive coping, blame and anger, wishful thinking and social withdrawal). This model indicates that potential targets for the acute post-disaster phase include increasing access to good social support and encouraging the use of positive coping strategies.

Vernberg (2002) has also conceptualised the delivery of post-disaster interventions using a chronological system in relation to the onset and cessation of disaster exposure. Interventions during each of these phases also typically fall within universal, selected and indicated categories with the aim of reducing or preventing long-term psychological difficulties. Universal interventions in the *preimpact, impact and recoil* phase may include ongoing communication regarding safety and coping and factual information regarding disaster events; selected interventions utilise psychological first aid and indicated interventions target individuals with acute distress and impairment. During the *immediate postimpact phase*, universal interventions need to be more present focused and crisis orientated and should aim to restore roles and routines, disseminate accurate disaster-related information and provide psychoeducation on psychological needs; selected interventions should involve assessment and brief interventions for acute stress reactions and psychological first aid, and indicated interventions should target children at high risk of PTSD using intensive treatment approaches. Universal interventions during the *recovery* and *reconstruction* phase include psychoeducation on mental health needs and resources available and manualised school-based curricular; selected interventions consist of identifying and treating children with persistent PTSS, and indicated interventions provide comprehensive integrated interventions for those at highest risk.

6.3 Preventative Early Intervention Approaches for PTSD in Children

There are now a growing number of empirically validated preventative early intervention materials and programs available to (1) minimise the impact of secondary PTEs after an initial traumatic event and (2) promote recovery and resilience and prevent the development of persistent traumatic stress following single-event trauma exposure during childhood. The majority of these interventions are in the area of medical traumatic stress developed for primary school-aged children and adolescents. In line with the models outlined above, this section will summarise the universal and selective/targeted evidence-based preventative interventions that can be delivered during the peri-trauma and acute phases following medical trauma and the immediate postimpact and short-term recovery and reconstruction phases following disasters. Of note, current guidelines state that psychological debriefing and pharmacotherapy should not be offered as a preventive intervention for children after trauma (Australian Centre for Posttraumatic Mental Health 2013; NICE 2005) and will therefore not be referred to throughout the rest of this chapter.

6.4 Universal Approaches

Trauma-Informed Care
After exposure to a traumatic event such as injury or a natural disaster, there are many PTEs that can follow (e.g. painful medical procedures, separation from caregivers, displacement). Therefore, the first goal for preventative universal interventions during the peri-trauma phase should be to minimise or prevent the potential for further PTEs and to increase feelings of safety and control (Kazak et al. 2007). This can be done by modifying children's and parents' subjective experiences of PTEs by providing trauma-informed care (Marsac et al. 2015). Trauma-informed care in a medical setting involves healthcare professionals understanding how trauma affects patients, family members and staff; minimising potential for medical care to be traumatic or trigger trauma reactions; assessing and addressing pre-existing stressors, risk factors, distress and family issues; and providing guidance and emotional support to promote a positive recovery for all involved (Marsac et al. 2015).

The Medical Trauma Working Group of the US National Child Traumatic Stress Network created the *"D-E-F" protocol* to give evidence-based guidelines for providing trauma-informed paediatric care during the acute phase of medical treatment (Stuber et al. 2006). The D-E-F model aims to reduce distress, provide emotional support and remember family. After the ABCs of physical care are met (i.e. airway, breathing and circulation), the following steps are recommended and can be provided by all paediatric healthcare professionals:

- D (distress): enquire about fears and worries, ensure that adequate procedural preparation and effective pain management is provided and ask about grief and loss
- E (emotional support): assess emotional support needs and identification of barriers
- F (family): address family distress and issues that may impede recovery

The toolkit contains a variety of resources that can be used in paediatric healthcare settings and further information on the D-E-F protocol can be accessed at: http://www.healthcaretoolbox.org/.

Psychological First Aid (PFA)
PFA is an evidence-informed modular approach that was developed for mental health and disaster response workers supporting children and adults who have recently experienced a natural disaster or terrorist attack. The Psychological First Aid Field Operations Guide (Brymer et al. 2006) was a joint collaboration between the US National Child Traumatic Stress Network (NCTSN) and US National Center for Posttraumatic Stress Disorder (NCPTSD) and aims to reduce initial distress and promote positive short- and long-term adaptive functioning across all age groups. The

five basic principles that are thought to promote positive adaption and therefore guided the selection of PFA strategies and techniques include (1) promoting a sense of safety, (2) utilising techniques to promote calming, (3) facilitating a sense of self- and community efficacy, (d) encouraging connectedness and (e) instilling hope (Brymer et al. 2006). PFA consists of eight modules, termed *core actions,* outlining specific goals, recommendations and interventions and are as follows (Brymer et al. 2006):

1. Contact and engagement – respond and initiate contacts in nonintrusive and compassionate ways
2. Safety and comfort – enhance individuals immediate and ongoing safety and offer both physical and emotional support
3. Stabilisation – help calm and orient individuals experiencing overwhelming emotions
4. Information gathering – identify immediate needs and concerns by gathering information about problems that require immediate attention, monitoring high-risk individuals and identifying potential target risk and resilience factors
5. Practical assistance – identify practical immediate needs and assist in prioritisation of action plans
6. Connection with social support – reduce stress by assisting access and connection with primary support persons
7. Information on coping support – provide psychoeducation regarding stress reactions and coping strategies to minimise distress and encourage adaptive functioning
8. Linkage with collaborative services – link or inform individuals about available services they may need in the future

The PFA Field Guide has also been adapted for use in schools. Both the PFA and PFA for Schools Field Operations Guides as well as online training in PFA can be accessed at: http://www.nctsn.org/content/psychological-first-aid.

Skills for Psychological Recovery (SPR)
The NCTSN and NCPTSD have also developed a second field operations guide, Skills for Psychological Recovery (SPR; Berkowitz et al. 2010), for use in the recovery phase following disasters. Similar to PFA, SPR is also an evidence-informed modular intervention that can be delivered by mental health professionals and disaster recovery workers in a variety of settings (e.g. schools, clinics, hospitals, community centres and homes) for all developmental levels across the lifespan. SPR is based on a secondary prevention model that utilises a skill-building rather than a supportive counselling approach. The specific aims of SPR are to promote skills to manage distress and help cope with post-disaster stress and adversity. The six components of SPR include:

1. Gathering information and prioritising assistance (e.g. identify primary concern and identify an action plan),
2. Building problem-solving skills,

3. Promoting positive activities (e.g. increase meaningful and positive activities),
4. Managing reactions (e.g. breathing, writing exercises, preparing for triggers),
5. Promoting healthy thinking (e.g. replacing unhelpful thoughts with helpful ones) and
6. Rebuilding health social connections (e.g. access social supports).

Each skill can be taught in one helping contact; however, ideally disaster survivors will participate in multiple contacts. The complete SPR Field Operations Guide and online training program can be accessed at http://www.nctsn.org/content/skills-psychological-recovery-spr.

School-Focused Training for Recovery

Teachers are in a unique and well-placed position to provide vital support to children following traumatic events. There are now many information-based post-trauma mental health resources that have been developed to facilitate recovery in school settings (Le Brocque et al. 2016). However, one such resource is both a set of materials that provide information to assist psychological recovery as well as a comprehensive training directed at teachers and those who will have responsibility for the care of children through schools (Le Brocque et al. 2016). The School-Focused Training for Recovery programme is evidence informed with components of the training that include (1) understanding of post-trauma responses in children, (2) the role of teachers and schools in promoting recovery following potentially traumatic events, (3) skills and tools to recognise children who may need further care and pathways for that care and (4) self-care (Le Brocque et al. 2016). The suite of resources as well as the training manuals and materials is available at www.som.uq.edu.au/childtrauma/post-disaster-resources/for-teachers.

Screening and Watchful Waiting

Most children experience a reduction in symptoms over time; thus current guidelines recommend a period of "watchful waiting" or monitoring before providing more intensive psychological intervention following trauma (Australian Centre for Posttraumatic Mental Health 2013; NICE 2005). Screening is recommended as a simple and cost-effective method for identifying children and parents who should continue to be monitored for risk or referred for more comprehensive targeted assessment or treatment (Australian Centre for Posttraumatic Mental Health 2013; NICE 2005). Screening is usually the first phase included in stepped-care intervention models. Refer to March, De Young, Dow and Kenardy (March et al. 2012) for a review of screening and assessment tools for PTSD.

Information Provision

Universal preventive interventions typically involve the provision of psychoeducation to children and their caregivers to assist in the prevention and/or reduction of traumatic stress symptoms and to promote a positive recovery following trauma. Information provision is often the first level in stepped-care models and is appropriate for all children and families after trauma. There are a now a number of information-based interventions that have been developed for different populations and presented in different formats (e.g. verbal discussion, print materials, self-directed websites, interactive online game) (Cox et al. 2010; Kenardy et al. 2008; Marsac et al. 2011). Guidelines suggest that the type of information provided should be of high quality and tailored to the type of trauma and individuals involved (Australian Centre for Posttraumatic Mental Health 2013). The type of information provided may include:

- Psychoeducation and normalisation of likely responses
- Reinforcement of existing and new coping strategies
- Encouraging enhancement of social supports
- Signs that indicate when further assistance may be needed
- Advice on how to seek further assistance

The advantages of information provision interventions are that they are generally inexpensive and require few resources and demands, can also include information for and about caregivers, siblings, health professionals and teachers and are unlikely to cause harm. However, research suggests that to optimise effectiveness and to reduce costs and burden of delivery, information provision interventions are best targeted towards children presenting with initial high levels of distress (Kassam-Adams et al. 2011; Kenardy et al. 2015). A number of good evidence-based information provision interventions for a variety of trauma types can be obtained from the following websites: CONROD http://www.conrod.org.au/cms/resources-and-tools/child-trauma-research-unit; After the Injury, https://www.aftertheinjury.org/; The National Child Traumatic Stress Network, http://www.nctsn.org/trauma-types; Phoenix Australia, http://phoenixaustralia.org/ and KidTrauma, www.kidtrauma.com.

6.4.1 Selected/Targeted Interventions

Selected/targeted preventative interventions are aimed at children who are identified as at risk (e.g. by screening tools) of developing persistent trauma reactions. This would typically be done in the second stage of a stepped-care approach (Kazak et al. 2006). Current guidelines suggest that TF-CBT-based early interventions may be useful in the acute period after a trauma (Australian Centre for Posttraumatic Mental Health 2013). A recent meta-analysis has recommended that targeted early interventions should include multiple sessions and the following components (Kramer and Landolt 2011):

- Psychoeducation
- Promotion of positive coping strategies
- Parental involvement
- Safe exposure to trauma-related reminders

Including parents as part of the early intervention is likely to be a key component in getting successful outcomes. The Child and Family Traumatic Stress Intervention (CFTSI; Berkowitz et al. 2011) is a four-session caregiver-youth preventative early intervention that has shown efficacy in preventing chronic PTSD. This intervention targets children who are screened as at risk and delivered within 30 days of the trauma. The intervention aims to (1) improve caregivers' support of their child by encouraging communication between the child and their caregivers about feelings, symptoms and behaviours and (2) provide targeted behavioural strategies to both child and caregiver to assist in adaptive coping to manage symptoms. For further information on CFTSI, see Chap. 7.

6.5 Special Considerations and Challenges

There are a number of important considerations and challenges that health professionals need to be mindful of when providing early intervention to children after exposure to a traumatic event. Each of these will be discussed below.

6.5.1 Developmental Stage

Although preschoolers, children and adolescents may present with a similar pattern of trauma symptoms; the way they process and respond to a traumatic event depends on their age and developmental maturity. Early childhood and adolescence are arguably the most important and vulnerable periods of development across the entire lifespan. It is therefore important to understand how a child's age and stage of development may affect their responses following a trauma and influence the way early intervention needs to be delivered. This section outlines the important considerations for each developmental phase and draws on Erickson's models of psychosocial development (Erikson 1950).

Infants and Toddlers (0–2 Years)
Infants are especially dependent on their caregivers to nurture them and meet their needs for physical contact, comfort, food, sleep and attention. Developing a secure attachment with a primary caregiver is a crucial task for this stage of development. However, after a trauma, it can be very challenging for a parent to meet their child's needs and maintain strong relationships. This can greatly affect a child's sense of trust in their parent's ability to protect them. Additionally, infants also have minimal skills to communicate or cope with pain or strong emotions, making them highly dependent on their parents to help them feel safe and secure and to regulate their emotions. This period is also when separation anxiety and fears of 'strangers' or unfamiliar people develop. Infants and toddlers may therefore be more aware of and frightened by separations from their caregivers and react fearfully around health professionals. In the early stages after a trauma, it is therefore best to minimise separations from parents wherever possible. Toddlerhood also represents a time

where children are struggling to gain a sense of autonomy and are learning new skills. Following trauma, toddlers may regress or show a delay in acquiring new developmental skills. Due to their limited verbal abilities, assessment and intervention strategies need to be done with parents.

Preschoolers (3–5 Years)
Preschoolers become more aware of how others think and feel and are therefore likely to notice and be sensitive to how their family members are responding to the event. Preschoolers are also more likely to develop false assumptions or magical thinking about the cause of the traumatic event (e.g. "The flood came because I was bad"; "The medical procedures are punishment for being bad"). They are also more likely to overgeneralise or catastrophise from the facts they have available (e.g. "All children die when they come to hospital"; "Nowhere is safe"). Further, young children are unlikely to understand the reason behind certain events (e.g. the need for painful medical procedures). Children of this age may also have more difficulties understanding that loss is permanent. Due to their limited communication skills, they may not be able to explain what is upsetting them or understand why their parents are distressed. Therefore, younger children's responses to traumatic events tend to be more behavioural. Direct observation of child behaviour and parent report are the best ways to assess the impact of trauma on young children. Preschoolers are still very reliant on adults to help them cope with scary or stressful experiences, and interventions need to be conducted mostly with parents. However, some strategies, such as using play or stories to process the event or relaxation strategies, can be completed with older preschool children.

Primary School-Aged Children (6–11 Years)
After a trauma, children often feel out of control and overwhelmed and are more likely to worry about the event and develop fears related to what happened. School-aged children have more coping skills available but will still observe adults to determine how serious the situation is and will often model their responses. They may discount verbal explanations if what they observe and notice does not match up with what adults are telling them. They will also use their imagination to "fill in the blanks" when they do not have realistic information. Intervention strategies can be targeted towards children (e.g. written materials, storybooks, coping skills); however, it is important to also include their parents in the assessment and treatment process.

Adolescence (12–18 Years)
Adolescents may feel self-conscious about their emotional responses at the time of the event or in the period after. PTSD reactions in this age group may be confused with the normal developmental demands of individuation and identify formulation. Social support and peer group are critical in this period; however, both may be

affected following a trauma. Thus adolescents are more likely to compare themselves to their peers and can feel particularly worried about being 'abnormal' or different or not having support from their friends. Further, trauma can shake their sense of safety and challenges their needs for independence, privacy, control and belonging. It continues to be important to involve parents in the assessment and intervention process; however, the focus of the intervention can be with the teenager. Interventions administered via web-based modalities may be particularly useful for this age group.

6.5.2 Role of Parents in Child Recovery

Parents play an important role in how well children respond to a traumatic event and need to be involved in the assessment and intervention processes. Studies have shown that caregivers also experience a range of psychological sequelae including PTSD, depression and anxiety following a child's trauma exposure (De Young et al. 2014). These adverse psychological responses can have a detrimental impact on the child's recovery process and can lead to deteriorations in the parent-child relationship and family relationships and functioning and, in turn, significantly influence the development and maintenance of trauma symptomatology in children (De Young et al. 2014). The impact of adverse parental psychological responses on the development of children's trauma symptoms, combined with parental distress in its own right, represents important reasons to identify and treat parental distress.

It is therefore important to also screen for parent distress and to include them in the provision of universal or targeted interventions as mentioned above. If parents are very distressed, it may be best to focus treatment with them first or to refer to own support pathways. Additionally, children depend on their parents to seek out and access treatment; therefore it is essential to engage with and maintain parent's involvement in the treatment process (Australian Centre for Posttraumatic Mental Health 2013). Parents need to be able to see the importance and be motivated to keep the child in therapy and to encourage them to use the recommended strategies. Parents of young children are usually the targets of the intervention, so their engagement with the process is particularly important.

6.5.3 Type of Event and Perceptions of Threat

Children's reactions to trauma may also differ depending on the nature of the traumatic event. For example, children who experienced flooding or destruction through gradual inundation (where they were able to safely remove themselves from the situation) may be more susceptible to reactions which focus around the loss of property and destruction of their homes. These children may be more likely to experience depressed mood, grief or simply withdraw following the disaster. Other children who were victims of sudden inundation or destruction (where the child or family's safety was at risk) may be more susceptible to reactions such as posttraumatic stress, anxiety and enhanced threat perceptions regarding their safety.

6.5.4 Feasibility, Timing and Ethical Issues

One of the most debated issues in the treatment of PTSD is the optimal time frame to provide early intervention. The issue is that we know the majority of individuals are resilient following trauma or recover within the first few months without needing professional help (Le Brocque et al. 2010). However, it is often not feasible to conduct interventions in the immediate time frame after a trauma because resources are not available and/or child and family members may be too distressed and not able to focus on their psychological recovery. Furthermore, many families and post-trauma care systems do not understand the appropriate means to screen for distress and do not have resources available to provide linked intervention at the right level for the child and their family. Screening instruments can be thought of as either risk screeners or concurrent screeners. Risk screeners are designed to detect those at risk for the development of ongoing problems, whereas concurrent screeners identify those with probable diagnosis. In the early intervention, this distinction is important, and more research is needed to both develop and validate effective screening tools, especially risk screeners.

The optimum timing for screening and intervention is not clear; however, it would appear that concurrent screens are more reliable when they are completed at, or greater than, 1 month after event as this allows for natural remission. However, it is often easier to identify at risk children and families and provide them with resources immediately following the event when they are more likely to be in the presence of health professionals. In contrast, it is much harder to follow up families after they are discharged from hospital as they are less likely to want to return when child's physically recovered, or families may be too focused on the recovery/reconstruction process after disasters. One possible model is to employ a rescreening approach where children are initially screened at a time close to the event and when screening is more easily administered, then to selectively follow up and rescreen those initially identified at risk at a later date (e.g. >1 month post-trauma) (March et al. 2015). Effective screening will not be sufficient as it is contingent for identification of children at risk to have a linked pathway of care including resourced intervention options. If screening occurs without these pathways being available, then the process of screening will potentially contribute to distress in the child and families without having any means to address this.

6.6 Research Evidence

In recent years, there has been a marked increase in the number of studies evaluating preventative early interventions for PTSD. However, currently there is limited and mixed evidence available on the efficacy and feasibility of providing early intervention, especially following mass disasters and for children under the age of 6 years (Kramer and Landolt 2011; La Greca and Silverman 2009). Nevertheless, the evidence base for early interventions for traumatised children is still promising and will be briefly reviewed here. Table 6.1 provides a summary of the known universal and selected/targeted early interventions that have been evaluated following single-event traumas during childhood.

PFA, SPR and School-Focused Training for Recovery are informed by evidence and theory; however, due to the challenges associated with doing research in a post-disaster environment, there are no RCTs to support their efficacy to date. Despite this, the programmes appear promising and are rated as acceptable and useful interventions by providers (Allen et al. 2010; Forbes et al. 2010; Le Brocque et al. 2016). Current guidelines state that PFA may be appropriate for all children when used as part of an immediate care model following a range of traumatic events (Australian Centre for Posttraumatic Mental Health 2013).

Screening following trauma exposure is widely recommended, and there are a number of screening tools now available for use with children and adolescents, including preschool age (Kramer et al. 2013; March et al. 2012). However, studies evaluating the feasibility and utility of screening programmes in paediatric settings are scarce. Charuvastra et al. (2010) implemented a screen-and-refer process in a school setting following a student suicide. The authors concluded that the direct in-school screening approach was feasible, was effective at identifying children who would not have received treatment and was well accepted by children, parents and school staff. Another recent school-based screening programme conducted 4 months after a wide-scale flood found screening was helpful in identifying children with clinical levels of distress and getting them access to treatment (Poulsen et al. 2015). Parents reported they were highly satisfied with the screening process (Poulsen et al. 2015). Recently, March et al. (2015) reported on the feasibility and utility of a large-scale multihospital site screening programme for children after injury. The screening process was accepted by children and parents and was successful at identifying children with PTSD and referring them to treatment. However, the feasibility of the programme was impacted by low uptake rates. An important finding was that the rescreening component reduced the numbers of children who needed to progress to diagnostic assessment. Thus, it was concluded that rescreening may save significant time and costs and should be considered in future screening programmes.

Two studies by Kenardy and colleagues have found that information-based universal prevention interventions provided within 2-week postaccidental injury were associated with reduced child anxiety symptoms, at 1 month (Kenardy et al. 2008) and 6 months post-injury (Cox et al. 2010), and reduced parental PTSS at 6 months (Kenardy et al. 2008). A moderator analysis of the RCT of the basic web-based early intervention developed by Cox and colleagues (http://conrod.org.au/cms/kids-accident-web-site) found that the intervention was most effective when given to children (aged 7–16 years) experiencing high levels of distress soon after the accident (Kenardy et al. 2015). Specifically, children in the intervention group that reported high levels of initial distress experienced a large reduction in PTSS, whereas children in the control group demonstrated an exacerbation in PTSS by

Table 6.1 Summary of universal and selected/targeted early interventions for preventing the development of PTSD in preschoolers, children and adolescents following single-event trauma

Author and year	Trauma	N	Age	Treatment	Timing	Design	Assessment	Findings
Universal prevention								
Kassam-Adams et al. (2015)	Medical trauma	72	8–12	Psychoeducation: self-directed web-based interactive game	w/n 2 weeks	RCT: intervention vs wait-list control (TAU)	Ax: 6, 12 and 18 wks Outcome: CPSS, PedsQL	Medium b/n group effect sizes were reported for PTSS change from baseline to 6 or 12 wks No significantly different group differences for 12-wk outcomes
Marsac et al. (2013)	Unintentional injury	100	6–17	Psychoeducation: directed web-based information provision	w/n 60 days	RCT: intervention vs control (TAU)	Ax: 6 weeks from baseline Outcome: PKQ-R, PCL-C/PR, PCL, CPSS	No differences in parent knowledge or PTSD between groups at 6-wk Ax
Zehnder et al. (2010)	RTA	99	7–16	One session delivered by psychologist: reconstruction of accident, identification of appraisals and psychoeducation	10 days	RCT: intervention vs control (TAU)	Ax: 2 and 6 months Outcome: IBS-KJ, CAPS-CA, CDI, CBCL	No significant differences for PTSS or other outcomes Effective for preadolescent children at reducing depressive symptoms and behavioural problems

Cox et al. (2010)	Unintentional injury	53	7–16	Psychoeducation: web-based and booklet information provision	2–3 weeks	RCT: intervention vs control (TAU)	Ax: 4–6 weeks and 6 months Outcome: TSCC-A, IES-R	Intervention group reported greater reductions in anxiety. No significant differences between groups for child or parent PTSS
Kenardy et al. (2008)	Unintentional injury	103	7–15	Psychoeducation: information brochure provision	72 h	Control (second hospital)	Ax: 1 and 6 months Outcome: CIES, SCAS, IES, DASS	Intervention group had greater reductions in child anxiety (but not PTSS) at 1 month and parental intrusion and PTSS at 6 months

Targeted preventative intervention

Kramer and Landolt (2014)	RTAs and burns	108	2–16	Two-session CBT interventions delivered by psychologist: 1. Reconstruction of accident, psychoeducation, general coping strategies 2. Specific coping strategies	Session 1–2 wks post-accident Session 2–4 wks post-accident	RCT: intervention vs control (TAU)	Screened for PTSD risk w/n 5–19 days post-injury. Screen: PEDS-ES or CTSQ Ax: 3 months, 6 months Outcome: PTSDSSI, CAPS-CA, CBCL, CDI	Intervention was ineffective in preschool children. For 7–16-year group, intervention resulted in significantly fewer internalizing problems and borderline less intrusion symptoms at 3 months

(continued)

Table 6.1 (continued)

Author and year	Trauma	N	Age	Treatment	Timing	Design	Assessment	Findings
Kassam-Adams et al. (2011)	Unintentional injury	85	8–17	Two sessions delivered by nurse or social worker: 1. Top concern identified, discussion of distress, support questions, psychoeducation workbook 2. Review progress and concerns, support, referral	Session 1 – during hospital ($M = 3$ days) Session 2–2 weeks post-discharge ($M = 23$ days)	Pilot RCT Intervention vs control (TAU)	Screened for PTSD risk w/n 2 weeks post-injury. Screen: STEPP, CPSS, CES-D Ax: 6 wks, 6 months Outcome: CPSS, CES-D, PedsQL	Both groups improved, but 10 % still had PTSD at 6 months. No significant differences between groups for PTSD, depression severity, or HR-QOL
Berkowitz et al. (2011)	Variety of PTE types	106	7–17	Four caregiver-child sessions delivered by clinician: 1. Parent: psychoeducation, protective role, Ax stressors 2. Child and parent: Ax, discussion about symptoms and psychoeducation, skill module for 1–2 problem areas 3. Child: Ax, review and practice 4. Child and Parent: Ax, review and practice, referral	Within 30 days	RCT: intervention vs supportive comparison condition	Screened for PTSD risk w/n 30 days Ax: 3 months Screen: PCL-C Outcome: PTSD-RI, TSCC	Treatment group had significantly fewer PTSD diagnoses and lower trauma and anxiety scores

Note: Ax assessment, *CAPS-CA* clinician-administered PTSD scale for children and adolescents, *CBCL* child behaviour checklist, *CBT* cognitive behavioural therapy, *CDI* children's depression inventory, *CIES* child impact of event scale, *CPSS* child PTSD symptom scale, *CTSQ* child trauma screening questionnaire, *DASS* depression anxiety stress scale, *HR-QOL* health-related quality of life, *IBS-A-KJ* interview for ASD, *IES* impact of events scale, *PCL* PTSD checklist, *PCL-C/PR* PTSD checklist for children-parent report, *PEDS-ES* pediatric emotional distress scale – early screener, *PedsQL* paediatric quality of life inventory, *PKQ-R* parent knowledge questionnaire-revised, *PTSD* posttraumatic stress disorder, *PTSD-RI* UCLA posttraumatic stress disorder index, *PTSDSSI* PTSD semi-structured interview and observational record for infants and young children, *PTSS* posttraumatic stress symptoms, *RCT* randomised control trial, *RTA* road traffic accident, *STEPP* screening tool for early predictors of PTSD, *TAU* treatment as usual, *w/n* within, *wks* weeks, *TSCC-A* trauma symptom checklist for children-A

6 months. If initial distress was not elevated, there were no significant differences observed between groups. These findings suggest that when costs and burden of delivery are important factors, then it may be best to only target children presenting with acute distress (Kenardy et al. 2015).

In contrast, an RCT of a web-based psychoeducational intervention for parents did not find any significant effects of the intervention on parent knowledge or PTSS at 6-week follow-up (Marsac et al. 2013). Recently, a novel self-directed interactive web-based game designed to prevent PTSS in school-aged children following acute medical events was developed and trialled in a pilot RCT (Kassam-Adams et al. 2015). Preliminary findings suggest that the intervention is feasible to deliver and engaging for children, and the effect sizes for reducing PTSS are promising. However, significant group differences on PTSS were not observed at 12 weeks.

To date, research has not found support for single-session early interventions for reducing PTSS. However, the intervention by Zehnder, Meuli and Landolt (Zehnder et al. 2010) was effective at reducing depressive symptoms and behavioural problems in a subsample of preadolescent children (7–11 years) involved in road traffic accidents (Zehnder et al. 2010).

Only three known published RCTs have assessed targeted preventive interventions for children. So far, only one early intervention, the CFTSI, appears to be effective at reducing child PTSD diagnoses and symptoms following exposure to PTEs (Berkowitz et al. 2011). Two other RCTs of two-session targeted preventative early interventions for injured children have not found intervention effects for reducing PTSD (Kassam-Adams et al. 2011; Kramer and Landolt 2014). Only one study has investigated any form of early intervention with injured children under 6 years of age (Kramer and Landolt 2014). Unfortunately, the intervention was not found to be effective at reducing the presence of child PTSD, PTSS or behavioural problems.

In sum, there are some promising, but not yet convincing, findings, for the role of early intervention at preventing trauma reactions following unintentional injury. All of the existing interventions include a psychoeducation component; however, they vary in the mode and timing of delivery, number of sessions and content. It is clear that further work is still needed to determine optimal timing and intensity of intervention needed to prevent the development of persistent PTSD among those at risk. Additionally, research is needed to ascertain the "active" component/s of the interventions that result in the psychological benefits. Further, work is still needed to determine when the best time is to screen children to identify risk status and what the best tools are to use. Finally, there is a pressing need for controlled trials examining the efficacy of early interventions for preventing the development of PTSD in young children.

6.7   Summary and Clinical Implications

Children of all ages are exposed to traumatic events on a regular basis, and the psychological, physical and social consequences can have serious short- and long-term implications and costs across the lifespan. Prevention or alleviation of persistent traumatic stress reactions and other psychopathologies for both children and their parents obviously has many benefits. However, as seen in this chapter, there are very few evidence-based interventions available, especially in the context of natural disasters and terrorism and for preschool-aged children. Based on the conceptual models and research evidence reviewed, a number of tentative recommendations can be made for the development and provision of preventative early interventions to children following single-event traumas. These include:

1. Wherever possible it is essential to minimise the potential for further secondary PTEs for the child and family through the provision of trauma-informed care.
2. Preventative early intervention programmes need to be age appropriate and developmentally sensitive and engage and support parents throughout the entire processes.
3. Interventions should incorporate a stepped-care approach that involves screening (ideally involving a rescreening process) and targeting resources towards those showing elevated acute levels of distress. However, any screening and intervention programme will need to be linked into a clinical service with the capacity to deliver appropriate care.
4. Intervention components most likely to be beneficial include providing psychoeducation, focus on supporting existing competencies and teaching coping skills and enhancing social supports.
5. Debriefing and pharmacological interventions should not be offered.
6. More high-quality research is still needed to determine the optimum time to provide screening and early intervention programmes and the duration and content of intervention materials, especially for children less than 6 years.

References

Alisic E, Zalta AK, van Wesel F, Larsen SE, Hafstad GS, Hassanpour K, Smid GE (2014) Rates of post-traumatic stress disorder in trauma-exposed children and adolescents: meta-analysis. Br J Psychiatry 204(5):335–340. doi:10.1192/bjp.bp.113.131227

Allen B, Brymer MJ, Steinberg AM, Vernberg EM, Jacobs A, Speier AH, Pynoos RS (2010) Perceptions of psychological first aid among providers responding to Hurricanes Gustav and Ike. J Trauma Stress 23(4):509–513. doi:10.1002/jts.20539

Australian Centre for Posttraumatic Mental Health (2013) Australian guidelines for the treatment of acute stress disorder and posttraumatic stress disorder. ACPMH, Melbourne

Berkowitz S, Bryant R, Brymer M, Hamblen J, Jacobs A, Layne C, et al (2010) Skills for psychological recovery: field operations guide. National Center for PTSD and National Child Traumatic Stress Network. Los Angeles, California, USA

Berkowitz S, Stover CS, Marans SR (2011) The Child and Family Traumatic Stress Intervention: secondary prevention for youth at risk of developing PTSD. J Child Psychol Psychiatry 52(6):676–685. doi:10.1111/j.1469-7610.2010.02321.x

Brymer M, Jacobs A, Layne C, Pynoos RS, Ruzek J, Steinberg A, et al (2006) Psychological first aid: field operations guide, 2nd edn. National Child Traumatic Stress Network, Los Angeles, CA, USA. Retrieved from: www.nctsn.org and www.ncptsd.va.gov.

Carrion VG, Weems CF, Ray R, Reiss AL (2002) Toward an empirical definition of pediatric PTSD: the phenomenology of PTSD symptoms in youth. J Am Acad Child Adolesc Psychiatry 41(2):166–173

Charuvastra A, Goldfarb E, Petkova E, Cloitre M (2010) Implementation of a screen and treat program for child posttraumatic stress disorder in a school setting after a school suicide. J Trauma Stress 23(4):500–503. doi:10.1002/jts.20546

Copeland WE, Keeler G, Angold A, Costello E (2007) Traumatic events and posttraumatic stress in childhood. Arch Gen Psychiatry 64(5):577–584. doi:10.1001/archpsyc.64.5.577

Cox CM, Kenardy JA, Hendrikz JK (2010) A randomized controlled trial of a web-based early intervention for children and their parents following unintentional injury. J Pediatr Psychol 35(6):581–592

Davis L, Siegel LJ (2000) Posttraumatic stress disorder in children and adolescents: a review and analysis. Clin Child Fam Psychol Rev 3(3):135–154

De Young AC, Hendrikz J, Kenardy JA, Cobham VE, Kimble RM (2014) Prospective evaluation of parent distress following pediatric burns and identification of risk factors for young child and parent posttraumatic stress disorder. J Child Adolesc Psychopharmacol 24(1):9–17. doi:10.1089/cap.2013.0066

De Young AC, Kenardy JA, Cobham VE, Kimble R (2012) Prevalence, comorbidity and course of trauma reactions in young burn-injured children. J Child Psychol Psychiatry 53(1):56–63. doi:10.1111/j.1469-7610.2011.02431.x

Erikson EH (1950) Childhood and society. Norton, New York

Forbes D, Fletcher S, Wolfgang B, Varker T, Creamer M, Brymer MJ et al (2010) Practitioner perceptions of Skills for Psychological Recovery: a training programme for health practitioners in the aftermath of the Victorian bushfires. Aust N Z J Psychiatry 44(12):1105–1111. doi:10.3109/00048674.2010.513674

Health Care Toolbox (2013) Basics of trauma-informed care. Children's Hospital of Philadelphia website. Retrieved from: http://www.healthcaretoolbox.org/

Kassam-Adams N, Felipe García-España J, Marsac ML, Kohser KL, Baxt C, Nance M, Winston F (2011) A pilot randomized controlled trial assessing secondary prevention of traumatic stress integrated into pediatric trauma care. J Trauma Stress 24(3):252–259. doi:10.1002/jts.20640

Kassam-Adams N, Marsac ML, Kohser KL, Kenardy JA, March S, Winston FK (2015) Pilot randomized controlled trial of a novel web-based intervention to prevent posttraumatic stress in children following medical events. J Pediatr Psychol 41(1):138–148. doi:10.1093/jpepsy/jsv057

Kazak AE (2006) Pediatric Psychosocial Preventative Health Model (PPPHM): research, practice, and collaboration in pediatric family systems medicine. Fam Syst Health 24(4):381–395. doi:10.1037/1091-7527.24.4.381

Kazak AE, Kassam-Adams N, Schneider S, Zelikovsky N, Alderfer MA, Rourke M (2006) An integrative model of pediatric medical traumatic stress. J Pediatr Psychol 31(4):343–355

Kazak AE, Rourke MT, Alderfer MA, Pai A, Reilly AF, Meadows AT (2007) Evidence-based assessment, intervention and psychosocial care in pediatric oncology: a blueprint for comprehensive services across treatment. J Pediatr Psychol 32(9):1099–1110. doi:10.1093/jpepsy/jsm031

Kenardy JA, Cox CM, Brown FL (2015) A web-based early intervention can prevent long-term PTS reactions in children with high initial distress following accidental injury. J Trauma Stress 28(4):366–369. doi:10.1002/jts.22025

Kenardy JA, Thompson K, Le Brocque RM, Olsson K (2008) Information-provision intervention for children and their parents following pediatric accidental injury. Eur Child Adolesc Psychiatry 17(5):316–325

Kramer DN, Hertli MB, Landolt MA (2013) Evaluation of an early risk screener for PTSD in preschool children after accidental injury. Pediatrics 132(4):e945–e951. doi:10.1542/peds.2013-0713

Kramer DN, Landolt MA (2011) Characteristics and efficacy of early psychological interventions in children and adolescents after single trauma: a meta-analysis. Eur J Psychotraumatol 2:7858. doi:10.3402/ejpt.v2i0.7858

Kramer DN, Landolt MA (2014) Early psychological intervention in accidentally injured children ages 2–16: a randomized controlled trial. Eur J Psychotraumatol 5. doi:10.3402/ejpt.v5.24402

La Greca AM, Silverman WK (2009) Treatment and prevention of posttraumatic stress reactions in children and adolescents exposed to disasters and terrorism: What is the evidence? Child Dev Perspect 3(1):4–10. doi:10.1111/j.1750-8606.2008.00069.x

La Greca AM, Silverman WK, Vernberg EM, Prinstein MJ (1996) Symptoms of posttraumatic stress in children after Hurricane Andrew: a prospective study. J Consult Clin Psychol 64(4):712–723. doi:10.1037/0022-006x.64.4.712

Landolt MA, Schnyder U, Maier T, Schoenbucher V, Mohler-Kuo M (2013) Trauma exposure and posttraumatic stress disorder in adolescents: a national survey in switzerland. J Trauma Stress 26(2):209–216. doi:10.1002/jts.21794

Le Brocque R, De Young A, Montague G, Pocock S, March S, Triggell N, Rabaa C, Kenardy J (2016) Schools and natural disaster recovery: the unique and vital role that teachers and education professionals play in ensuring the mental health of students following natural disasters. Journal of Psychologists and Counsellors in Schools, 1–23. doi: 10.1017/jgc.2016.17 (in press).

Le Brocque RM, Hendrikz J, Kenardy JA (2010) The course of posttraumatic stress in children: Examination of recovery trajectories following traumatic injury. J Pediatr Psychol 35(6):637–645

March S, De Young AC, Dow B, Kenardy JA (2012) Assessing trauma-related symptoms in children and adolescents. In: Beck GJ, Sloan DM (eds) The Oxford handbook of traumatic stress disorders. Oxford University Press, New York

March S, Kenardy JA, Cobham VE, Nixon RD, McDermott B, De Young A (2015) Feasibility of a screening program for at-risk children following accidental injury. J Trauma Stress 28(1):34–40. doi:10.1002/jts.21981

Marsac ML, Hildenbrand AK, Kohser KL, Winston FK, Li Y, Kassam-Adams N (2013) Preventing posttraumatic stress following pediatric injury: a randomized controlled trial of a web-based psycho-educational intervention for parents. J Pediatr Psychol 38(10):1101–1111. doi:10.1093/jpepsy/jst053

Marsac ML, Kassam-Adams N, Delahanty DL, Widaman KF, Barakat LP (2014) Posttraumatic stress following acute medical trauma in children: a proposed model of bio-psycho-social processes during the peri-trauma period. Clin Child Fam Psychol Rev 17(4):399–411. doi:10.1007/s10567-014-0174-2

Marsac ML, Kassam-Adams N, Hildenbrand AK, Kohser KL, Winston FK (2011) After the injury: initial evaluation of a web-based intervention for parents of injured children. Health Educ Res 26(1):1–12. doi:10.1093/her/cyq045

Marsac ML, Kassam-Adams N, Hildenbrand AK, Nicholls E, Winston FK, Leff SS, Fein J (2015) Implementing a trauma-informed approach in pediatric health care networks. JAMA Pediatr 170(1):70–77 . doi:10.1001/jamapediatrics.2015.22061-8

NICE (2005) Post-traumatic stress disorder (PTSD): the management of PTSD in adults and children in primary and secondary care. NICE Clinical Guideline 26 Available at http://guidance.nice.org.uk/CG26.

Nugent NR, Goldberg A, Uddin M (2015) Topical review: the emerging field of epigenetics: informing models of pediatric trauma and physical health. J Pediatr Psychol 41(1):55–64. doi:10.1093/jpepsy/jsv018

Poulsen KM, McDermott BM, Wallis J, Cobham VE (2015) School-based psychological screening in the aftermath of a disaster: are parents satisfied and do their children access treatment? J Trauma Stress 28(1):69–72. doi:10.1002/jts.21987

Price J, Kassam-Adams N, Alderfer MA, Christofferson J, Kazak AE (2015) Systematic review: a reevaluation and update of the Integrative (Trajectory) Model of Pediatric M*edical Traumatic Stress*. J Pediatr Psychol 41(1):86–97. doi:10.1093/jpepsy/jsv074

Stuber ML, Schneider S, Kassam-Adams N, Kazak AE, Saxe G (2006) The medical traumatic stress toolkit. CNS Spectr 11(2):137–142 Retrieved from http://europepmc.org/abstract/MED/16520691

Vernberg EM (2002) Intervention approaches following disasters. In: Greca AML, Silverman WK, Vernberg EM, Roberts MC (eds) Helping children cope with disasters and terrorism. American Psychological Association, Washington

Vernberg EM, La Greca AM, Silverman WK, Prinstein MJ (1996) Prediction of posttraumatic stress symptoms in children after Hurricane Andrew. J Abnorm Psychol 105(2):237–248. doi:10.1037/0021-843X.105.2.237

Zehnder D, Meuli M, Landolt MA (2010) Effectiveness of a single-session early psychological intervention for children after road traffic accidents: a randomised controlled trial. Child Adolesc Psychiatry Ment Health 4:7. doi:10.1186/1753-2000-4-7

The Child and Family Traumatic Stress Intervention

Carrie Epstein, Hilary Hahn, Steven Berkowitz, and Steven Marans

7.1 Theoretical Underpinnings

The Child and Family Traumatic Stress Intervention (CFTSI) is a brief evidence-based, trauma-focused mental health treatment that was developed at the Childhood Violent Trauma Center at the Yale Child Study Center. CFTSI grew out of more than two decades of closely observing and learning about the phenomena of trauma from children and families impacted by abuse, violence, and other potentially traumatic events. In addition, the developers of the CFTSI model learned a great deal from colleagues in multiple disciplines, including mental health, social work, public health, law enforcement, child welfare, pediatrics and emergency medicine, and other professions serving children and families during all phases of the trauma response.

Since the early 1990s, clinicians at the Yale Childhood Violent Trauma Center have collaborated with law enforcement and child protective service partners to respond to over 20, 000 children and adults impacted by traumatic events, including physical and sexual abuse, neglect, domestic violence, murders, murder-suicides, sexual assaults, suicides, and motor vehicle accidents, as well as school shootings, terrorist attacks, airplane crashes, house fires, and hurricanes. As part of this work, clinicians have conducted acute, on-scene interventions, as well as longer-term clinical treatment, and have coordinated care for children and families impacted by traumatic events. This work led to a deeper appreciation of the details of traumatic reactions, including the fact that children's symptoms are often not recognized by caregivers upon whom they rely for support. Through this extensive and often extended clinical work, it also became increasingly clear that these children not only suffered alone, but were at great risk for longer-term posttraumatic disorders. In addition to direct clinical observations of numerous traumatized children and families and research on risk and resilience, CFTSI is richly informed by psychoanalytic, behavioral, and cognitive theories of development and human functioning.

7.1.1 The Traumatic Situation and Its Subsequent Phases

The traumatic situation may be defined as one in which the individual experiences an unanticipated, overwhelming danger or an immediate threat to physical and/or emotional safety that leads to: (1) the subjective experience of helplessness and loss of control; (2) immobilization of usual methods for decreasing danger and anxiety; and (3) neurophysiological dysregulation that compromises affective, cognitive, and behavioral responses to stimuli.

Posttraumatic reactions fall into three phases. The clinical phenomena of each phase provide indications about the appropriate clinical responses:

- *The acute phase* refers to the immediate period (moments and hours) that follows a traumatic event. Sudden dysregulation in thinking, affect, and physiology is frequently exacerbated by the chaotic external circumstances that often accompany and follow the child's traumatic exposure. Thus, the phenomena of acute traumatization would suggest that immediate interventions focus on identifying high-risk children and families, ensuring immediate stabilization and prioritizing additional assistance.
- *The peritraumatic phase* refers to the days and weeks following a traumatic event. In the peritraumatic period, the degree of chaotic dysregulation seen in children during the acute phase gives way to a presentation of more organized signs and symptoms that reflect neurophysiologic changes, as well as efforts to reverse accompanying feelings of helplessness, loss of control, and isolation. This phase offers an opportunity for early intervention, with the goal of helping children and their caregivers achieve greater control and mastery over symptoms before those symptoms become entrenched and part of longer-term, established posttraumatic disorders and symptomatology.
- *The posttraumatic phase* refers to the months following a traumatic event. In this phase, traumatic symptoms have become entrenched and may reflect a failure of recovery that can lead to alterations in the developmental trajectory, impacting functional adaptation and views of self, world, and others, as well as unfolding personality organization (Foa and Meadows 1997).

In this chapter, we will focus on the peritraumatic phase, opportunities for early intervention, and the development of CFTSI, a treatment model that maps onto the clinical phenomena of traumatic reaction in this phase.

7.1.2 Peritraumatic Focus on Symptoms

Symptoms in the peritraumatic period reflect continued neurophysiologic, emotional, cognitive, and behavioral dysregulation and may also serve as organized attempts to protect against the perception that the original, real danger persists (Marans 2013; Southwick and Charney 2012). However, the symptoms themselves perpetuate the experience of loss of control, predictability, and order that are so essential for successfully navigating tasks of daily life. As such, symptoms constitute a threat to tasks involved in progressive development, and may add to preexisting deficits in mastering these tasks. For example, the avoidant child may be unable to engage in social interactions and activities that are critical to the developing sense of autonomy and personal success. Similarly, the inability to concentrate in school because of intrusive thoughts and hyperarousal may lead the affected child to fall behind both in reality and in his/her own sense of competence. Withdrawal, irritability, and anxiety may interrupt close relationships at a time when social support is critical to recovery. It is also important to note that in addition to the suffering that occurs, the degree and severity of symptoms in the peritraumatic period is predictive of longer-term posttraumatic disorders (Ozer et al. 2003). Intervening in this phase therefore serves several important functions, namely: (1) helping the child and family to achieve control over symptomatic responses; (2) decreasing suffering and interference with current adaptation and progressive development; and (3) decreasing the perpetuation or development of long-term, established posttraumatic symptoms (Marans 2013).

7.1.3 Key Risk and Protective Factors

There are multiple risk factors that can contribute to the level of symptomatology and the extent to which either recovery or the development of long-term disorders occurs (see Chap. 2). These factors include physical proximity to the index event (Pynoos et al. 1987), emotional proximity (i.e., the degree to which the threat or danger is directed at the child or at those to whom the child is close), preexisting vulnerabilities in psychological functioning (Breslau et al. 1998), previous traumatic experiences (Davidson et al. 1991), the failure of recognition by adults of the child's distress, and the lack of family and other social supports (Hill et al. 1996; Ozer et al. 2003). Of these factors, two of the key predictors of poor posttraumatic outcomes are (1) the failure to recognize the child's posttraumatic distress (Hill et al. 1996; Kliewer et al. 2004) and (2) the absence of social (i.e., family) support (Trickey et al. 2012). It is well established that social support and communication are critical in helping children mediate their traumatic experiences (Salmon and Bryant 2002), and that these are central protective factors in preventing longer-term posttraumatic disorders (Ozer et al. 2003; Trickey et al. 2012).

When children are alone with and do not have words for their traumatic reactions, then symptomatic behavior may be their only means of expression. To recover, children need recognition and understanding from the most important source of support in their lives – their caregivers. However, caregivers are frequently unable to appreciate the connections between their child's traumatic experience and the ensuing symptoms and behaviors (Kassam-Adams et al. 2006; Shemesh et al. 2005). Children need help to identify, articulate, and communicate their traumatic stress reactions and emotions, and to learn and employ coping strategies to reduce traumatic stress reactions. While children may rely on caregivers as the optimal source of support in these efforts, caregivers may also require education, support, and practical skills to help them manage their children's traumatic reactions.

In acknowledgment of what is known about key risk and protective factors, CFTSI focuses on: (a) increasing caregivers' understanding of their children's posttraumatic reactions, as well as their own; (b) improving children's observation and recognition of their own posttraumatic reactions; (c) facilitating the child and caregiver's communication about the child's symptoms; (d) teaching coping strategies to support children and caregivers in gaining mastery over traumatic reactions; and (e) assessing the need for longer-term treatment, for both posttraumatic and previously unidentified preexisting disorders.

7.2 CFTSI in Clinical Practice

7.2.1 Overview and Goals

CFTSI is a five- to eight-session evidence-based, peritraumatic mental health treatment model developed by Steven Berkowitz of the University of Pennsylvania, Perelman School of Medicine, and Carrie Epstein and Steven Marans of the Yale Child Study Center, Yale University School of Medicine. A model with demonstrated effectiveness in reducing children's trauma symptoms in the aftermath of traumatic experiences and reducing or interrupting PTSD and related disorders in children (Berkowitz et al. 2011), CFTSI was specifically developed for implementation with children aged 7 years and older during the peritraumatic period. CFTSI is manualized (Berkowitz et al. 2012) and a standardized training protocol has been developed. A treatment application of CFTSI for young children (ages 3–6 years old) has also been developed (Marans et al. 2014), as well as a treatment application for children recently placed in foster care (Epstein et al. 2013). Please refer to Table 7.1 at the end of this chapter for basic overview of the CFTSI sessions, including content, participants, duration, and timing of sessions.

With careful attention to structure and pacing, CFTSI aims to replace the chaos, dysregulation, and isolation of the posttraumatic experience with structure, language, and an opportunity for recognition from, and close connection with, caregivers. Implemented with the child and the non-offending caregiver, CFTSI focuses on increasing communication between child and caregiver about the child's traumatic stress reactions, providing clinical strategies to reduce traumatic stress symptoms and increase self-regulation. In this way, CFTSI not only offers the opportunity for early symptom reduction but also helps the child and caregiver regain control through reduction and mastery of symptoms. CFTSI also provides a seamless introduction to longer-term treatment and other mental health interventions when needed.

CFTSI is the right match for a child when there is a recent traumatic event. In order to identify children who could benefit from CFTSI, a brief standardized trauma-focused assessment instrument is administered to screen for trauma symptoms as reported by the child and separately as reported by the caregiver. The intensity of children's symptomatic responses can vary widely during the peritraumatic

7 The Child and Family Traumatic Stress Intervention

Table 7.1 CFTSI session outline

CFTSI session	Participants	Timing	Duration	Content
Screening	Clinician Caregiver Child	Conducted as soon as possible after the event or formal disclosure of physical or sexual abuse	One client hour	Administer standardized trauma symptom assessment instrument as a clinical interview with caregiver and with child separately to assess child's level of trauma symptoms
Session 1	Clinician Caregiver	Conducted as soon as possible after screening	One client hour	Provide psychoeducation about trauma and trauma symptoms Assess caregiver's trauma history Assess caregiver's trauma symptoms by administering a standardized trauma symptom assessment instrument. Obtain caregiver's report of child's trauma history and symptoms by administering standardized instruments Address case management and care coordination issues
Session 2	Clinician Child	Conducted within a week or less after Session 1	One client hour	Provide psychoeducation about trauma and trauma symptoms Assess child's trauma history and trauma symptoms by administering standardized instruments
Session 3	Clinician Caregiver Child	Conducted within a week or less after Session 2	One client hour	Begin discussion by comparing caregiver and child's reports about trauma history and trauma symptoms Identify and provide specific trauma reactions to be the focus of clinical interventions and introduce coping strategies
Session 4	Clinician Caregiver Child	Conducted 1 week after Session 3	One client hour	Point out, encourage, and support communication attempts Reassess child's symptoms Practice coping strategies, support efforts
Session 5	Clinician Caregiver Child	Conducted 1 week after Session 4	One client hour	Follow same format as Session 4 Review progress made and identify additional case management or treatment needs
Post-assessments	Clinician Caregiver Child	Conducted same day after completion of Session 5		Administer standardized trauma symptom assessment instrument as a clinical interview with caregiver and with child separately to assess child's level of trauma symptoms Administer standardized trauma symptom assessment instrument as a clinical interview with caregiver to assess caregiver's level of trauma symptoms Client completes consumer satisfaction survey

phase. For that reason, and because CFTSI is an early treatment model, if either the child or caregiver endorses one new trauma symptom or reports an exacerbation of an existing symptom(s) following the recent traumatic event, CFTSI may be a good match for the child. Involvement of a non-offending caregiver in CFTSI is essential and is discussed below.

As described, the traumatic experience is one that includes a lack of control, lack of predictability, and sense of chaos that may continue unabated after the precipitating traumatic event is over. The symptoms themselves perpetuate the original traumatic loss of control and dysregulation. CFTSI offers an alternative to these painful/disturbing reactions by providing order and predictability, as well as strategies to gain mastery and control over symptoms of traumatic dysregulation. The highly structured format of CFTSI was developed to address precisely the dysregulation of cognitive, affective, somatic, and behavioral processes that is central to the traumatic situation. The CFTSI model uses standardized clinical assessment instruments to facilitate clinical dialogues that focus on increasing the child and caregiver's recognition, discussion, and mastery of trauma symptoms. In this way, CFTSI helps to offset the deficits that result from traumatic dysregulation.

Illustrating the CFTSI Model: The Case of Mia

The case described below is an example of one of the thousands of cases that have received CFTSI in the Child Advocacy Center (CAC) setting. CACs promote a child-friendly, safe, and neutral location in which law enforcement and child protective service investigators conduct and observe forensic interviews with children who are alleged victims of crimes (including physical and/or sexual abuse) and where the child and non-offending family members receive support, crisis intervention, and referrals for mental health and medical treatment. CFTSI has been effective in the CAC setting, where treatment has been provided to children and families either internally within the program or by an agency that partners with the CAC to provide mental health treatment.

Mia was an 11-year-old girl who had been physically abused by her father. Mia's parents had been separated for many years and Mia lived with her mother, spending weekends with her father. Frightened by threats that he would hurt her siblings if she told anyone, Mia had successfully hidden evidence of her father's abuse. However, following a weekend visit with her father, staff at Mia's school noticed severe bruising and contacted Child Protective Services, who subsequently brought Mia to a CAC. During a forensic interview at the CAC, Mia disclosed that her father had beaten her.

When the abuse was reported, Child Protective Services made the determination that Mia could no longer live with her father and needed to live full time with her mother, Regina. Regina was upset to learn about Mia's abuse, but she also made it clear that she was resentful about suddenly being solely responsible for Mia's care. As a single mother of four children, Regina already felt overwhelmed and expressed frustration about what she saw as the additional burdens of Mia's mental health treatment.

Pre-treatment screening for trauma symptomatology was conducted separately with Mia and with Regina in a clinical interview format, using a standardized trauma symptom assessment instrument. Mia reported clinically significant levels of symptoms, while her mother reported Mia having relatively few symptoms. Regina's own experience of distress and aggravation about the additional burdens she anticipated for herself may have resulted in the discrepancy between her report of symptoms and those reported by Mia. This discrepancy may also have reflected Regina's minimal awareness of her daughter's symptoms and lack of attunement to her daughter's feelings.

7.2.2 Session 1: Meeting Individually with the Caregiver

During the first session of CFTSI, the clinician meets individually with the primary caregiver(s) and begins by providing education about trauma and common traumatic stress reactions, as well as discussing the typical impact of traumatic experiences on children. As part of this discussion, the clinician explains that, like the traumatic experience, the resulting symptoms continue the sense of loss of control and lack of predictability, and CFTSI focuses on strategies for reestablishing a sense of control. The clinician then provides an outline of the sessions and explains the reasons that communication about symptoms and skills for managing reactions should result in a diminution of symptoms.

It is important to point out that although psychoeducation about trauma is provided during Session 1, there are many opportunities to link the observable phenomena that emerge in subsequent sessions back to themes of trauma psychoeducation. By returning to and referencing the earlier discussions about trauma, the clinician establishes a shared frame of reference with the caregiver and child that gives a context for CFTSI specifically, as well as for the coping strategies focused on reducing trauma symptoms that are introduced during CFTSI.

As part of Session 1, the clinician next conducts a brief assessment of the caregiver's trauma symptomatology, by administering a standardized trauma symptom assessment instrument. This helps to identify when adults may need additional care in their own right, as well as inform ways in which the caregiver's symptoms may come into play when addressing their children's symptoms. A case management survey provides an opportunity to discuss external stressors affecting the family and make referrals to appropriate community resources. The clinician then gathers a developmental history of the child, including an assessment of the child's trauma history. Using a standardized approach to provide structure in the discussions, the clinician assesses the caregiver's impression of the child's level of trauma symptoms. As the clinician gathers the caregiver's report of the child's symptoms, the clinician explores with the caregiver how the caregiver became aware of these symptoms (i.e., Did the caregiver observe the symptom? Did the child tell the caregiver about the symptom?). This also becomes an opportunity to convey that it is not uncommon for caregivers to be unaware of the full scope and impact of the child's traumatic experience. This discussion can be helpful to the clinician in forming a baseline assessment of the caregiver's observational capacities and the current level of caregiver-child communication about symptoms.

> **Case Example Mia: Session 1**
>
> At the start of CFTSI, it was clear that Regina would need a great deal of support to develop an understanding of how she could be of help to her child. In addition to the anger and resentment she expressed, Regina also indicated that she felt quite overwhelmed. She also spoke about her negative sense that her life was now an "open book" due to her current involvement with Child Protective Services. At the same time, Regina also stated that she wanted to support her daughter. Expression of this latter sentiment created a key moment in the initiation of the CFTSI treatment that was crucial to engaging this mother.
>
> Initially, the clinician experienced Regina as insensitive and distant and an unlikely ally or authentic source of support for Mia. However, the clinician did not simply give up on Regina's capacity to help Mia recover from significant trauma symptoms. Instead, the clinician capitalized on the first CFTSI session as a structured opportunity to turn full attention to Regina and toward what might be underlying contributions to her apparently unsympathetic attitudes. Regina, in turn, seemed to appreciate being heard, and the clinician was subsequently able to engage her with greater empathy. This led to an empathic shift in Regina's appreciation of Mia's traumatic experience and increased her concern about her daughter's emotional well-being.
>
> Providing psychoeducation about trauma helped to deepen Regina's appreciation of Mia's experience. At first, Regina minimized the damaging impact of corporal punishment, reporting that she herself was raised in a home in which beatings were commonplace, and that she had not been adversely affected. However, following a more general discussion of trauma, Regina was able to consider how Mia's experience of severe physical abuse might be adversely impacting Mia on multiple levels. In fact, Regina was able to recognize the link between the abuse and the symptoms that Mia was reporting, including physical reactions (i.e., heart racing, stomach aches), emotional reactions (i.e., depression, anxiety), behavioral reactions (i.e., withdrawal, eating and sleeping difficulties), and cognitive reactions (i.e., feelings of guilt for disclosing).
>
> The psychoeducation component of Session 1 also provided Regina with a better understanding of the impact of trauma and trauma symptoms on the family as a whole, including how they might lead a caregiver to feel overwhelmed. This discussion gave Regina an opportunity to express feelings of anger and resentment toward Mia's father more directly, as well as to recognize the ways in which these feelings were being displaced and misdirected toward Mia. As a result, Regina's initial insensitivity was able to evolve into an increased appreciation of her daughter's experience.

7.2.3 Session 2: Meeting Individually with the Child

In the second session of CFTSI, the clinician meets individually with the child and, in a similar fashion to Session 1, begins by providing education about trauma and reviewing possible reactions that children commonly experience following a traumatic event. Again, by creating frame of reference and by creating this anchor in psychoeducation, the therapist has an opening to segue into talking about why the child is coming to therapy, the rationale for CFTSI, and what the goals of the treatment will be. In this way, the clinician helps the child begin to organize his/her experience of posttraumatic events and gives the treatment a structure that is important to both children and families impacted by trauma.

Using standardized instruments to provide structure in the discussions, the clinician gathers information from the child about their trauma history and assesses the child's understanding of his/her level of trauma symptomatology. As part of the discussion with the child, the clinician explores with the child whether or not he/she has communicated with the caregiver or anyone else about his/her trauma symptoms. The clinician ensures that the child understands that the clinician will be comparing the child's assessment of his/her trauma history and trauma symptoms to the caregiver's report and that they will all be reviewing and discussing them together in Session 3. The clinician explains that communicating feelings and symptoms to the caregiver will help the caregiver identify ways to support the child. In addition, the clinician emphasizes that the coping strategies that they will implement during the next session will help decrease the child's symptoms and increase his/her sense of control.

> **Case Example Mia: Session 2**
> At the start of CFTSI Session 2, Mia was guarded and anxious. In response to questions assessing her trauma symptoms, Mia reported struggling with anxiety, a strong startle response, and difficulty concentrating, as well as frequent nightmares and intrusive thoughts. Mia described feeling overwhelmed with sadness at times, profound loneliness, and the belief that she was doing everything wrong. Mia reported that at other times she felt irritable and very sensitive. Mia was experiencing significant levels of self-blame, guilt, and regret about disclosing the abuse. Mia expressed feelings of ambivalence toward her father: she was mad at him but stated that she was sad about the situation as well.

7.2.4 Session 3: Meeting Together with the Child and Caregiver

CFTSI Session 3 is held with the child and caregiver together to review, compare, and contrast the observations and responses that each reported with respect to the child's trauma history and symptoms. Goals for this session are to increase caregiver support by initiating a discussion between the child and caregiver about the child's trauma reactions, to help the child communicate about reactions and feelings more effectively, and to increase the caregiver's appreciation of the child's experience. In this session, the child and caregiver have an opportunity to "compare notes" and come to a greater understanding of one another's observations about the child's traumatic stress symptoms and level of distress.

During this session, the clinician begins a discussion between the child and caregiver by reviewing traumatic reactions in general. The clinician then walks the child and caregiver through each of their reports about the child's trauma history and symptoms, comparing responses and making observations about what each has reported. As part of this discussion, the clinician explores ways in which the child and caregiver can use each other's observations and identification of symptoms to increase communication about the child's struggles. The clinician encourages a greater awareness of the specific timing and circumstances in which the child's symptoms occur, which may include the identification of trauma reminders that are causing symptoms to occur. The goal here is to improve their ability to anticipate and more readily recognize when symptoms are occurring. This is a first step toward managing and reducing symptoms and returns the locus of control over symptoms to the child and caregiver. As part of this process, the clinician helps the child and caregiver identify new ways to communicate about the occurrence of symptoms, with an emphasis on sensitivity and directness. Following this, the clinician helps identify the most concerning, specific trauma symptoms that will be the focus of clinical interventions, such as anxiety, intrusive thoughts, aggressive or oppositional behaviors, depressive withdrawal, or issues with sleeping. Next, the clinician introduces coping strategies to reduce symptoms and help return the child to optimal levels of control. Strategies may include helping the family reestablish daily routines, as well as learning relaxation and stress management techniques, affective regulation skills, cognitive processing techniques, and behavior management techniques, often coupled with effective parenting skills. After introducing the specific coping skills and strategies that will be used to manage and master the identified symptoms, the clinician engages the child and caregiver in practicing them in the session.

Case Example Mia: Session 3
During the previous CFTSI session, Mia had expressed anxiety about meeting together with her mother in the upcoming session, including the concern that her mother would react to her in unsupportive, critical ways. When Mia and Regina came into the room for Session 3 and sat down on the couch, the physical distance between them was notable. Mia's mother sat rigidly on the couch showing no warmth toward her daughter, while Mia appeared anxious, looking down at her lap. Aware of the tension in the room, the clinician began by reviewing the goals of the session, pointing out that children and caregivers frequently have concerns about discussing upsetting symptoms and feelings. The clinician then discussed with Mia and Regina what each had reported about Mia's trauma history and trauma symptoms, noting where they reported

similar levels of symptoms and where there were discrepancies. Both Mia and Regina responded well to this approach and became engaged in the discussion. After collaboratively identifying some of Mia's most concerning symptoms, the clinician began introducing coping strategies aimed to help reduce the most troubling of these symptoms.

In spite of Regina's readiness to participate initially, her apparent irritation about engaging in the process resurfaced when the clinician introduced coping strategies. In response to the demonstration of focused breathing and an invitation to practice this technique, Regina responded disdainfully, asking, "Do *I* have to do focused breathing?" Undeterred, the clinician used sympathetic humor along with a reminder to Regina about her importance in her child's recovery as a way of encouraging her to participate. Regina seemed surprised as she reported her own experience of the technique's calming effects. The moment when Mia described similar effects was the first time in quite a while that the two shared a sense of connection, relief, and joint accomplishment. This would become the first in a series of positive interactions that Mia and her mother were able to share, as the clinician introduced additional coping strategies of guided imagery and progressive muscle relaxation. The resulting interactions were far less tense and provided opportunities for Mia to experience her mother's clear investment in her well-being and as a central support in her efforts to gain mastery over her trauma symptoms and recover.

7.2.5 Session 4: Meeting Together with the Child and Caregiver

In CFTSI Session 4, the clinician meets again with the child and caregiver to discuss the experiences of the previous week and to support communication attempts around the identified trauma symptoms. The clinician reassesses the child's symptoms from the perspectives of both child and caregiver, asking first for the child's report and then for the caregiver's. The clinician also asks both about the use and usefulness of the coping strategies that were discussed and practiced in the previous session. Based on that discussion, the clinician may suggest modifications to the coping strategies and/or introduce additional approaches to lowering the child's symptoms.

Case Example Mia: Session 4
In Session 4, Regina was much more emotionally present and connected with Mia than in previous sessions. In fact, she was now openly supportive and encouraging. When the clinician inquired about the previous week and whether Mia's symptoms had decreased since the last session, Mia's mother proudly reported several examples of effective communication, times they practiced the coping strategies, and times during the week when they had spent quality time together. Mia appeared less anxious and made eye contact more frequently with both her mother and the clinician.

7.2.6 Session 5: Meeting Together with the Child and Caregiver, Including Case Disposition and Recommendations

The final session of CFTSI has the same structure as Session 4 with the key addition of making disposition decisions and discussing next steps at the end of the session. Similar to Session 4, the clinician meets with the child and caregiver to discuss the experiences of the previous week and assess current status of trauma symptoms. The clinician points out and supports demonstrations of concordance regarding to the child's trauma symptoms which are the result of better communication, reviews the coping strategies discussed in previous sessions, and introduces additional strategies to further lower the child's trauma reactions, if necessary. In addition, the clinician assesses whether there is a need for further trauma-focused treatment or treatment for any previously unidentified preexisting disorders uncovered during CFTSI. Recommendations and plans are made to address any additional treatment needs that have been identified.

Post-CFTSI Assessments
While disposition planning in Session 5 is based on the current status of the child's symptoms, the original screening instrument is also re-administered following the conclusion of CFTSI. The comparison between the pre- and post-screening assessments has been useful to both clinicians and families in confirming successful mastery of posttraumatic reactions, as well as identifying areas that may remain problematic and require further intervention. Additionally, comparing pre- and post-assessments can serve an important function for clinicians, supervisors, and their agencies in tracking the effectiveness of the treatment, as well as helping to identify challenges to implementation that may require further consideration. In addition, caregivers complete a consumer satisfaction survey to indicate the extent to which different elements of CFTSI were helpful.

> **Case Example Mia: Session 5**
> By the last CFTSI session, Mia's symptoms had decreased significantly. Perhaps as a result of having achieved greater symptomatic control, Mia was now in a better position to focus on her continuing thoughts/feelings of self-blame. In their discussion, the clinician suggested that focusing the blame on herself offered Mia an alternative to the reality of loss of control that occurred in the original traumatic experience. Slowly, Mia could begin to appreciate that her wish for a sense of control and her need to reverse feelings of helpless were leading to a distorted view of herself as the focus of blame. In other words, if the abuse was her fault, Mia could fantasize that she had control in a situation where, in fact, she had not. Mia could also recognize that this was an emotionally costly strategy. With her greater appreciation of her distorted views of herself, Mia became more receptive to strategies that would help her to interrupt her repetitive, intrusive thoughts of self-blame. Notably, this was

supported by her mother who turned to Mia, put her arm around her, and said warmly, "Mia, I know it's not your fault. I love you and I'm here to help you." In response to this genuine, heartfelt statement, Mia visibly relaxed. After this interaction, Mia was much more open and able to talk with her mother about her worries and her symptoms, including the occurrence of self-blaming intrusive thoughts.

Following the completion of CFTSI Session 5, which included case disposition and recommendations, the clinician re-administered the original symptom screening instrument in order to make a final evaluation of the status of Mia's posttraumatic symptoms. Both Mia and her mother reported a major decrease in Mia's symptoms, and the symptoms were, in fact, below clinically significant levels. They expressed great pleasure in what they now recognized as a shared achievement. Relieved of the feeling that she was only a burden to her mother and with lines of communication more open, Mia was now able to experience her mother as a source of help and support.

These sessions are added if more time is needed to focus on addressing the following:

(a) Helping the caregiver manage and decrease their own trauma symptomatology through the introduction of coping strategies
(b) Engaging a caregiver who is initially less supportive of the child (e.g., is angry at the child, initially blames the child for the traumatic event, etc.)
(c) Ensuring that a child or caregiver with cognitive limitations or developmental delays is fully engaged and understands the focus of the clinical work
(d) Addressing the concerns of a child who is initially hesitant to communicate with the caregiver about his/her traumatic stress reactions or other issues that may arise

While CFTSI is generally conducted in five treatment sessions, it is not uncommon for one to three additional CFTSI sessions to be added as needed.

7.2.7 Skill Level of Clinicians

CFTSI is provided by Master's, Ph.D., or MD level mental health clinicians. Training in CFTSI assumes that clinicians already have training in the phenomena of trauma and trauma reactions, child development, as well as client engagement skills

7.3 Special Challenges in Implementing CFTSI

In order to successfully implement CFTSI, the clinician must be able to recognize and meet challenges that may arise when conducting an early, brief intervention such as CFTSI. Several of these challenges are described below.

7.3.1 Children Who Are Hesitant to Communicate with Their Caregivers About Their Trauma Symptoms

It is not uncommon for children to be hesitant about communicating with their caregivers about their trauma symptoms. Some children are concerned that by revealing their symptoms, they are also revealing their own unwanted sense of feeling small, helpless, and needy. Other children may be concerned that if they discuss their symptoms, they will further burden caregivers who are already impacted by the traumatic event. For yet other children, especially adolescents, communicating about symptoms reflects neediness and feels contrary to normal strivings for autonomy and independence. These same children may even project a host of reactions onto their caregiver, including increased upset, anger, intrusive overprotectiveness, and even blame for the precipitating events.

The CFTSI model anticipates these potential concerns in several ways. Having conducted the first session with the caregiver, the clinician has some sense of the caregiver's initial attitudes about the traumatic event, the child's presenting symptomatology, and about their child more generally. In the next CFTSI session, the clinician has the opportunity to review the child's experience of his/her symptoms, as well as to directly raise the question with the child about whether he/she has any concerns about their caregiver's reactions. Within this context, the clinician can discuss with the child the idea that alerting the caregiver to the child's experience of symptoms and concerns, which will happen in Session 3, has the advantage of decreasing isolation and increasing the role of the caregiver as a supportive ally in the child's mastering of distressing symptoms. Furthermore, the clinician can also consider whether the child's concerns are part of a recognized pattern of avoidance: that is, whether reluctance to discuss symptoms with the caregiver is grounded in an attempt to avoid acknowledging and reflecting on the child's symptoms or, alternatively, reflects valid concerns about the caregiver's response. In either case, the clinician's work with the child and caregiver attempts to identify and decrease the sources of these concerns as part of the CFTSI process. By helping the child convey these concerns openly with the caregiver in the third session of CFTSI, the clinician helps both the child and caregiver appreciate key factors contributing to the child's behavior and symptoms. Key factors may include: the caregiver's inaccurate expectations and/or real reactions that may inhibit child-caregiver communication; and the caregiver's capacity to support the child's mastery of distressing symptoms.

7.3.2 Traumatized Caregivers

In many CFTSI cases, caregivers have been traumatized by the same precipitating events that have overwhelmed their children. Some affected adults are able to mobilize their highest levels of functioning in support of their children. Others, however, are less able to contain their own traumatic dysregulation and may therefore be less able to attend to the symptoms or feelings of their children, or they may at times be unable to distinguish between their reactions and those of their children. Similarly, traumatic events that impact children may also arouse reactions in caregivers that derive from the caregiver's own trauma history. For many, the unconscious nature of the link between past and current experiences can contribute to caregiver's difficulties in distinguishing between their own aroused feelings and those of their children. When caregiver's distress and the sources thereof go unidentified and unaddressed, adults may not only suffer more than is necessary, but they may also unwittingly expose their children to continued insecurity at a time when children are most in need of emotional stability, predictability, and support from caregivers.

CFTSI addresses the challenge of implementing CFTSI with traumatized caregivers beginning in the first session by first reviewing caregivers' own ideas about trauma and then providing information about the impact of traumatic events that applies equally to children and adults. Using a standardized assessment tool, clinicians ask caregivers about their own current symptoms. This provides clinicians with the opportunity to explore the historical context of these symptoms with regard to both previous traumatic events and possible long-standing symptoms. The aim of these inquiries is twofold: (1) to determine what intervention strategies might be useful in addressing the caregivers' symptoms above and beyond what might be gained from participation in CFTSI (including a referral for caregiver's own treatment, if indicated); and (2) to help caregivers more clearly recognize ways in which their own reactions may be coloring their experiences of, and response to, their child's reactions. With these goals in mind, an additional individual meeting with the caregiver may be scheduled in preparation for, or as an adjunct to, the joint sessions with the child. Identifying their own posttraumatic reactions heightens caregivers' abilities to observe, monitor, and respond to their child's symptoms and can simultaneously increase conscious awareness of the need to get help in managing their own traumatic dysregulation. In many situations, caregivers also benefit from learning and practicing coping skills intended for their child.

7.3.3 Angry, Child-Blaming Caregivers

It is not uncommon for clinicians to encounter caregivers who are angry at, and even blame, the child for the occurrence of the traumatic events themselves. This is especially challenging for clinicians whose successful implementation of CFTSI is based on enhancing and capitalizing on a caregiver's greater appreciation of and support for the child's experience. When the clinician is confronted with the discrepancy between what the clinician believes the child needs and what is seen as the caregiver's unhelpful, unsupportive attitudes, the clinician may experience a range of reactions. Without conscious recognition and control, the clinician's human reaction of frustration and annoyance may undermine the basic aims and approaches of CFTSI. For example, a clinician may feel frustrated with the caregiver and may inadvertently express anger by defending the child or lecturing at the caregiver. Similarly, the clinician may prematurely determine that there is no possibility of mobilizing the caregiver's productive participation in CFTSI. Before doing either, it is incumbent on the clinician to explore what might be interfering with the caregiver's capacity and motivation to engage in CFTSI.

Toward this end, the clinician must first be able to recognize the extent to which identification with the child is narrowing clinical perspective and biasing reactions. When the clinician is able to appreciate and observe this potential area of vulnerability, he/she is in a much better position to return to the role of therapist – that is, to step back and consider the source(s) of the caregiver's angry and/or blaming attitude toward the child. For example, the child's symptomatology may remind the caregiver of his/her own traumatic experience and may trigger his/her own posttraumatic symptoms. Similarly, the caregiver may become angry and blaming when the child's symptomatic behaviors are experienced as a current challenge to the caregiver's sense of efficacy and control, so dramatically interrupted by the traumatic event. As such, getting angry and blaming the child for the precipitating traumatic events may be the caregiver's unconscious attempt to undo his/her own original and continued experience of loss of control and helplessness.

In order to address these challenges, CFTSI clinicians are able to use findings from their structured assessment of the caregiver's posttraumatic reactions and trauma history, as well as the child's developmental and trauma histories to inform discussions with the caregiver about their angry and blaming attitudes. When caregivers express and hold on to these attitudes firmly during the first CFTSI session, it is often helpful for the clinician to schedule an additional meeting with the caregiver in order to explore these issues more fully. The aim of such a meeting is to decrease the automatic nature of unhelpful responses to the child by increasing the caregiver's recognition and understanding of the factors that contribute to these attitudes and how they can interfere with recovery for both the child and caregiver. Identifying any of the child's long-standing, preexisting difficulties with which the caregiver has been challenged in the past may offer a chance to establish an empathic connection.

Helping the caregiver to identify ways in which their own posttraumatic symptoms may be impacting the child's recovery can help the caregiver to better address their child's needs as they are better able to appreciate the difference between their own reactions and those of their child. The recognition of this distinction can also increase the caregiver's capacity for their own self-care. At times, referring the caregiver for his/her own treatment may allow greater engagement in CFTSI.

7.4 Research on the CFTSI Model

Research on clinical interventions affords the opportunity to explore a host of questions. While it is essential to demonstrate efficacy in randomized trials, it is also critical to demonstrate effectiveness in real-world settings. In addition, it is crucial to understand which elements are central mechanisms of therapeutic action. CFTSI research strategies will seek to address all of these questions. To date, there have been several methodological approaches taken in the development of the evidence base for CFTSI, including a randomized clinical trial and a chart review of CFTSI cases completed in community settings. On the basis of the research to date, CFTSI has been included in the US Substance Abuse and Mental Health Services Administration's (SAMHSA) National Registry of Evidence-based Programs and Practices (NREPP), as well as in the California Evidence-Based Clearinghouse for Child Welfare.

7.4.1 Randomized Control Trial

A randomized clinical trial (RCT) was conducted from 2007 to 2009 (Berkowitz et al. 2011) and involved participants aged 7–17 who were referred by a hospital-based child abuse program or an urban police department or recruited from a pediatric emergency department after a potentially traumatic event. Children and parents were screened by phone or in person using the PTSD Checklist-Civilian (PCL-C) (Weathers et al. 1994) and were initially determined eligible if either caregiver or child endorsed at least one PTSD symptom. Eligible participants were randomized using a block design to CFTSI or the comparison condition. Children in the CFTSI condition ($N = 53$) received the four-session version of the CFTSI model as it was protocolized at that time.[1] Children in the comparison condition ($N = 53$) received a protocolized four-session intervention that included psychoeducation and both individual caregiver and child meetings as well as meetings with the child and caregiver together. The study focused on the diagnosis of PTSD immediately after the intervention and 3 months post-intervention. PTSD was measured using the UCLA PTSD Reaction Index for DSM IV (Pynoos et al. 1998). Logistic regression was performed to examine group differences in PTSD diagnosis at 3 months following the end of treatment ($N = 82$), while controlling for new potentially traumatic events. CFTSI reduced the odds of a full PTSD diagnosis by 65 % and a partial diagnosis by 73 % (see Fig. 7.1). PTSD was applied as a dichotomous variable. Logistic regression was used, and any new potentially traumatic event was controlled for in both groups: Investigators found an odds ratio of .345. Thus, youth receiving CFTSI were 65 % less likely to have PTSD at the 3-month follow-up than youth in the comparison condition. Subsequent analyses demonstrated an effect size was 0.4 ($p < .03$) (Carla Stover, personal communication, June, 2011).

---

[1] The original model as evaluated in the RCT was described as having four sessions with the possible addition of two to three sessions, when indicated, to address additional needs of the child, caregiver, or both. In this earlier version of CFTSI, what are now Sessions 2 and 3 were conducted on the same day. As CFTSI was disseminated into a broader array of clinical settings, clinicians found it was less problematic logistically to schedule these two sessions on separate days. As a result, CFTSI is now described as a five- to eight-session model.

Fig. 7.1 Percent of youth meeting PTSD criteria at baseline and 3-month follow-up

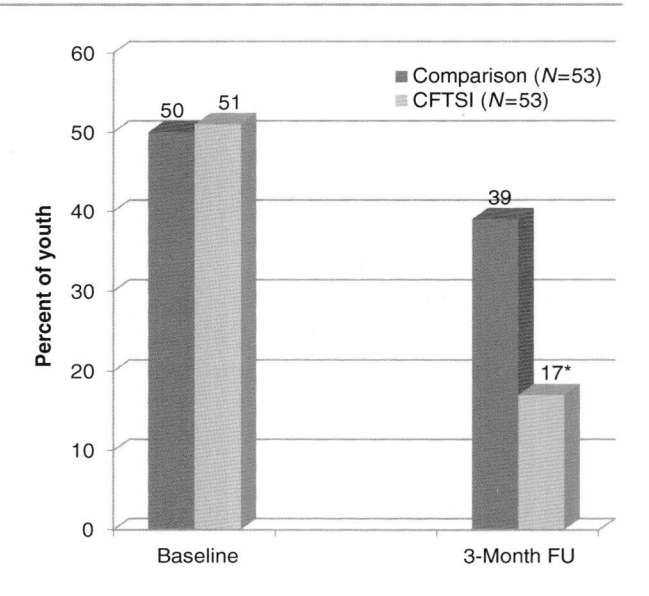

7.4.2 Chart Review

In addition to the RCT, two additional studies of CFTSI have utilized a chart review approach to examine CFTSI cases completed at the Safe Horizon CACs in New York City. The first study (Oransky et al. 2013) examined caregiver and child agreement regarding child exposure to potentially traumatic events, children's PTSD and mood symptoms, and children's functional impairment while controlling for caregivers' PTSD symptoms. Samples for both studies included 114 caregiver-child dyads that completed CFTSI following disclosure of sexual abuse in a forensic setting. Participating caregivers were predominantly mothers ($N = 99$); in a small number of cases, the participating caregiver was the father ($N = 6$) or another family member ($N = 9$). Child PTSD symptoms were measured using Part I, and functional impairment was measured using Part II of the Child PTSD Symptom Scale (CPSS) (Foa et al. 2001); mood symptoms were assessed using the Short Mood and Feelings Questionnaire (MFQ) (Angold and Costello 1987); exposure to potentially traumatic events was measured using the Trauma History Questionnaire (THQ) (Berkowitz and Stover 2005); and caregiver PTSD symptoms were assessed using the PCL-C (Weathers et al. 1994). At baseline, children reported significantly higher rates of PTSD and mood symptoms as compared to caregivers, and discrepancies were significantly, positively correlated with children's greater reported levels of PTSD and depressive symptoms ($p < .05$) as well as functional impairment ($p < .001$). In addition, investigators found that caregiver PTSD symptom severity was significantly and positively associated with caregiver reports of children's PTSD symptoms, depressive symptom severity, and youth functional impairment (Oransky et al. 2013).

The second chart review study examined the outcomes of CFTSI when implemented in the CAC setting following sexual abuse (Hahn et al. 2015). This study evaluated whether the findings of the RCT demonstrating a reduction of traumatic stress symptoms immediately following the intervention were replicated in a real-world setting. In addition, the relationship between child and caregiver symptomatology at baseline and the effectiveness of CFTSI was examined in order to assess for whom CFTSI was most beneficial. De-identified data was extracted from charts of 114 CFTSI cases completed at Safe Horizon's CACs in New York City. Paired sample t-tests found significant differences between child traumatic stress symptoms pre- and post-CFTSI using the CPSS (Foa et al. 2001) (t(117) = 11.07, $p < .001$) (see Fig. 7.2). Caregiver and child ratings of child's symptom severity as measured by the CPSS were compared at baseline and post-intervention in order to assess change in the concordance between child and caregiver's ratings of child traumatic stress symptom severity, with children reporting higher levels of traumatic stress symptoms as compared to caregivers (t(106) = 3.55, $p < 01$). No significant difference was found between child and caregiver ratings of child traumatic stress symptom severity post-intervention. Child's baseline symptom severity (CPSS) and trauma history as measured using the THQ (Berkowitz and Stover 2005) were found to be significantly, positively associated with symptom severity following CFTSI (both $p \leq .01$), while caregiver's baseline PTSD symptoms as assessed using the PCL-C (Weathers et al. 1994) were not associated with child's post-intervention symptom severity. This finding demonstrates the ability of CFTSI to interrupt the natural course of symptom development in children whose caregivers demonstrate posttraumatic symptomatology (Hall et al. 2006; Kassam-Adams et al. 2006; Nugent et al. 2007; Shemesh et al. 2005). Additional research is needed to understand the mechanisms of action and the effectiveness of distinctive components of the CFTSI model on the child's peritraumatic stress symptoms and thereby upon the course of a child's posttraumatic recovery (Shemesh et al. 2005).

The limitations of the chart review methodology are well recognized; however, these chart reviews provide important support for the CFTSI model and in particular the model's capacity to meaningfully affect posttraumatic symptomatology and

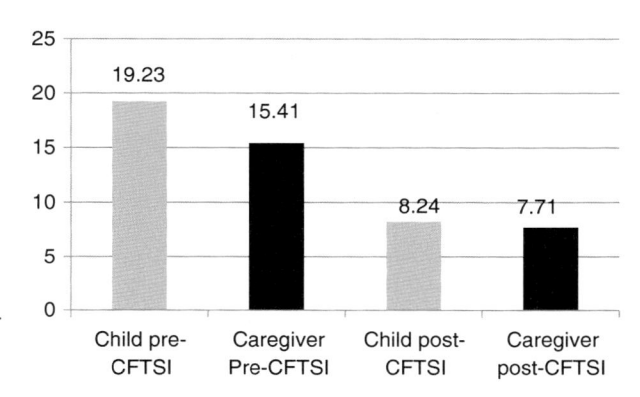

Fig. 7.2 Child and caregiver CPSS ratings pre- and post-CFTSI

	Child pre-CFTSI	Caregiver Pre-CFTSI	Child post-CFTSI	Caregiver post-CFTSI
	19.23	15.41	8.24	7.71

caregiver-child communication, when implemented in a real-world setting. By demonstrating the feasibility of implementing and evaluating CFTSI at Safe Horizon's CACs, we hope to begin the process of establishing CFTSI as being effective in community programs.

7.4.3 Open Trial

While additional large-scale randomized trials would be invaluable to answer questions about the intervention, significant challenges to funding clinical trials have proven a considerable impediment. At the same time, CFTSI investigators have recognized the opportunity for evaluation that is created through the process of CFTSI dissemination and implementation. CFTSI includes standardized symptom assessments as an integral part of the clinical intervention and provide support and structure to clinicians as they provide analogous support and structure to traumatized children and families As such, implementation of the CFTSI protocol automatically yields information through which investigators can continue to learn about the intervention.

The CFTSI Site Sustainability Project (CSSP) was created as a mechanism to simultaneously support agencies in their implementation of the CFTSI model and allow for ongoing development of the model's evidence base. Agencies are asked to join the CSSP at the time of clinical training. Utilizing a web-based data collection platform in real time, CFTSI providers enter limited demographic information and pre-intervention symptom information on all cases that are screened for CFTSI and limited additional information for all cases that start the intervention. Conceptualized to serve dual functions, the CSSP operates as a quality assurance system for users, while offering investigators a mechanism for gathering data about large numbers of CFTSI cases as they are completed in a variety of treatment settings. All information entered into the system is collected in the course of screening for and implementing the CFTSI model. This information is used to generate implementation metrics that are reported back to agency teams each month and are utilized as part of a continuous quality improvement process. In addition, the system has been designed to support fidelity to the model, following the intended path of the clinical intervention, and agency participation is in turn supported by offering specific benefits to participants at all levels, including automated scoring and graphic representations of symptom assessments for clinicians; feedback about status of model implementation for supervisors; and data about the impact of CFTSI at the agency level, including the metric of consumer satisfaction, for agency leaders.

At the same time, collecting de-identified client level information that emerges naturally from implementation of the clinical intervention, CFTSI investigators have the opportunity to examine pre-, post-, and follow-up data on significant numbers of cases and ultimately to move beyond the question of *Does CFTSI work?* to *How well does CFTSI work in different settings and with different populations?* This question is of particular interest because it redresses a key weakness of RCT methodology, which has the capacity to demonstrate significance, but often is very selective with respect to eligibility criteria and imposes strict protocol adherence, which frequently results in a considerable diminution of RCT effects when translated into real-world settings.

7.4.4 Future Directions

In addition to pursuing further investigations with RCT and chart review methodologies, the CSSP and open trial approach to studying CFTSI offer exciting prospects for expanding the current evidence base in real-world settings in which this brief treatment model is being introduced. The use of standardized measures and the entering of clinical data into the centralized CSSP for all CFTSI cases is leading to a constantly growing n that will not only continue to address outcome and efficacy but will afford the opportunity to explore the details of CFTSI's mechanisms of therapeutic action as well as challenges to implementing early trauma-focused treatment for children and families.

The excitement that CFTSI has generated among agency leaders and mental health professionals serving children and their caregivers following traumatic events has been significant, as evidenced by the continuous and growing demand for training in the clinical model. In addition to its role in evaluating and further refining the CFTSI model, the CSSP offers support for these teams of dedicated mental health professionals as they undertake the tasks of adopting and sustaining CFTSI implementation within their agencies.

References

Angold, A., Costello, E. J., Messer, S. C., Pickles, A., Winder, F., & Silver, D. (1995). The development of a short questionnaire for use in epidemiological studies of depression in children and adolescents.International Journal of Methods in Psychiatric Research, 5, 237–249.

Berkowitz S, Epstein C, Marans S (2012) The child and family traumatic stress intervention implementation guide for providers. Childhood Violent Trauma Center, New Haven, CT.

Berkowitz S, Stover CS (2005) Trauma history questionnaire parent and child version. Questionnaire. Childhood Violent Trauma Center, New Haven, CT.

Berkowitz S, Stover CS, Marans S (2011) The child and family traumatic stress intervention: secondary prevention for youth at risk of developing PTSD. J Child Psychol Psychiatry 52(6):676–685. doi:10.1111/j.1469-7610.2010.02321.x

Breslau N, Kessler RC, Chilcoat HD, Schultz LR, Davis GC, Andreski P (1998) Trauma and post-traumatic stress disorder in the community: the 1996 detroit area survey of trauma. Arch Gen Psychiatry 55(7):626–632

Davidson JR, Hughes D, Blazer DG, George LK (1991) Post-traumatic stress disorder in the community: an epidemiological study. Psychol Med 21(3):713–721

Epstein C, Marans S, Berkowitz S (2013) The child and family traumatic stress intervention treatment application for children in foster care. Childhood Violent Trauma Center, New Haven, CT

Foa EB, Johnson KM, Feeny NC, Treadwell KR (2001) The child PTSD symptom scale: a preliminary examination of its psychometric properties. J Clin Child Psychol 30(3):376–384. doi:10.1207/s15374424jccp3003_9

Foa EB, Meadows EA (1997) Psychosocial treatments for posttraumatic stress disorder: a critical review. Annu Rev Psychol 48:449–480. doi:10.1146/annurev.psych.48.1.449

Hahn H, Oransky M, Epstein C, Smith Stover C, Marans S (2015) Findings of an early intervention to address children's traumatic stress implemented in the child advocacy center setting following sexual abuse. J Child Adolesc Trauma 1–12. doi: 10.1007/s40653-015-0059-7

Hall E, Saxe G, Stoddard F, Kaplow J, Koenen K, Chawla N, Lopez C, King L, King D (2006) Posttraumatic stress symptoms in parents of children with acute burns. J Pediatr Psychol 31(4):403–412. doi:10.1093/jpepsy/jsj016

Hill H, Levermore M, Twaite J, Jones L (1996) Exposure to community violence and social support as predictors of anxiety and social and emotional behavior among African American children. J Child Fam Stud 5(4):399–414

Kassam-Adams N, Garcia-Espana JF, Miller VA, Winston F (2006) Parent-child agreement regarding children's acute stress: the role of parent acute stress reactions. J Am Acad Child Adolesc Psychiatry 45(12): 1485–1493. doi: 10.1097/01.chi.0000237703.97518.12 00004583-200612000-00011 [pii]

Kliewer W, Cunningham JN, Diehl R, Parrish KA, Walker JM, Atiyeh C et al (2004) Violence exposure and adjustment in inner-city youth: child and caregiver emotion regulation skill, caregiver-child relationship quality, and neighborhood cohesion as protective factors. J Clin Child Adolesc Psychol 33(3):477–487

Marans S (2013) Phenomena of childhood trauma and expanding approaches to early intervention. Int J Appl Psychoanal Stud 10(3):247–266. doi:10.1002/aps.1369

Marans S, Epstein C, Berkowitz S (2014) The child and family traumatic stress intervention treatment application for young children. Childhood Violent Trauma Center, New Haven, CT

Nugent NR, Ostrowski S, Christopher NC, Delahanty DL (2007) Parental posttraumatic stress symptoms as a moderator of child's acute biological response and subsequent posttraumatic stress symptoms in pediatric injury patients. J Pediatr Psychol 32(3):309–318. doi:10.1093/jpepsy/jsl005

Oransky M, Hahn H, Stover CS (2013) Caregiver and youth agreement regarding youths' trauma histories: implications for youths' functioning after exposure to trauma. J Youth Adolesc 42(10):1528–1542. doi:10.1007/s10964-013-9947-z

Ozer EJ, Best SR, Lipsey TL, Weiss DS (2003) Predictors of posttraumatic stress disorder and symptoms in adults: a meta-analysis. Psychol Bull 129(1):52–73

Pynoos R, Frederick C, Nader K, Arroyo W et al (1987) Life threat and posttraumatic stress in school-age children. Arch Gen Psychiatry 44(12):1057–1063

Pynoos R, Rodriguez N, Steinberg AM, Stuber M, Frederick C (1998) The UCLA PTSD reaction index for DSM IV (Revision 1). Univerity of California/Trauma Psychiatry Program, Los Angeles

Salmon K, Bryant RA (2002) Posttraumatic stress disorder in children. The influence of developmental factors. Clin Psychol Rev 22(2):163–188

Shemesh E, Newcorn JH, Rockmore L, Shneider BL, Emre S, Gelb BD et al (2005) Comparison of parent and child reports of emotional trauma symptoms in pediatric outpatient settings. Pediatrics 115(5):582–589. doi:10.1542/peds.2004-2201

Southwick SM, Charney DS (2012) Resilience: the science of mastering life's greatest challenges. Cambridge University Press, New York

Trickey D, Siddaway AP, Meiser-Stedman R, Serpell L, Field AP (2012) A meta-analysis of risk factors for post-traumatic stress disorder in children and adolescents. Clin Psychol Rev 32(2):122–138. doi: http://dx.doi.org/10.1016/j.cpr.2011.12.001

Weathers F, Litz B, Herman D, Huska J, Keane T (1994) The PTSD checklist-civilian version (PCL-C). National Center for PTSD: Boston, MA

Trauma-Focused Cognitive Behavioral Therapy

Matthew D. Kliethermes, Kate Drewry, and Rachel Wamser-Nanney

8.1 Theoretical Underpinnings

Trauma-Focused Cognitive Behavioral Therapy (TF-CBT; Cohen et al. 2006a) is the most widely used and disseminated treatment for children and adolescents who have been exposed to traumatic events (Cohen et al. 2010). TF-CBT is appropriate for children ages 3–18 who have experienced a trauma and are subsequently exhibiting significant trauma-related difficulties such as post-traumatic stress disorder (PTSD), depression, and behavior problems. TF-CBT is a components-based treatment model that includes individual child and caregiver sessions, as well as conjoint child-caregiver sessions designed to support the child's relationship to his/her caregiver within the context of coping with trauma. For the past 25 years, TF-CBT has been evaluated, and the research conducted to date demonstrates that TF-CBT is effective for children of different developmental stages, cultures, and those who have experienced different traumatic events. Indeed, TF-CBT has amassed the most extensive empirical support of all interventions for treating childhood trauma (Cohen et al. 2010) and has been deemed a Model Program by the US Substance Abuse and Mental Health Services Administration (SAMSHA 2015).

M.D. Kliethermes (✉)
Children's Advocacy Services of Greater St. Louis,
Department of Psychological Sciences, University of Missouri-St. Louis (UMSL),
St. Louis, MO, USA
e-mail: kliethermesm@umsl.edu

K. Drewry
Children's Advocacy Services of Greater St. Louis,
University of Missouri-St. Louis (UMSL), St. Louis, MO, USA
e-mail: drewryk@umsl.edu

R. Wamser-Nanney
Department of Psychological Sciences, University of Missouri-St. Louis (UMSL),
St. Louis, MO, USA
e-mail: wamserr@umsl.edu

As the name indicates, TF-CBT is a cognitive behavioral intervention at heart. Yet, in many ways TF-CBT is a "hybrid" intervention. TF-CBT predominantly combines trauma-sensitive interventions with cognitive behavioral principles but also includes "dashes" of attachment, developmental neurobiology, family, empowerment, and humanistic theory in order to best meet the various needs of traumatized children and families (Cohen et al. 2006a). In the following section we discuss the theoretical underpinnings of TF-CBT and describe how CBT principles are used to address trauma-related symptoms in children.

8.1.1 Stress Management

The initial TF-CBT components originate from stress management models, such as stress inoculation therapy (SIT; Meichenbaum 1985), in order to prepare children for subsequent exposure to trauma-related memories. Stress management techniques including education about stress and trauma as well as relaxation, affect regulation, and cognitive skills are implemented in early sessions to increase the child's ability to tolerate the trauma processing that occurs throughout TF-CBT (Cohen et al. 2006a). Education about trauma normalizes trauma exposure and reactions and establishes the rationale for trauma processing. Relaxation provides the child with the ability to better regulate emotional and physiological arousal during trauma processing. Affect regulation and cognitive coping skills help the child better identify, express, and modulate the emotions and thoughts he/she experienced during the trauma and in their daily life. The early TF-CBT components begin the gradual exposure process as discussing trauma, and learning skills to manage stress require that the child begins to indirectly process his/her trauma experiences, a critical aspect of TF-CBT.

Using the analogy of teaching a child to ride a bike, the stress management aspect of TF-CBT is like the preparation that occurs before the child actually gets on the bike. The child may be taught the basics of how to pedal, steer, and brake and may be provided with necessary safety equipment (e.g., helmet, pads) before riding the bike. The child may also be taught the "rules of the road" and how to safely ride a bike. Rather than just putting the child on a bike and saying, "Okay, go!" preparing a child decreases the child's anxiety about riding the bike (and the caregiver's!) and increases the child's likelihood of success.

8.1.2 Gradual Exposure to Traumatic Content

A core principle of TF-CBT is the use of gradual exposure (Cohen et al. 2006a). Gradual exposure involves progressively exposing the child to trauma reminders and memories of increasing intensity. Trauma is discussed in every TF-CBT session. During the initial components of treatment, the child identifies his/her trauma reminders and plans ways to cope with them. In the trauma narration component, the child begins by describing less upsetting parts of the trauma and gradually begins to discuss the most distressing aspects. The child eventually experiences less distress in response to trauma-related content. Successfully tolerating this distress helps the child develop a sense of mastery over traumatic memories, by breaking the association between traumatic memories/reminders and strong emotional or physiological reactions. Gradual exposure also allows the child to learn that thinking about or talking about his/her trauma can be done safely.

It is important to highlight the benefits of *gradual* exposure as opposed to "flooding" the child with trauma content. Gradually exposing the child to trauma content ensures that his/her coping resources are not overwhelmed. Alternately, exposing the child to overwhelming trauma content might cause the child to deteriorate in session and/or fall back on maladaptive coping strategies (e.g., dissociation, self-injury, substance abuse). Neither of these outcomes helps accomplish the goal of breaking the child's mental associations between traumatic memories and current distress.

The value of gradual exposure over flooding can also be illustrated using the example of learning to ride a bike. A child who is initially afraid of riding a bike will begin to lose that fear once he/she has successfully ridden a bike for the first time. They will then naturally and gradually take on more challenging bike-riding activities without significant distress. However, if the first time a child rides a bike, the parent pushes them down a steep hill and the child crashes at the bottom, the child's fear of riding a bike will remain the same or increase; and it will be much harder to get back on the bike. Exposure work in TF-CBT is also done gradually to prevent this sort of "crash." Possession of well-developed coping skills decreases the likelihood of the child and caregiver of being overwhelmed during gradual exposure.

8.1.3 Cognitive Interventions

Cognitive-based interventions are another core mechanism of TF-CBT. An increase in negative and/or inaccurate beliefs about the self (e.g., self-blame, incompetence), others (e.g., people are untrustworthy), and the world (e.g., the world is a dangerous place) is commonly associated with trauma (Brewin and Holmes 2003). Per cognitive theory, beliefs of this nature can lead to a variety of negative outcomes including PTSD symptoms, depression, anxiety, and aggressive or self-destructive behaviors (Beck 1976). In TF-CBT, cognitive interventions are used to prevent or ameliorate these difficulties by improving the child's ability to monitor cognition and develop more accurate, healthy beliefs (Cohen et al. 2000).

Returning to the bike-riding analogy, a child who successfully learns to ride a bike may later crash and scrape his/her knee. The child may then start to doubt his/her abilities and avoid bike riding. If a parent reminds the child of all the times he or she has successfully ridden a bike before, the child may regain his/her confidence and ride the bike again. In the context of trauma, following sexual abuse by a man, a child may develop the belief that all men are dangerous and untrustworthy. The child may then experience anxiety around and avoid future contact with men. In TF-CBT, cognitive interventions are used to help the child understand the impact of this thought on his or her feelings and behaviors, become aware of cognitive distortions, and develop the ability to evaluate his/her thoughts and beliefs.

8.1.4 Caregiver Involvement

Although TF-CBT is inherently child focused, the model recognizes the critical impact that caregivers have on their children, particularly as models for coping with trauma. Caregiver involvement in TF-CBT is paramount for two primary reasons. First, following a trauma children often look to their caregiver to determine how to respond. Children may learn both adaptive and maladaptive reactions to trauma through observational learning from their caregivers (Deblinger and Heflin 1996). Ideally the caregiver's involvement in treatment would focus on increasing the extent that they model adaptive coping strategies and decrease their use of maladaptive strategies. Second, there are clear indications that adaptive caregiver functioning has a significant positive impact on children's trauma-related symptoms (Cohen and Mannarino 2000). The inclusion of caregivers in TF-CBT is therefore conceptualized to be a key mechanism for recovery (Cohen et al. 2006a).

The main goals of caregiver involvement are to increase the caregiver's ability to effectively parent the child, ensure that the caregiver recognizes the need for gradual exposure, and address the caregiver's own distress and cognitive distortions related to the child's trauma. This allows the caregiver to more effectively model trauma-related coping and support the child. These goals are accomplished in a parallel fashion to that used with the child. Caregivers learn effective parenting skills and stress management, engage in gradual exposure, and identify and correct trauma-related cognitive errors. For example, the therapist educates the caregiver about the importance of helping the child "face" their traumatic memories and helps the caregiver practice the skills needed (e.g., empathic listening) to support the child's trauma processing. The therapist also "coaches" the caregiver to use these skills in conjoint sessions, so that the caregiver will be able to continue implementing the skills after treatment has ended. The child and caregiver are brought together during conjoint parent-child sessions at regular intervals so that the caregiver can model adaptive communication and coping skills for dealing with post-traumatic reactions and provide emotional support to aid the child's recovery from trauma.

Returning to the analogy of learning to ride a bike a final time, the caregiver teaching a child to ride a bike may also be anxious about the child falling down or doubt that the child will ever be successful. That anxiety may result in the caregiver delaying bike-riding lessons or being reluctant to let go and allow the child to ride independently. The child may sense the caregiver's anxiety, become anxious as well, and also avoid riding the bike. Conversely, if the caregiver models riding a bike for the child, communicates confidence in the child's ability, maintains a calm demeanor, and runs alongside shouting encouragement while prepared to steady the child if he/she should start to wobble, this will increase the odds of success. A particularly anxious caregiver may need external support in order to be an effective model. They would likely benefit from talking to other caregivers who have successfully taught their children to ride a bike and to learn particular strategies that were most effective.

8.2 How to Do TF-CBT

8.2.1 Overview of the TF-CBT Model

The TF-CBT model consists of nine components which can be summarized by the acronym PRACTICE: **p**sychoeducation and **p**arenting, **r**elaxation, **a**ffective expression and modulation, **c**ognitive coping, **t**rauma narrative and processing, **i**n vivo mastery, **c**onjoint parent-child sessions, and **e**nhancing future safety and development (see Cohen et al. 2006a for further details). The PRACTICE acronym also serves as a reminder for the child, family, and therapist of the value of practicing these skills during and after treatment. Although the PRACTICE components are consistent across trauma types, TF-CBT values flexibility and creativity. Thus, the components are tailored to the characteristics of the child (e.g., age, interests, strengths, and difficulties) and to the type(s) of trauma the child has experienced. Sessions are structured such that, in each session, the therapist meets individually with the child and his/her caregiver(s) to provide the TF-CBT content to the child and caregiver in a parallel fashion. Caregivers also receive additional intervention to increase their use of effective parenting skills. The entire TF-CBT model is trauma focused, with exposure to trauma-related content included in every session. Perfect mastery of skills is not required; however, children should exhibit significant gains in each component prior to beginning the next. At the end of each component, the therapist facilitates conjoint work in which the child and caregiver review the content covered in the completed component. Therapists have the opportunity to exercise flexibility in determining the length and pace of treatment. In general, however, TF-CBT sessions last 50–60 min and include individual time for the child and caregiver. Standard TF-CBT lasts 8–16 treatment sessions, with one-third of the time working on the stabilization skills, one-third for trauma narration and processing, and one-third for conjoint work, in vivo mastery, and safety. In some cases of complex trauma (as is illustrated in the case study in this chapter), treatment may last 16–24 sessions, with one-half of treatment devoted to stabilization skills, one-fourth spent in trauma narration and processing, and one-fourth in conjoint, in vivo mastery, and safety.

Overview of the PRACTICE Components

- *Psychoeducation* is the first component and is key in enhancing engagement, reducing stigma, and modeling non-avoidance of trauma-related content. Psychoeducation begins during the feedback session following a trauma-focused assessment. The caregiver and child are provided information regarding the trauma(s) (e.g., prevalence rates, who typically experiences it, common myths), as well as common reactions to trauma such as PTSD, emotional and behavioral difficulties, and feelings of guilt and shame. The clinician tailors the content to the particular client and includes the assessment results to describe the child's trauma reactions. Information regarding the child's diagnosis should be provided in an honest but digestible manner without a lot of clinical jargon. For instance, reexperiencing and avoidance symptoms of PTSD can be described as upsetting reminders of the trauma, and, because of this distress, the child tries to avoid those reminders. Normalization of trauma-related responses can be a very powerful intervention. The clinician also discusses how trauma can impact caregivers. For some caregivers, children's trauma disclosure can actually be a traumatic event. Further, many caregivers of abused children may have experienced negative interpersonal interactions after the abuse is discovered (e.g., "How could you not have known he was abusing your daughter?"). Some caregivers would benefit from their own individual therapy to support their recovery from their child's trauma. Referring caregivers for their own treatment should be done sensitively and conveyed not as a punishment but as recognition of how distressing it is when one's child experiences trauma. The therapist also provides an overview of the TF-CBT model. For trauma-exposed children and their caregivers, psychoeducation regarding the empirical support for TF-CBT can instill hope. Finally, both children and caregivers should receive information about the specific type(s) of trauma experienced by the child. For example, a child exposed to sexual abuse may benefit from learning about what constitutes sexual abuse, the prevalence of sexual abuse, and feelings and thoughts commonly experienced by sexual abuse survivors. This content serves to demystify the specific trauma type, normalize the child's reactions, and gradually expose the child to direct discussion of trauma. The material covered in this component can also be referenced during later cognitive processing.

- *Parenting training* is also initiated at the outset of treatment and continues throughout the model. Parental support and effective parenting are critical predictors of children's recovery from trauma (Cohen and Mannarino 2000; Deblinger et al. 1996), and parents often find it challenging to manage children's difficult behaviors that might have developed or intensified in the aftermath of trauma. Parenting skills emphasized in TF-CBT include praise, selective attention, time-out, contingency reinforcement programs (e.g., sticker charts), and effective commands and consequences. Functional behavioral analyses can be conducted to gain valuable information regarding the child's behavior to maximize treatment success. In individual sessions with the caregivers, therapists can engage the caregivers in role-plays or discuss specific behavioral examples to give the caregiver practice using these skills in session. The therapist can also model these skills for the caregiver during conjoint parent-child sessions.
- *Relaxation* techniques help children reduce their bodies' physiological response to stress- and trauma-related cues. It is often useful to begin with differentiating between normal and traumatic stress responses and help the child understand the rationale for relaxation. The therapist and child should identify times when relaxation skills are necessary to use, including scenarios in which trauma-related cues are present. As different relaxation strategies are effective for different people, the therapist and child should engage in a variety of adaptive relaxation skills to build their coping "toolkit" such as focused breathing, mindfulness, meditation, guided imagery, and progressive muscle relaxation. Some children may resist traditional relaxation activities and instead may engage in

exercise, yoga, or relaxation activities such as listening to music, art, and gardening. The caregiver also learns relaxation skills to manage their own stress as well as to be able to reinforce those skills in their child.
- *Affective expression and modulation* helps increase children's ability to identify feelings, especially trauma-related feelings (e.g., shame, rage, terror, helplessness). Trauma-exposed children often have overwhelming and painful trauma-related feelings, which they may struggle to identify, express, and modulate. Here, the therapist helps the child recognize, label, and express a range of feelings while reinforcing the fact that all feelings are valid. Activities used to engage children in building these affective identification and expression include games, feelings charades, books, and art therapy techniques. The therapist helps the child link emotions with trauma reminders. Children are taught skills to help manage their emotions more effectively such as positive self-talk, thought interruption, and problem-solving with the goal of building a "toolkit" with which they can manage difficult emotions.
- *Cognitive coping* facilitates children's ability to identify their thoughts and understand the relationship between thoughts, feelings, and behavior. Children initially learn how to identify their thoughts. Thoughts can be described to younger children as "our brains talking to us" and illustrated through the use of games such as playing twenty questions, guessing the number the child is thinking, and singing songs in their head. Children then learn to distinguish between thoughts and feelings. The therapist explains the cognitive triangle to demonstrate the relationship between thoughts, feelings, and behaviors using scenarios that are tailored to the child's development and interests. During this discussion, the therapist should reiterate the idea that it is possible to change one's feelings and behaviors by altering one's thoughts. The therapist can present examples of cognitive distortions such as all-or-nothing and catastrophic thinking in developmentally sensitive ways. These skills will be eventually used to challenge and correct trauma-related cognitions that are inaccurate and/or unhelpful.
- *Trauma narration and processing* is when the child focuses on the specific trauma(s) experienced in the form of gradual exposure. The therapist begins by explaining the rationale for gradual exposure to the caregiver and child. Then the therapist assists the child in identifying a narration format. Trauma narration can take many forms; some children choose to write and draw about their experiences in a storybook, while others might create a timeline, perform a skit or puppet show, or write a poem. The goal is for the child to recount their traumatic memories while experiencing safety and support in the context of the therapeutic relationship, thereby unpairing the memories from overwhelming or distressing feelings. The final product is much less important than the process. Once the child has completed their base account of the traumatic event, the therapist and child review it to add additional details as well as thoughts and feelings the child had during the time of the trauma. The child's level of distress should be monitored throughout trauma narration to avoid overwhelming the child, recognizing that manageable levels of distress are an expected part of trauma processing.

After the child has directly discussed the trauma, the therapist helps the child identify, analyze, and revise any trauma-related cognitive distortions or thoughts that are inaccurate or unhelpful. These distortions often become evident during the child's trauma narration and processing. They might also be uncovered by asking the child to engage in meaning-making discussions or activities. Common trauma-related cognitive distortions include self-blame, overestimation of danger, or that the child is damaged due to the trauma. Once distorted thoughts are identified, the therapist can use cognitive processing techniques such as Socratic questioning, responsibility pie, or the best friend role-play, to help the child explore and revise them.

While the child is engaged in trauma narration and processing, the caregiver should also be directly discussing the trauma in sessions with the therapist. As long as it is clinically indicated, the therapist reviews the child's trauma narrative or similar product individually with the caregiver as it is being created. At the end of this component, children generally share their narrative with their caregiver in a conjoint session during which the caregiver provides support and reinforces healthy trauma-related cognitions.

- *In vivo mastery* helps children master innocuous trauma-related cues (e.g., a child who experienced a dog attack becoming fearful and avoidant of all dogs) occurring in the "real world" and decreasing dysfunctional avoidant behaviors. Children learn to "face their fears" of trauma-related cues through the use of gradual exposure in real-world settings. The exposure plan should be as detailed as possible with gradually increasing amounts of exposure to the feared stimulus. As these exposures generally occur outside of treatment, it is critical that the caregiver is actively involved and in agreement with the exposure plan to ensure the child's success.
- *Conjoint parent-child sessions* are intended to occur in most TF-CBT components and are designed to facilitate positive communication and parental support. These sessions are utilized to help children and their caregivers practice the skills learned in TF-CBT and communicate more openly about the traumatic event. For conjoint work, 60-min sessions can be divided so that the therapist meets with the child for 15 min, then with the caregiver for 15 min, and then all together for 30 min. During PRAC conjoint sessions, the caregiver, child, and therapist will review the skills learned in the component in an engaging, family-oriented manner. For example, psychoeducation material can be reviewed while playing a psychoeducation bingo game.
- *Enhancing future safety and development* typically occurs at the end of TF-CBT and is intended to provide the child and caregiver with the necessary skills to safely cope with future stressors. This component may also be used earlier in treatment should immediate safety concerns arise (as is illustrated in the case study). Although we cannot assure the child will never be revictimized, we can teach children personal safety skills designed to increase feelings of preparedness and reduce risk for revictimization. The child can practice personal safety skills in role-plays with the clinician. Depending on the child's particular trauma and developmental stage, other content commonly covered in this component

includes sex education, healthy versus unhealthy relationships, and violence prevention. Clinicians can also provide the child education regarding risky behaviors such as substance use and sex. Finally, caregivers should be encouraged to consider future potential parenting situations such as dating and substance use and develop trauma-informed parenting responses. The therapist should also help the child and caregiver identify possible future trauma reminders and plan for ways of coping with them. Finally, the therapist reviews the skills learned and progress made during the course of treatment and works to prepare the caregiver and child for graduation.

8.2.2 Case Study

Jenny Smith is a 14-year-old biracial female living with her biological mother, Ms. Smith, and her stepfather. Jenny experienced multiple traumas including domestic violence between her biological parents from ages 0–5, severe emotional abuse by her stepmother from ages 5–8, multiple episodes of sexual abuse including vaginal penetration by her stepmother's older son (age 8), the imprisonment of her biological father on drug-related charges (ages 12 to present), and severe bullying at school, particularly during the fifth grade.

Upon initiation of services, the therapist completed clinical interviews and trauma-focused assessment measures with Jenny and Ms. Smith. Assessment results indicated that Jenny exhibited significant symptoms of PTSD (e.g., frequent flashbacks, psychological distress triggered by trauma reminders, avoidance of trauma reminders, severe hyperarousal), depression, and social anxiety. Jenny and Ms. Smith reported that these symptoms began at the time Jenny had contact with her stepmother (age 5–8) but had been exacerbated by subsequent exposure to bullying. Jenny frequently spent the majority of each day alone in her room and avoided most social interactions. Due to her chronic emotional distress, she often used a variety of maladaptive coping strategies, primarily self-injury and marijuana, to aid in emotional regulation. Jenny had worked with multiple therapists prior to the TF-CBT provider and had been hospitalized multiple times due to suicidal ideation and self-injury (i.e., cutting herself on her legs with broken glass). The TF-CBT provider discussed concerns regarding initiating TF-CBT in the context of ongoing self-injurious behavior. However, Jenny expressed a strong need to resolve the PTSD symptoms that she was experiencing and indicated a willingness to discontinue self-injury. Jenny and the TF-CBT therapist agreed to a safety contract that Jenny would discontinue self-injurious behavior and that the provider would assess for self-injury in each session. They agreed that if self-injury requiring medical attention recurred, progress through the TF-CBT components would be discontinued until sufficient safety and stability could be restored.

Psychoeducation The clinician began psychoeducation during the assessment process. When providing assessment feedback and discussing the treatment plan, the therapist took care to help Jenny and Ms. Smith connect Jenny's emotional and behavioral difficulties to her past trauma experiences. In particular, the therapist noted that Jenny's exposure to chronic trauma and stress throughout early childhood had impacted her ability to self-regulate, especially her emotions. Over the course of the next three sessions, the TF-CBT provider explained this to Jenny and Ms. Smith using the concept of "survival brain." Jenny learned how post-traumatic stress reactions could be conceptualized as an individual being "stuck" in survival brain. That is, even though she was not currently in actual life or death situations, her brain was reacting as though she was. Jenny was exhibiting frequent "survival responses" such as fighting (e.g., frequent arguments with her stepfather), escaping (e.g., withdrawing to her room, substance use), freezing (e.g., shutting down in social situations), giving up (e.g., no longer attempting to make friends, not giving effort on schoolwork), and crying for help (e.g., suicidal threats, self-injurious behavior, clinging to her mother).

During the psychoeducation component, the therapist initiated the typical TF-CBT session structure of individual work with both Jenny and Ms. Smith and subsequent conjoint work focused on facilitating trauma-focused communication between them. Jenny was initially highly resistant to remaining in the waiting room while the therapist met with Ms. Smith, stating that "people were looking at her" and predicting that she would have a panic attack. Jenny requested to join the therapist and Ms. Smith or remain in an unoccupied room near the therapist's office. The therapist explained to Jenny that this was an example of "survival brain," whereby her brain was operating as though danger was present without any observable evidence.

During the conjoint psychoeducation session, Jenny and Ms. Smith played a game of "trauma trivia" with questions focused on the occurrence and impact of trauma in general and the specific traumas that Jenny had experienced. The activity encouraged collaboration and communication between Jenny and Ms. Smith in a playful, enjoyable manner. Upon reflection, Jenny commented that, prior to starting TF-CBT, she never would have believed that she and Ms. Smith could have a positive conversation about these topics.

Parenting Parenting education also began during the assessment process and continued throughout the remainder of treatment. During the assessment, Ms. Smith and the therapist discussed various behavior management strategies that Ms. Smith had attempted and Jenny's reactions to those efforts. The concept of "survival brain" was also used to assist Ms. Smith in understanding the emotional and behavioral difficulties that Jenny was experiencing during interactions with Ms. Smith and her stepfather. This led to discussions regarding how common parenting practices such as threats of consequences, expression of anger, and judgmental statements might be a "trigger" for Jenny, or an event reminiscent of previous trauma, therefore causing a trauma reaction. During one session early in treatment, Ms. Smith practiced de-escalation techniques such as speaking in a low, calm voice, using validation and empathy in response to Jenny's outbursts. The therapist encouraged Ms. Smith to use these strategies during conjoint sessions and checked in with her throughout treatment on the use of the strategies at home.

Relaxation Due to Jenny's high level of dysregulation and history of self-injury, the clinician spent four sessions working in this component. As Jenny had previously participated in non-trauma-focused therapy, she had been exposed to multiple forms of relaxation but suggested that they were unhelpful. The therapist explained the rationale for relaxation, noting that due to being stuck in survival brain, Jenny's body was primed for survival responses, which are counter to being relaxed. The therapist explained that relaxation techniques are one way to help "turn off survival brain." The clinician also determined that one reason Jenny had limited success with previous relaxation work was due to her having limited awareness of her arousal level. She would either fail to recognize the need for using relaxation skills or would attempt to implement them when she was already in an extreme state of arousal. The therapist taught Jenny a modified version of a Subjective Units of Distress Scale (SUDS), which included both her current level of distress (from 0 to 10, with 10 indicating extreme distress) and her current level of self-control (from 0 to 10, with 10 indicating complete lack of control). Of note, Jenny reported increased self-regulation simply from monitoring her level of distress. The therapist explored her current methods of relaxation. She reported currently using aromas and visual images to aid in relaxation and meditation. Therefore, the therapist encouraged Jenny to utilize sensory-based relaxation strategies (e.g., scented candles, lava lamp) in combination with more traditional techniques such as focused breathing, mindfulness, and progressive muscle relaxation.

During caregiver sessions, the therapist introduced Ms. Smith to the rationale for relaxation and familiarized her with the techniques that Jenny found most helpful. At the end of this component, Jenny and her mother completed conjoint work during part of a session where Jenny taught Ms. Smith the mindfulness strategies that she had learned, which they then practiced together. Ms. Smith and Jenny discussed how they could implement mindfulness activities at home.

Affect Expression and Modulation Jenny presented with a well-developed vocabulary of "feeling words" and exhibited a solid ability to identify and express her emotions. She demonstrated a tendency to "wallow" in her emotions rather than to avoid them. Thus, the therapist focused on helping Jenny understand the role of emotions in "survival brain." Over the course of two sessions, Jenny learned that the primary functions of emotions are to help us understand our environment, to help communicate how we are doing to others, and to motivate action. She began to understand that when in survival brain, emotions may be triggered by relatively innocuous events in the present that in some way resemble past trauma. Jenny had historically responded to these emotions with some form of maladaptive coping response, such as marijuana or self-injury. The therapist and Jenny discussed that emotions can be tolerated without action and they will eventually dissipate. She practiced this "emotional tolerance" skill along with previously honed relaxation strategies. Jenny also developed behavioral strategies focused on changing her surroundings and becoming active (e.g., going for a walk) to help her break out of mood states.

During the same two sessions, the therapist taught Ms. Smith the concept of "emotion coaching," that is, focusing on helping Jenny label her emotions and accepting her emotions in a validating fashion. Ms. Smith initially struggled with this type of interaction, having a tendency to focus on her own emotions and become defensive and blaming. The therapist helped Ms. Smith identify this pattern and engaged her in role-plays to practice responding empathetically to Jenny's feelings. Ms. Smith became gradually more adept at this process and was able to successfully use them in a conjoint session, largely focused on Jenny's feelings about her father's upcoming release from prison.

Cognitive Coping The therapist spent four sessions addressing this component as many of Jenny's difficulties appeared tied to inaccurate and unhelpful beliefs related to her trauma. Jenny had previously frequently articulated negative beliefs about herself and others. She often expressed that she was worthless or deficient in some way and that other people were predatory or otherwise untrustworthy. Although these beliefs seemed related to Jenny's trauma history, they influenced her current relationships with family and peers. The therapist introduced her to the cognitive triangle to help her understand the connection between thoughts, feelings, and behaviors. For example, Jenny recognized that her frequent thoughts about people being dangerous resulted in periods of intense anxiety that caused her to distance herself even further from the people around her.

The therapist also explained the concept of thinking errors, highlighting Jenny's emotional reasoning and mind reading. As homework, Jenny began tracking her thoughts using thought records and ultimately practicing the process of testing and correcting her thinking errors. The term "thought balancing" was used to highlight that Jenny's beliefs tended to focus on the most negative interpretation of events and that they needed to be "balanced" by including all available information. For example, Jenny reported frequent thoughts that "she wasn't good enough" to be successful at her schoolwork. In reaching that conclusion, she focused on a specific situation in which she was having difficulty with an assignment, and her teacher commented that she was "slacking." Jenny "balanced" this thought by paying attention to other "evidence," such as the fact that she recently received high grades on multiple assignments and that all students struggle with schoolwork on occasion. This led to the balanced belief that although she was struggling on the current assignment, by and large she was successful academically.

Meanwhile, Ms. Smith also learned the cognitive concepts and skills Jenny learned. She practiced applying the cognitive triangle and thought balancing to her own experiences. The therapist encouraged Ms. Smith to assist Jenny in thought balancing at home and conducted a conjoint session in which Ms. Smith helped Jenny identify a recent thinking error and walk through the process of thought balancing.

Although many of the beliefs that Jenny expressed appeared to be related to past trauma, the therapist did not actively attempt to identify and correct trauma-related distortions (e.g., "It's my fault my stepmother abused me") at this time. Within TF-CBT, cognitive restructuring of trauma-related beliefs ideally is delayed until after completion of the child's trauma narrative. This allows the therapist to have an optimal understanding of the child's traumatic experiences prior to helping them develop more accurate and helpful beliefs.

Enhancing Safety and Future Development In the typical progression through TF-CBT, enhancing safety and future development is the final component, although this component can be implemented earlier if significant safety or stability concerns arise. At this point in treatment, Jenny reported increased conflict with her stepfather, which escalated until Jenny became physically aggressive with him after he verbally degraded her. She became increasingly depressed and subsequently engaged in her first incident of self-injury since beginning TF-CBT. Jenny was hospitalized for a week, and changes were made with regard to her medications. Subsequently, Jenny's depressive symptoms decreased significantly, and she reported no longer experiencing urges to self-harm.

Following her release from the hospital, the clinician resumed services with Jenny. However, as stipulated in the safety contract initiated at the beginning of treatment, typical progression through TF-CBT was temporarily discontinued, and the enhancing safety component was prioritized. For approximately 1 month, sessions were focused on assessing her current stability, revisiting previously learned coping strategies, and assessing the appropriateness of resuming TF-CBT progression. It became evident that Jenny was experiencing a significant benefit from her new medication regimen and that her mother and stepfather had made efforts to decrease the amount of conflict in the home. She expressed the desire to resume TF-CBT, stressing that the early components had been helpful despite her self-injurious behavior. Ms. Smith also noted that Jenny seemed to be functioning much better after her discharge from the hospital as demonstrated by her reduced symptoms of depression. Therefore, the therapist resumed TF-CBT with Jenny, with frequent monitoring of any suicidal ideation and urges to self-harm.

When TF-CBT restarted, the therapist briefly reviewed the previously learned cognitive coping skills. In a conjoint session, Jenny and Ms. Smith discussed a recent thinking error that Jenny had experienced and developed a more balanced belief by exploring the evidence for and against the initial belief. Jenny continued practicing cognitive coping skills via thought tracking homework throughout the remainder of TF-CBT. She began exhibiting independent application of these skills, such as self-correcting a thought (i.e., "My mom doesn't love me") that she experienced during an argument with Ms. Smith. The therapist determined that Jenny had sufficiently mastered the PRAC skills to begin direct gradual exposure in the trauma narration and processing component.

Trauma Narration and Processing Given the complexity of Jenny's trauma history, the therapist decided to work with Jenny to develop a timeline of critical events, including traumatic ones that she had experienced during her life. This approach allows the trauma narrative process to capture all events that might have an impact on the child's current functioning, without requiring detailed processing of each event. A timeline also allows for the therapist to gradually increase the intensity of trauma exposure. Processing can begin by talking about traumatic events generally but then shift to more detailed discussion of specific events that are most distressing.

Over the course of six sessions, Jenny recognized that the emotional abuse by her stepmother and the sexual abuse by her stepmother's son caused her the most distress. The therapist assisted Jenny in processing these experiences in greater detail, with Jenny describing specific incidences of each, focusing on sensory detail and her emotional and cognitive experiences of the trauma. Jenny initially found this process distressing, reporting distress levels reaching an "8" or "9" on the SUDS scale. When these periods of distress occurred, the therapist reminded Jenny that her distress was a normal manifestation of "survival brain" and encouraged her to use her coping skills to help calm her brain's "survival response." When necessary, Jenny took brief breaks to implement one or more of these skills and then resumed trauma exposure and processing. By the end of this component, Jenny found that she could tolerate extended periods of trauma processing with only mild to moderate levels of distress.

While constructing her timeline and engaging in detailed processing of emotional and sexual abuse experiences, it became evident that two cognitive themes were consistent across many experiences. Jenny had developed persistent beliefs that she is worthless and that other people are inherently dangerous. The therapist initiated cognitive processing work related to these themes. She explored how the various events on her timeline contributed to the development of these beliefs. For example, Jenny's feelings of worthlessness corresponded to the emotional abuse by her stepmother. She came to realize that her negative beliefs about herself and others were the by-product of her past trauma and not accurate in a broader context. This ultimately led her to develop two balanced beliefs. Jenny concluded, "Although people have tried to convince me I was worthless, my view of myself does not have to be based on their opinion." She also determined, "Some people have tried to hurt me in my life, but many people have not. I don't have to be afraid of everyone."

During this component, the therapist shared Jenny's work on her trauma narrative with Ms. Smith and discussed how to provide appropriate support and empathy during discussions about trauma. This process was difficult for Ms. Smith. She experienced significant guilt related to Jenny's exposure to domestic violence and emotional abuse. Ms. Smith struggled with a tendency to want to tell Jenny how to cope with her experiences more effectively, rather than empathizing with the emotional pain Jenny was experiencing. Ms. Smith also engaged in cognitive processing regarding her beliefs about her level of responsibility for Jenny's trauma exposure. This work helped her recognize the difference between being *responsible* for an outcome versus *regretting* an outcome and to respond to Jenny in a less defensive manner. After the narration and processing was complete, Jenny shared her timeline and her "lessons learned" with Ms. Smith in a conjoint session. Ms. Smith was able to remain present and supportive in the conjoint trauma narrative session, during which she served as an empathetic witness to Jenny's traumatic experiences.

In Vivo Mastery The in vivo component was especially beneficial for Jenny due to her difficulties with social anxiety. In vivo exposure started early in treatment to help her overcome her avoidance of social interactions, particularly with groups of unfamiliar people. Jenny initially requested to remain in an empty room near the therapist's office while the therapist met individually with Ms. Smith, rather than staying in the waiting room. The therapist encouraged Jenny to remain in the waiting room for gradually increasing periods of time while the therapist met with Ms. Smith. Over time, she began tolerating remaining in the waiting room for 30 min with minimal distress. To further address her social anxiety, the therapist assigned Jenny homework to explore safe social settings in her daily life (e.g., sitting in a coffee shop). Ms. Smith played an important role in this process. For example, she initially stayed with Jenny in the coffee shop and then gradually moved further away from Jenny until she was outside of the building. Jenny eventually became able to remain in some public places on her own for up to 30 min. No further in vivo exposure work was required following the trauma narration component.

Enhancing Safety and Future Development Although safety served as an ongoing focus during the entire course of TF-CBT with Jenny, the therapist revisited the enhancing safety and future development at the conclusion of treatment. Here, the focus of the component shifted from addressing present concerns to considering how Jenny might maintain her current level of safety and stability in the future. Over the course of four sessions, the therapist devoted significant time to helping Jenny identify potentially triggering situations that she might experience in the future such as intimate relationships and criticism from teachers or employers. Jenny planned to use the skills she had mastered earlier in treatment in future situations. Given her tendency toward cognitive errors, the therapist focused on cognitive coping skills that Jenny had learned in prior sessions, stressing the importance of checking and balancing her thoughts on a regular basis. Jenny decided to hang a picture of the cognitive triangle in her room to remind her to check her thoughts on a regular basis. Jenny also worked to develop assertiveness and communication skills to ensure that she would be able to effectively advocate for herself as needed. The therapist encouraged Ms. Smith to consider difficult parenting situations (e.g., dating, substance use, conflict between Jenny and her stepfather) that might arise and to develop potential trauma-informed parenting approaches (e.g., negotiation, developmentally appropriate limit setting) that she might implement in response to those challenges.

Toward the end of treatment, Jenny and Ms. Smith completed the assessment measures to reevaluate Jenny's level of trauma-related difficulties. Both reported that Jenny was exhibiting significantly reduced symptoms of PTSD and depression. Ms. Smith noted that Jenny was functioning well at school and appeared less withdrawn at home. Jenny noted that she was not experiencing ongoing flashbacks or intrusive thoughts and reported a decrease in negative thoughts about self and others. She also stated that she had not engaged in any further self-injurious behavior since the incident that occurred mid-treatment and that she had significantly decreased her marijuana use. Having completed all PRACTICE components, and based on Jenny's improved functioning, Jenny, Ms. Smith, and the therapist determined that Jenny had successfully completed TF-CBT. Jenny and her mother both participated in a "graduation" session that focused on celebrating Jenny's progress during TF-CBT. Ms. Smith conveyed her pride in Jenny's accomplishments. More importantly, Jenny expressed feeling proud of herself and communicated her strengthening belief that she was competent to face her future.

8.3 Special Challenges

8.3.1 Lack of Caregiver Engagement

As discussed, caregiver engagement is a critical ingredient of TF-CBT. When TF-CBT is implemented optimally, therapists spend approximately one-half of therapy time working with caregivers in parallel individual sessions and periodic conjoint caregiver-child sessions. Research findings show that TF-CBT is more effective when caregivers are engaged (Cohen et al. 2006a). Caregiver participation in TF-CBT is associated with greater reductions in children's externalizing and depressive symptoms (Deblinger et al. 1996) as well as increased parenting efficacy and reduced trauma-related distress and depressive symptoms in caregivers (Cohen et al. 2004a). Unfortunately, many TF-CBT providers struggle with caregiver engagement and treatment buy-in (Hanson et al. 2014). The failure to effectively engage caregivers may be due to therapists' lack of understanding of the importance of caregiver participation or concrete barriers experienced by caregivers that limit their ability to participate in treatment.

The literature on treatment engagement identifies concrete (e.g., lack of transportation or child care) and perceptual (e.g., beliefs about therapy) barriers to engaging families in child mental health services (Gopalan et al. 2010). McKay and colleagues have developed manualized engagement strategies in which clinicians directly elicit and address possible concrete and perceptual barriers during a pretreatment phone call and during part of the first session (McKay and Bannon 2004). In a randomized trial, children and foster parents who participated in TF-CBT plus the engagement intervention were less likely prematurely terminate treatment (Dorsey et al. 2014). TF-CBT providers looking to increase caregiver engagement might consider implementing evidence-based engagement strategies to use during initial phone and in-person contacts.

The ultimate goal of engagement, of course, isn't just for caregivers to attend sessions but for them to actively collaborate in the therapy process, implement new strategies, and follow therapeutic recommendations. TF-CBT therapists can set the stage for this by working to ensure caregivers, many of whom have likely felt judged or blamed by other professionals, feel heard, respected, and valued. As part of the engagement intervention, McKay recommends identifying the caregiver's own greatest concern about the child, even when it differs from the referral reason (McKay and Bannon 2004). Therapists can then provide concrete strategies or resources to address the caregiver's identified concern (e.g., sleep issues, behavior problems, school refusal) at the outset of treatment (or highlight how it will be targeted later in the TF-CBT model).

8.3.2 Insufficient Gradual Exposure in Early Components

Inadequate gradual exposure in the early TF-CBT components is another common implementation barrier. Beginning TF-CBT clinicians may mistakenly believe that the model is divided into two halves: the skill-building components (P-P-R-A-C) and the trauma-focused components (T-I-C-E). In fact, the entire model is trauma focused, with gradual exposure to trauma reminders incorporated into every session. For example, during the psychoeducation phase, the clinician should refer to the specific trauma type the child experienced by its correct name (e.g., "the domestic violence" rather than "that thing that happened") and provide basic information about its prevalence, impact, and so forth. Since this information is communicated in a developmentally appropriate and engaging way, the child is unlikely to experience distress despite the activation of trauma memories; instead, he or she begins to make new associations between the trauma memories and feelings of safety and empowerment (Cohen et al. 2012). Through gradual exposure, the child learns from the outset of treatment that he or she can grow stronger from confronting trauma reminders.

Without sufficient gradual exposure in the P-P-R-A-C components, the therapist is (often unwittingly and unknowingly) reinforcing the child's traumatic avoidance. This makes the child's (and the therapist's) job much harder when it comes time for the trauma narration and processing. Without the "baby steps" that gradual exposure affords, the child has not had the opportunity to learn experientially that addressing trauma reminders is a manageable, safe, and helpful activity. Completing the narration and processing may therefore seem like a bigger deal than it is, and the child may be more reluctant to begin or require a slower pace, prolonging treatment unnecessarily. As attrition from therapy is common, many children who start TF-CBT will be unable to finish treatment, often for reasons beyond their control. For those who terminate prematurely, many may do so before they start or complete the trauma narration and processing; for these clients, the gradual exposure in the P-P-R-A-C components is the only exposure they will experience in a therapeutic setting.

8.3.3 Crises of the Week

Crises of the week (COW) are another often encountered TF-CBT implementation barrier. When therapists consistently sacrifice gradual exposure or skill building to attend to COW, they are undermining the effectiveness of the model by interfering with its continuity and progression (Cohen et al. 2006a). Instead, therapists should use their clinical judgment and creativity to respond to families' concerns and practical needs in ways that do not slow down treatment or reinforce traumatic avoidance. When children or caregivers experience a significant stressor (e.g., death of a loved one, change in placement) during treatment, it is generally appropriate for the therapist to provide supportive listening to maintain the therapeutic alliance (Cohen et al. 2010). These events can also be used to reinforce psychoeducation (especially when the stressor involves a trauma-related adversity) and the use and generalization of coping skills (Cohen et al. 2010). Thus, whenever possible, the COW become grist for the therapeutic mill, working in service of, rather than counter to, the goals of P-P-R-A-C components.

In other cases, a TF-CBT therapist might consider reserving a small amount of time (no more than 10 or 15 min) at the beginning or end of the session for problem-solving about a child or caregiver's identified COW (e.g., school-related issue, relationship breakup). Again, the therapist should look for ways to review and reinforce concepts and skills covered in prior components. Alternatively, the therapist could spend the last few minutes of a session working to link a family with community resources. The key is that the therapist does not allow too much time to be diverted from the model's trauma focus. If the COW are too significant or distracting to allow for discussion of trauma-related material in every session, alternate treatment approaches should be considered (Cohen et al. 2010).

8.4 Research and Empirical Support

The initial efficacy for the TF-CBT extends into the early 1990s, when the TF-CBT developers began independently conducting intervention studies for sexually abused children (Cohen and Mannarino 1993; Deblinger et al. 1990). Over the past two decades, TF-CBT has become the first-line treatment for childhood trauma and is the most extensively researched treatment for trauma-exposed children (Cohen et al. 2010). Numerous randomized clinical trials have demonstrated that TF-CBT is effective at reducing the impact of trauma in children ages 3–17 exposed to wide variety of traumatic events in the United States (Cohen et al. 2004a, b) and around the world (Murray et al. 2013; O'Callaghan et al. 2013). TF-CBT has been observed to have superior outcomes in relation to community treatment as usual (Deblinger et al. 1996), nondirective supportive therapy (Cohen and Mannarino 1996), child-centered therapy (Cohen et al. 2004a, b), and wait-list control (King et al. 2000). TF-CBT is effective at mitigating the adverse impact of trauma for a variety of traumatic events including intimate partner violence (Cohen et al. 2011) and traumatic grief (Cohen et al. 2004b, 2006b).

Importantly, TF-CBT is able to address the myriad of adverse consequences that can follow exposure to trauma. Children who have received TF-CBT exhibit improvements in anxiety, depression, sexual problems, dissociation, feelings of shame, and PTSD symptoms (Cohen and Mannarino 1996; Cohen et al. 2004a, b). Children's caregivers have also been observed to benefit from TF-CBT and exhibit lower levels of abuse-related distress, improved parenting skills, and increased supportive parent-child interactions following TF-CBT. Further, treatment gains have been observed to be maintained at 1-year follow-up (Cohen and Mannarino 1997;

Deblinger et al. 2006). In a recent meta-analysis of TF-CBT, TF-CBT was observed to significantly improve PTSD, depressive symptoms, and behavior problems at posttreatment and throughout 1 year posttreatment (Carey and McMillen 2012).

In summary, TF-CBT is an effective treatment for children ages 3–18 who have experienced trauma and is viewed as a "first-line" treatment for reducing trauma-related symptoms. TF-CBT has been widely disseminated to community sites through numerous statewide learning collaboratives (Cohen and Mannarino 2008). Even though the evidence supporting TF-CBT continues to mount, the research literature regarding the TF-CBT model is still developing. Work is needed to examine predictors of positive treatment response and for whom TF-CBT will be most effective. Studies investigating the timing and dosing of the PRACTICE components may provide new insights regarding effectively delivering TF-CBT. Dismantling studies regarding the need for each of the PRACTICE components would also prove useful. Finally, in light of the significant efforts to disseminate TF-CBT, dissemination research is needed to determine the best method for learning the model and how to support new TF-CBT clinicians' use of the TF-CBT model with adequate fidelity.

References

Beck AT (1976) Cognitive therapy of the emotional disorders. Penguin, New York

Brewin CR, Holmes EA (2003) Psychological theories of posttraumatic stress disorder. Clin Psychol Rev 23:339–376

Cary CE, McMillen JC (2012) The data behind the dissemination: a systematic review of trauma-focused cognitive behavioral therapy for use with children and youth. Child Youth Serv Rev 34(4):748–757

Cohen JA, Mannarino AP (1993) A treatment model for sexually abused preschoolers. J Interpers Violence 8:115–131

Cohen JA, Mannarino AP (1996) A treatment outcome study for sexually abused preschool children: Initial findings. J Am Acad Child Adolesc Psychiatry 35:42–50

Cohen JA, Mannarino AP (1997) A treatment study for sexually abused preschool children: outcome during a one-year follow-up. J Am Acad Child Adolesc 36:1228–1235

Cohen JA, Mannarino AP (2000) Predictors of treatment outcome in sexually abused children. Child Abuse Negl 24:983–994

Cohen JA, Mannarino AP (2008) Disseminating and implementing trauma-focused CBT in community settings. Trauma Violence Abuse 9:214–226

Cohen JA, Mannarino AP, Berliner L, Deblinger E (2000) Trauma-focused cognitive behavioral therapy: an empirical update. J Interpers Violence 15:1203–1223

Cohen JA, Deblinger E, Mannarino AP, Steer RA (2004a) A multi-site, randomized controlled trial for children with sexual abuse-related PTSD symptoms. J Am Acad Child Adolesc Psychiatry 43:393–402

Cohen JA, Mannarino AP, Knudsen K (2004b) Treating childhood traumatic grief: a pilot study. J Am Acad Child Adolesc Psychiatry 43:1225–1233

Cohen JA, Mannarino AP, Deblinger E (2006a) Treating trauma and traumatic grief in children and adolescents. The Guildford Press, New York

Cohen JA, Mannarino AP, Staron VR (2006b) A pilot study of modified cognitive-behavioral therapy for childhood traumatic grief (CBT-CTG). J Am Acad Child Adolesc Psychiatry 45:1465–1473

Cohen JA, Bukstein O, Walter H, Benson RS, Chrisman A, Farchione TR, Hamilton J, Keable H, Kinlan J, Schoettle U, Siegel M, Stock S, Medicus J, AACAP Work Group On Quality Issues

(2010) Practice parameter for the assessment and treatment of children and adolescents with posttraumatic stress disorder. J Am Acad Child Adolesc Psychiatry 4:414–430

Cohen JA, Mannarino AP, Iyengar S (2011) Community treatment of posttraumatic stress disorder for children exposed to intimate partner violence: a randomized controlled trial. Arch Pediatr Adolesc Med 165:16–21

Cohen JA, Mannarino AP, Deblinger E (eds) (2012) Trauma-focused CBT for children and adolescents: treatment applications. Guilford Press, New York

Deblinger E, Heflin AH (1996) Treating sexually abused children and their nonoffending parents: a cognitive behavioral approach. Sage, Thousand Oaks, CA

Deblinger E, McLeeer SV, Henry D (1990) Cognitive behavioral treatment for sexually abused children suffering post-traumatic stress: preliminary findings. J Am Acad Child Adolesc Psychiatry 29(5):747–752

Deblinger E, Lippman J, Steer R (1996) Sexually abused children suffering posttraumatic stress symptoms: initial treatment outcome findings. Child Maltreat 1:310–321

Deblinger E, Mannarino AP, Cohen JA, Steer RA (2006) A follow-up study of a multisite, randomized, controlled trial for children with sexual abuse-related PTSD symptoms. J Am Acad Child Adolesc Psychiatry 45(12):1474–1484

Dorsey S, Pullmann MD, Berliner L, Koschmann E, McKay M, Deblinger E (2014) Engaging foster parents in treatment: a randomized trial of supplementing trauma-focused cognitive behavioral therapy with evidence-based engagement strategies. Child Abuse Negl 38:1508–1520

Gopalan G, Goldstein L, Klingenstein K, Sicher C, Blake C, McKay MM (2010) Engaging families into child mental health treatment: updates and special considerations. J Can Acad Child Adolesc Psychiatry 19:182–196

Hanson RF, Gros KS, Davidson TM, Barr S, Cohen J, Deblinger E, Mannarino AP, Ruggiero KJ (2014) National trainers' perspectives on challenges to implementation of an empirically-supported mental health treatment. Adm Policy Ment Health Ment Health Serv Res 41:522–534

King NJ, Tonge BJ, Mullen P, Myerson N, Heyne D, Rollings S et al (2000) Treating sexually abused children with posttraumatic stress symptoms: a randomized clinical trial. J Am Acad Child Adolesc Psychiatry 39:1347–1355

McKay MM, Bannon WM Jr (2004) Engaging families in child mental health services. Child Adolesc Psychiatr Clin N Am 13(4):905–921

Meichenbaum D (1985) Stress inoculation training. Pergamon Press, New York

Murray LK, Dorsey S, Skavenski S, Kasoma M, Imasiku M, Bolton P et al (2013) Identification, modification, and implementation of an evidence-based psychotherapy for children in a low-income country: the use of TF-CBT in Zambia. Int J Ment Heal Syst 7:24

O'Callaghan P, McMullen J, Shannon C, Rafferty H, Black A (2013) A randomized controlled trial of trauma-focused cognitive behavioral therapy for sexually exploited, war-affected Congolese girls. J Am Acad Child Adolesc Psychiatry 52(4):359–369

Substance Abuse and Mental Health Services Administration (SAMHSA) (2015) SAMHSA's national registry of evidence-based programs and practices. Retrieved 29 Oct 2015, from http://www.nrepp.samhsa.gov/

Cognitive Therapy for PTSD in Children and Adolescents

9

Sean Perrin, Eleanor Leigh, Patrick Smith, William Yule, Anke Ehlers, and David M. Clark

9.1 Theoretical Underpinnings

This treatment is based on a developmentally sensitive adaptation of Ehlers and Clark's (2000) model of PTSD, empirical evidence and our own clinical experience. Central to this model is the experience of a sense of current threat despite the fact the traumatic event happened in the past and which arises from two sources:

- First, the worst moments of the trauma are poorly elaborated in memory, being inadequately integrated into their context both within the event and within the context of previous and subsequent experiences/information. This has the effect that people with PTSD remember the trauma in a disjointed way. While they recall the worst moments, it may be difficult for them to access other information that could correct impressions they had or predictions they made at the time. In other words the memory for these moments has not been updated with what the person knows now. Because of a predominance of sensory processing during the event, the trauma memories of individuals with PTSD are heavily laden with the most distressing visuo-sensory aspects of the event (pain sensations, the sight of blood, the sound of loved ones screaming). Intrusion symptoms are frequent because the individual has a low threshold for perceiving trauma-related stimuli (perceptual priming) that activate the trauma memory. These include stimuli that are not meaningfully linked to the trauma in any way and only share common sensory characteristics such as specific colours, sounds, smells, tastes or bodily sensations.

- The second source of current threats is idiosyncratic (person-specific) appraisals (personal meanings) about the trauma and its consequences for the individual that go beyond what everyone would find threatening about the trauma. Such appraisals may include overestimating the frequency of traumatic events, holding mistaken beliefs about the causes of the trauma (excessive guilt) or negatively evaluating their reactions during the trauma (weakness, shame, embarrassment). It also includes 'frozen meanings' of particular moments of the trauma that did not come true (I am going to die, I will never see my loved ones again), as these meanings have not been updated due to the disjointed nature of the memory. Very common are appraisals about the meaning of PTSD and related symptoms, e.g. intrusive symptoms may be interpreted as signs that the person is losing control of their mind, is permanently damaged and can no longer cope with adversity or as a form of punishment for causing the trauma.

Frequent PTSD symptoms, a sense of current threat and trauma-related appraisals motivate a wide range of dysfunctional coping strategies, i.e. suppressing traumatic intrusions, trying not to think/talk about the event, avoiding traumatic reminders, hypervigilance and ruminating about the causes of the trauma. Such strategies may be either intentional or habitual and often make sense to the individual, i.e. they are meaningfully linked to appraisals and may provide short-term symptom relief. Unfortunately these strategies bring unintended consequences. Hypervigilance and suppression can increase the frequency of traumatic intrusions. Avoidance may prevent changes to problematic appraisals and keep the person from elaborating the trauma memory in ways that would make involuntary activation of the trauma memory less frequent.

An important aspect of the model as applied to children is the role of parents' appraisals of the trauma (and the child's reaction to it) in their ability to help their child recover from the trauma. Seeing their child suffer from PTSD, parents may develop beliefs that their child is permanently changed and unable to cope with intense emotions (either the child's or their parents'). Common in parents are the dual beliefs that they are responsible for their child's trauma *and* that their child is more vulnerable to harm going forward. Such beliefs may cause the parents to become *overprotective*, shadowing or checking up on the child, discouraging the child from returning to the full range of pre-trauma activities, discouraging conversation about the trauma or confrontations with reminders and voicing fearful thoughts about the likelihood of further harm. This overprotectiveness (and modelling of anxiety) may lead to fewer opportunities for the child to talk about the trauma, to confront reminders and to test the validity of trauma-related appraisals. Despite the parents' best efforts to mask their own reactions, the child may interpret their parents' reactions as further evidence that everything has changed for the worse and they (the child) are at fault.

9.2 How to Do Cognitive Therapy for PTSD in Children and Adolescents

9.2.1 Model-Derived Targets of Therapy

The model of PTSD developed by Ehlers and Clark (2000) provides clear treatment targets that are the focus of this cognitive therapy (CT) approach. First, the trauma memory needs to be elaborated and developed into a coherent account. Second, problematic appraisals of the trauma and its consequences need to be identified and updated. Third, unhelpful cognitive and behavioural strategies need to be dropped. In addition when working with children and young people, CT for PTSD may include work with parents or caregivers. They may be recruited as co-therapists, or a more substantial piece of work may be indicated to help modify any relevant beliefs about the trauma and its effects and their parenting style.

9.2.2 Treatment Components

The treatment components flow from the model of PTSD (Ehlers and Clark 2000) and are administered in a flexible and developmentally sensitive manner. They do not follow a prescribed session-by-session approach; the components are used throughout treatment as necessary to address the model-derived targets. Unlike other approaches to PTSD, this treatment does not involve training in relaxation, positive self-talk or any other form of anxiety management to reduce the upset that accompanies re-experiencing symptoms or contact with reminders. While such interventions have proven useful as part of other CBT interventions for PTSD, they can be seen as running counter to the cognitive model presented to the child and parents at the start of treatment. A fuller description of the components and materials that can be shared with the family can be found in Smith et al. (2010).

Psychoeducation At the first treatment session, the child and usually the parents are provided information about what is commonly known about PTSD. We then use the cognitive model to explain why symptoms persist in some children longer than others. First, the child's symptoms are reviewed with emphasis on how the 'here and now' quality of traumatic intrusions or becoming emotional for no apparent reason is a hallmark of PTSD. Second, the child is helped to identify strategies they have been using to deal with traumatic intrusions and upset and to recognise that while these may have been useful for coping with milder upsetting experiences, these strategies may be helping to maintain their symptoms. Third, it is explained that the treatment involves fully processing the trauma and reversing their particular maintaining factors. To help the child understand the model, we use the cupboard and puzzle metaphors described by Ehlers and Clark (2000) in our case study below. Written, age-appropriate information about PTSD and treatment are also provided.

Reclaiming Your Life In the first or second treatment session, the child and parents are asked to identify activities that give the child a sense of fun, social connectedness and meaning that they may have dropped after the trauma because of fears that arise from the trauma or the parents being excessively wary. It is explained that such withdrawal can give the trauma more prominence in the child's life and leave them feeling stuck and unable to move on from the trauma. The child is encouraged, with support from the parents, to identify and return to normal activities and to explore new avenues for social connectedness right from the beginning of therapy. The therapist returns to this topic throughout treatment to promote the sense of moving forward from the trauma.

Reliving After psychoeducation and reclaiming your life, the child is guided through an imaginal reliving to help access the moments in the trauma memory that are linked to the problematic meanings of the trauma. Where necessary the child may be guided through the initial living by writing out a narrative of the trauma. For younger children the therapist may use cartoon strips or storyboards which the therapist helps the child to complete. The use of reliving overlaps with reliving in prolonged exposure (PE, see Chap. 10) but also differs in important ways. Like PE, it is explained to the child that reliving can be difficult and it is natural to get upset or scared, but such reactions will diminish as they work on the memory. No instruction is given to engage any form of relaxation or anxiety management strategies either prior to or during reliving. Where there is an unwillingness to proceed because of fear/upset, the therapist provides empathy and encourages the child to talk about their feelings, normalising these within the context of the cognitive model. The child is then asked to talk about the trauma from its beginning until the point when they felt safe again in the first-person present tense. During reliving the therapist will ask the child to say what they can see, smell and hear and what they are thinking and feeling. Unlike standard PE, the therapist does not ask the child to repeatedly describe the traumatic experience. Instead from the first reliving onwards, the primary focus is to identify in the trauma memory areas of confusion or that lack narrative clarity and that involve emotional 'hotspots.' These aspects of the trauma memory can sometimes change in a beneficial way just through reliving, but in CT they are directly targeted by other techniques as well. When looking for hotspots, therapists prompt for greater detail and meanings to the child at points in the narrative that appear to be particularly stressful or where the child seems to miss parts out or rush through the memory. The therapist may ask the child to 'rewind and hold' or 'stop the tape' so they can describe what they see, feel and think at particularly fragmentary, confusing or upsetting parts of the narrative and identify negative appraisals that usually accompany such moments. Following the reliving the child and therapist may update the draft of the written narrative (or cartoon strips/storyboards).

9 Cognitive Therapy for PTSD in Children and Adolescents

Cognitive Restructuring It is sometimes possible for the child to experience a change in trauma-related appraisals simply from doing explorative reliving with the therapist (and as homework). However in CT the therapist devotes considerable time to helping the child identify idiosyncratic appraisals about the trauma and/or their reactions. Maladaptive appraisals are modified by the provision of more accurate information either from the therapist, parents and/or friends, behavioural experiments, stimulus discrimination or a site visit.

Updating the Trauma Memory Hotspots in the narrative are often accompanied by appraisals about feared outcomes (I am thinking I will never see my mother again) or the meaning of physiological sensations or behaviours to the self (I am paralysed watching my mother struggling to get out of the car and I am a coward for not helping her). Such appraisals can intrude into the present when the memory is activated, contributing to the current sense of threat and other intense emotional reactions (e.g. guilt, anger, disgust). The therapist discusses these hotspots with the child outside of reliving and helps them to identify alternative and more functional appraisals that are then incorporated into the reliving. This is done by asking the child to include the new information in the trauma narrative by speaking it out loud during imaginal reliving of the hotspot or writing it into the relevant spot in the narrative script (e.g. I am thinking I will never walk again *but now I know that I will*). We have found that cognitive restructuring is much more potent if it is integrated into the memory in this way. Therapists may deploy a number of techniques to help identify appraisals and to then update the trauma memory such as writing and/or drawing the event, using imagery techniques (e.g. flying above the scene of the accident to gather information from a different perspective) and using information gathered from parents or newspaper/police accounts (see Smith et al. 2010 for a description).

Working with Triggers (Stimulus Discrimination) A key feature of the model is that a wide range of stimuli that resemble cues present during the trauma (including low-level cues such as colours and sounds) can easily trigger the trauma memories in a way that makes it seem as though the trauma is happening again. CT uses a distinctive technique to deal with this problem. First the therapist and child work like detectives to identify the various stimuli that trigger unwanted intrusions. Often these stimuli come as a surprise as they may have no obvious meaning link to the trauma but are just a perceptual similarity (e.g. a colour or sound that was present in trauma and triggers the memory even when part of an innocuous object that has no other relation to the trauma). Second, the child is encouraged to confront these triggers, allowing the trauma memory to be activated, and then to make a conscious effort to focus on everything about the present which is different from the memory while remaining aware of the present. We call this the '*Then* versus *Now*' technique. This is done initially in session with the guidance of the therapist and then practised as homework.

Site Visit Another very important technique for updating the trauma memory is the site visit. Returning to the site of the trauma (when it is safe to do so) is a helpful way of enabling the child to see that the trauma is over. The first time the site visit is carried out, the therapist is present and usually the parents. To help facilitate their understanding that the trauma is over, the child is asked to remind themselves of the trauma while at the site and then to look around and notice everything that has changed since the trauma. Revisiting the site often provides invaluable information to help further modify the trauma-related appraisals that accompany hotspots in the trauma memory.

Parent Work Parents of younger children are always involved in treatment, and the extent to which they are involved in each session will depend on clinical need. Older adolescents may present for treatment without their parents and parental involvement is then negotiated. All parents should be provided with psychoeducation and a description of the treatment. They should be encouraged not to pressure their child to talk about the trauma or to immediately drop avoidance behaviours. Instead they should be encouraged to help their child re-engage with previously enjoyed activities, to complete homework assignments and later to accompany the child during site visits. During therapy the parents are invited to the room at the end of sessions to discuss their child's progress and reclaiming your life activities. Parents may be more closely involved with frequent joint parent-child sessions, particularly where the child is younger or has significant separation anxiety. A few joint sessions can be helpful if they involve the parents modelling talking about the trauma, providing more accurate information about the trauma and helping their child challenge any appraisals about the causes/effects of the trauma and the parents' ability to keep the child safe.

Some parents will find exposure to traumatic reminders very upsetting and will have difficulty refraining from catastrophic statements in front of their child or refraining from overprotective behaviours more generally. Under such circumstances the therapist will meet with the parents separately to address such issues, framing them in an empathic way as part of the traumatic response. Parents and siblings should be screened for PTSD and where necessary referred to treatment. However the child's treatment need not be delayed until after the parents have started/completed their own treatment. In our experience children with PTSD often make clinically significant and durable treatment gains despite parents or siblings continuing to suffer from PTSD. Furthermore, problematic trauma-related appraisals held by the parents and overprotective behaviours often diminish as the child's symptoms improve in treatment and the child displays a greater willingness to confront traumatic reminders.

9.2.3 Structure of Treatment

CT for PTSD symptoms tied to a single event trauma typically involves 10–12 weekly sessions lasting 60–90 min. Longer sessions are usually held when carrying out work on the trauma memory, out-of-the-office behavioural experiments and site visits or when additional parent work is needed. The first treatment session is a cognitive assessment in which a shared formulation is developed, goals of treatment are agreed upon and PTSD symptoms are normalised. Subsequent sessions involve (flexibly administered) reclaiming your life assignments, reliving and identifying hotspots, cognitive restructuring and updating of the trauma memory, working with triggers, revisiting the trauma site and parent work. In the final session, a detailed 'therapy blueprint' is developed with the young person as part of relapse prevention.

9.2.4 Case Report

Assessment
Jenny (age 11) was referred by social services for treatment of PTSD and low mood. Her mother and father were being supported by social services because both suffered from physical and mental health problems and the mother had learning difficulties. When Jenny was 7 years of age she saw her mother collapse into a state of unconsciousness as a result of alcohol intoxication. Jenny telephoned emergency services and an ambulance came and took her and her mother to hospital. Jenny was collected from the hospital by her grandmother and spent the next 3 months moving between her grandmother and other relatives while her father looked after her mother. Once her mother was well enough, Jenny returned home to her parents but spent weekends with her grandmother.

In the first few days after her mother collapsed, Jenny began having frequent nightmares and prominent intrusive images of the sound and then the sight of her mother choking and collapsing, telephoning the ambulance and trying to explain what had happened and of her mother lying in the hospital and overhearing the doctor commenting on her condition. These images were currently triggered by thoughts about her parents' ongoing health problems or when she heard people coughing, sirens, or saw ambulances or news items about hospitals or doctors. People drinking alcohol also served as a trigger. She avoided any and all reminders. Jenny blamed herself for the incident and felt responsible for her parents' safety, and this caused significant restriction in her activities and chronically low mood.

Jenny completed two questionnaires that would be used at the start of every treatment session to monitor progress: the 8-item Children's Revised Impact of Event Scale (CRIES-8, Yule 1997) and the 9-item Patient Health Questionnaire, Adolescent Version (PHQ-A; Johnson et al. 2002). At the start, midpoint and end of treatment, Jenny also completed the 25-item Posttraumatic Cognitions Inventory, Child Version (cPTCI; Meiser-Stedman et al. 2009).

Formulation
Based on the interview, Jenny met DSM-IV and ICD-10 criteria for PTSD (chronic) and major depression (moderate). She scored in the clinical range on the measures of PTSD and depression. On the cPTCI she endorsed strongly held beliefs that the trauma had caused her frightening symptoms that were permanent and impacted every aspect of her life and indicated that she now felt more vulnerable to harm and unable to cope. Her memory of the incident was disjointed and laden with the

sounds of her mother choking and hitting the floor, sirens and doctors talking, as well as images of her mother unconscious on the floor and on a hospital bed. She had difficulty accessing the sequence of events. Intrusive imagery was involuntarily triggered by a wide range of matching cues, e.g. coughing, sirens and people looking unwell.

Several prominent appraisals were identified during the course of treatment. First, when she heard and then saw her mother choking and collapsing she thought, 'My mum will die and I'm going to be alone forever'. Second, when she telephoned for an ambulance Jenny thought her mind had gone blank for a moment and she thought, 'I can't do it. I can't get anyone to understand me and mum will die because of me'. Third, Jenny believed her mother would die and she would never see her again when she heard medical staff comment that her mother was in critical condition. Jenny had overgeneralised fears for the health and safety of her parents and an inflated sense of responsibility for protecting them (I have to be on guard all the time). At night she would check and would look in on her parents to make sure they were still breathing and during the day search the house for evidence they were drinking excessively. She appraised her own PTSD reactions negatively (I can't cope anymore). Avoidance prevented her testing these appraisals and so symptoms persisted. Family factors included her father's avoidance of talking about the incident. An individualised version of the cognitive model is shown below. The formulation is developed with and shared with the client, and thus it is important that the elements in the model be described in an age-appropriate and concrete manner (see Fig. 9.1).

Course of Treatment

The initial formulation pointed to a number of treatment targets. The first was to gather information about the incident to reduce disjointedness in the memory. The second was to identify appraisals of the event and its aftermath and update the trauma memory. The third was to identify and drop dysfunctional coping strategies. The fourth was to work with family members to support Jenny's treatment. Jenny was usually brought to treatment sessions from school by her grandmother as her father would remain at home to care for her mother who was frequently unwell. However her parents were also able to attend for the second session, and they were met with separately to discuss ways in which they could help Jenny overcome the effects of the trauma.

Sessions 1–2 The focus of these sessions was psychoeducation and reclaiming your life and involved her parents and grandmother. During the psychoeducation component, Jenny learnt that even police and paramedics develop PTSD. This surprised her and helped to shift her belief that her own PTSD symptoms meant she was weak and could not cope with stress anymore. Jenny was also seen alone and helped to identify the strategies she currently used to cope with the trauma memory and how these might be backfiring. This was illustrated through a thought suppression experiment where she was asked to imagine and then suppress the image of a

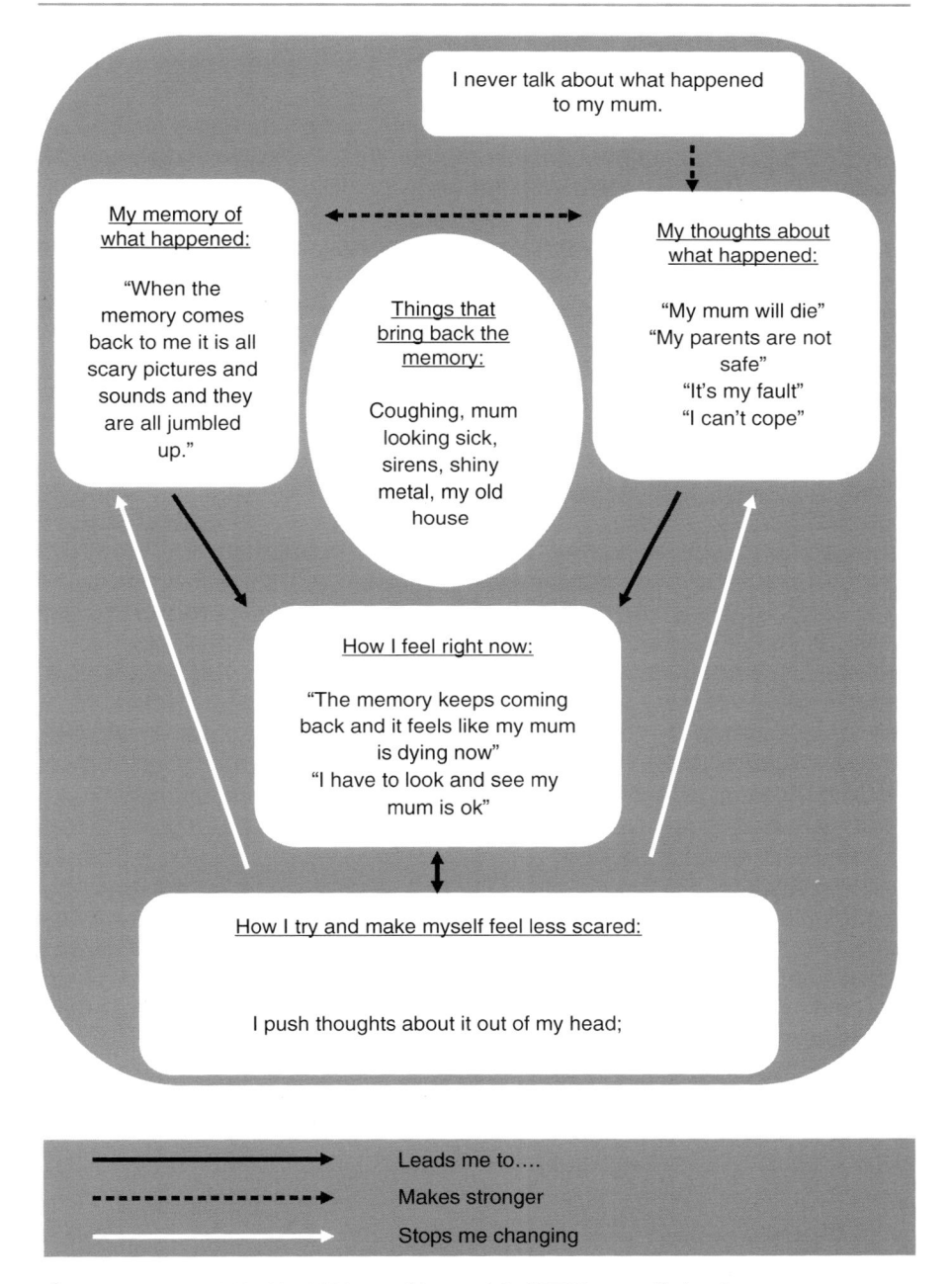

9 Cognitive Therapy for PTSD in Children and Adolescents

My memory of what happened:

"When the memory comes back to me it is all scary pictures and sounds and they are all jumbled up."

I never talk about what happened to my mum.

Things that bring back the memory:

Coughing, mum looking sick, sirens, shiny metal, my old house

My thoughts about what happened:

"My mum will die"
"My parents are not safe"
"It's my fault"
"I can't cope"

How I feel right now:

"The memory keeps coming back and it feels like my mum is dying now"
"I have to look and see my mum is ok"

How I try and make myself feel less scared:

I push thoughts about it out of my head;

⟶ Leads me to....
⇢ Makes stronger
⟹ Stops me changing

Fig. 9.1 Ehlers and Clark's (2000) cognitive model of PTSD as applied to Jenny

bright pink bunny sitting on therapist's head. Jenny laughed as soon as the experiment began as the only thing she was able to think about was the pink rabbit.

During the reclaiming your life component, Jenny indicated that her day-to-day activities were very limited; she went to school and came home to be near her parents. At home she stayed in her bedroom reading with the door open, often coming out to check on her parents. She often turned down her grandmother's suggestions for doing something fun after school. On weekends with her grandmother she found it hard to concentrate because her thoughts drifted to her parents' safety and she wanted to see/call them. Socratic questioning identified Jenny's strongly held belief that she was responsible for keeping her parents safe at all times and this prevented her from attending after-school clubs or accepting invitations from friends. Jenny was helped to recognise the link between her low levels of activity and her low mood, and she agreed to try 'beating the mood bully'. With input from her parents, grandmother, social worker and school, a number of possible activities were identified during schooldays and at the weekends. These activities were described as a series of behavioural experiments wherein Jenny would take part in activities with the support of adults (to start) and test the effect on her mood.

Finally, the therapist introduced the notion of dropping avoidance behaviours in response to traumatic intrusions. As a homework assignment Jenny was asked to think of her intrusions as trains trying to pass through a station. As the train approaches, it can be rather noisy and scary and the platform may shake, but the best thing to do is to just watch it pass and not try and stop it. This homework assignment was linked into the next key point that from the next session treatment would involve fully processing the trauma and reversing the maintaining factors. In order to explain the point that treatment involves voluntarily activating and then elaborating the trauma memory, she was asked to visualise a cupboard whose doors wouldn't close because the contents had just been thrown in loosely and were jumbled. Trying to push the doors closed (analogous to suppressing the memories) didn't work as they just spring open again. However, opening the doors, taking all the contents out, sorting them and putting them back (analogous to updating the trauma memory) allowed the doors to close and stay shut.

Sessions 3–9 Sessions always begin with completion of brief measures of PTSD and depression and a review of homework. Jenny was slowly increasing her participation in activities arranged by and involving her parents and grandparents, and she felt her mood starting to lift. She was keen to try some after-school activities with her friends.

The primary focus of these sessions was updating the trauma memory. Jenny was again introduced to the concept of reliving, and she expressed her fear that she could not be able to cope with anxiety she would experience during the reliving. She was helped to operationalise this fear in the form of a prediction wherein during reliving she would become so scared that she would lose control, run out of the room and end up in hospital. She rated belief as an 8 on a 10-point scale (10 = completely believe). The therapist validated and normalised her fears. So for the first reliving Jenny agreed to try it out as an experiment to see if her prediction would come true.

Jenny undertook the first reliving in the first person and stayed in the present tense for most of it. She was asked to rate her anxiety on a 10-point scale (10 = highest level of anxiety) throughout and these ratings were charted by the therapist. Her first account of the trauma was fragmented and with considerable sensory detail. After the reliving Jenny acknowledged that although she had been very anxious, she did not in fact run out of the room, or even get out of her chair, nor did she end up in hospital. Furthermore as she sat talking with the therapist after the reliving, she noticed that her anxiety had come down. She was asked to predict whether she would 'lose control and go mad' if she did the reliving again, and she now rated this belief as 0/10 (*reappraisal*).

After this first reliving, Jenny acknowledged an urge to call her parents. She was helped to see that this urge was linked to the current sense of threat activated with the trauma memory. She was also helped to see that sometimes checking on her parents also triggered an intrusion. The therapist explained how the senses of a current threat would reduce with further work on the trauma memory and this would help reduce her worries about her parents so she could stop checking on them and spend more time with friends away from home (*dropping unhelpful strategies*).

Jenny was assisted in making a written narrative of the trauma and this was transferred to a whiteboard in the therapy room. Jenny was surprised at how much of the trauma she could recall, but there were aspects of the event that remained unclear, e.g. how long it took for the ambulance to arrive. Jenny's grandmother was invited into the session, and she provided new information that helped Jenny to fill some of the gaps in her memory and discovered that the ambulance had reached the home within 15 min.

Jenny was asked to look at the trauma narrative and to identify the worst or most scary moments. The therapist would then rewrite these sections using a different coloured marker and identify these as potential 'hotspots'. Three hotspots were identified: (1) when she heard and then saw her mother choking and collapsing and believing her mother was dead on the kitchen floor, (2) when she telephoned the emergency services and she thought she could not make herself understood and that her mother would die as a result and (3) when she was in the hospital and Jenny overheard a staff member say her mother was in critical condition and Jenny took this to mean her mother would die and that it would be her fault if her mother died. These appraisals were written out on a form so that Jenny could see how more accurate information is incorporated into the trauma memory (see Table 9.1).

Each hotspot was then worked on in turn. Attached to the first hotspot was the appraisal that Jenny's mother was dead when she found her on the kitchen floor. To modify this appraisal, Jenny was then asked to describe times she had spent with her mother recently. She was then asked to produce a recent picture of her and her mum together from her mobile phone and to look at this in the session. A second appraisal during the first hotspot was that her mother could not possibly survive given the sounds she was making and how she seemed to stop breathing. A member of the clinic staff who was a medical doctor joined the session and she talked Jenny through what happened to her mother in clear factual detail. This provided Jenny

Table 9.1 Record for updating peri-traumatic appraisals

Situation	What I thought at the time	Feeling (0–10)	What I know now New information	Feeling (0–10)
Hearing and seeing my mum choke and collapse	My mum will die, and I'm going to be alone forever	Scared 10	My mum survived; I like sitting and chatting with her mother in the evenings about her schoolwork and books she enjoyed. The noises mum made showed she was still breathing and a sign she was still alive	Relief 10
Trying to call an ambulance	I can't do it, I can't get anyone to understand me, and mum will die because of me	Scared 10 Helpless 10 Angry with myself 10	My mum survived and is still alive. I was really brave in the moment and did more than most 7-year-olds would be able to do. I helped save my mum's life	Relief 8 Proud 8
A member of hospital staff saying 'she's in a critical condition'	My mum will die, and I'll never see her again	Scared 10 Sad 10 Alone 8	My mum survived. 'Critical condition' is a medical term for people who are very ill. It doesn't mean they are going to die, but they need lots of help	Relief 8

with helpful information to understand that the noises her mother had made were because she was still breathing and a sign she was still alive (*reappraisal*).

After restructuring these appraisals around the first hotspot, Jenny asked to add the new information into her written narrative using a red pen. She was then asked to sit with her mobile phone on her lap with the recent picture of her and her mum displayed and to bring that image to mind. She then read the hotspot out loud identifying her appraisal at the time, 'I think my mum is going to die…', and then specified the new information out loud '…and now I know she did not die. She was very unwell, but she recovered, and we enjoy spending time together, sitting and talking about books and my lessons'.

For the second hotspot it was important to restructure her appraisal, 'I can't do it, I can't get anyone to understand me, and mum will die because of me'. First, Jenny was asked whether her request for an ambulance was successful or if her mother had survived. Jenny agreed but still thought she had not done enough to make herself clear to the emergency worker on the phone. Jenny was asked to remember how old she had been at the time of the incident and whether she knew any children of the same age now and to describe them. Jenny talked about a cousin who was a boisterous little girl always running and wanting to play. The therapist asked whether she would expect her 7-year-old cousin to be able to telephone an ambulance, discuss symptoms and manage an emergency situation. By taking this perspective Jenny was able to realise that what she had done was very brave and may have saved her mother's life. This information was entered on her record form (see Table 9.1). Again, the trauma memory was updated by helping Jenny place this new information in her written narrative and saying this new information aloud at the relevant hotspot with a photo of her mother on her lap, 'I am talking on the phone to the emergency operator, and I am thinking I can't get anyone to understand me and mum will die because of me…but now I know the operator understood me very well, the ambulance came, and my mum did not die'.

For the third hotspot Jenny's appraisal was that the term 'critical condition' meant her mother would die and it would be Jenny's fault. Jenny was encouraged to bring to mind an image of her mother from recent times to confirm that her mother was alive. The medical doctor joined the session and explained to Jenny that 'critical condition' meant her mother was very ill but did not necessarily mean she would die. This new information was incorporated into the hotspot in her trauma memory, 'I hear the doctor say critical condition, and I am thinking that my mum is going to die, but now I know that critical condition means mum was very sick and she is not dead'.

Around the sixth session, Jenny was asked to recomplete the measure of trauma-related beliefs (cPTCI). The therapist scored the measure and then went through some of the individual items with Jenny. There had been a significant shift in her appraisals about the meaning of her symptoms such that she no longer believed that she was permanently changed in a negative way, or that the future only held frightening or negative consequences for her, or that she was unable to cope or prevent bad things from happening. However Jenny still had a moderately strong belief that she needed to be vigilant for danger, and with further exploration this belief was linked to her worries that if she did not monitor her parents' safety and wellbeing, something bad might happen to them. We talked about the fact that this worry had begun immediately after the trauma and was a natural reaction to that event. Jenny was helped to identify all of the people and services now involved in supporting her mother and how the level of support had actually increased since the trauma. We talked about how her checking up on her mother made sense at the time of the trauma, but doing so now (repeatedly) was only making her worry and preventing her from moving forward from the trauma. She was again encouraged to consider/test whether checking up on her parents really made them any safer or made her feel less worried.

At the end of each treatment session, Jenny's grandmother joined the session and her progress and homework assignments were discussed. This involved helping Jenny and her grandmother to identify possible pleasant activities for reclaiming her life. We also discussed how Jenny could work on dropping any unhelpful behaviours like avoiding reminders and checking up on her parents, and these would be planned in the form of behavioural experiments, i.e. to test whether checking up on her mum made her worry more or less about her.

Session 10 There had been considerable progress in processing the trauma memory; it was less disjointed, and peri-traumatic appraisals had been identified and restructured and more accurate appraisals incorporated into the memory. Jenny was now able to go through her trauma narrative at a steady pace, with little distress and a stronger sense of the trauma being in the past. Over the course of these sessions, there had been a sharp decline in the frequency of her traumatic intrusions, but she still reacted to some reminders with some degree of intrusion, distress and avoidance (or checking). Thus the focus of this session was working with triggers (traumatic reminders) and planning a site visit.

The first step was to carefully map out where and when any remaining intrusions occurred in order to identify triggers. Jenny was encouraged to be Sherlock Holmes as many triggers are sensory and can be difficult to detect. Jenny identified hospitals, ambulances, sirens, the sound of coughing, gurneys, shiny metal (Jenny had been at head height with the metal of the gurney her mother lay on), and the house where the family used to live where the incident occurred.

The second step involved 'breaking the link' between the triggers and the trauma memory (*stimulus discrimination*). To do this Jenny first learned to distinguish 'Then' (the time of the trauma) from 'Now'. Next, intrusions were intentionally triggered, and Jenny worked on using 'Then versus Now' discriminations. For example, Jenny brought a shiny piece of metal from home that reminded her of the metal guardrail around her mother's hospital bed. Jenny held the pipe and looked at it, allowing the image of her mother on the hospital bed to appear in her mind and then to describe the image to the therapist. Jenny was asked to describe any similarities/differences between the shiny metal pipe in her hand and the guardrail of the hospital bed. Jenny immediately spotted the differences, 'The metal in my hand is just a bit of piping, not a guardrail. I am sitting with my therapist in the clinic; it is sunny outside. I am not sitting next to my mother's bed in a hospital room at night'.

As homework Jenny was encouraged to do these 'Then versus Now' exercises whenever she encountered a reminder of the trauma or had an intrusion. We also discussed a trip to the house where the trauma had occurred for the next session so that Jenny could repeat the 'Then versus Now' exercise with her therapist and grandmother (*site visit*). Jenny indicated that she was prepared to do so and grandmother was invited into the room and plans were made for the visit.

Session 11 As planned, the therapist met Jenny and her grandmother outside of her old house. Jenny gave examples of the trigger work she had done as homework, saying: 'I am just upset because I am thinking about what happened to my mum. It's not happening all over again. My mum is ok'. Jenny was then asked to activate the trauma memory and then look around the outside of the house and street and notice similarities/differences between then and now. Jenny noticed the curtains had changed, a small playground had been built opposite the house, and there were new flowers planted. Jenny recalled that where the ambulance and a police car had been parked on the night of the trauma there were now cars parked. She noted how dark it had been the night of the trauma that the people on the street were watching all of the commotion. Now the street was empty except for a few people walking by and it was still light out. Jenny recalled that after the ambulance arrived, she stood for a few moments watching her mother be lifted into the ambulance. She noticed that her mother was not moving at all despite how much the gurney was being moved about. She thought her mother must be dead and would never be coming home again. We discussed what Jenny knew now, that her mother was in fact only unconscious and was strapped tightly in the gurney and could not move. She knew now that her mother didn't come home to this house because the whole family was moved while her mother was in the hospital. She knew now that her mother had not died and she and Jenny spent time together recently doing fun things.

Jenny was asked whether the incident involving her mother still felt like it just happened or was happening again when she thought about it standing outside of the house. Jenny said that she had a feeling that something really awful happened to her mum at this place but that it was something in the past and she knew her mum was home waiting for her right now. Jenny was asked to describe the difference in her feelings when she talked about the trauma now from the start of treatment. She said it was the worst and scariest day of her life but thinking about it now did not make her feel like it was happening all over again or that she needed to check up on her mum. The therapist and Jenny's grandmother commented on Jenny's extraordinary progress. We agreed to meet once more at the clinic to formally review her progress and plan a follow-up meeting.

Session 12 (End of Treatment) Jenny completed the brief measures of PTSD (CRIES-8) and depression (PHQ-A) and the cPTCI. The therapist also asked about the DSM-V symptoms of PTSD and major depression. Jenny no longer met criteria for either disorder. She was in the normal range on the self-report measures of PTSD and depression. The therapist then showed Jenny graphs comparing her pretreatment, session-by-session and post-treatment scores on the self-report questionnaires. The therapist again went through several of the items on the cPTCI Jenny had just completed to show how her self-blame for the trauma and her beliefs that she was permanently damaged and that she was vulnerable to harm had all changed for the better.

Review of the symptom data was followed by a discussion of the types of things Jenny had done to reclaim her life from the trauma. Jenny was able to say that she could be in the house separate from her parents and without feeling a constant pressure to check up on them. She felt better about going to school and spending time with friends and her grandparents because she was not constantly having intrusive thoughts or wanting to contact her parents. She looked forward to going to sleep at night after a busy day because she was no longer having nightmares.

The conversation then moved to what Jenny had learnt in treatment. Jenny was able to say that pushing thoughts out of her head did not work and that constantly checking up on her parents only made things worse. She felt strongly now that what happened to her mother was not her fault and that for a 7-year-old she had been incredibly brave on the day her mother collapsed. She felt more confident in herself, as well as in school and with friends. The therapist then helped Jenny to write down what she had learnt in treatment as her 'blueprint for the future.' It was explained to Jenny how she could use this blueprint to remind herself what she had learnt if she started having intrusions again or felt the urge to check on her parents.

It was agreed that this was good time to stop treatment. Jenny's grandmother was then invited into the room and asked to give her view about what had changed since the start of treatment. She explained that Jenny seemed like a completely new person. She could not remember Jenny ever being so confident, independent or smiling as much. She remarked that Jenny was now offering to help her around the house and suggesting fun things they could do together. She said that Jenny's parents were extremely pleased about and proud of her progress. A plan was made to review Jenny's progress in 6 months with Jenny or the family contacting the clinic in the interim if there were any concerns.

Some Additional Comments on Family Work

Just after the first assessment of Jenny, and in agreement with Jenny's father, the therapist referred the father to adult services for individual treatment of PTSD. He was supported throughout this process. In addition, both parents were able to come for a family session near the start of treatment. The parents were asked about how the trauma had affected Jenny and in turn their parenting of her. Both parents were surprised by the extent of the symptoms reported by Jenny to the therapist as she had not told them how much she was thinking about (and still upset) by the trauma. They were very much aware, however, that Jenny seemed less confident than she had been before the trauma as she now seemed to shadow them and was reluctant to leave the house. Their response to these behaviours was to reassure her that they were okay and to encourage her to spend more time with her friends and grandmother. This prompted a discussion of hypervigilance in PTSD and Jenny's overgeneralised fear of her parents becoming seriously ill.

The parents indicated that they were willing to try anything to help Jenny overcome her hypervigilance and regain her confidence. So we discussed how Jenny would be asked to undertake a series of experiments through which she would learn that her checking behaviours caused her anxiety and prevented her from learning that her parents were capable of managing their own health and her parents would refrain from providing her reassurance on their health. For example, Jenny often checked her parents' medication to make sure they had taken their dose. It was agreed that they would purchase a locked medicine cabinet with the key held by the parents. Once this cabinet was in place, Jenny regularly fed back to her therapist that her parents took their medication without her intervention and she felt less worried and anxious about this issue.

Additional behavioural experiments were planned specifically targeting Jenny's belief 'If I am not with my parents, they will become ill'. These included a series of trips outside the home to local shops and to see friends. Jenny resisted the urge to cut her trips short or to contact her parents on their mobile phone (text messages), and her parents refrained from providing her reassurance about their health on the phone or at home. Instead her parents would praise Jenny for spending time with them talking about issues other than their health, for playing and for spending time with her friends and family. In our individual sessions, Jenny was asked about these experiments and said that her parents had good support systems in place for themselves and did not need her to constantly monitor them. She began to enjoy her time with her parents more and to engage in enjoyable activities with her friends and grandparents.

Outcome

Jenny is an 11-year old girl who started treatment with severe and chronic PTSD and secondary depression in the moderate range of severity. At the first meeting she came across as mature beyond her years and inhibited. She would not allow herself to take part in fun activities, as she felt responsible for others, particularly her parents. Over the course of 12 weekly sessions, she engaged well with the various treatment components, and as a result she no longer met diagnostic criteria for PTSD or depression. Jenny was now engaging in independent play and after-school clubs and taking part in the school play. These gains were subsequently maintained at a pre-planned, 6-month follow-up interview.

Direct depression treatment was minimal, primarily involving a few techniques to increase the frequency of pleasant activities (*reclaiming your life*) and cognitive restructuring to modify negative, trauma-related appraisals that were depressive either in nature or impact. Consistent with our own experience, we expected that the updating of the trauma memory and modification of trauma-related appraisals would lead to a significant reduction in intrusive memories and this in turn would lead to a further weakening of her trauma-related beliefs, as well as improvements in mood, sleep, energy and concentration. Jenny responded extremely well to this PTSD-specific treatment despite the presence of a comorbid depressive disorder and significant psychosocial adversity in the form of parental physical/mental health problems and maternal learning disability. The involvement and ongoing support of her parents and carers were all important in her recovery.

9.3 Special Challenges

Issues of safety, the family environment and informed consent/assent weigh upon treatment decisions for all children with mental health difficulties and no more or less so with those who have PTSD. Safety is always the primary concern, and if there is evidence that the young person or a parent is planning (or has recently engaged in) acts of extreme self-harm, or there is ongoing violence/abuse in the family, or there is an imminent risk of harm to the child from some other source, or there is evidence of emerging and untreated symptoms of psychosis, then these are the appropriate targets for further assessment and treatment. Work with traumatic memories and reminders can be anxiety provoking, but such procedures are not inherently unsafe, even if the trauma was sexual in nature or involved the death of loved ones. Careful use of the procedures described here under supervision from a clinician experienced in the cognitive behavioural treatment of PTSD, and with routine monitoring of symptoms, is highly unlikely to produce a worsening of the child's condition.

It will be obvious to the reader that no child fully overcomes their symptoms of PTSD being dragged along unwillingly to therapy sessions by a parent. Nor can a therapist or parent *push* a child into recovery by repeated admonitions to talk about the trauma or forcing confrontations with traumatic reminders. It should be expected that the child will have high levels of anticipatory fear about the treatment and about possible stigmatisation from peers for attending treatment. Such fears should be acknowledged by the therapist and dealt with using information, empathy and support. Making the young person aware that PTSD symptoms occur even among the heroes in our society (emergency service workers, soldiers, sports figures) and they too seek treatment can go a long way to reduce fears of being labelled as crazy or weak. Engagement with the treatment can be facilitated with the judicious use of age-appropriate metaphors that can help the child understand treatment will involve them moving at their own speed to piece together the fragments of their trauma memory. Motivation may be further enhanced by helping the child to recall the pleasant aspects of their life that were lost following the trauma and that these will return with treatment.

Age and Developmental Difficulties Sometimes when child mental health professionals hear the term 'cognitive therapy', they assume that younger children or those with developmental difficulties will have great difficulties identifying appraisals or engaging with verbal change techniques. Our own experience is that age or the presence of developmental difficulties is not the primary issue. Rather it is the skill of the therapist in adapting their language and the pacing of treatment to help the child access and describe the content of their thoughts, to draw links between thoughts and other aspects of functioning and to consider the costs/benefits of holding on to certain beliefs. Items from the cPTCI can be read aloud to help the child identify trauma-related appraisals that help maintain symptoms. Younger children and those who struggle to speak can be engaged through the use of toys, cartoon strips or storyboards with which the therapist helps the child to identify the details of the trauma, correct appraisals and add new information to the trauma memory. Sometimes younger or less verbal children are more willing to speak to a parent than the therapist. In such instances, the parent is asked to join sessions and supported in taking the role of co-therapist.

Contextual and Comorbidity Issues PTSD is a chronic condition that often drives comorbidity and wider difficulties in the family and school and yet often goes untreated because clinicians prioritise the treatment of secondary disorders like depression or family issues at the expense of PTSD. Likewise the presence of certain symptoms (e.g. school refusal, self-harm, substance use) and/or unresolved medical or asylum issues is often viewed as precluding treatment of the child's PTSD. As the current case demonstrates, significant comorbidity or psychosocial adversity need not preclude a successful outcome. We have experience of successfully delivering this treatment, often with only minor variations, to children and adolescents with severe health difficulties, children in refugee camps and post-war/disaster settings, via translators, and to refugees who have only temporary leave to remain in the country.

Parental Psychopathology Another concern sometimes raised by therapists is whether it is possible or appropriate to successfully treat the child's PTSD when the parents have significant and untreated symptoms of PTSD, anxiety or depression.

There is considerable evidence that parental symptoms are significant risk factors for the child developing PTSD and for the severity of their PTSD symptoms. However the severity of the trauma itself, trauma-related beliefs, rumination and thought suppression play an even stronger role in risk for and severity of PTSD in children. At present there is no evidence from randomised controlled trials (RCTs) to suggest that the presence of parental symptoms prevents the child from making a significant and lasting recovery with a course of trauma-focused cognitive behavioural therapy. In our own experience, successful treatment of the child's PTSD (and comorbid symptoms) is often associated with marked reductions in the parents' own symptoms and improvement in family functioning more broadly. Nevertheless family factors need to be assessed in each case and where necessary parents offered separate treatment sessions or referral to their own treatment.

Finally, therapists familiar with evidence-based, cognitive behavioural approaches should recognise that shifting focus to acute comorbid problems does not necessitate a new form of treatment or abandoning work on PTSD. The interventions that comprise this PTSD-specific treatment include psychoeducation, routine symptom monitoring, activity scheduling, cognitive restructuring, avoidance-reduction techniques, parent training and liaison work, all of which form the basis of evidence-based approaches for a wide range of internalising and externalising problems. This treatment is not a prescriptive, session-by-session approach but a collection of theoretically and empirically supported components that are administered in a flexible, developmentally sensitive manner. Nevertheless we do not recommend that the therapist omits one or more of the various components to accommodate comorbidity. Rather the spacing between interventions can be increased or decreased to deal with situational difficulties (rescheduling sessions around school exams/holidays) or comorbidity (school refusal). Likewise, parents, teachers and social services can be engaged to deal with comorbid problems in parallel treatments, while the therapist continues to focus on the PTSD.

9.4 Research Evidence

There is substantial evidence in support of the model that underpins this treatment. As predicted by the Ehlers and Clark's (2000) model, studies have found that aspects of the trauma memory, peri-traumatic appraisals and dysfunctional cognitive strategies are significant risk factors for the development and for the severity of PTSD in children (e.g. Ehlers et al. 2003; Meiser-Stedman et al. 2007, 2009, 2014; Salmond et al. 2010; Stallard 2003). In a recent longitudinal study of adolescents exposed to a car bomb, Duffy et al. (2015) found that the cognitive factors specified by the Ehlers and Clark model contributed significantly to prediction of PTSD and accounted for the largest proportion of variance in symptoms. The impact of parents' trauma-related appraisals on their child's symptoms of PTSD is under-investigated, but there is evidence that parental symptoms of PTSD and parental overprotectiveness may increase the child's risk for developing PTSD (Trickey et al. 2012).

Direct support for the current treatment can be found in our randomised controlled trial (RCT) with clinically referred children and adolescents (aged 8–18 years) with a primary diagnosis of DSM-IV PTSD linked to a single-incident trauma (Smith et al. 2007). Ninety-two percent of the children in the treatment condition lost their PTSD diagnosis at post-treatment compared to only 42 % in the delayed treatment group, and these gains were maintained at the 6-month follow-up. Moreover changes in PTSD symptoms were mediated by changes in trauma-related beliefs as measured by the cPTCI. An RCT examining the effectiveness of this cognitive approach for PTSD relative to treatment as usual in children aged 3–8 years is currently under way (Dalgleish et al. 2015). RCTs involving adults show that this treatment yields marked and durable reductions in PTSD diagnoses and the severity of PTSD and related symptoms relative to wait-list, self-help, repeated assessments and active treatment not focused on the trauma (Duffy et al. 2007; Ehlers et al. 2003, 2014). Furthermore changes in trauma-related appraisals have been found to precede and predict changes in PTSD symptoms over the following week for adults undergoing this treatment (Klein et al. 2012).

References

Dalgleish T, Goodall B, Chadwick I, Werner-Seidler A, McKinnon A, Morant N, Schweizer S, Panesar I, Humphrey A, Watson P, Lafortune L, Smith P, Meiser-Stedman R (2015) Trauma-focused cognitive behaviour therapy versus treatment as usual for post-traumatic stress disorder (PTSD) in young children aged 3 to 8 years: A randomised controlled trial. Trials 16:116

Duffy M, Gillespie K, Clark DM (2007) Post-traumatic stress disorder in the context of terrorism and other civil conflict in Northern Ireland: randomised controlled trial. BMJ 7604:1147

Duffy M, McDermott M, Percy A, Ehlers A, Clark DM, Fitzgerald M, Moriarty J (2015) The effects of the Omagh bomb on adolescent mental health: a school-based study. BMC Psychiatry 15:18

Ehlers A, Clark DM (2000) A cognitive model of posttraumatic stress disorder. Behav Res Ther 38(4):319–345

Ehlers A, Clark DM, Hackmann A, McManus F, Fennell M, Herbert C, Mayou R (2003a) A randomized controlled trial of cognitive therapy, a self-help booklet, and repeated assessments as early interventions for posttraumatic stress disorder. Arch Gen Psychiatry 10:1024–1032

Ehlers A, Hackmann A, Grey N, Wild J, Liness S, Albert I, Deale A, Stott R, Clark DM (2014) A randomized controlled trial of 7-day intensive and standard weekly cognitive therapy for PTSD and emotion-focused supportive therapy. Am J Psychiatry 3:294–304

Ehlers A, Mayou RA, Bryant B (2003b) Cognitive predictors of posttraumatic stress disorder in children: results of a prospective longitudinal study. Behav Res Ther 41(1):1–10

Johnson JG, Harris ES, Spitzer RL, Williams JB (2002) The patient health questionnaire for adolescents: validation of an instrument for the assessment of mental disorders among adolescent primary care patients. J Adolesc Health 3:196–204

Kleim B, Grey N, Wild J, Nussbeck FW, Stott R, Hackmann A, Clark DM, Ehlers A (2012) Cognitive change predicts symptom reduction with cognitive therapy for posttraumatic stress disorder. J Consult Clin Psychol 3:383–393

Meiser-Stedman R, Dalgleish T, Smith P, Yule W, Glucksman E (2007) Diagnostic, demographic, memory quality, and cognitive variables associated with acute stress disorder in children and adolescents. J Abnorm Psychol 116:65–79

Meiser-Stedman R, Smith P, Bryant R, Salmon K, Yule W, Dalgleish T, Nixon R (2009) Development and validation of the Child Post-Traumatic Cognitions Inventory (CPTCI). J Child Psychol Psychiatry 50(4):432–440

Meiser-Stedman R, Shepperd A, Glucksman E, Dalgleish T, Yule W, Smith P (2014) Thought control strategies and rumination in youth with acute stress disorder and posttraumatic stress disorder following single event trauma. J Child Adolesc Psychopharmacol 24:47–51

Salmond CH, Meiser-Stedman R, Glucksman E, Thompson P, Dalgleish T, Smith P (2010) The nature of trauma memories in acute stress disorder in children and adolescents. J Child Psychol Psychiatry 5:560–570

Smith P, Perrin S, Yule W, Clark D (2010) Post traumatic stress disorder: cognitive therapy with children and young people. Routledge, Lonndon

Smith P, Yule W, Perrin S, Tranah T, Dalgleish T, Clark D (2007) Cognitive behavioral therapy for PTSD in children and adolescents: a preliminary randomized controlled trial. J Am Acad Child Adolesc Psychiatry 46(8):1051–1061

Stallard P (2003) A retrospective analysis to explore the applicability of the Ehlers and Clark (2000) cognitive model to explain PTSD in children. Behav Cogn Psychother 31:337–345

Trickey D, Siddaway AP, Meiser-Stedman R, Serpell L, Field AP (2012) A meta-analysis of risk factors for post-traumatic stress disorder in children and adolescents. Clin Psychol Rev 32(2):122–138

Yule W (1997) Anxiety, depression and post-traumatic stress in childhood. In: Sclare I (ed) Child psychology portfolio. Windsor, NFER-Nelson

10. Prolonged Exposure Therapy for Adolescents with PTSD: Emotional Processing of Traumatic Experiences

Sandy Capaldi, Laurie J. Zandberg, and Edna B. Foa

10.1 Theoretical Underpinnings

Prolonged exposure therapy for adolescents (PE-A; Foa et al. 2008) is an adaptation of the widely studied, empirically validated adult protocol of prolonged exposure (Foa et al. 2007). The treatment is based on emotional processing theory (EPT; Foa and Kozak 1986; Foa et al. 2006), which provides a framework for understanding the factors that contribute to the development and maintenance of post-traumatic stress symptoms, the mechanisms underlying natural recovery from these symptoms, and the amelioration of these symptoms via exposure treatments. EPT proposes that emotions like fear are represented in memory as a cognitive structure (i.e., information network) which serves as a blueprint for action. A fear structure is a specific type of cognitive structure that includes representations of the feared stimuli (e.g., a bear) and the associated physical responses (e.g., sweating, shaking), as well as the meanings associated with the stimuli ("bears are dangerous") and responses ("sweating means I'm afraid"). When a fear structure represents realistic threat, it guides effective response. For example, if approached by a bear (a feared stimulus), the fear structure would be activated, and the meaning of the feared stimulus ("bears are dangerous") would promote a response (such as sweating or shaking). Thus, EPT states that cognitive structures of emotions include representations of the meaning of the stimuli that give rise to the emotion as well as the emotion-related responses and their meaning. A fear structure becomes pathological,

---

S. Capaldi, Psy. D • L.J. Zandberg, Psy. D • E.B. Foa, Ph. D (✉)
Perelman School of Medicine, Department of Psychiatry, University of Pennsylvania, 3535 Market Street, Philadelphia, PA 19104, USA
e-mail: foa@mail.med.upenn.edu

however, when elements of the fear structure are erroneous or unrealistic, evoking fear of and escape from harmless stimuli.

According to EPT, a traumatic memory is a specific cognitive structure that contains representations of the stimuli that were present during the trauma, responses (fear, shame, guilt, anger) that were present during the trauma, and the meaning of these stimuli and responses. A trauma memory structure underlying post-traumatic stress disorder (PTSD) contains a large number of stimuli that are erroneously associated with the meaning of danger. For example, an adolescent who was sexually assaulted may associate related but harmless stimuli, such as men with similar builds as the perpetrator or small, enclosed spaces, with the meaning of danger. As a result, individuals with PTSD are likely to perceive the world as entirely dangerous. In addition, representations of the individuals' responses during and following the trauma often become associated with the meaning of incompetence (e.g., "I failed to save my friend"; "My PTSD symptoms mean that I am a weak person"). These two perceptions – that the world is entirely dangerous and the person is very incompetent – serve to maintain PTSD symptoms.

While PTSD symptoms are common immediately following a traumatic event, most people manifest a decline in these symptoms over time without treatment. EPT suggests that natural recovery occurs through repeated activation of the trauma memory in daily life, as the person engages with trauma-related thoughts and feelings, shares the traumatic event with others, and confronts situations that are reminders of the trauma. These experiences provide information that disconfirms the perception that the world is entirely dangerous and that the person is entirely incompetent. For individuals with PTSD, however, avoidance of trauma-related thoughts, feelings, and situations impedes activation of the trauma memory and integration of disconfirming information that would alter the pathological elements in the fear structure.

For example, if an adolescent girl who experienced childhood sexual abuse avoids all men with body types similar to the perpetrator, she never learns that the majority of men who are physically similar to the perpetrator are safe. Additionally, by avoiding thinking about what happened, this adolescent's memory will often remain fragmented and poorly articulated, and the erroneous perception that she was responsible for the abuse will remain unquestioned. The adolescent's avoidance behaviors are negatively reinforced because they temporarily reduce distress and so become habitual in similar circumstances. While avoidance reduces distress in the short term, it perpetuates PTSD by blocking experiences that would otherwise modify the pathological elements in the fear structure.

Effective PTSD treatment modifies the pathological elements of the fear structure and reduces pathological reactions by simulating natural recovery. In order to achieve this, two conditions are necessary. First, the fear structure must be activated (i.e., feared stimuli must be approached). Second, new information that is incompatible with the unrealistic elements in the fear structure must be available and incorporated. When this new learning (or emotional processing) takes place, stimuli that used to evoke pathological responses will no longer do so.

PE-A aims to promote emotional processing by encouraging patients to talk about the trauma, referred to as revisiting and recounting the trauma memory (imaginal exposure), and to approach objectively safe situations that are trauma reminders, referred to as real-life experiments (in vivo exposure). By deliberately confronting safe but avoided trauma-related thoughts, feelings, and situations, the pathological fear structure is activated, and erroneous elements are modified through corrective experiences. Repeatedly recounting the traumatic memory reduces the anxiety associated with thinking about the trauma, provides opportunities to organize and better understand what happened, and helps the individual to explore and disconfirm other erroneous perceptions (e.g., that the adolescent's actions mean he/she is incompetent or at fault for the trauma). Confronting trauma reminders and situations that are erroneously perceived as dangerous via real-life experiments reduces PTSD symptoms by breaking the habit of avoidance, promoting recognition that these situations are not harmful, and increasing the adolescent's confidence in his or her ability to cope.

10.2 How to Do Prolonged Exposure for Adolescents

Prolonged exposure for adolescents (PE-A; Foa et al. 2008) is a manualized, symptom-focused treatment designed to target PTSD symptoms in the aftermath of all types of trauma. It is accompanied by a workbook for clients to use along with the treatment sessions (*Prolonged Exposure Therapy for PTSD: Teen Workbook;* Chrestman, Gilboa-Schechtman, & Foa, 2008). PE-A was developed and tested with adolescents ages 12–18 and includes four phases (pretreatment preparation, psychoeducation and treatment planning, exposures, and relapse prevention/treatment termination), each comprised of several modules that emphasize a specific therapeutic task or goal. It is delivered in an individual format and is intended to be flexible, providing for an optional pretreatment preparation phase, inclusion of parents/caregivers in portions of sessions, and varying lengths of sessions as well as the ability to complete a single module over one or several sessions, based on the developmental needs of the adolescent. The typical course of treatment occurs over 10–15 weekly sessions of 60–90 min length.

Case Illustration
Bella was a 14-year-old girl who lived with her mother, stepfather, and stepsister (age 16). She was in eighth grade in an online school and had been in an emotional support classroom for the 2 years prior. She was brought into treatment by her mother and reported a trauma history that involved her father's suicide attempt when she was 8, a motor vehicle accident at age 10, and sexual abuse by her older brother from the ages of 11 to 13. Bella had been hospitalized 6 months prior to her initial evaluation due to suicidal ideation immediately following disclosure of the sexual abuse to a school counselor. She had been prescribed and was regularly taking psychiatric medications since that hospitalization. She reported severe PTSD symptoms at her evaluation as well as moderate depressive symptoms. Bella had also been struggling with

trichotillomania since the sexual abuse began, which had worsened to the point of her being unwilling to go to school in the prior 2 years and led to her enrollment in online classes. During assessment, Bella, her mother, and the therapist agreed that PTSD was Bella's primary problem (with depression and trichotillomania being secondary to PTSD), that the sexual abuse was the trauma that was distressing her the most, and that Bella would participate in PE-A.

10.2.1 Phase 1: Pretreatment Preparation

The pretreatment preparation phase consists of two modules (the motivational interview module and the case management module). This phase usually takes 1–2 sessions, depending on the developmental level and motivation of the adolescent, as well as the presence of other factors that might interfere with treatment. The motivational interview module is designed to assess the adolescent's motivation and willingness to commit to treatment as well as serve to increase motivation if it is lacking. The case management module aims to address other obstacles to treatment (such as pre-existing mental health or other issues) as well as the level of parental involvement in the treatment, limits of confidentiality, and further assessment of risk.

Case Illustration
In her first session, Bella was asked to describe why she was seeking treatment now, how she felt about beginning treatment, and to rate her level of motivation for treatment. Bella related that it had not been her idea to seek treatment, but that she was here at her mother's behest. She told the therapist that she was interested in feeling better but was not sure if therapy would actually be helpful for her. Because of her ambivalence toward treatment, Bella and the therapist discussed the impact the trauma had on her life (feeling more afraid of things, feeling sick more often, difficulty going to school because of hairpulling, feeling different from friends, and her mother being much more protective of her) as well as the potential benefits of participating in treatment. She was asked to identify potential costs of therapy and noted that she might lose the special treatment she received from others, feeling that others might not be as nice to her if she was feeling better. The therapist and Bella discussed the benefits of relinquishing this special treatment, and how reducing her PTSD symptoms could be a bigger benefit than getting special treatment. They then completed a list of pros and cons about engaging in the treatment. Once complete, Bella looked over the list and concluded that there were more pros than cons. The therapist revisited the question of her motivation for therapy, and Bella stated that she was willing to give therapy a try because the benefits far outweighed the drawbacks.

Case Illustration
Since there was still time left in the session, the therapist proceeded to the case management module by asking about Bella's current family situation and other potential stressors or obstacles to treatment. Bella reported a good relationship with her mother and stepfather and a difficult relationship with her biological father because he did not believe that his son had sexually abused her. Her parents were divorced and Bella had little contact with her father. Bella's brother had been sent to a juvenile detention facility for treatment after the investigation of her sexual abuse allegations, where he had resided since. In this session, Bella reported that their family, in conjunction with her brother's treatment providers, was planning for reunification of Bella and her brother in a few months. At the time, neither Bella nor her mother knew exactly what the plan or ultimate goals for reunification would entail, but Bella reported that she was open to it. She had some sense that the result would involve deciding where her brother would live when he was released, and although she did not want to live in the same home with him again, she was willing to consider having him live with her father. The therapist inquired about how Bella wanted her mother to be involved in the treatment, and she expressed that she did not want her mother to know the specifics of the sexual abuse. The therapist explained that a portion of each session could be devoted to having her mother in the room to discuss progress and/or concerns and that the therapist could also provide her mother with psychoeducational handouts and general updates. Bella did not want to include her mother in the sessions on a regular basis, but was open to periodically include her on an as-needed basis. She explained that her mother worked and would likely not accompany her to every session anyway. Bella and the therapist agreed to this plan, with the caveat that her mother would be informed of any risky or dangerous behaviors (suicidal/homicidal ideation, self-injury, substance use, or any other kinds of abuse), just as they had discussed during the assessment when reviewing the limits of confidentiality.

The therapist then conducted a risk assessment for suicidality, self-injury, substance use, and the presence of any other dangerous behaviors. Bella denied all of these. They discussed Bella's previous hospitalization and how she felt that she could no longer live now that her family knew about the sexual abuse. Although Bella had thought about suicide at that time, she had not made an attempt, but instead told her mother about it. Since Bella had this history of suicidality, they developed a crisis coping plan that specifically listed the actions Bella agreed to take if she began to have suicidal thoughts in the future, including telling her mother, engaging in pleasurable activities (listening to music, calling a friend, skateboarding, etc.), and calling the therapist. The session ended by meeting together with Bella and her mother to discuss her mother's level of involvement in treatment and to review the crisis coping plan together. Her mother introduced other barriers to treatment, including Bella's difficulty going out in public due to her hair loss as well as a problematic pattern of staying up all night and sleeping during the day. Plans for these difficulties were discussed, and the session ended with assignment of homework, which was to review the crisis coping plan completed in session each day.

10.2.2 Phase 2: Psychoeducation and Treatment Planning

Phase 2 is comprised of three modules (the treatment rationale module, the gathering information module, and the common reactions to trauma module). Phase 2 typically requires 2–3 sessions. This phase allows the therapist to discuss with the adolescent the reasons for confronting fears instead of avoiding them, the factors that maintain post-trauma difficulties, and the reactions the adolescent has experienced in response to the trauma.

Module 1: Treatment Rationale The goals of this module are to describe the structure of the treatment to the adolescent, introduce the rationale for treatment, and teach the adolescent a breathing retraining technique. Although the goals of this module are psychoeducational, it is designed to be an interactive discussion.

> **Case Illustration**
> This session began with a review of homework. Bella had reviewed her crisis coping plan and even added several other pleasurable activities to her list. After praising her for completing homework, the therapist discussed the rationale for treatment with Bella. The therapist explained that it is typical to experience difficulties in reaction to trauma in the immediate aftermath, but that continued avoidance of trauma-related thoughts and situations can in part explain the development and maintenance of PTSD symptoms such as nightmares and difficulty sleeping. The therapist explained the two major reasons that PTSD symptoms persist: (1) avoidance of thoughts, feelings, and situations related to the trauma and (2) the presence of unhelpful thoughts and beliefs. The therapist made it clear that avoidance only works in the short term to reduce distress, but that in the long term, it could make it more difficult to get past her post-trauma reactions. They discussed the techniques that would be used during treatment to target the two kinds of avoidance present in PTSD: recounting the memory (where Bella would repeatedly remember and talk about the trauma) and real-life experiments (where Bella would be encouraged to face safe but avoided situations). Bella was able to give an example in her own life that demonstrated her understanding of the rationale. She explained that she had been afraid of riding in cars after the accident she experienced when she was 10 years old and that her mother had gradually gotten her to be able to do this again by taking her on longer and longer drives. She expressed that she had felt very frightened and upset about the accident at first, but that it became much easier to deal with as she became more comfortable in cars. The therapist praised her understanding of how the treatment would work and, since there was time left in the session, moved on to module 2.

Module 2: Gathering Information The goal of this module is to complete the trauma interview, found in the therapist guide for PE-A (*Prolonged Exposure Therapy for Adolescents with PTSD: Emotional Processing of Traumatic Experiences;* Foa et al. 2008). The trauma interview allows the therapist and adolescent to choose an index trauma, decide upon the start and end points of the trauma account, and identify unhelpful beliefs about the trauma.

> **Case Illustration**
> The therapist began the trauma interview with Bella by asking her to briefly describe the trauma that was currently the most distressing to her. Although Bella had experienced several traumas during the course of her life, she quickly identified the sexual abuse by her brother as the worst trauma. The therapist explained that treatment would focus on a single incident that occurred and that it was most effective and efficient to focus on the most distressing incident. Although there were many instances where her brother would touch her inappropriately or sneak into her room at night, on one occasion he escalated his behavior and tried to rape her. This incident was the most distressing for Bella, and she was asked to describe it in as much detail as she felt comfortable giving. The therapist then asked about Bella's feelings during and after the trauma, any injuries that resulted from the trauma, and any changes in her beliefs after the trauma.
>
> After completing the trauma interview, the therapist taught Bella about breathing retraining, a technique to help her slow down her breathing. The therapist talked Bella through repetitions of the breathing retraining cycle for 3 or 4 min while audio recording the instructions so she could practice at home. Bella's homework for this session included reading the accompanying chapter of the *Prolonged Exposure Therapy for PTSD: Teen Workbook* (Chrestman et al. 2008), listening to the recording of the breathing retraining, and practicing the breathing retraining three times per day.

Module 3: Common Reactions to Trauma The goal of this module is to identify the reactions to trauma that the adolescent is experiencing and explain that many people have similar reactions after experiencing a traumatic event. The intention is to aid the adolescent in understanding that his/her reactions are common and understandable for individuals with PTSD and not a sign of personal failure to cope or irreparable damage. This discussion is interactive, and the adolescent is asked to write down the reactions they have experienced while the discussion is ongoing.

> **Case Illustration**
> After reviewing Bella's homework, the therapist began the discussion by asking how Bella felt she had changed since the trauma. Bella talked about increased fear and anxiety, feeling on edge, reexperiencing (intrusive thoughts, nightmares,

and flashbacks), avoidance of trauma-related thoughts and situations, emotional numbness, anger, guilt, shame, feelings of losing control, changes in her perceptions of herself and the world, and hopelessness. The therapist put these reactions in the context of common responses to a traumatic experience, in an attempt to help Bella understand how these changes were related to her trauma. Bella said that it made her feel somewhat better to know that she was not the only one who had experienced such changes after a traumatic event. Since there was time left in the session, the therapist moved on to module 4.

10.2.3 Phase 3: Exposures

Phase 3 is comprised of three modules, the real-life experiments module, the recounting the memory module, and the worst moments module. Phase 2 typically requires 7–10 sessions. This phase focuses on the two conditions necessary for emotional processing of the trauma: encouraging the adolescent to face their fears instead of avoiding them and ensuring that these exposures provide corrective information (i.e., that an avoided situation is actually safe and that the adolescent can talk about the trauma without falling apart).

Module 4: Real-Life Experiments The goals of this module are to discuss the rationale for real-life experiments, explain the procedure for completing real-life experiments, build a hierarchy of avoided situations, and prepare the adolescent for real-life experiment homework. At times, parental involvement is required for the planning and execution of real-life experiments, either because the adolescent wants a coach or helper when beginning certain real-life experiments or because the adolescent may need a parent in order to achieve the logistics of a real-life experiment (e.g., needing a ride to the mall).

Case Illustration
The therapist discussed the rationale for real-life experiments with Bella by explaining that while avoiding trauma reminders feels better temporarily, it also keeps her from doing all the activities she wants to do, which can make her feel worse overall. By practicing real-life experiments, Bella would get the chance to experience the situation, gather evidence like a scientist, and see how safe the situation really was. The therapist assured Bella that she would never be asked to try out a situation that was actually dangerous, but that they would work on situations that only feel dangerous now because of the trauma she experienced. The therapist also explained the ways that real-life experiments would help to reduce Bella's symptoms (by breaking the habit of avoiding, by helping her get used to the situation so that it becomes less upsetting over time, by helping her learn that the situation can actually be safe, by helping her realize that her uncomfortable feelings will not last forever, and by helping her to feel more in control of and better about herself).

The therapist and Bella then discussed a way to measure her upset feelings by using a "stress thermometer" that goes from 0 to 10, with 0 being not feeling upset at all and 10 being the most upset Bella has ever felt in her life. The therapist elicited examples of situations from Bella that represented a 0, 5, and 10 to ensure understanding of the stress thermometer. They then built the real-life experiment hierarchy together by identifying situations and activities that Bella was avoiding. Once this list had been generated, Bella rated the degree of distress each of the items would cause using the stress thermometer ratings. The following are selected items from Bella's hierarchy:

The final part of this session focused on assignment of homework. Homework for this session included reading the accompanying chapters of the workbook, listening to the recording of the session, and practicing the breathing retraining three times per day. Additionally, the first two real-life experiments were assigned for homework. Bella agreed to begin reading a book about a girl who was sexually abused that she had been wanting to read but avoiding for 30 min each day as well as to get a sample of the cologne her brother wore and leave it open near her for 30 min each day.

Stress thermometer ratings	Real-life experiments
10	Taking a shower at home with the door unlocked
9	Being in the dark in my room alone
9	Looking at pictures of my brother
7	Using the toilet at home with the door unlocked
7	Being upstairs by myself at home at night
7	Sitting on a bench at the mall with mom, with people behind me
6	Being downstairs by myself at home
5	Walking without looking over my shoulder in public
5	Smelling the cologne my brother wore
4	Reading a book about sexual abuse

Module 5: Recounting the Memory The goals of Module 5 are to discuss the rationale for recounting the trauma memory, to engage in recounting the trauma through "memory talk" (or imaginal exposure), and to have a discussion that will help the adolescent to process the traumatic memory after completing memory talk. This module is repeated in successive sessions before moving on to the next module and usually takes 2–5 sessions. Memory talk is most often accomplished through imaginal exposure to the trauma memory, but can be done in several ways depending on the developmental level of the adolescent. If the adolescent is unable to verbally recount the memory, other options such as writing the memory, drawing it, or recounting through stories are also available. The goal in each session of memory

talk is to have the adolescent recount the memory repeatedly and in as much detail as possible for 20–40 min. After memory talk is complete in each session, time is devoted to emotionally process the trauma through discussion with the therapist about the adolescent's thoughts and feelings not only about the memory talk in that session but also about the trauma itself. Through these discussions, it is expected that the adolescent will begin to gain a different perspective on the trauma (e.g., "what happened was not my fault"). Memory talk is audio recorded in each session and the adolescent is asked to listen to the recording each day.

Case Illustration

This session began with homework review, and Bella reported success with the first two real-life experiments she attempted. She had begun to read a book about sexual abuse and had gotten a sample of the cologne her brother wore and practiced these three to four times each. She reported that both were easier the last time than they were the first time. The therapist praised Bella for her efforts and then discussed the rationale for recounting the trauma memory. The therapist normalized Bella's urges to avoid thinking about the trauma while at the same time pointing out that trying not to think about it had not made it any easier to deal with. The therapist explained that the purpose of recounting the memory was to allow Bella to organize and digest what happened so that it would not feel so overwhelming or confusing. The therapist discussed how recounting the memory would allow Bella to see that thinking about the trauma and having actually experienced it are two very different things, that she would not fall apart while talking about it, and that she was competent and strong.

Bella was given instructions about how to recount the memory. She was asked to close her eyes and tell the story of the trauma from the beginning of the event to the end and told that she would work on it for approximately 30 minutes, repeating the narrative as necessary until the time was up. In order to get in touch with her memory emotionally, she was asked to recount the memory in the present tense and to include as many details as possible, including thoughts, feelings, and sensations during the trauma. Bella was also told that the therapist would check in on her stress thermometer ratings every 5 minutes and might ask questions to help elicit more details so that Bella could sufficiently engage with the trauma memory. Bella began memory talk hesitantly and spoke slowly and carefully throughout the next 25 minutes. During this time, she repeated the memory twice. Her affect was relatively flat throughout and she reported the events that occurred as if giving a police report, with very little emotion. While she gave the basic details of what happened, she skipped over or rushed through what may have been the most difficult parts of the event, particularly what her brother had said and did when he attempted to penetrate her. Since this was Bella's first session of memory talk, the therapist did not push for more details but instead was supportive and encouraging of Bella's efforts. Bella's stress thermometer rating started at an 8 and ended at a 6.

After memory talk was over, the therapist processed the trauma with Bella via discussion. The therapist first congratulated and praised Bella for her courage in doing the memory talk. They then discussed the experience of recounting the memory, how it had gotten a little bit easier the second time through, and explored her thoughts and beliefs related to the trauma and its aftermath. Bella brought up feelings of shame and guilt about the trauma, feeling as if she were a "freak" because her brother was the perpetrator of the trauma and that it was her fault it had gone as far as it did because she had not told anyone about it. The therapist allowed Bella to talk about these feelings and was empathic, but did not try to change her thinking. After this processing of the trauma, the therapist discussed new real-life experiments for the week and assigned Bella homework for this session, which included listening to the recording of the memory talk and practicing her assigned real-life experiments daily.

This module was repeated with Bella for three more sessions. In the beginning of each of these three sessions, the therapist checked on Bella's completion of homework. Bella practiced her real-life experiments almost daily and worked her way up her hierarchy as she mastered each item. She also listened to the audio recording of her memory talk from the previous session nearly every day. After homework review in each session, Bella completed memory talk for 20–40 minutes. The therapist encouraged her to talk about the trauma in more detail during these sessions, which helped her to emotionally engage with the memory. Her rather flat affect faded, although she was still very controlled during the memory talk. She never cried or let too much emotion show. Her peak stress thermometer ratings during memory talk fell to a 4 by session 6. After memory talk in each session, the therapist would process the trauma with Bella by asking how it was for her that day, which would lead into a discussion of how Bella was thinking and feeling about the trauma. Processing during these sessions focused on Bella's sense of guilt about the trauma. In particular, Bella felt that since this trauma had been ongoing for several years, the index trauma where she was nearly raped was her fault because she should have disclosed the abuse sooner. During these first sessions of processing, the therapist simply allowed Bella to discuss why she felt guilty and how it had affected her since her disclosure of the abuse.

Module 6: Worst Moments As the adolescent begins to experience habituation to the trauma memory, the therapist and adolescent will begin working on the most distressing parts of the memory, or the "worst moments," in order to intensify emotional processing. This module is typically introduced after 2–5 sessions of recounting the memory (module 5) and repeated for the remainder of phase 3, remaining the focus until the adolescent is nearing the end of treatment and relapse prevention is introduced. The worst moments module is identical to the previous module in terms of structure (homework review, 20–40 minutes of memory talk, processing, and homework assignment), with the exception that memory talk focuses on only a small segment of the full trauma memory, the worst moment.

In the first session of this module, the therapist explains that while the adolescent has been recounting the entire memory of the trauma up to that point, the task is now to narrow the focus to only the very worst parts of the memory. The therapist and adolescent choose the worst moments together (based on stress thermometer ratings and the adolescent's subjective report), and the adolescent is instructed to focus memory talk on just this piece of the memory. The adolescent is asked to repeat the "worst moment" as many times as necessary in the allotted 20–40 minutes. If more than one worst moment is identified, memory talk focuses repeatedly on the most difficult of the worst moments, and other identified worst moments are worked on sequentially in the order of difficulty after the first one has been processed. Focusing on only the very worst parts of the memory gives the adolescent the opportunity to more closely examine what happened at the times and to elaborate on details that he or she might still be avoiding. In addition, the worst moment sessions allow for a greater number of memory talk repetitions per session, to facilitate greater habituation to even the most difficult parts of the trauma.

Case Illustration
After reviewing Bella's homework, the therapist and Bella chose the worst moment of the trauma memory and discussed how recounting just the worst moment in greater detail would help her. Bella chose only one worst moment, which was when her brother put a pillow over her head and attempted to penetrate her. The therapist explained that memory talk would focus on just this piece of the memory so that she would get to repeat it many times in a single session. As in previous sessions, time was devoted to processing the trauma memory after memory talk was completed.

This module was completed with Bella for four sessions. During these sessions, Bella continued to consistently complete her homework of practicing more and more difficult real-life experiments and listening to the audio recording of her memory talk. In session, while completing memory talk to her worst moment, the therapist encouraged Bella to talk in more and more detail about this worst part. The therapist asked for details about what Bella was thinking and how she was feeling as her brother attempted to penetrate her, asked questions about the physical sensations that occurred at the time, and encouraged Bella to describe what had happened moment by moment. While Bella found it difficult, particularly in regard to describing her brother's physical actions during the attempted rape, she was able to eventually say these things out loud. She continued to be emotionally engaged with the memory, as evidenced by her expressions and body language during memory talk, but she remained controlled throughout, never breaking down or sobbing. Her stress thermometer ratings went from a peak of 9 in the first worst moment session to a peak of 3 by the last worst moment session.

During processing, the therapist focused on asking Bella questions related to her feelings of guilt that could help her to see that there might have been reasons or justifications for why she had not told about the abuse as soon as it started occurring. The most fruitful discussions for Bella stemmed from questions about what her brother had been like as a person and what the family dynamic had been like in the home at the time. Through these discussions, Bella related that her brother had ruled the family with his behavior and tantrums even from an early age and that she had learned that going against him would result in consequences, whether from her brother or her father who always sided with him. As she related this, Bella began to see that she did indeed have reasons for not disclosing the abuse when it started or any time thereafter. She was eventually able to let go of her guilt around not disclosing sooner and began instead to feel anger toward her brother for the first time. Bella was encouraged to acknowledge and sit with her angry feelings, as it was normal to feel angry in a situation like this, but soon let go of the anger as she began to feel pity for her brother instead and to hope that the treatment he was receiving was helping him to overcome whatever difficulties he had been experiencing that may have led to him abusing her.

10.2.4 Phase 4: Relapse Prevention/Treatment Termination

Module 7: Relapse Prevention When the adolescent's functioning has sufficiently increased, the memory of the trauma is easier to think about, PTSD symptoms have decreased satisfactorily, and the next module is begun. The goals of module 7 are to identify potential future triggers and the tools the adolescent has learned to deal with these triggers.

Case Illustration
After four sessions of worst moments, Bella had conquered nearly all of her real-life experiments, was no longer avoidant of thoughts or feelings about the sexual abuse, and was showing a significant decrease in self-reported PTSD symptoms. Bella and the therapist decided that her treatment was winding down and moved on to the relapse prevention module. For Bella, reunification with her brother was the foremost topic during this module, which consisted of two sessions. During these sessions, the therapist and Bella discussed the process of reunification, her willingness to engage in the process, and her expectations about the process. The reunification process would be gradual, beginning with an exchange of letters and phone calls and moving to supervised visitations. Ultimate placement of her brother after his release from his program was undecided. Bella restated her desire to have her brother in her life again. She expressed that she was hoping to get some answers from him about why he had abused her. She and the therapist discussed the likelihood that this would occur or that any answers she received would be satisfactory. Bella was able to use what she learned from the therapy about the abuse not being her fault to understand that there was likely no answer to why her

> brother had abused her. She also likened the process of gradual reunification to her real-life experiment work and so felt confident it would be successful. The start of the reunification process was planned for several months after treatment would be terminating, so Bella was also assured that she could schedule future sessions as the time drew near if she felt she needed it.

Module 8: Final Session In this module, the adolescent recounts the memory one last time, using the entire memory and not just the worst moments that have been the focus of the recent sessions. Processing involves comparing how the adolescent feels now as compared to the start of treatment. Items from the real-life experiment hierarchy are re-rated and changes in ratings are discussed. The discussion also includes identifying the most and least helpful parts of treatment. Finally, a celebratory activity chosen by the adolescent is completed.

> **Case Illustration**
> In Bella's final session, she recounted the entire trauma memory that she had worked on in treatment, with a peak stress thermometer rating of 3. During processing, Bella discussed how overwhelmed and confused she had felt about the abuse prior to treatment and how she could now see that the abuse was not her fault, and there were very limited choices she felt she had in terms of telling someone about it. She expressed that she felt much safer in general and not as apprehensive. When re-rating her real-life experiment hierarchy, it was discovered that all items had reduced to a 3 or lower. She was able to see that confronting the situations and practicing them are what led to this change. Bella said that talking about what happened was the most helpful part of treatment, with facing her fears in real life coming in at a close second place. She and the therapist discussed how to utilize the skills she learned in treatment going forward. Bella had decided that she wanted to enjoy some snacks with the therapist and her mother as a celebratory activity, so her mother was brought into the session. While snacking, they discussed Bella's progress and the changes her mother had noticed in her. The therapist also presented Bella with a certificate of achievement to highlight her success. The session ended with plans to meet in the future if needed regarding the reunification process with her brother.

10.3 Special Challenges

A number of challenges may arise when implementing PE-A with an adolescent. The following addresses some of the most commonly encountered difficulties. The first challenge lies in assessing appropriateness for PE-A. It is important to remember that PE-A is a treatment for PTSD symptoms and not a treatment for trauma. As such, it is critical to carefully assess PTSD symptoms. If PTSD symptoms are present and interfering in the adolescent's life, it is also essential to determine that PTSD symptoms are the primary target of treatment. If comorbid conditions exist, these comorbidities should be secondary to PTSD symptoms in order for PE-A to be the treatment of choice. Note that full criteria for a diagnosis of PTSD are not a requirement for appropriateness for PE-A. If an adolescent is experiencing subthreshold PTSD (e.g., meets criteria for reexperiencing, avoidance, and increased arousal symptoms, but does not meet full criteria for cognition/mood symptoms), PE-A may still be appropriate as long as the symptoms experienced are distressing, interfering, and primary.

PE-A may not be recommended if the adolescent is at imminent risk of suicide or homicide, engaging in extensive self-injury, experiencing psychotic symptoms which are not well managed by medication, or living in an environment where there is very high risk of an assault. These situations or comorbidities should be addressed and stabilized prior to beginning PE-A, just as with any other treatments. Additionally, if other disorders are causing more functional interference for the adolescent, these primary diagnoses should be addressed before implementing PE-A. These issues underscore the importance of careful assessment both before and during treatment with both interview and self-report clinical measures.

It is also important to ensure that the adolescent has a sufficient memory of the traumatic event. A sufficient memory has a beginning, middle, and end and can be visualized and described by the adolescent. In the cases of head injury, intoxication, or dissociative amnesia where the adolescent does not remember the entire event, PE-A can still be appropriate if the adolescent can remember the circumstances prior to and after the lapse in memory. In this way, short, disconnected moments of a trauma that are remembered can be sufficient for participating in PE-A.

Another challenge that is frequently encountered when implementing PE-A is maintaining focus on the trauma work. Adolescents with PTSD are often dealing with other life stressors related to their trauma, such as legal or court involvement, being in foster care, dealing with physical injuries, and loss of family or other supportive people in their lives. These stressors may make it difficult for adolescents to engage in treatment. A strong therapeutic alliance can be helpful in mitigating the effects of these stressors. The groundwork for a good therapeutic alliance is supported by many PE-A techniques, including providing rationales for the treatment and its techniques and discussion of common reactions. The therapist should also remember that maintaining focus on the trauma work is often far more helpful than getting distracted by some of these other stressors. These stressors should not be ignored; rather, time should be set aside in each session (10–15 min at the end) to discuss these other issues. Of course, true crises or risks of harm should be addressed immediately and may require a session or two of management.

It is also important for therapists to tailor treatment to the developmental level of the adolescent. PE-A allows for flexible implementation of treatment techniques, such as using role-plays, stories, or games to explain therapeutic concepts or using writing or drawing to recount the trauma memory. PE-A's modular format also allows for shorter or longer sessions, with presentation of a single or multiple modules in each session depending on the adolescent's attention span. Therapists should be careful to use vocabulary and examples appropriate to the adolescent's developmental level to ensure understanding of and buy-in to the treatment rationale. It should also be noted that PE-A has been used with children younger than 12, but has not yet been empirically validated for these ages.

Therapists implementing PE-A may also encounter challenges related to parental involvement in the treatment. While it is often important for parents to understand the rationale for the treatment and be supportive of their child's efforts to face his or her fears, adolescents are often struggling with issues of independence and privacy from parents. PE-A incorporates both of these goals by offering psychoeducational materials for all parents and allowing adolescents to choose the level of involvement their parent will have. Additionally, while a supportive parent is ideal, some adolescents may have complicated or estranged relationships with parents, or there may be no parental involvement in treatment. Developmental level can play a part in parental involvement as well. For example, younger adolescents may need parental assistance in order to achieve the logistics of any given real-life experiment (e.g., being driven to the mall). In other cases, parents may encourage their adolescent's avoidance, and so educating them about the rationale for real-life experiments and getting their input on items to be included on the hierarchy can be important.

Difficulties with engagement during recounting the memory may also present challenges. While it is expected that adolescents can become upset while recounting their trauma and in fact signals that they are engaging with the memory, over-engagement sometimes occurs. Over-engagement includes extreme emotional distress or severe dissociation during recounting, such that the adolescent is no longer processing the memory in a way that promotes learning. Helping the adolescent to titrate his or her engagement (by recounting with eyes open, writing the memory, etc.) is helpful when this occurs. Under-engagement during recounting the memory can also be especially challenging. Under-engagement occurs when the adolescent is unable to connect to the memory emotionally. Again, the therapist's task here is to assist the adolescent in titrating the recounting (by coaching or role-playing, reiterating the rationale, asking questions about details of the memory, etc.).

10.4 Research/Evidence

The research literature supporting the use of PE in the treatment of PTSD among adults is extensive. PE has been studied for over two decades in both research and non-research clinical settings and has been shown to produce rapid and large reductions in PTSD symptoms secondary to a range of trauma types (see for review: Powers et al. 2010) that are maintained up to 10 years after treatment (Resick et al. 2012). PE benefits extend beyond PTSD symptoms and include significant reduction in depression and general anxiety (Powers et al. 2010), anger (Cahill et al. 2003), and guilt (Resick et al. 2002), as well as improvement in social functioning (Markowitz et al. 2015) and physical health problems (Rauch et al. 2009). Based on this confluence of research support, numerous treatment guidelines recommend the use of PE and exposure-based treatment for PTSD, including the Institute of Medicine (2008) and National Institute for Health and Care Excellence (2005).

Studies of PE-A in adolescent populations, while more limited in number, have demonstrated its effectiveness and its superiority to comparison therapies. For example, in a randomized controlled trial, PE-A demonstrated superiority to time-limited dynamic psychotherapy (TLDP) in reducing PTSD and depression severity and elevating global functioning among adolescents with PTSD related to a single event trauma (n = 38, ages 12–18; Gilboa-Schechtman et al. 2010). After treatment, 73.7 % of PE-A patients met the criteria for good end-state functioning (compared to 31.6 % in TLDP), and 68.4 % of PE-A patients no longer met diagnostic criteria for PTSD. These symptom improvements were maintained at both 6- and 17-month follow-up.

In a second randomized controlled trial, PE-A was compared to client-centered therapy (CCT), a form of supportive counseling that focuses on alliance building and problem-solving daily stresses. Participants in this study were adolescent females with PTSD related to sexual abuse presenting for treatment at a community mental health clinic (n = 61, ages 13–18; Foa et al. 2013). Following treatment, adolescents who received PE-A exhibited greater reductions in symptoms of PTSD and depression and greater improvements in global functioning compared to CCT. Additionally, 83.3 % of adolescents receiving PE-A no longer met the criteria for PTSD at posttreatment, compared with 54 % of adolescents receiving CCT. Consistent with the Gilboa-Schechtman et al. (2010) study, symptom change following PE-A was maintained at 12-month follow-up. Although further research is needed, the evidence to date supports the effectiveness of PE-A for adolescent PTSD as exemplified by its designation in 2011 as "well-supported by research evidence" (California Evidence-Based Clearinghouse for Child Welfare), the highest designation a treatment program can receive.

References

Cahill SP, Rauch SA, Hembree EA, Foa EB (2003) Effect of cognitive-behavioral treatments for PTSD on anger. J Cogn Psychother 17:113–131. doi:10.1891/jcop.17.2.113.57434

California Evidence-Based Clearinghouse for Child Welfare (2011) Retrieved 27 Jan 2016, from http://www.cebc4cw.org/program/prolonged-exposure-therapy-for-adolescents/detailed

Chrestman K, Gilboa-Schechtman E, Foa EB (2008) Prolonged exposure therapy for PTSD: teen workbook. Oxford University Press, New York

Foa EB, Chrestman K, Gilboa-Schechtman E (2008) Prolonged exposure therapy for adolescents with PTSD: emotional processing of traumatic experiences. Oxford University Press, New York

Foa EB, Hembree EA, Rothbaum BO (2007) Prolonged exposure therapy for PTSD: emotional processing of traumatic experiences therapist guide. Oxford University Press, New York

Foa EB, Huppert JD, Cahill SP (2006) Emotional processing theory: an update. In: Rothbaum BO (ed) Pathological anxiety: emotional processing in etiology and treatment. Guilford Press, New York, pp. 3–24

Foa EB, Kozak MJ (1986) Emotional processing of fear: exposure of corrective information. Psychol Bull 99:20–35. doi:10.1037/0033-2909.99.1.20

Foa EB, McLean CP, Capaldi S, Rosenfield D (2013) Prolonged exposure vs. supportive counseling for sexual abuse-related PTSD in adolescent girls: a randomized controlled trial. JAMA 310:2650–2657. doi:10.1001/jama.2013.282829

Gilboa-Schechtman E, Foa EB, Shafran N, Aderka IM, Powers MB, Rachamim L, Rosenbach L, Yadin E, Apter A (2010) Prolonged exposure versus dynamic therapy for adolescent PTSD: a pilot randomized controlled trial. J Am Acad Child Adolesc Psychiatry 49:1034–1042. doi:10.1016/j.jaac.2010.07.014

Institute of Medicine (2008) Treatment of posttraumatic stress disorder: an assessment of the evidence. National Academies Press, Washington, DC

National Institute for Health and Care Excellence (2005) Retrieved 2 Dec 2016, from https://www.nice.org.uk/guidance/CG26/chapter/1-Guidance#the-treatment-of-ptsd

Markowitz JC, Petkova E, Neria Y, Van Meter PE, Zhao Y, Hembree E, Lovell K, Biyanova T, Marshall RD (2015) Is exposure necessary? a randomized controlled trial of interpersonal psychotherapy for PTSD. Am J Psychiatry 172:430–440. doi:10.1176/appi.ajp.2014.14070908

Powers MB, Halpern JM, Ferenschak MP, Gillihan SJ, Foa EB (2010) A meta-analytic review of prolonged exposure for posttraumatic stress disorder. Clin Psychol Rev 30:635–641. doi:10.1016/j.cpr.2010.04.007

Rauch SAM, Grunfeld TEE, Yadin E, Cahill SP, Hembree E, Foa EB (2009) Changes in reported physical health symptoms and social function with prolonged exposure therapy for chronic posttraumatic stress disorder. Depress Anxiety 26:732–738. doi:10.1002/da.20518

Resick PA, Nishith P, Weaver TL, Astin MC, Feuer CA (2002) A comparison of cognitive-processing therapy with prolonged exposure and a waiting condition for the treatment of chronic post-traumatic stress disorder in female rape victims. J Consult Clin Psychol 70:867–879. doi:10.1037/0022-006X.70.4.867

Resick PA, Williams LF, Suvack MK, Monson CM, Gradus JL (2012) Long-term outcomes of cognitive-behavioral treatments for posttraumatic stress disorder among female rape survivors. J Consult Clin Psychol 80:201–210. doi:10.1037/a0026602

Narrative Exposure Therapy for Children and Adolescents (KIDNET)

11

Maggie Schauer, Frank Neuner, and Thomas Elbert

11.1 Theoretical Underpinnings of Narrative Exposure Therapy (NET)

Children and adolescents become traumatized when they are repeatedly exposed to negative experiences that are intense enough to trigger an alarm response or another strong reaction of the defense cascade (Schauer and Elbert 2010). The consequences are particularly devastating for mental health if the pain and fear are caused by the attachment figure, because caregivers are meant to provide the opposite of this: safety, reassurance, and calm. Children who experience one type of adversity also frequently experience other forms of stress, which may include emotional neglect, social rejection, and physical or sexual abuse, either within the family or externally.

Multiple experiences of severe stress form building blocks for trauma-related suffering (Neuner et al. 2004; Schauer et al. 2003) that leave their survivors vulnerable into adulthood (Kolassa et al. 2010). Consequently, new traumatic experiences are most devastating when they affect those who have had to endure childhood adversities (Nandi et al. 2015) that have led to permanent changes in implicit memory.

Narrations from child survivors who have experienced severe and often ongoing stress describe immense pain and sadness. These children desperately seek emotional closeness and meaning-making (Schauer et al. 2004, 2005; Onyut et al. 2005; Catani et al. 2009; Hermenau et al. 2011). For survivors of multiple and complex traumatization, stabilization therapies that involve active detachment from the

---

M. Schauer (✉) • T. Elbert
University of Konstanz, Constance, Germany
e-mail: maggie.schauer@uni-konstanz.de; thomas.elbert@uni-konstanz.de

F. Neuner
University of Bielefeld, Bielefeld, Germany
e-mail: frank.neuner@uni-bielefeld.de

memory of the trauma, or therapies which only attend to the trauma incidentally, or select an isolated traumatic event as the target of therapy, have not proven to reduce the resulting suffering in its entirety in these children. Such therapies are insufficient to modulate maladaptive changes in neural and epigenetic organization and will not redirect development toward functionality (Lindauer 2015; Jongh and Broeke 2014; Neuner 2012; Beutel and Subic-Wrana 2012; Elbert and Schauer 2014).

Humans with broken lifelines need a comprehensive approach of narrative restructuring and in sensu exposure not only of their trauma memories but also of their entire biography. Children and adolescents need support to be able to reflect on their life stories and process the traumata as well as their empowering life experiences. *Narrative exposure therapy* (NET; Schauer et al. 2005/2011) focuses on the elaboration of the autobiography, including integration of both the traumatic experiences and other highly arousing events. KIDNET has been designed for minors affected by multiple and continuous exposure to traumatic stressors, such as abuse, social disadvantage, and/or repeated experiences of organized violence. Chronologically guided narration along the timeline with a focus on the most arousing events can be sufficient to provide considerable relief and reinstate individual functioning, even in children who suffer from severe and complex traumatization (Catani et al. 2009; Ruf et al. 2010). Storytelling is universal in child-rearing across cultures. When combined with imaginal exposure, it will allow meaning-making and location of the cascade of traumata in context (Ruf and Schauer 2012). With its testimony approach, NET also aims to document children's rights abuses, within the family and in war.

In traumatized individuals, memory functions have lost their orchestration. Their own biographies seem fragmented, without coherence (e.g., Brewin et al. 2010). Therefore a core component of KIDNET is to assign each traumatic event a corresponding spatial and temporal context (*where* and *when* did things happen?). This autobiographical information is referred to as "cold memory" (Elbert and Schauer 2002). It is verbally accessible and hence supports communication and reappraisal. This allows an adjustment in the meaning of events to occur. Cold memory contains records of conscious experiences that assign context to hot memories, which are the sensory, cognitive, and emotional traces of arousing experiences. In trauma-related disorders, the key problem is the failure of proper connections to the associative hot memories including when and where the experience happened, resulting in feelings of impending threat and helplessness. This leads to lasting posttraumatic stress, anxiety, and depression (Brewin et al. 2010; Brewin 2014; Schauer et al. 2011). As a consequence, the attachment-seeking system in children is overly activated. Their ability to adequately regulate emotions and their motivation to explore and learn are jeopardized because of their decontextualized "hot memories" (Table 11.1).

Emotionally arousing events result in detailed sensory and perceptual images tied together in associative networks (Schauer et al. 2011). Arousing memories – for example, one's first romantic kiss – may be activated by sensory cues such as the *scent of a given perfume* or invoke physiological responses such as *heart pounding* in pleasant anticipation. In addition to sensations and emotions, hot memories also include a cognitive component – *am I dating the right boy? My parents will be angry with me....* For traumatic experiences, hot memories may involve features of the past scene: the sound of bullets, the smell of fire (sensory elements), fear and panic (emotions), thoughts of helplessness (cognition), sweating, and heart palpitation (physiological memories). In traumatized survivors, these memories can only be accessed involuntarily, forming the basis for flashbacks and nightmares related to the traumatic moments themselves. With an increasing number of experiences, more and more sensory elements become associated to this memory (this phenomenon is called a "fear network") and thus act as cues that increase the likelihood that the core feelings of trauma (fear, helplessness, arousal) will become activated. This hot memory network is the result of experiences that were made at different times, in different places, and thus do not share a common cold memory. Consequently, with increasing exposure to stressors, the fear network becomes larger while these hot traumatic memories lose their connections to spatial and temporal information (Schauer et al. 2011). When cues trigger these hot memories, there is no connection to a single episode, and the experience is erroneously located in the here and now.

These cold memory deficits pave the way for frequent arousal peaks and cause nightmares and flashbacks. Children relive events and may replay them over and over again. Therefore in narrative exposure therapy, the survivor constructs a chronological narrative of her/his life story with the assistance of the therapist and with a focus on emotionally arousing experiences. The associative entanglement of the traumatic experiences will be transformed into a coherent narrative, whereby the facts are embedded in the emotions and cognitions that they have elicited in the past and their memory activates in the here and now. Hot and cold memory contents become reconnected (see Table 11.1). Empathic understanding, active listening, congruency, and unconditional positive regard are key components of the therapist's behavior.

Table 11.1 Hot and cold memory

Cold memory (context: time and place of episodic events)	Hot memory (sensation-cognition-emotion-physiological responding)
Abstract, flexible, contextualized representations	Inflexible, sensory-bound representations
Verbally accessible – support communication, reappraisal, and consequent alteration of life goals	Detailed sensory and perceptual images that can be accessed only involuntarily and that form the basis for flashbacks and nightmares
Contains records of distinct conscious experiences that can be activated by both voluntary and involuntary retrieval	Memory is associative and not contextualized, hence traumatic moments experienced as happening again in the present
Can situate information in its appropriate spatial and temporal context – *allocentric*	Supports *egocentric* view only

> Brewin and colleagues (2010; Brewin 2014) point out that evidence from both cognitive psychology and neuroscience confirms distinct neural bases to abstract, flexible, contextualized representations and to inflexible, sensory-bound representations. The latter is primarily supported by areas of the brain directly involved in perception (e.g., representational cortex) rather than in higher-order cognitive control. The lack of involvement of structures such as the hippocampus results in a non-contextualized memory that is experienced as reoccurring in the present. Contextualized representations contain records of conscious experience that can be activated by both voluntary and involuntary retrieval and also support communication, reappraisal, and the consequent alteration of life goals. This system can situate such information in its appropriate spatial and temporal context. Verbal expression supports the ability to deliberately retrieve and reorganize memory representations and reconstruct them from the low-level sensation-based memory and its corresponding representations.

In this way, the method of narrating those experiences that have the highest arousal peaks across one's entire life does not require the individual to select a single traumatic event from their multifold history of trauma. It rather acknowledges their human life as a whole and helps a child to reclaim ownership of their autobiography. Instead of focusing on an index trauma, KIDNET embraces a life-span perspective. Severe trauma, whether it is the result of an act of nature or deliberate human cruelty, challenges basic assumptions about the world and our expectation to have control over our lives. In developing individuals, repair of attachment wounds can occur, while the emotional networks are activated during narration, if the child encounters a therapeutic contact that guarantees warmth and empathy. KIDNET helps children to chase their ghosts away. They are able to put good and bad into perspective within their stories, experience reparative adult emotional support, and put their thoughts and feelings into words in order to heal the trauma. Instead of therapeutic neutrality, KIDNET promotes advocacy and children's rights for survivors.

11.2 How to Do KIDNET

The classical narrative exposure therapy (Schauer et al. 2005) approach is divided into three parts, and so is KIDNET (for details see Schauer et al. 2011):

> **KIDNET Treatment Plan Overview**
> - Part 1: *Assessment and psychoeducation*: Structured diagnostic interview including *trauma event checklists*, followed by a *brief psychoeducation* for the child and the caregiver in one or two sessions (each about 90 min)

- Part 2: *Lifeline exercise*: Laying out the lifeline as an overview of the highly arousing positive and negative life events along the biographic timeline (done in one session with about 90–120 min)
- Part 3: *Narrative exposure*: Chronological narration of the whole life story including imaginal exposure of the traumatic events (90 min sessions, number of sessions should be determined after the lifeline excercise and typically may range from five to ten). At the end of the treatment, rereading of the whole testimony in a final session and signing of the document by all witnesses and the survivor or laying out a final lifeline including symbols for hopes and wishes for the future. Handing over the life story to the survivor (and his/her non-offending parent)

11.2.1 Part 1: Assessment and Psychoeducation

11.2.1.1 Step 1 (Optional Component for Preschool and Primary School Children, Without Parent)

Build rapport and assess what is immediately on the child's mind – grasping implicit, sensory memories ("hot" memories)

To build rapport with a child, it is often helpful to ask the child to draw a picture or arrange small toys and play with them. When asked to draw a picture, a traumatized child frequently presents an image of its associative trauma memory – that is, the picture fuses elements from various traumatic experiences, sometimes combined with monsters from the fantasy world.

A therapist may introduce her/himself by saying:

> My name is Nell. I am a psychologist (doctor, nurse, social worker etc.) from the (clinic, university, school, etc.). I am here to help children who have experienced extremely bad things such as (use example as useful: war, rape, forced migration, torture, massacre, accidents etc.) and to write down what happened. Before I talk to you about your experiences and the pain that children feel when bad events happen, I was wondering if you could draw a picture about whatever is on your mind or bothering you right now.

The therapist stays in close emotional contact with the child and verbalizes what a child draws or displays with materials. If the child shows something that is obviously related to a bad experience, the therapist tells the child that she/he wants to know more about the bad things that have happened. They may continue with step 2 (a checklist) by explaining that people may experience many bad things and that it is good to know what has upset the child and is probably still bothering her/him. If the child draws something that is not likely to be related to a trauma, the therapist also validates the child and shows interest by asking about the content of the picture before continuing with step 2.

11.2.1.2 Step 2 (Mandatory): Structured Diagnostic Interview Including Event Checklists with the Child (Without the Parent)

KIDNET allows a stepwise approach to disclosure of trauma material. At the beginning of treatment, survivors of trauma are typically avoidant of reminders of their traumatic experiences. However, simply agreeing or disagreeing to an item list, and indicating *when* and *where* things happened, is possible for the majority. An allocentric position (external viewpoint asking for cold facts and context information) will allow the child to feel in control and will not be overwhelming. A thorough and engaged clinical interview (assessment) is essential and will begin the process of establishing a therapeutic relationship.

We recommend using a checklist for assessing both traumatic experiences and other stressors that the child might have experienced within and outside the family. For typical events, the "pediatric Maltreatment and Abuse Chronology of Exposure" (pediMACE; Isele et al. 2016, available in English and German from the authors upon request) has been proven to be a useful tool for schoolchildren of all ages. Introductory items provide information about the familial constellation and the living environment of the child. The child is then asked to respond with "yes" or "no" if he or she has experienced any adverse social situations. Depending on available time and resources, experiences are temporally anchored within lifetime periods – for instance, stages of formal education (kindergarten, primary school, etc.), places of living (my hometown, refugee camp, etc.), or other suitable references. Similar experiences at different ages can be ranked. Inclusion of positive formulated items complements this list in order to remind the child that there were not only bad moments in life. In this way, the pediMACE is a list of typical adversities that normalizes the child's experiences (since they become "known" to the therapist) and legitimizes the reactions to traumatic stressors. The measure asks for the following interpersonal events that are relevant for trauma treatment: parental emotional violence (adults living in the household), parental physical violence (adults living in the household), emotional violence by siblings (children living in the household), physical violence by siblings (children living in the household), emotional neglect, physical neglect, witnessing interparental violence (adults living in the household), witnessing violence to siblings (children living in the household), peer abuse (physical and emotional), sexual violence, and parental loss.

For children who have additionally been exposed to organized or community violence and/or other traumatic experiences such as natural disasters, corresponding checklists should be used. If the child reports stressful experiences, a diagnostic instrument for PTSD such as the UCLA Child PTSD Reaction Index (DSM-5 version: Pynoos and Steinberg 2013) should be applied. Depressive symptoms and suicidality must also always be considered.

Case: T. was 15 years old when she was referred from the school psychologist to a child psychiatric ward because of her eating disorder and, from there, to our outpatient clinic. She was clearly underweight when she first presented. Her school performance had worsened over the course of the last year, with impairment in cognition and memory as well as learning functions, and she had begun to skip more and more school days. She was unfriendly to teachers and peers, was using cannabis, and was uninterested in social activities. She presented at our unit together with her mother, who was seeking close contact to the staff and was very emotional and overly grateful for the possibility of treatment. The mother was suffering from borderline personality disorder and had occasionally been in psychological treatment at other institutions.

The event checklist revealed that T. had been left alone and neglected many times at a preschool age by her mother and later had been sexually abused by her father who was divorced from the mother. In addition, due to the unsettled life of the mother, the family moved many times during her childhood. She had also suffered a severe car accident. After the structured interview, T. was diagnosed with PTSD, depression, and suspected cannabis use disorder.

11.2.1.3 Step 3 (Mandatory Step, with the Presence of a Non-offending Caregiver): Psychoeducation

In KIDNET, psychoeducation is an ongoing companion to treatment, framing the experiences and increasing understanding of symptoms and the rationale for treatment. It is typically repeated briefly and focused on the area of difficulty. After completing the assessment, trauma reactions are explained to the child and his/her caregivers in an open and transparent manner. Introducing the trauma checklist and explaining why it is useful to know what trauma does to the individual, the family and the community informs the child and the caregiver about why they are suffering from distressing events and what can be done about this. This allows the family to regain a sense of control over the symptoms and hope for change.

The therapist provides a detailed explanation of the symptoms using age and education appropriate language and without using medical or scientific terms.

Example:

After the many events you have experienced, most children would be upset. This aftershock is known as a post-traumatic reaction. Our mind and body are designed to notice and remember dangerous information since when there are lots of scary things happening, it may be better for us to be too careful and very aware of what might be happening nearby, in order to keep safe. This survival strategy has become part of yourself, but it is painful and extremely tiring, as you know.

A psychoeducation introducing KIDNET could be as follows:

In order to successfully control the terrible memories from moments when you were fearful in your life or got hurt, we need to gain access to these past events. Together, we want to look at the thoughts, feelings and bodily sensations you had when you experienced … (incidents). I'll help you tell your life story and write everything down. When exploring these bad moments in slow motion, they will lose their power and remain where they belong: in the past. We call what has happened to you a violation of your child rights. You should know that nobody is allowed to violate or harm a child.

Adolescents will need a clear and full explanation about their trauma experience and the treatment plan (which can be given in the presence of their caretakers). Example for psychoeducation with adolescents:

No matter how hard survivors of such terrible experiences try to push them away, memories come back: they intrude into their lives, during the day and in dreams at night. All of a sudden, the person may become upset, scared or detach herself from reality. All of this happens without really knowing 'why'. During a terribly horrifying moment, our mind cannot understand what is going on. It is just too much. We become highly aroused in order to react quickly and make sure we survive if we can, or we feel like fainting, but we have no time in these moments to process any of this information. However, our memory brings up these feelings and fragments later on in order to understand, digest and put together all of this until it makes sense. Reliving those feelings, pictures, and bodily sensations shows that the mind is trying to process this horrible event, to make it understandable – because this may be vital throughout life.

What we want to do now is to give them room here during therapy. We want to explore them together so that they lose their horror in the presence.

For small children the therapist can use metaphors for "cleaning up" the memory to help children understand the rationale for the therapy: like the example of a "stuffed wardrobe," where things pop out (intrusions) and will only stay inside, when the items are taken out, sorted, and folded back in, or the example of a wound that is infected and hurts when touched, which needs to be opened up again, disinfected, and then healed. Sometimes, it might even be helpful during psychoeducation to draw the associations of the child's fear network (Schauer et al. 2011) and see how the different sensory elements (seeing, hearing, touch, etc.), thoughts, feelings, bodily reactions, and meanings are connected to each other.

The psychoeducation should result in the child obtaining the following:

- A helpful explanation about their suffering
- A clear understanding of what will happen during treatment and that she/he is invited to participate voluntarily
- An explanation of what is expected of him/her in the process of KIDNET
- Answers to any remaining questions the child may have about the therapy

In older children it is important to explain why talking about the traumatic event can help to overcome the person's suffering and that giving testimony is an important step in documenting the violation of children's human rights and gaining dignity.

11 Narrative Exposure Therapy for Children and Adolescents (KIDNET)

Case report (cont.): In the case of T., it became apparent that the mother did not know about the sexual abuse her adolescent girl had suffered as a child. Together with T., we thoroughly prepared how we wanted to tell this information to the mother. After that, the mother was invited into the room.

During the psychoeducation step, we explained to the girl and her mother what we had found in the diagnostic interview, normalizing the reactions to the childhood stressors and the current behavioral problems of T. Afterward, we assured the caregivers' support for the planned trauma-focused treatment and detailed the concept of KIDNET and the rationale for treatment.

The mother agreed to take the topic to her own therapist in order to come to terms with the disclosure of her daughter.

11.2.2 Part 2 (Characteristic Part of KIDNET): *Lifeline*

In the next session (allow about 90 min, without the presence of the caregiver), the child's individual life history will be displayed on a timeline, by taking a bird's-eye view of his or her life. This step, also performed in an allocentric position, helps structure the fragmented memory by organizing the life experiences as symbols chronologically along the timeline.

A piece of rope or ribbon is put to the floor or on a table (for physically challenged children) and unfolded by the individual. One end of the rope represents "birth," the unfolded line itself represents the course of life, and the other end should be rolled up to indicate the future yet to come. With the help of the therapist, the young person starts to place natural items that represent memories of significant emotional events along the lifetime periods on the *lifeline* (see Fig. 11.4). In this way they systematically organize all of the memorable biographical events (see Schauer et al. 2011; Schauer and Ruf-Leuschner 2014): "stones" represent moments of negative valence (e.g., fear, horror, sadness, loss) and "flowers" represent moments of positive valence (e.g., joy, love, achievements, important people). In addition, there are two more symbols representing distinct dynamics: sticks for active involvement in aggressive acts (*acts of violence or appetitive aggression* like, e.g., perpetrating acts, fights, delinquency, killing, combat) and, if desired, candles for moments in life when the child experienced a loss (i.e., *grieving*).

The therapist accompanies the process by empathically verbalizing what is being laid down, finding suitable labels (titles, descriptions) for the symbols, and making sure that the cold memory system is activated and contextual information is added during this exercise: "what happened?" (e.g., death of my mother in the hospital);

"when did this happen? how old were you?"; and "where did this happen?". Hot memory information is not requested during the lifeline exercise. Gentle encouragement by the therapist is necessary to clearly frame the different events in this manner.

The *lifeline* exercise should be completed in one 90-min session followed by a brief review of the session. The therapist may take a picture of the completed *lifeline* or let the child make a drawing on a piece of paper with colored pencils and note the text of the labels (title, age/year, and place).

> *Case report (cont.)*: The therapist placed a flower symbolizing T.'s birth at the beginning of her lifeline. (Note that all other symbols are placed by the client herself). T. explained that she was born to a family with mother (name), father (name), and brother (name and age) and they lived in (name of town). She placed a flower for her brother, who she loved a lot. At the age of 3 years, there was a stone for her witnessing domestic violence. At 5 years old, her parents got divorced and T. had to spend weekends with her abusive dad. She remembers crying when she had to see him. T. placed a stone for the first event of sexual abuse at this age and two more events for which she had distinct memories. Then, she put a flower for pleasant memories in school, followed by a stone for when the family moved to another country, cutting her off from her friends. This was followed by two flowers for her two dogs whom she loved a lot and then later, at the age of 10 years, two stones because the dogs were put down when the mother again moved with her to a different country. Another stone for the time when she was hit by a car (stone, 11 years old). Every now and then she had been sent to her father, having to spend holidays with him. The father introduced his daughter to child pornography and sold her at sex parties. T. placed different big stones for discrete memories and dates of such violent events at that age. With her brother T. started to smoke cannabis when she was 12 years old. Another stone was placed 1 year later, representing when the police came to their home to arrest her brother. At the age of 13, she joined a gang and they started to rob petrol stations and old people on the street (sticks). T. laid down a stone for a very emotional moment at this age: her mother severely beat her, shouted at her, and called her bad names when the girl tried to tell her mother about the sexual abuse. After the beating, the mother broke into tears and apologized. T. began to starve herself, losing more and more weight. A stone was placed for when she was admitted to a psychiatric hospital (age 14). The mother and her boyfriend smoked cannabis in the house and offered the substance to T. because they believed that this would increase her feeling of hunger and make her eat. T. felt betrayed (stone). Her school performance worsened. An edgy stone for her first romantic experience that failed (15 years) and, as a consequence, massive intrusions and flashbacks of the sexual abuse started. Finally, a flower was laid for the

> very kind and understanding school psychologist who listened to T. for the first time in her life. On the future part of the rope, she placed flowers for the "hope to overcome her trauma symptoms" and her "wish to play more guitar music" and develop a vision for a good future.

11.2.3 Part 3: Narrative Exposure (Mandatory)

In the next step, the core procedure of KIDNET begins. The survivor (without the presence of the caregiver) starts narrating his/her whole life over several treatment sessions (allow 90+ min per session) along the chronology of the *lifeline*. The sessions with narrations may begin with another brief psychoeducation:

> As you know, we want to construct a detailed, comprehensive and meaningful narrative of your good and bad experiences. We want to fill in all the gaps until the testimony is complete, the bad feelings and the pain dissolve and the fear goes down. Our experience is that the more complete the narration gets, the more you can understand about what happened to you and the more the suffering will decrease. We will always go along your life's timeline: we will proceed step by step as the event unfolds. After this, we might go over it again, correct and complete things if we need to, until we reach a final version within a few sessions. However, each individual session will always be taken to the end of the event. It will last about one-and-a-half hours each time. We will take enough time at the end of each session to make sure you are comfortable.

The therapist might want to provide a much simpler explanation for younger children, for example:

> You are already 8 years old now and you have listened to and watched many stories about others. These stories are exciting or wonderful, but also scary, wild and dangerous sometimes. Have you ever told your own story? I would like you to tell me what happened in your life. You report your events and I will imagine what it must have been like to experience these moments. I'll write it down and then you can listen to it and even correct it. We'll make a little book about you, with the picture of your lifeline on the front cover. We'll talk about all the good and the bad experiences to make the bad dreams go away. Later, we can see together whom you will allow to read the book.

The different symbols – which were previously placed on the *lifeline* – each represent a specific event. Now, during the *narration* part, the individual is asked to elaborate on the different situations of fear, joy, aggression, or grief. The therapist's intervention differs with the type of symbols:

1. *Stones*, the representatives of traumatic events, are the focus of the therapeutic attention in KIDNET. Each scene gets processed using imaginal exposure.

Negative arousal needs to be low at the completion of a successful session dealing with a "stone."
2. *Flowers*, symbolizing important relationships, joyful experiences, achievements, and other resources, are closely described and partially relived, although not in as much detail as stones. Positive arousal may carry on at the end of the session.
3. *Sticks*, representing one's own aggressive acts, are processed with a full imaginal exposure in order to contextualize the aggressive acts and explore the associative network. The therapist searches for mixed feelings, moments of ambivalence, and emotional arousal. The therapist fully accepts the reported feelings, even when positive. Role changes and moral systems need to be discussed after completion of the narration (see FORNET, Elber et al. 2012; Hecker et al. 2015).
4. *Candles* for situations of losses and social pain or rejection are reported and mourning is assisted. Such narratives resolve an important paradox: stable contact to the lost one is achieved (through use of reliving and rituals), while at the same time a "letting go" process is facilitated.

Narrating a highly arousing event means continuously exploring different levels of experience with the support of the therapist while the report progresses (for details, see Schauer et al. 2011): sensations ("what did you see, hear, feel, smell perceive, etc.), cognitions ("what did you think when you experienced …?"), emotions ("what did you feel when you were sensing, thinking…?"), physiology ("what was your bodily reaction when you experienced…?"), and meaning ("what did these sensations, thoughts, emotions, bodily reactions mean to you?"). At the same time, continuous explicit verbalization of the experiences in the "here and now" needs to be enabled while narrating (Fig. 11.1).

In every *narrative exposure* procedure and especially when survivors are prone to dissociate, the here-and-now sensations and experiences need to be reinforced and consciously made tangible *while talking about the past*. This is a crucial step to ex-posure (lat.: step out of) from the past event and to enhance the contrast between the trauma material and the present. Often, sensations, thoughts, emotions, and physiological responses are similar or the same as they were in the past when the associative memory network is triggered in the present. Therefore, the therapist can stimulate talking about the trauma material by drawing from the current bodily responses when thinking about it in the here and now. At the same time, it is made clear that these sensations come from the past, they just feel as if it is happening in the here and now. The child is encouraged to continuously experience with dual awareness: switch between the past tense : "what did you experience then (on the different levels)…" and the present tense: "what do you experience in the here and now when you think and talk about the past event?". Counteracting shutdown responses and a guided pendulum motion between the contexts is advisable if a child is prone to dissociate (see Schauer and Elbert 2010). This creates a sense of safety and allows detailed exploration of the trauma material and full imaginal exposure.

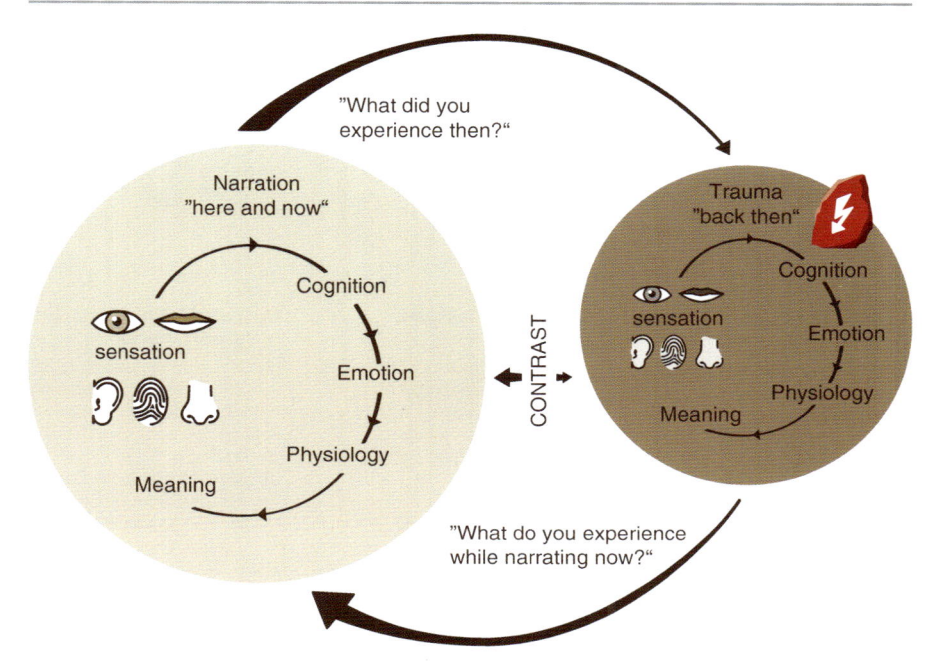

Fig. 11.1 The method of the NET narration procedure. During the imaginal exposure, the different levels of experiencing are continuously explored in detail while the child tells the story. Every now and then, the therapist invites contrasting the past (trauma) context from the current context (Schauer et al. 2011)

The therapist makes sure to support the young individual in the following two ways:

- Allowing time to fully activate the emotional network associations of the hot memories and helping to put the experiences into words
- Conscious contrasting (time, place, setting, sensations, cognitions, bodily responses, emotions, etc.) of the two levels of living through these experiences (level "then," the past event, versus level "now," the imaginal exposure to the memory) is key for integrating the experience.

In this way, a thorough narration of the young person's biography is constructed which is very detailed for highly arousing moments in life and briefly summarizes life in between. The therapist supports the imaginary reliving and emotional processing of the traumatic events and the chronological structuring of the fragments, taking an empathic and accepting role. The therapist writes down the child's testimony. In the subsequent session, the material is read to the client, and the child is asked to correct it and to add further details (Fig. 11.2).

Children enjoy talking about joyful moments from their childhood. For many people who have been exposed to childhood abuse, organized violence, and war, the

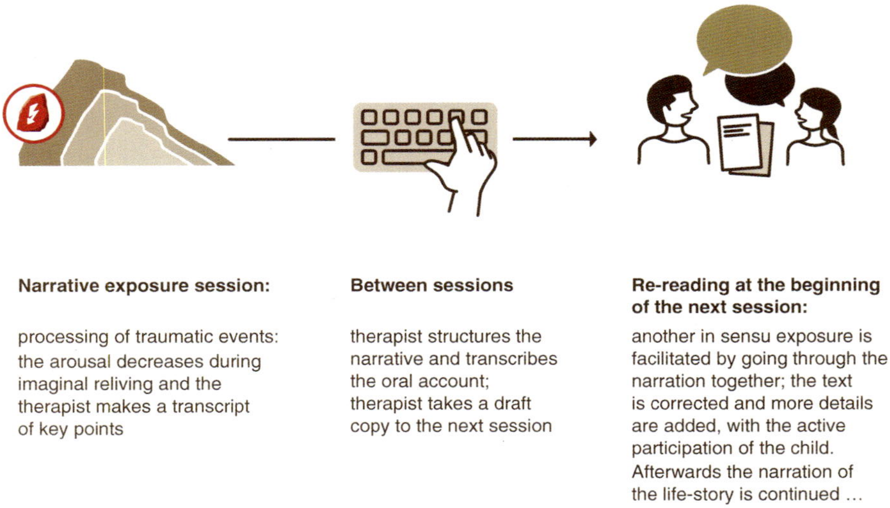

Narrative exposure session:

processing of traumatic events: the arousal decreases during imaginal reliving and the therapist makes a transcript of key points

Between sessions

therapist structures the narrative and transcribes the oral account; therapist takes a draft copy to the next session

Re-reading at the beginning of the next session:

another in sensu exposure is facilitated by going through the narration together; the text is corrected and more details are added, with the active participation of the child. Afterwards the narration of the life-story is continued …

Fig. 11.2 The process of narrative exposure: Imaginary exposure session, writing down the narration after the session and rereading the text and providing another possibility for exploring the content in the consecutive session (see Schauer 2015). After the rereading, the narration is continued chronologically along the timeline

memory of good moments in their life has largely disappeared. Remembering and reliving memories of positive experiences, moments of mastery, or important relationships can mean a lot to survivors of adversities. The therapist should include accounts of the "flowers" of life as well as all the other important experiences. Situations involving social pain, grief, and loss receive particular consideration, respect, and warmth. The experiences are explored in the same way by asking for sensations, cognitions, emotions, bodily responses, and meaning while the narrative evolves. It is important to show empathy and allow for corrective relationship experiences. The child is aided in keeping in mind the distressing and painful details of the memory until the physiological arousal decreases. In this way, a detailed report about the traumatic event is constructed in chronological order (Fig. 11.3). The child/adolescent needs continuous positive validation for his/her courage to work through these highly arousing events.

During the narrative process the attention of the therapist focuses on the following:

- *Time*: Establish *when* the incident took place. Begin with the lifetime period (e.g., *when I was going to primary school*). Then, proceed to the particular moment of the hot spot. Spend most of the exploration narrating around the highest arousal until it decreases.
- *Location*: In parallel with the time, establish *where* the incident took place (e.g., *when I was still living in my hometown*). Where was the person at that time? Then proceed to the specific location (e.g., *when I was passing in front of the town hall…*).

- *Arousal*: Start working through the incident as arousal rises, viewing all of it in sequence. Go in "slow motion" as the arousal gets higher. Make sure that any fear-provoking associations do not overwhelm the child nor that the individual is under-engaged. It is necessary that the child is emotionally activated and involved. The physiological arousal should stay within an optimal window of tolerance and functionality. During high arousal, the hot memories will be detailed; these must be explored and connected to the contextual, cold facts. Therapists may use a rough drawing of the situation or figurines to replay the scenes that had happened during the traumatic events (an allocentric view on the scene engages the cold memory system). The therapist, in alliance with the young survivor, needs patience and tenacity to explore the hot spots and their significance on the different levels (sensations, cognitions, emotions, physiology, behavior, etc.). Arousal should decrease for each trauma scene (processed chronologically), and the reporting of traumatic moments becomes increasingly tolerable. In this way the child is soon able to hold the traumatic event in mind and talk about it in a comprehensive manner and listen to the narration while all aspects are illuminated. The therapist should not allow a reduction in tension to occur just because the child avoids parts of the event that are painful. Quite the opposite: Allow enough time to explore the meaning of the worst moments. Often, the factual report about the course of the event does not automatically reveal what it meant for the survivor and how it impacted on the mind. However, detailed analysis of the meaning of the event should not distract from continuing to talk through the stone. Verbalizing the painful injury of the person that took place on the level of meaning requires the full support of the therapist.
- *Awareness – then and there vs. here and now* (*dual awareness*): When the child is recalling the event, help him/her to focus on what they perceived at that time (e.g., senses, thoughts, actions at the time), and contrast it to what they are experiencing now during the narration (see Fig. 11.1).
- *Reinforce reality*: Prevent avoidance, dissociation, or flashbacks by orienting and grounding the child to the present with the help of sensory cues, such as "can you feel the chair you are sitting on… touch the texture," "while you think about the past now, can you briefly tell me what is in the picture in our therapy room here – describe items in room," "outside there are people walking in the aisle, please tell me what you can hear," etc. Short interventions of this kind should not prevent continued exploration of the event: "Good, you can hear people having a conversation outside the room in our clinic here in Konstanz. But at the time, when you were hiding in your house in Idlib during the war, you could hear the sound of explosions…" (Fig. 11.1).

In this manner, the life review moves forward until a full version of the individual's biography is complete and the story has reached the present day (Fig. 11.3). In the last session, the whole narration is reread to the child, or a final overview *lifeline* is laid out (Fig. 11.4). In the case of multiple (different) traumatic events, a rereading of the whole document makes sense.

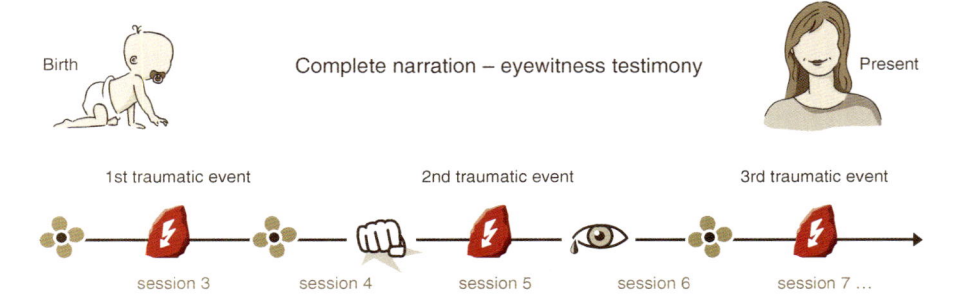

Fig. 11.3 In NET/KIDNET, the whole life of the individual is chronologically narrated from birth to the present time, highlighting the highly arousing moments of positive and negative valence including traumata, achievement/resources, loss/grief, and one's own aggressive acts

Case report (cont.): When T. started telling her life story, she was very excited and interested to explore all the details of the incidents. She was well able to tolerate all the feelings that came up during the narration and quickly learned to pay attention to the different levels of processing (sensations, cognitions, emotions, physiology, meanings of these sensory experiences, thoughts, feelings, bodily responses) as well as contrasting "then and there" with "here and now." She enjoyed the unconditional attention of the therapist guiding the session. The narration of each last session was reread each time at the beginning of the next session, allowing further completion and giving a natural chance for a second reliving and meaning-making. In this way, the therapeutic process progressed smoothly.

T. showed up punctually to her treatment sessions until we came close to the events of the sexual abuse by her father. The first time she talked about the sexual violence, she avoided the start of the narration and involved the therapist in a discussion about false memories. After some time, the therapist gave a brief psychoeducation and gently directed the attention of T. back to the task of exploring the traumatic event. Concrete contextual questions helped get this started. "On which day did your father first violate you?", "Can you describe the room, the time of day, the beginning of the event – were you already wearing your night gown when he came to your bedside?..."

Slowly and precisely, T. started narrating the scene. Whenever her memory went blank and she was unable to retrieve pictures, focusing on her bodily arousal and sensations helped to tell the story and allow progress. T. started crying when she remembered the helplessness and pain she felt at the time and she could feel some of the anger now, which she had to suppress in the presence of her father at the time. The story was taken to the moment after the abuse had ended when her father had left the bedroom in the past event and a point of relative safety and relief was reached.

Although physically tired at the end of the session, T. expressed her surprise about the clarity of the recovered memories and felt unsure of whether she should be embarrassed or relieved. The witness gave personal feedback and normalized feelings of shame and guilt.

The next session was canceled by T. because she had confronted her mother with the sexual abuse for the first time. This was very frustrating for her, since initially the mother claimed her experiences were only fantasies. However, the more elaborate and precise her memories became, the more safe T. felt. In the following weeks, the girl started to trust her assignment of bodily reactions to their emotional memories, and over time, she developed a stable sense of self.

At the end of T.'s treatment, both mother and child were invited to decide how to go about the testimony document and juridical case of child abuse and to talk about T.'s future.

However, in the case of complex trauma with many of the same events (such as sexual abuse), the detailed rereading at the very last session can be replaced in favor of a final *lifeline* session. Alternatively, both can be done: the child places the symbols on the *lifeline* one after the other and the therapist chronologically rereads the according parts of the narration. In a final *lifeline* session at the end of treatment, the child may want to place flowers for hopes and wishes for the future on the *lifeline* ("I hope to see my family again after the war," "I wish that my sister would recover from her illness," "I want to graduate well from school and become a doctor," etc.).

In any event, the child survivor and all witnesses such as the therapist, interpreter, or co-therapist sign the final testimony in the last session. The eyewitness report may serve as a document for child rights and human rights violations or be used for juridical and awareness-raising purposes or be electronically archived for later use.

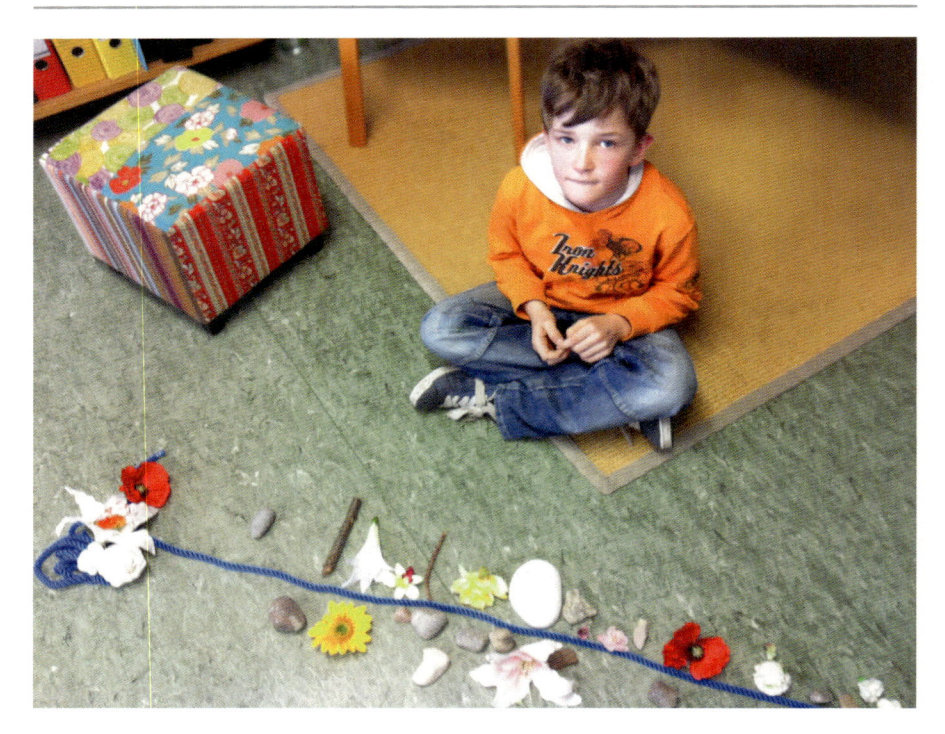

Fig. 11.4 *Lifeline* with symbols for specific experiences and with flowers for hopes and wishes concerning the future

> *Case report* (*cont.*): Initiated through the lifeline approach and continued with the biographical narration, T. could reflect on her life as a whole and recognized recurrent themes and patterns, such as the neglect and pain she had endured and how she had started suffering and coping with emotional and behavioral responses. Activating her terrifying lifetime memories in the safe and empathetic encounter with a caring listener, T. experienced corrective relationship contact and felt emotionally supported.

> Over the course of the coming year, T. was invited every 3 months for a follow-up interview at our clinic. The interviewer observed that her motivation for school performance significantly increased in parallel with the remission of trauma symptoms and her ability to feel and act progressively independent from the emotional state of her mother. Her intrusive symptoms (terrifying nightmares and genital pains) remitted together with the nausea (feelings of disgust) and her inability to consciously recall the sexual abuse (avoidance). Even her feelings of estrangement toward other people decreased,

and she started experiencing a sense of belonging. T's environment responded positively to her changes, and she felt more and more integrated and accepted in her peer group.

For the last appointment, she surprisingly brought her guitar and sang a self-composed song called "Worte finden" (transl: finding words) to her therapists about the loneliness and entanglement of maltreated children who love and hate their abusive parents and do not know how to reach independence, since they are caught up in such guilt and shame. Upon leaving, she expressed once again her gratitude and surprise about this new experience of not having to fight her own inner world, but actually receiving support from another human in the presence of strong emotions – both good and bad.

11.3 Special Challenges

Trauma-related suffering results from the cumulative exposure to traumatic stress, and as we indicated above, the logic of KIDNET requires reprocessing (contrasting the imaginal reliving with the feelings in the here and now through narration) of all major "stones" and "flowers" in a person's life. Children have a shorter lifeline, generally with fewer traumas, and their brains are also more plastic. Therefore, treatment may seem easier than with adults. On the other hand, the imaginal exposure may be more challenging in smaller children, since they very actively have to expose themselves to the memory in their imagination. In addition, meaning-making requires insights into life and knowledge of perpetrators' motivations that a child may not easily have. For instance, a 7-year-old cannot understand the meaning of sexual abuse and its effects this trauma may have later in life. The therapist is particularly challenged to respond to the individual development stage and to explain things in simple words and a transparent manner without avoiding (Ruf and Schauer 2012). A seventeen-year-old, on the other hand, may want to seek justice and revenge, again without fully comprehending what it may mean to go to court against, for example, a family member. Therefore, the use of the testimony cannot simply be left to the child without further counseling. In KIDNET, the therapist may need additional sessions to discuss what the experience of, for example, sexual and gender-based violence means in general and to the child in particular. Based on this knowledge, the child, the caregiver (if appropriate), and the therapist may discuss how to use the testimony. The therapist, for instance, may suggest that the testimony only be used in an anonymous form so that others are protected from experiencing such a fate.

PTSD in childhood is particularly harmful, as it is associated with behavioral disorders, learning difficulties, and crime-related conduct throughout life. Within a healthy family, the parents and siblings may provide useful resources to cope with this problem once the PTSD symptoms have dissipated. Family members may be instructed accordingly, indicating, for example, that externalizing behavior is a consequence of traumatic experiences rather than a basic trait of the child. Parental psychopathology results in a more difficult situation and has been found to impact the parent-child interaction and the infant's development. Emotional neglect, abuse, and inconsistent parenting by distressed caregivers play a key role in lifelong mental health problems, health risk behavior, and psychopathology in the parents of tomorrow who are raised under conditions of continuous trauma. Narrations – even transgenerational ones (those that start with the time before the child was born) – can be helpful for children to find an explanation for their caregiver's reactions.

11.3.1 When Parent and Child Are Both Traumatized

When both parent and child present with PTSD, several components of treatment may be carried out with both (non-offending) parent and child being present. In such cases, the focus of the treatment is the dyad (parent-child) that is needed to reconstruct a *lifeline* starting from the moment of their common life experience and thus the moment of the child's birth. Therefore, the caregiver is the one that starts the *lifeline* and she/he is asked to place the events she/he has experienced since the child was born up to the moment the child has its first memory on the line. Then, the child is asked to participate in the reconstruction of the lifeline. The procedure must be dynamic and permit parent-child interaction while placing the common events on the *lifeline*. The parent is instructed to intervene in a non-invasive manner; thus, repeated interruption of the reconstruction must be avoided, and the child in return needs to be allowed greater initiative to reconstruct the lifeline. Parts 1 and 2 of the treatment can be carried out together with the parent-child dyad.

At present, there are only a few unpublished case reports suggesting that a child's narration can also be observed by a parent who does not intervene, but complements the narration whenever the child is confused or not certain about the course of some events. Often though, it is useful to process this part of the treatment in separate sessions for the parent and the child.

A parent-assisted narrative can be useful if the caregiver is a non-offender and sensitive and able to help the child reconstruct events that have been experienced in early childhood and if improvements in the parent-child relationship as a subordinate treatment effect is desirable. Furthermore, this is the case if a framework is offered in which both are invited to share experiences that have been a subject of avoidance. The dyad also allows for the modification of dysfunctional meanings of the events together with facilitation of cognitive strategies and challenging of maladaptive behavior. In this way the trauma-focused treatment would naturally combine with cognitive interventions for parent and child. A conjoined narration will result from the narration of common experiences.

11.3.2 Prevention and Community Work

Short-term trauma-focused public mental health interventions on a larger scale are required at the community and societal level (Schauer and Schauer 2010) in order to (1) reach an even greater number of survivors and their families and (2) stimulate a societal change that helps prevent further child abuse and other atrocities. Individual narrations (testimonies) detailing acts of violence are potentially of significant value in holding accountable those who are ultimately responsible. Such testimonies have not only been instrumental in international and domestic tribunals specially constituted to tackle war crimes and crimes against humanity but are also of potential use for changing the behavior of the communities at large. KIDNET can produce detailed written testimonies that may serve as an intervention on the community level, helping to assemble collective narratives. In this way, trauma and suffering will be acknowledged (an important healing agent common to all evidence-based individual trauma therapies; Schnyder et al. 2015), and reintegration of both perpetrators and victims may be facilitated, where otherwise both may be treated with suspicion or rejected.

The enormous impact of violence and trauma spectrum disorders on populations drives mass refugee migration (Schauer 2016). The inclusion of robust, low-threshold, and efficient treatment modules like KIDNET in resource-poor environments or countries that host high numbers of refugees is an indispensable component within task shifting "screen and treat" cascade models of care (Schauer and Schauer 2010). Children and their families (Schauer et al. 2014) involved in war, flight, or continuous trauma scenarios (e.g., townships, reservations, or refugee and detention camps) need to translate their experiences into transgenerational narratives in order to avoid haunting legacies and allow healing and integration.

11.4 Research Evidence

The first case of a child war survivor treated with KIDNET was described by Schauer et al. (2004), and further cases with excerpts from narrations and a pilot study were presented by Onyut et al. (2005). Results showed a substantial reduction in trauma-related symptoms at the end of treatment. Clinically significant depression had remitted to nonclinical levels.

Evidence for the effectiveness of KIDNET in children, adolescents, and young adults is summarized in Schauer et al. (2011) and includes randomized controlled trials with between-group design. Superiority was demonstrated in comparison to active (e.g., Catani et al. 2009, Sri Lanka; Ertl et al. 2011, Uganda) and inactive (e.g., Crombach and Elbert 2015, Burundi; Ruf et al. 2010, Germany) control conditions in regard to the reduction of PTSD severity/diagnosis and related disorders. Within the group, effect sizes were large, ranging from a Hedges $g = 1.3$ (Ruf et al. 2010) to a Cohen's $d = 1.8$ (Catani et al. 2009), whereby about 80% (Catani et al. 2009) no longer fulfilled PTSD criteria following treatment. Thus, the family of NET therapies has proven to be effective in quite different cultural settings.

Dissemination and re-dissemination trials, including multilayered stepped-care models for large population sizes, have been effectively implemented since 2003 for NET (Neuner et al. 2008; Jacob et al. 2014; Köbach et al. 2015) and KIDNET (Schauer 2008).

Finally, Hermenau and team (Hermenau et al. 2011) treated orphaned children who had been traumatized by domestic violence in the family and also institutional care. Using a long baseline, results showed that KIDNET produced a significant reduction in symptoms which could be sustained, while a new and nonviolent instructional system was introduced in the orphanage in response to the content of the narrations. In young adult orphans who had survived mass human rights violations and genocide, KIDNET showed significant reductions in symptoms of PTSD, depression, and guilt (Schaal et al. 2009). Currently there are multicenter RCTs in usual care settings under way to study the effectiveness and mechanisms of change caused by KIDNET (e.g., Kangaslampi et al. 2015).

KIDNET is a useful and evidence-based intervention that therapists can adapt to fit to the individual needs of a traumatized child. It can be combined with other forms of assistance. However, to use just parts of it, such as the lifeline as a stand-alone technique, is neither justified by evidence nor by the theoretical background. In fact, we recommend orienting individual treatment toward the theoretical goal, tying each cue of the trauma-associated memory with the context and meaning.

Acknowledgment We thank Dr. Katy Robjant (vivo international) and Dr. James Moran (University of Konstanz) for helpful input and comments on this chapter.

References

Beutel ME, Subic-Wrana C (2012) Stabilization for complex post-traumatic stress disorder preparation or avoid the trauma confrontation? Psychotherapeut 57(1):55–57

Brewin CR (2014) Episodic memory, perceptual memory, and their interaction: foundations for a theory of posttraumatic stress disorder. Psychol Bull 140(1):69–97

Brewin CR, Gregory JD, Lipton M, Burgess N (2010) Intrusive images in psychological disorders: characteristics, neural mechanisms, and treatment implications. Psychol Rev 117(1):210

Catani C, Kohiladevy M, Ruf M, Schauer E, Elbert T, Neuner F (2009) Treating children traumatized by war and tsunami: a comparison between exposure therapy and meditation-relaxation in North-East Sri Lanka. BMC Psychiatry 9(1):22

Köbach A, Schaal S, Hecker T, Elbert T. (2015) Psychotherapeutic intervention in the demobilization process: addressing combat-related mental injuries with narrative exposure in a first and second dissemination stage. Clin Psychol Psychother. doi: 10.1002/cpp.1986. [Epub ahead of print]

Crombach A, Elbert T (2015) Controlling offensive behavior using narrative exposure therapy: a RCT of former street children. Clin Psychol Sci 3(2):270–282

Elbert T, Schauer M (2002) Psychological trauma: Burnt into memory. Nature 419(6910):883–883

Elbert T, Hermenau K, Hecker T, Weierstall R, Schauer M (2012) FORNET: behandlung von traumatisierten und nicht-traumatisierten gewalttätern mittels narrativer expositionstherapie. In: Endrass J, Rossegger A, Urbaniok F, Borchard B (Hrsg.) (eds) Interventionen bei

Gewalt- und Sexualstraftätern: Risk-Management, Methoden und Konzepte der forensischen Therapie. Berlin: Medizinisch Wissenschaftliche Verlagsgesellschaft. p 255–276

Elbert T, Schauer M (2014) Epigenetic, neural and cognitive memories of traumatic stress and violence. In: Cooper S, Ratele K (eds) Psychology serving humanity: Proceedings of the 30th International Congress of Psychology: Volume 2: Western Psychology. Psychology Press, East Sussex/New York

Ertl V, Pfeiffer A, Schauer E, Elbert T, Neuner F (2011) Community-implemented trauma therapy for former child soldiers in Northern Uganda: a randomized controlled trial. JAMA 306(5):503–512

Hecker T, Hermenau K, Crombach A, Elbert T (2015) Treating traumatized offenders and veterans by means of narrative exposure therapy. Front Psych 6:80. doi:10.3389/fpsyt.2015.00080

Hermenau K, Hecker T, Ruf M, Schauer E, Elbert T, Schauer M (2011) Childhood adversity, mental ill-health and aggressive behavior in an African orphanage: changes in response to trauma-focused therapy and the implementation of a new instructional system. Child Adolesc Psychiatry Ment Health 5:29

Isele D, Hecker T, Hermenau K, Ruf-Leuschner M, Schauer M, Moran J, Teicher MH, Elbert T (2016) (in press). Assessing exposure to adversities in children: the pediatric maltreatment and abuse chronology of exposure interview. Submitted for publication

Jacob N, Neuner F, Mädl A, Schaal S, Elbert T (2014) Dissemination of psychotherapy for trauma-spectrum disorders in resource-poor countries: a randomized controlled trial in Rwanda. Psychother Psychosom 83:354–363

Jongh AD, Broeke ET (2014) Response to "Treatment compliance and effectiveness in complex PTSD patients with co-morbid personality disorder undergoing stabilizing cognitive behavioral group treatment: a preliminary study." Eur J Psychotraumatol 5:23498. doi: 10.3402/ejpt.v5.23489

Kangaslampi S, Garoff F, Peltonen K (2015) Narrative exposure therapy for immigrant children traumatized by war: study protocol for a randomized controlled trial of effectiveness and mechanisms of change. BMC Psychiatry 15:127

Kolassa IT, Ertl V, Eckart C, Kolassa S, Onyut LP, Elbert T (2010) Spontaneous remission from PTSD depends on the number of traumatic event types experienced. Psychological Trauma: Theory, Research, Practice, and Policy 2:169–174

Lindauer RJL (2015) Trauma treatment for children and adolescents: stabilizing or trauma-focused therapy? Euro J Psychotraumatol 6, doi:10.3402/ejpt.v6.27630. http://doi.org/10.3402/ejpt.v6.27630

Nandi C, Crombach A, Bambonyé M, Elbert T, Weierstall R (2015) Predictors of post-traumatic stress and appetitive aggression in active soldiers and former combatants. Euro J Psychotraumatol 6:2655

Neuner F, Schauer M, Karunakara U, Klaschik C, Robert C, Elbert T (2004) Psychological trauma and evidence for enhanced vulnerability for PTSD through previous trauma in West Nile refugees. BMC Psychiatry 4(1):34

Neuner F (2012) Safety first? Trauma exposure in PTSD. In: Neudeck P, Wittchen HU (eds) Rethinking the model – refining the method. Springer, New York

Neuner F, Catani C, Ruf M, Schauer E, Schauer M, Elbert T (2008) Narrative exposure therapy for the treatment of traumatized children and adolescents (KidNET): from neurocognitive theory to field intervention. Child Adolesc Psychiatr Clin N Am 17(3):641–664

Onyut PL, Neuner F, Schauer E, Ertl V, Odenwald M, Schauer M, Elbert T (2005) Narrative Exposure Therapy as a treatment for child war survivors with posttraumatic stress disorder: two case reports and a pilot study in an African refugee settlement. BMC Psychiatry 5:7

Pynoos RS, Steinberg AM (2013) UCLA PTSD reaction index for children/adolescents – DSM-5. University of California, Los Angeles

Ruf M, Schauer M, Neuner F, Catani C, Schauer E, Elbert T (2010) Narrative Exposure Therapy for 7 to 16-year-olds – a randomized controlled trial with traumatized refugee children. J Trauma Stress 23:437–445

Ruf M, Schauer M (2012) Facing childhood trauma: narrative exposure therapy within a cascade model of care. In: Murray J (ed) Exposure therapy: new developments. Nova Science Publishers, New York

Schaal S, Elbert T, Neuner F (2009) Narrative exposure therapy versus interpersonal psychotherapy: a pilot randomized controlled trial with Rwandan genocide orphans. Psychother Psychosom 78:298–306

Schauer E (2008) Trauma treatment for children in war: build-up of an evidence-based large-scale mental health intervention in North-Eastern Sri Lanka. Dissertation University of Konstanz. http://nbn-resolving.de/urn:nbn:de:bsz:352-opus-54249

Schauer M, Neuner F, Karunakara U, Klaschik C, Robert C, Elbert T (2003) PTSD and the "building block" effect of psychological trauma among West Nile Africans. ESTSS (European Society for Traumatic Stress Studies). Bulletin 10(2):5–6

Schauer E, Neuner F, Elbert T, Ertl V, Onyut PL, Odenwald M, Schauer M (2004) Narrative Exposure Therapy in Children – a Case Study in a Somali Refugee. Intervention 2(1):18–32

Schauer M, Neuner F, Elbert T (2005). Narrative exposure therapy: a short-term intervention for traumatic stress disorders after war, terror, or torture. Göttingen: Hogrefe & Huber Publishers

Schauer M, Elbert T (2010) Dissociation following traumatic stress: etiology and treatment. J Psychol 218(2):109–127

Schauer M, Schauer E (2010) Trauma-focused public mental-health interventions: a paradigm shift in humanitarian assistance and aid work. In: Martz E (ed) Trauma rehabilitation after war and conflict. Springer, New York

Schauer M, Neuner F, Elbert T (2011) Narrative Exposure Therapy (NET). A short-term intervention for traumatic stress disorders, 2nd edn. Hogrefe & Huber Publishers, Cambridge/ Göttingen

Schauer M, Jongedijk R, Kaiser E (2014) Narrative exposure therapy for children and families – integrating memories of trauma, war and violence. (Narratieve exposure therapie voor kinderen en families). In: E. Captain, T. Mooren (eds), Family, generations and war. Historical, psychological and artistic views. Conference Proceedings. Amsterdam: National Committee for 4 and 5 May, 2014, pp 81–96

Schauer M, Ruf-Leuschner M (2014) Die Lifeline in der Narrativen Expositionstherapie (NET). Psychotherapeut 59:226–238

Schauer M (2015) International encyclopedia of social & behavioral sciences. In: Wright JD (ed) Narrative exposure therapy, 2nd edn. Elsevier, Amsterdam

Schauer M (2016) The mass refugee movement – better reframed as mental health crisis? Global perspectives of the International Society for Traumatic Stress Studies ISTSS Stress Points, 2016: http://dx.doi.org/10.13140/RG.2.1.4113.1926

Schnyder U, Ehlers A, Elbert T, Foa EB, Gersons BP, Resick PA, Cloitre M (2015) Psychotherapies for PTSD: what do they have in common? Eur J Psychotraumatol 6. doi:10.3402/ejpt.v6.28186

STAIR Narrative Therapy for Adolescents

12

Omar G. Gudiño, Skyler Leonard, Allison A. Stiles, Jennifer F. Havens, and Marylène Cloitre

12.1 Introduction

Skills Training in Affective and Interpersonal Regulation (STAIR) plus Narrative Therapy – Adolescent Version (SNT-A; Cloitre et al. 2014) is an evidence-based psychosocial intervention for adolescents with trauma-related difficulties. As its name suggests, STAIR emphasizes the development of emotional and interpersonal skills that can support present functioning and enhance future resilience. In some settings, due to limited amounts of time available (e.g., inpatient stays), only the skills training component of the treatment (STAIR-A) is implemented. However, in other settings, such as in outpatient services or school-based programs, the treatment is extended to include review of traumatic events and the creation of a trauma narrative in the context of developing a life story (SNT-A). This chapter provides an overview of the rationale for SNT-A as well as a session-by-session overview accompanied by an illustrative case example to highlight how this approach is applied in real-world practice. We subsequently review typical challenges that can arise when implementing the treatment and discuss how to address them. Finally, we provide a brief summary of the evidence base supporting the use of SNT-A.

O.G. Gudiño (✉) • S. Leonard • A.A. Stiles
Department of Psychology, University of Denver, Denver, CO, USA
e-mail: Omar.Gudino@du.edu

J.F. Havens
Department of Child & Adolescent Psychiatry, New York University School of Medicine & Bellevue Hospital Center, New York, NY, USA

M. Cloitre
Division of Dissemination and Training, National Center for PTSD, Menlo Park, CA, USA

Departments of Psychiatry and Child & Adolescent Psychiatry, New York University School of Medicine, New York, NY, USA

12.2 Theoretical Underpinnings

The specific skills included in STAIR-A to target emotional and social competencies were selected based on difficulties observed in adolescents and the challenges of the adolescent years, including difficulties with impulse control, concerns about self-identity, problems with appropriate and effective socializing, and engagement in school. STAIR was initially developed to address impaired emotional and social competencies among adult survivors of childhood abuse (see Cloitre et al. 2006). However, many adult patients reported that the "turning point" in the downward trajectory of their lives began during adolescence, which involved escalation in risky behaviors, drug use, and violence either as victim or perpetrator. These personal reflections by patients are supported in the empirical literature. Furthermore, studies examining the prevalence of trauma exposure across the lifespan suggest that adolescents are at high risk of exposure. Nearly two thirds of adolescents 13 to 17 have been exposed to at least one potentially traumatic event (McLaughlin et al. 2013), and adolescents are at greater risk of experiencing a traumatic event compared to children and adults (Breslau et al. 2004; Nooner et al. 2012).

Such exposure places adolescents at increased risk of developing a wide range of trauma-related problems, including internalizing and externalizing disorders (Kilpatrick et al. 2003; Layne et al. 2014). Equally important, exposure to trauma is associated with a wide range of risky and impairing behaviors beyond diagnostic status, such as running away and self-harming behaviors (e.g., Havens et al. 2012; Mueser and Taub 2008). Consistent with these data and perhaps not surprisingly, parent-rated functional impairment appears to be a key factor driving referrals for services (Gudiño et al. 2009).

Exposure to trauma and its associated psychological and behavioral problems can adversely affect the development of important social and emotional capacities. Adolescence is a time of revision in self-definition and sense of self-worth and a time of both growth and challenge in managing peer relationships and social networks. These tasks can be particularly challenging among youth with trauma-related difficulties. Trauma has been associated with weakened emotional, social, and cognitive skills and can lead to greater difficulties integrating well into supportive and healthy social networks and greater challenges coping effectively with future trauma exposure (APA 2002).

Thus, the underlying rationale for SNT-A centers on the notion that exposure to trauma hinders the development and effective use of emotional and social capacities that can support present-day functioning, protect against the adverse effects of future stressors, and stop the "downward cycle" of trauma and resource loss. The treatment is intended to provide awareness of the impact of trauma on adolescents' *emotional* and *social* experience, provide more effective options for managing difficult situations, and enhance their sense of control and mastery. The treatment also reduces trauma-related symptoms, including post-traumatic stress disorder (PTSD), anxiety, and depression symptoms. Narrative therapy (NT) further helps adolescents to make sense of traumatic experiences, further reduces PTSD and related symptoms, and provides an experience that reinforces a sense of mastery. Below we describe the specific nature of compromised emotional and social competencies that informed the development of STAIR.

Development of Emotional and Social Capacities in the Context of Trauma Exposure

Maltreated youth experience difficulties *identifying and managing emotions* as well as *understanding the interpersonal causes of emotion* (e.g., Shipman et al. 2003). Emotion regulation abilities are also compromised due to neurobiological alterations resulting from chronic exposure to trauma (DeBellis et al. 1999). As a result, understanding, describing, and managing emotional experiences can be significantly compromised. Exposure to trauma results in a loss of resources to effectively regulate emotions, a problem independent of difficulties associated with specific disorders (Kim and Cicchetti 2010; Lansford et al. 2002), yet this ability is central to promoting adaptive functioning and preventing maladaptive behavior (Cicchetti et al. 1995; Eisenberg et al. 2001). Loss of this important resource is therefore viewed as a significant factor limiting well-being.

Childhood maltreatment and trauma also have adverse effects on interpersonal and social development. For example, adolescents exposed to trauma are more likely to experience hostile, aggressive, or easily disrupted peer and romantic relationships (Kim and Cicchetti 2010; Cantrell et al. 1995). A sense of connectedness to others and social support can be important determinants of resilience following trauma exposure (e.g., Nooner et al. 2012). These abilities to build and maintain relationships and to draw support from social networks are therefore seen as important resources that can significantly impact current functioning and recovery from trauma.

Developing a cohesive sense of self is also a major task of adolescence, yet a history of trauma can create a diminished sense of self and substantial feelings of shame and guilt. However, the malleability of a sense of self during adolescence is also an opportunity to reframe future possibilities for the adolescent. One function of the narrative therapy is to support the development of a balanced perspective that acknowledges the history of trauma but also invites the adolescent to consider who they wish to be and clarifies a positive imagined future for themselves. The skills training phase begins by having the adolescent identify goals for himself or herself; the skills development that follows is shaped around practicing the skills in a way that supports the attainment of these goals. The narrative work is conducted so that the trauma is placed in the context of a developing autobiography, which includes reference to the strong and positive self that is growing, with progress during STAIR as evidence of this growth.

12.3 How to Do STAIR Narrative Therapy for Adolescents (SNT-A)

12.3.1 Protocol Description and Application

SNT-A is a cognitive behavioral intervention that begins with a skills training (STAIR) module, which can range from 8 to 12 sessions, followed by the addition of 4 to 8 sessions of a narrative therapy module, during which STAIR work continues. The total duration of SNT-A therefore ranges from 12 to 20 weekly sessions.

Skills training first targets emotion management and subsequently targets social competencies while continuing to incorporate and build on the emotion management skills. SNT-A has been used with boys and girls ages 11 and older who have experienced a wide range of traumas. Given the focus on supporting adolescent functioning, youth with emotional and interpersonal difficulties impairing their functioning and those with diagnoses of PTSD, depression, and other trauma-related symptoms are most likely to benefit from the intervention. The treatment has been empirically evaluated in a group format both with and without the narrative component. However, the manual was developed to allow for delivery of SNT-A in individual therapy.

The skills training in STAIR uses a strength-based approach in that it identifies skills that the adolescent brings to the treatment and then strengthens and builds on them. The purpose of skills development includes (a) helping the adolescent better manage trauma-related symptoms and problems, (b) functioning more effectively and with more confidence in daily life, (c) supporting the adolescents' emotional and social maturation, and (d) building resilience in the face of future exposures. The narrative work is introduced after eight to ten skills sessions and the skills work continues. Many effective trauma-focused interventions include exposure to and processing of traumatic memories (National Research Council 2014). SNT-A proposes a balance between skill development and exposure-based interventions. On the one hand, skills training interventions can provide important life skills to help adolescents manage day-to-day experiences; on the other hand, the narrative therapy allows the adolescents to look back on past experiences and reappraise their meaning, particularly in light of emotional, social, and personal development demonstrated through the skills work.

STAIR prioritizes the development of a strong therapeutic alliance and flexible and personalized delivery of the intervention. The treatment is illustrated below through the presentation of a clinical case example and a session-by-session description of the intervention in practice. A list of interventions and their rationale is included in Table 12.1. The treatment manual (Cloitre et al. 2014), including additional materials detailed below, can be obtained by contacting the authors of this chapter.

12.3.2 Case Description

Teresa, a 16-year-old Latina in the tenth grade, presented with ongoing difficulties getting into verbal altercations at school and conflict with her biological mother, and her foster mother was concerned about extended periods of irritability, anger, withdrawal, and sadness. Teresa had lived with her birth mother until the age of 8 but had subsequently been removed by child protective services due to a history of physical abuse, exposure to domestic violence, and neglect. Teresa was placed with her maternal grandmother, with whom she had a good relationship. When Teresa was 11, however, her grandmother passed away suddenly and Teresa moved into a foster home. At the time of intake, Teresa was in her third foster placement. Teresa

Table 12.1 STAIR-A/SNT-A interventions and rationale by session

Session	Interventions	Rationale
1. Introduction to treatment	Psychoeducation about common reactions to trauma Treatment rationale Personal goals	Normalize client's experience and build rapport Provide hope and facilitate investment Personalize treatment and shared understanding of treatment outcomes
2. Identification and labeling of feelings/safety plan	Psychoeducation about impact of trauma on coping with feelings Labeling and self-monitoring of feelings Deep breathing exercise Safety planning	Normalize client's experiences and develop common language for feelings Provide a technique for regulating uncomfortable emotions Development of safety plan to detail personalized menu of effective skills and plan for addressing safety concerns
3. Coping with upsetting feelings: self-care and relaxation	Psychoeducation about coping with upsetting feelings Identification and evaluation of current coping skills Self-care and self-soothing strategies	Build understanding of effective and maladaptive coping skills in response to upsetting feelings Demonstrate that emotions can be regulated with coping skills Emphasize the importance of self-care
4. Coping with upsetting feelings: cognitive coping	Cognitive coping skills: thought stopping, attention shifting, and positive self-statements	Increase client's sense of agency and control over thoughts/feelings
5. Dealing with upsetting situations	Psychoeducation about dealing with upsetting situations Focus on achieving goals Coping strategies: pros vs. cons	Utilize strategies other than avoidance for dealing with upsetting feeling and situations Use personal goals to determine appropriate responses to upsetting situations
6. Coping strategies for dealing with upsetting situations	Coping strategies: "feel good" activities	Encourage client to be open to experiencing greater range of feelings Establish situations that encourage positive emotions and reduce distress
7. Using positive imagery to deal with upsetting feelings	Rationale for positive imagery Positive imagery activities	Utilize positive images to produce feelings of calm and relaxation Use imagery to identify and organize positive image of self
8. Relationship between feelings and self-talk	Psychoeducation about self-talk Attending to self-talk Coping with upsetting self-talk	Develop client understanding and awareness of self-talk Provide client with coping strategies for dealing with upsetting self-talk

(continued)

Table 12.1 (continued)

Session	Interventions	Rationale
9. Skills for clear communication	Introduction of skills for clear communication	Develop strategies for effective communication and improved relationships
10. Introduction to role-playing feelings vs. behavior	Introduction to role-playing Role-playing practice	Provide safe environment to practice reacting in different ways to upsetting situations Opportunity for therapist to share observations, feedback, and suggestions for improving communication and outcomes
11. Role-playing with focus on assertiveness	Defining assertiveness Identification of current difficulties with assertiveness Psychoeducation about effective assertiveness Role-playing situations requiring assertiveness	Provide an opportunity to practice being assertive, experience success in communication, and handle unsuccessful interactions effectively
12. Transition to narrative storytelling (NST)	Rationale for NST Address concerns about transition to NST Initial storytelling (neutral and traumatic memories) Debriefing	Normalize fears and anxiety about new stage of treatment and invest client in the importance of NST Provide opportunity for client to access trauma-related feelings/thoughts and manage emotions with effective coping skills Practice with less stressful memories Illustrate that avoidance is not the only way client can manage memories of trauma
13–15. Continued work on storytelling	Continued NST NST with multiple traumas	Support habituation to trauma memories Support development of cohesive life story that includes, but is not defined by, trauma
16. Reviewing progress and termination	Review progress Identification of future goals Termination of treatment	Review treatment to highlight what has been accomplished and what needs continued work in the future Support client's sense of efficacy and hope moving forward

had been seeing a psychiatrist on a monthly basis for approximately 2 years, but they were concerned that Teresa was not very forthcoming during sessions and that her academic and interpersonal functioning remained impaired. Teresa's foster mother was also concerned about Teresa's longstanding difficulties managing her emotions and the impact these difficulties were having on Teresa's ability to get along with others at home and school. Everyone agreed that Teresa could benefit from additional services to address these difficulties.

Teresa was seen for an initial evaluation, where she completed a trauma history checklist and measures of PTSD, depression, anxiety, and externalizing problems. On these measures, Teresa also disclosed that she had been raped by a male acquaintance when she was 13 years old. Although Teresa had disclosed this to her caseworker and an investigation was conducted, charges were never filed and Teresa had never spoken about this event again. Results suggested that Teresa had clinically significant symptoms of PTSD and depression. While she did not meet criteria for an externalizing disorder, Teresa did experience frequent and impairing anger outbursts and interpersonal conflict that contributed to her mood difficulties.

Introduction to Treatment and Setting Personal Goals (Session 1)
The first session sets the groundwork for treatment by fostering a therapeutic alliance, normalizing Teresa's experience, facilitating engagement, and instilling hope. The therapist provided opportunities for Teresa to ask questions or share concerns. Teresa's only question was about the evaluation results. This provided a key opportunity to use information gathered during the evaluation to orient her to SNT-A. The therapist also got to know Teresa better by asking her about her goals. Achieving Teresa's goals was seen as a key way to increase Teresa's motivation and engagement with therapy and to help her see therapy as a resource for increasing her strengths, not just getting rid of her "bad behavior."

The therapist began by noting, in a matter-of-fact way, that Teresa endorsed several traumatic or stressful experiences in her lifetime. While reviewing a worksheet listing common reactions to trauma, Teresa noted that she didn't realize these were "common reactions people have when they go through something like what I went through." The therapist also used this worksheet to help Teresa focus on how trauma may impact her emotions and relationships. Here, Teresa was able to clarify that she often felt overwhelmed by emotions or alternatively didn't know what she was feeling. She also noted a strong desire to avoid emotions when possible. In terms of relationships, Teresa noted that she felt distant and different from those around her, didn't trust others, and preferred avoiding becoming "too close" with people. She also noted that she was easily irritated by others and often got into verbal arguments with family and friends because of this.

Given the important focus on the therapeutic alliance, the therapist used this opportunity to discuss the client-therapist relationship with Teresa. The therapist noted that given the common concerns Teresa shared about difficulty trusting others and concerns about becoming "too close" to others, it was important to acknowledge that Teresa may have concerns about the therapist or about therapy. Teresa noted, "I don't know you, so yeah I don't trust you." The therapist validated this as a response that made a lot of sense both given that they have not known each other for long and that Teresa has had many experiences that have helped her learn to be wary of trusting others. The therapist noted that developing a trusting relationship was something that would take ongoing effort by the therapist and client but that with time and experience, the relationship between the two could support Teresa's progress in therapy.

Without delving into the details of the client's trauma history, the therapist provided psychoeducation about PTSD, depression, and anger, linking the evaluation results to the discussion. The therapist also provided an overview of SNT-A, reviewing the rationale for the two phases of treatment. Teresa noted that she was hesitant to try therapy again but was attracted to the idea of a time-limited intervention that was focused on developing skills.

Finally, the therapist guided Teresa in developing personal goals for treatment. Here, the therapist attempted to elicit goals related to emotions ("I want to be less angry all the time") and relationships ("I wish I could trust people") but also more practical goals to support a sense of mastery and positive sense of self. With much scaffolding, Teresa was able to identify wanting to become "a better cook" as a personal goal. Teresa shared that her birth mother taught her to cook and that her foster family often praised her cooking. She specifically wanted to expand her skills by mastering new recipes.

Unfortunately, Teresa's foster mother was unable to attend sessions regularly but could occasionally join part of a session by telephone or in person. The therapist and Teresa discussed how it would be helpful for her foster mother to have a general sense of what SNT-A would entail. Together, they decided that it would be important for her foster mother to understand how trauma impacts emotions and relationships generally and to receive an overview of SNT-A. The therapist and Teresa called her foster mother to review this.

Identification and Labeling of Feelings and Safety Plan (Session 2)

Session 2 provided an opportunity to normalize and better understand Teresa's difficulties with emotional coping and to begin developing strategies for managing uncomfortable emotional responses. After briefly checking in about Teresa's reactions to the first session, the therapist introduced a "safety plan" as an important tool to be used throughout treatment.

Therapist Okay, when we talked last time, you mentioned that sometimes you get upset when your birth mom is late or does not attend a visit.

Teresa Yes! That really gets on my nerves! I was mad the rest of the day the last time that happened.

Therapist It sounds like that is a really tough situation and I'm sorry that that has happened many times. Unfortunately, when upsetting things like this happen to us, it can be hard to figure out how to cope with them. This safety plan is one tool that can help us plan for dealing with upsetting situations. Look at this first column (references safety plan). What are some "warning signs" that you are getting upset? What happens in your body, thoughts, or behavior that lets you know you are getting upset?

Teresa I've never really thought about it. I'm not sure.

Therapist Well, if I was there what would I see you doing? How would I know that you are starting to get upset?

Teresa Well, I guess I start to pace a lot. My foster mom always points that out when I'm waiting for a visit with my birth mom. Oh, and I fidget with my hands too!

The therapist worked with Teresa to also elicit bodily (e.g., face feeling hot) and cognitive (e.g., "Who does she think she is!") "warning signs." The therapist then guided Teresa in identifying effective coping strategies she already utilizes.

Therapist Even though you face many challenging situations, you already have skills that help you deal with them. What are some things you do that help you feel better when something upsetting happens?

Teresa I'm not sure. I guess I just hang out with my best friend.

Therapist Is there anything you do when you're with your best friend that is helpful?

Teresa Well, sometimes I just talk about how messed up everything is. She's a really good listener so sometimes it's just nice to get things off my chest. Other times we just watch movies or do our nails. It just depends.

Therapist Great! It sounds like you have some really good coping strategies that you find useful. You get support from a trusted friend or you try activities that are fun (watching a movie) or help to get your mind off of things (doing your nails).

At this early stage, the goal is to start building a menu of coping resources. The therapist highlights that Teresa already has some effective coping strategies and reminds her that throughout treatment she will develop additional ones. Those that are effective for Teresa will be added to the safety plan, so that this document represents an accurate summary of current skills at her disposal. The therapist also notes that at times the coping strategies may not be sufficient and it is important to have an emergency "backup" plan. If Teresa has tried all of the strategies on her safety plan and she is still in distress or feels like she is a danger to herself or others, she can then follow the emergency plan. The therapist works with Teresa to identify talking to her foster mother, calling the therapist's emergency line, and calling emergency services (e.g., 911) as three emergency action steps she can take if needed. The therapist explained that this safety plan will be reviewed and revised at each session.

After developing an initial safety plan, the therapist provided psychoeducation about how traumatic events can impact what one feels and how one expresses feelings. Teresa was also introduced to the notion that feelings are useful guides for action and provide us with important information. In order to effectively use information from feelings to plan how to behave, Teresa was first taught to identify and name feelings. Since Teresa noted in the first session that knowing what she was feeling was a challenge, the therapist provided Teresa with a list of feelings and used a handout to practice labeling feeling states described in images or vignettes. This provided opportunities for the therapist to scaffold and support Teresa's ability to use the feeling list to identify and verbalize how a character in a picture might feel in a given situation.

The therapist then introduced a self-monitoring of feelings worksheet to further support Teresa's ability to make connections between situations and feeling states. Using an example of a mildly distressing situation from the past week, the therapist helped Teresa briefly describe the situation (e.g., I got in trouble for not cleaning my room), how she felt (annoyed), the intensity of the feeling (somewhat strong), what she thought ("I wish she would leave me alone!"), and what she did to cope (went to bedroom and listened to music). The therapist explained that self-monitoring was an important tool for helping Teresa and the therapist understand her emotional experiences and that the worksheet would form the basis for future sessions. Lastly, the therapist introduced a deep breathing technique to help Teresa regulate feelings of anxiety, anger, and irritability. After practicing the technique in session, Teresa agreed to add deep breathing and listening to music (identified when completing the self-monitoring worksheet) to her safety plan. At the end of the session, Teresa was asked to complete the self-monitoring of feelings worksheet at least twice before the next session.

Coping with Upsetting Feelings: Self-Care and Relaxation (Session 3)
Subsequent sessions focused on utilizing the self-monitoring worksheet to organize discussions of events occurring between sessions. Each new session focused on introducing new skills and building on previous skills by revising the safety plan at the end of each session. In session 3, the therapist expanded on previous discussions of how trauma impacts feelings by introducing the idea of more and less helpful coping strategies. The therapist began by reminding Teresa that she already had helpful coping strategies and encouraged a more extensive discussion of these strategies, beyond what was already documented on the safety plan. The goal here was for Teresa and her therapist to obtain a clear understanding of the range of coping options Teresa uses as well as their effectiveness.

Of note, Teresa discussed some coping strategies which were questionable. This provided an important opportunity to highlight the distinction between effective and maladaptive coping strategies while validating Teresa's efforts to deal with overwhelming emotions.

Teresa Sometimes I get so mad that I go to my friend's house and we drink some of her dad's alcohol. I've only done it a couple of times but just wanted to feel better and that's all I could think of.

Therapist It sounds like you were so upset that this seemed like a good option at the time. As we talk about coping strategies, it's important that we talk about all strategies we can use. Some will be more or less helpful, so now is a great time for us to really think about which ones we should keep in your toolbox.

Teresa (smiling) Let me guess; drinking is not one we get to keep.

Therapist Well, yes. Drinking is not one we should keep on the list, but it's important to talk about why it might not be the most helpful strategy. What about it is helpful and what about it is not?

Teresa I guess I like that it just helps me stop thinking about what made me mad, but if my foster mother found out, I could get in real trouble. Plus people in my family have problems with drinking, so I don't want that to happen to me.

Therapist So you like that it gets your mind off of what happened, but at the same time, there could be negative consequences. If getting your mind off of what happened is the helpful part, are there other things you could do that get your mind off of things?

Teresa I've never thought of it, but sometimes when I go for a run, I feel so focused on what I'm doing that it's hard to think about anything else.

After developing an inventory of current effective coping strategies, the therapist introduced additional strategies Teresa could practice and eventually incorporate into her repertoire, if she found them helpful. These included self-care strategies (e.g., getting enough sleep) as well as self-soothing strategies targeting all five senses (e.g., paying attention to the way ingredients smell when she is working on a new recipe or putting on her favorite comfy sweatshirt). For homework, Teresa was asked to continue using the self-monitoring worksheet, to practice some of the new skills discussed in this session, and to continue practicing new recipes to build a sense of mastery.

Coping with Upsetting Feelings: Cognitive Coping (Session 4)
In session 4, Teresa continued to develop a sense of agency by learning new emotion regulation skills. This time, however, the session focused on cognitive skills including thought stopping/attention shifting, positive self-statements, and "emotion surfing." Before introducing and practicing these skills, the therapist facilitated a discussion about how and when coping skills can be useful. In particular, the therapist wanted to make it clear that coping skills were not designed to cover up or avoid important feelings. Rather, they were viewed as a way that Teresa could gain more control over her emotions and decide when and how to express them in the most helpful way. For example, the therapist worked with Teresa to develop a list of positive self-statements that she could say to herself to counter self-critical thoughts. Teresa had a very difficult time generating such statements but was able to recall positive things others have said to her. Similarly, the therapist used the "emotion surfing" handout to guide Teresa in using mindfulness techniques as another strategy for regulating emotions. With this exercise, Teresa was able to practice using mindfulness to notice and describe her emotional experience. Teresa was asked to practice cognitive coping skills between sessions so that the strategies she found most helpful could be added to her safety plan.

Dealing with Upsetting Situations (Session 5)
In the fifth session, Teresa learned about confronting challenging emotions in order to attain one's goals (distress tolerance). First, the therapist highlighted how emotional avoidance is common following traumatic events, and yet, avoiding emotions entirely could deprive Teresa of important information (e.g., when negative feelings point to areas of our lives that need to change) or important experiences (e.g., full experience of positive feelings). Thus, Teresa was introduced to the idea of utilizing one's goals to determine when facing emotions one would rather avoid is important.

The therapist recalled that Teresa wanted to avoid visits with her birth mother because they often make her upset, yet she also expressed a desire to improve her relationship with her. Using the "Dealing with Upsetting Situations" handout, Teresa was able to gain some clarity on her goal of improving her relationship with her birth mother as well as the pros/cons of visiting with her. In the end, Teresa was tasked with determining how to proceed. Teresa decided that despite potential cons, like possible arguments, improving her relationship with her mother and finding a way to feel connected to her were more important than avoiding possible conflicts. She was also hopeful that the use of skills learned in therapy could mitigate the likelihood of conflict. This practice of writing out goals and pros/cons when facing upsetting situations was added to the between-session work.

Coping Strategies for Dealing with Upsetting Situations (Session 6)
In session 6 Teresa continued to build skills, with a specific focus on increasing the experience of feelings at the positive end of the spectrum. For example, the therapist worked with her to develop a list of "feel good" activities that Teresa can use to cope with upsetting situations or to enhance her mood. Using a list provided by the therapist, Teresa identified potential "feel good" activities she wanted to try during the coming week. Some activities (writing poetry) were familiar to Teresa, yet she had never considered them emotion regulation strategies. Others were relatively simple strategies that she had always wanted to try but had yet to (e.g., going to the local art museum). This also provided an opportunity for the therapist to discuss Teresa's experience developing her cooking skills, trying new recipes, and building an enhanced sense of mastery. Teresa described a recent time when she cooked dinner for her foster family. She was proud that her cooking was lauded and smiled as she recalled what a good time the family had. She was motivated to continue improving her cooking skills and wondered whether she might want to be a chef in the future.

Using Positive Imagery to Deal with Upsetting Feelings (Session 7)
In session 7, Teresa continued developing skills by focusing on positive imagery as a method for increasing feelings of calmness and relaxation. Fortunately, Teresa had attended the local art museum as a "feel good" activity, and she had many examples of how much she enjoyed looking at works of art. The therapist expanded on these observations by noting that images (whether we see them or simply visualize them in our mind) of positive people, places, things, or words can make us feel happy or

calm. To experience this even further, Teresa worked with the therapist to create a "positive image collage" in session. She cut words, images, and designs that she liked or that made her feel good from magazines and arranged them in a collage. The therapist encouraged Teresa to focus on positive images when constructing the collage and periodically facilitated discussion about the meaning or relevance of an image. Teresa was especially drawn to images of exotic dishes and those of families cooking together. She discussed many positive memories of cooking alongside her birth mother and grandmother. As she worked on this project, Teresa noted that she might enjoy looking at pictures of friends or family members or visualizing special days (e.g., when she and her grandmother made a birthday cake for her mother).

Relationship Between Feelings and Self-Talk (Session 8)
By session 8, Teresa had developed a diverse set of emotion regulation strategies and was becoming more adept at identifying which strategies were particularly helpful for her. In this session, the therapist taught Teresa cognitive coping strategies to supplement her emerging skills. The therapist introduced the concept of "self-talk" – the automatic thoughts we have about ourselves or about situations. The therapist first guided Teresa to identify her "self-talk" using an example from the previous week (receiving a poor grade on a math exam). With scaffolding, Teresa was able to verbalize thoughts such as "I can never do anything right" and "nothing ever works out the way I want." Then, Teresa and the therapist discussed specific cognitive coping strategies to directly challenge negative self-talk (e.g., looking at evidence for/against or generating alternative explanations) as well as using previously learned skills (e.g., positive self-statements) to cope with negative self-talk. For practice outside of session, Teresa was asked to complete a modified version of the self-monitoring of feelings worksheet that emphasizes the identification of self-talk and practice of cognitive coping strategies.

Skills for Clear Communication (Session 9)
While prior sessions primarily targeted emotion regulation skills, remaining skill sessions focused on interpersonal functioning. In session 9, Teresa learned strategies that can help her express her needs and desires clearly and build stronger relationships. First, the therapist introduced "I messages" as a communication tool that can support us in communicating our feelings and needs to others in a way that is clear and less likely to make others feel blamed or attacked. Teresa used sentence frames to generate "I messages" that applied to a range of hypothetical situations. As Teresa mastered this skill, the therapist worked with her to practice generating statements that she could use during visits with her mother. For example, Teresa rehearsed saying, "When you do not show to a visit (behavior), I feel disappointed (feeling) because I won't get to see you for another few weeks (result)." She noted that it felt "awkward" to talk in this way, yet she was able to explore how statements such as these might help her improve communication with her mother – one of her relational goals.

Additional communication skills included saying "no" in a respectful and firm tone and making requests of others. The therapist and Teresa discussed how experiences of trauma can make it difficult for us to set limits, assert our needs, or request something from others. Teresa has previously mentioned that she avoids interactions with boys at her school because she feels that they "just don't listen" and she is worried about having more verbal altercations at school. To assist in these situations, Teresa practiced saying "no" in a role-play where a boy insisted that she sit with him at lunch using the "broken record" technique, which included repeatedly saying "no" in an assertive manner. Teresa also practiced making requests of others in a manner that increases the likelihood that the request will be met. This included helping Teresa identify what her goal or need is and then considering who to make the request to, the timing of the request, and the specific wording of the request in order to communicate her need effectively.

Introduction to Role-Playing Feelings Versus Behavior (Session 10)
Teresa returned to session excited to report that she had tried the broken record technique with a boy at school who asked her to copy her homework. While she stated that it felt weird to just say "no" to him, she was surprised that it had actually worked. In session 10, the therapist presented role-playing as a way to continue developing interpersonal skills. Importantly, Teresa would have the opportunity to consider the perspective of others, to consider how she wanted to respond to situations that did not go as she planned, and to benefit from learning these skills in a safe environment where the therapist could model behavior and also provide immediate feedback. Following each role-play, Teresa and the therapist identified aspects of the interaction that worked well and practiced ways to improve aspects that had been less successful.

To provide scaffolding, the role-playing moved from an easy, everyday situation (e.g., talking with a teacher about a missed assignment) to more challenging situations (e.g., talking with her birth mother about missing a scheduled visit) that provided opportunities for Teresa and the therapist to switch roles several times. The therapist found that role-playing allowed them to observe Teresa's behavior firsthand, to identify interpersonal strengths, and to provide constructive and supportive feedback while modeling good communication skills.

Role-Playing with Focus on Assertiveness (Session 11)
In session 11, Teresa engaged in role-plays to practice assertiveness, to experience additional success in interpersonal communication, and to practice using more challenging, and sometimes unsuccessful, interactions. Using examples that occurred over the course of therapy, Teresa and the therapist identified challenges that Teresa faced when asserting herself (e.g., being unclear about what it was that she wanted or being aggressive rather than assertive). Teresa then had the opportunity to build her interpersonal competency by participating in role-plays of increasingly challenging situations that require assertiveness. These exercises provided opportunities for discussion of how assertiveness may not guarantee that others will respond positively, yet assertive behavior may lead to more successful interactions overall.

Narrative Therapy (Sessions 12–16)

Over the course of the skills training phase, Teresa was able to demonstrate improved competency in her ability to manage her emotions and get along with others. She reported fewer negative interactions with her mother, and interpersonal conflicts at school were virtually eliminated. However, Teresa continued to report significant distress about intrusive thoughts related to her sexual assault and experiences with domestic violence, avoidance of traumatic reminders, and ongoing irritability, trouble sleeping, and hypervigilance. The narrative therapy phase thus focused on helping her talk about and process her traumatic experiences in a safe environment. Teresa was reminded about the rationale for using narrative therapy as a way to access feelings and thoughts related to the traumatic experiences and to practice effective coping skills to manage distressing emotions.

Given that Teresa experienced multiple traumas, it was important for the therapist to understand which memories Teresa found the most distressing at present. Thus, the therapist had Teresa use a 0–100 scale to indicate the current level of distress associated with specific memories. Teresa began by practicing telling a neutral memory and then telling a moderately upsetting memory (rated 20) about a time her mother and a boyfriend had a verbal altercation. Teresa was asked to tell the story of what occurred using the present tense while the therapist took brief notes about the different parts of the memory. During this initial storytelling, the therapist utilized active listening skills while minimally probing for detail. The goal at this stage was to allow Teresa to habituate to the memory. Rather than avoiding or becoming overwhelmed by thoughts of the event, Teresa began to see that she was able to think and talk about the experience without intense emotional reactions.

In the subsequent session, Teresa was asked to repeat the narration of the event. During these repetitions, the therapist was increasingly active in guiding Teresa through the exposure. At times the therapist would gently refocus Teresa when she avoided the event, provided support during especially difficult parts of the narrative, elicited descriptions of thoughts and feelings experienced at the time, and assessed the level of distress by asking Teresa to use the 0–100 scale. The therapist also praised Teresa for her bravery and highlighted reductions in Teresa's distress over repeated storytelling (e.g., visible signs of decreased anxiety and graphing of distress ratings). Teresa and her therapist also discussed the experience of telling her story, encouraged the use of coping skills as needed, and discussed Teresa's reactions to or thoughts about the content of those stories. Upon terminating the exercise, Teresa was coached to use deep breathing and mindfulness exercises to ensure that she was calm and grounded in the present.

In this manner, narrative therapy gradually progressed to more distressing memories of a severe incident of domestic violence that led to her mother being hospitalized as well as the memory of her sexual assault. As she became less distressed by a specific memory, the therapist empowered her to decide when it was time to move to a new memory. After the first storytelling of a new memory, the therapist typically became more actively involved in guiding the storytelling by asking probing questions and identifying "hot spots" (i.e., the most distressing parts of a memory).

As Teresa became accustomed to narrating memories and evidenced increased habituation to the memories, session time following the exposures focused more on exploring the thoughts and feelings elicited by the narrative. Here, the therapist focused on highlighting the interpersonal and emotional content of the narrative and in helping Teresa develop a new understanding of the meaning of the traumatic events. Over the course of sessions 12–16, Teresa developed a more integrated "life story" where she was able to acknowledge and discuss painful past experiences while feeling more empowered and in control of her future.

Finally, session 16 provided an opportunity for Teresa and the therapist to review her progress and celebrate her effort and accomplishments. To celebrate, Teresa wanted to bake a special desert she had recently mastered and to share it during the final session. The therapist helped Teresa identify future personal goals and discussed additional supports or resources that Teresa could rely on. Teresa noted that she was surprised by how new skills that she thought could not "fix things" actually made things much better over time. She was especially happy that her relationships at home and school improved and she no longer saw these interactions as a source of daily stress. Teresa's functioning had improved significantly and she was feeling "like I can be okay even with everything that has happened in the past."

12.4 Special Challenges

Therapists will find that the manual is structured while leaving room for adaptations due to individual differences in symptoms and existing skills. Nonetheless, clinicians implementing SNT-A flexibly across a wide range of adolescents may encounter special challenges. Below we list common challenges that therapists may encounter, and we provide guidance on how to address these challenges.

12.4.1 Limited Skills

Some adolescents will present with very few adaptive skills or will have a wide range of "maladaptive" skills. In such instances, we recommend balancing validation of the adolescent's attempts at coping coupled with more direct guidance from the therapist. For example, when a client has a difficult time generating examples of adaptive coping skills they use or has difficulty labeling basic feeling states, the therapist may find it useful to rely closely on the handouts and examples provided in the manual. The intervention is designed so that adolescents build on existing skills each week, so the client and therapist can look forward to increasing the effective tools at the client's disposal over the course of treatment.

A related challenge includes adolescents primarily relying on maladaptive coping strategies. In these instances we recommend taking a nonjudgmental approach that attempts to balance validation of the adolescent's experience and needs with support in identifying new, more adaptive strategies. Approaching these challenges in a flexible manner that helps adolescents learn to make choices in the real world can be especially helpful. Rather than discounting maladaptive strategies outright, the therapist can contrast the fit between the coping strategy and the adolescent's personal goals (see example above). The therapist can thus validate the reason the client continues to use the maladaptive strategy while facilitating a fruitful discussion of how a behavior may nonetheless interfere with other goals the client has for themselves. In this manner, therapists can help adolescents work through real-world life decisions, and open and honest discussion may further enhance client-therapist alliance.

Adolescents may also experience hopelessness or discount the potential benefit of a new skill. For example, adolescents will often note that "breathing doesn't work!" or that relaxation strategies "won't fix it!" In these instances, we suggest clarifying the role of relaxation strategies (e.g., helping us feel calm, giving us time to think about what to do next). Active coaching of skill use in session can also be an effective way to increase the likelihood of attempting new skills. For example, the client and therapist can conduct a simple "experiment" where the therapist actively coaches the client in the use of deep breathing when the client is becoming agitated. Rather than focusing on convincing the client that existing skills are maladaptive or that new skills can be helpful, this provides an important opportunity for the client to experience for themselves how something as simple as deep breathing can be a powerful tool to support functioning.

12.4.2 Uncertainty About How to Use a Flexible Implementation Strategy

While the flexibility of the manual is appealing, it also means that there will not always be direct guidance on how to implement an intervention for a specific client or how to handle new client issues that emerge on a weekly basis. By remembering the core elements and rationale for SNT-A, particularly the STAIR phase, therapists can make key decisions about how to handle a challenging new situation. For example, many stressful or emergent situations arising in a given week can be discussed by highlighting how emotion regulation, interpersonal skills, and past traumatic experiences may have contributed to the experience of the stressor and/or can be used to support current functioning. Thus, challenges that could have interfered with a planned session can instead be used as a way to teach about and practice the skills that the therapist had planned for a given session. Furthermore, the ongoing use of the self-monitoring of feelings worksheet and the client's safety plan can be used to organize how emergent issues are examined and how to address them, respectively.

The client's personal experiences can also be used to help the therapist bring the SNT-A manual to life. For example, as the client describes real-life situations they are facing, the therapist can help the client view these situations through the framework of SNT-A. In this manner, the client obtains exposure to the content of the protocol in a manner that is personally relevant. Furthermore, by focusing on emotional and interpersonal competencies, the therapist can provide coaching and support practice of skills the client can use to address actual challenges in their life in more skillful ways.

12.4.3 Discomfort with Skills Practice

A skills training approach may be new to clients and therapists. As a result, there may be a pull for sessions to focus on *talking* about skills rather than active practice and coaching of skill use. For example, both clients and therapists may begin discussing how they might approach an interpersonal situation. Because role-playing can feel new and awkward, however, role-playing may be less likely to be included in the session. Therapists may find it helpful to openly acknowledge any uncomfortable thoughts and feelings associated with role-playing. Furthermore, therapists can remind clients about the rationale for conducting role-plays. While discussions about interpersonal situations can provide new insight and knowledge, role-plays can provide useful information about the client's skill level and effectiveness in using skills outside of sessions. Role-plays can also provide clients with opportunities to test and refine new behaviors in a safe and supportive environment. To decrease the difficulty for the client, the therapist may elect to play the more challenging role in the role-play initially, or the client can be given the option of responding in a less-than-ideal manner purposely. Once the therapist has coached the adolescent to use a new behavior effectively in session, the therapist can be certain that the client can demonstrate good use of the new skill and may be more likely to use the skill effectively outside of session.

12.4.4 Discomfort with Narrative Work

Similarly, clients and therapists may have concerns about openly discussing traumatic memories during the narrative therapy phase of treatment. Here again it can be helpful for the therapist to be confident in the rationale for narrative therapy and research evidence supporting its role in trauma-focused treatments. The therapist can then use this knowledge to remind the client about why narrative therapy is an important part of the intervention. Therapists may also find it helpful to think about how exposure to trauma is embedded throughout the intervention. From the first session, the therapist and client openly acknowledge that traumatic events have occurred, and while they may not delve into details about the trauma, avoidance is not encouraged. Thus, the therapist and client have had repeated exposure to talking about the traumatic experiences prior to the second phase of treatment. The transition to narrative therapy can therefore be framed as a change in the relative amount of exposure within a session rather than a qualitative shift in the treatment. Narrative therapy can also be framed as a way to provide the client with opportunities to practice STAIR-A skills under increasingly challenging situations. By expressing confidence in the adolescent's ability to engage in narrative work and modeling confidence in the utility of narrative work, the therapist can support the client in gradually facing traumatic memories. Successful initial narrative sessions that provide the client with an opportunity to try a challenging task in a controlled and safe environment for a limited time can provide the client with the evidence they need to successfully engage in future narrative work.

12.5 Evidence Base for SNT-A

Five studies of adults and two studies of adolescents provide evidence for the efficacy of SNT. In a quasi-experimental study of adolescent girls ($N = 46$; ages 11–16) of racial/ethnic minority background who had experienced multiple stressful or traumatic events over their lifetime, Gudiño et al. (2016) examined the effectiveness of SNT-A relative to a matched assessment-only comparison group. Girls in the intervention condition ($n = 23$) received 16 sessions of SNT-A in a school-based group format, whereas girls in the matched comparison condition ($n = 23$) only completed assessments at scheduled intervals. Relative to girls in the assessment-only condition, girls participating in SNT-A evidenced statistically and clinically significant improvements posttreatment on indicators of resiliency, including improved social engagement ($d = .65$) and locus of control ($d = .46$), and marginally significant improvement in interpersonal relations ($d = -.46$). Girls receiving the intervention also evidenced significant reductions in depressive symptoms ($d = .58$) posttreatment and marginally significant reductions in anxiety symptoms ($d = .42$) relative to the assessment-only group. Treatment gains were largely maintained after 3 months, with scores for depression, anxiety, and social stress remaining significantly improved relative to baseline.

While no significant overall differences were found between groups on symptoms PTSD, post hoc analyses revealed a trend whereby girls who had clinically elevated levels of PTSD at baseline and showed higher levels of engagement with the trauma narrative (i.e., completed the homework and were willing to talk about their reactions during sessions) experienced reductions in PTSD symptoms relative to girls who were less engaged. Taken as a whole, results from this study suggest that SNT-A delivered to high-risk girls can successfully enhance resilience and reduce symptoms of psychopathology.

The efficacy of an abbreviated version of SNT-A, which used a skills only and shortened version of STAIR (called Brief STAIR-A), was examined in an open trial of adolescent psychiatric inpatients exposed to multiple traumatic events (Gudiño et al. 2014). This study, as far as we know, is one of only two studies available about trauma treatments for adolescents in inpatient settings. Boys and girls ($N = 38$; ages 12–17) received a three-module repeatable group version of STAIR-A. Participants received a median of six skills training sessions delivered by clinical staff of the inpatient unit. From pre- to posttreatment, participants exhibited significant decreases in PTSD and depressive symptoms as well as significant increases in coping effectiveness. Effect sizes for symptom reduction ($d = .65–.67$) and coping effectiveness ($d = .75$) were moderate. Results from this study suggest that participation in STAIR-A is associated with significant reductions in symptoms as well as improved coping effectiveness, even in adolescents with significant trauma-related difficulties.

Additional evidence for the efficacy of the SNT comes from studies of adults. These studies include an initial randomized controlled trial (RCT) of SNT for adult survivors of childhood abuse with PTSD ($N = 58$) relative to a waitlist control condition, a follow-up component RCT of SNT with adult survivors of childhood abuse, a benchmark study of SNT for survivors of the World Trade Center attacks of 9/11 treated by community providers with flexible implementation, and a comparison study of STAIR alone as a group treatment for individuals who have experienced a range of traumas and suffer from comorbid PTSD/schizoaffective disorders compared to a treatment as usual (supportive) therapy (see Cloitre & Schmidt, 2015 for review). In addition, STAIR and SNT delivered in an individual format in an outpatient clinic have been found beneficial to both male and female veterans with PTSD and military sexual trauma (Cloitre et al. 2016).

Thus, STAIR narrative therapy is an efficacious treatment that has demonstrated evidence for enhancing client functioning, improving indicators of resiliency, and decreasing symptoms of psychopathology across a wide range of individuals with trauma-related difficulties. It has been effective for individuals with childhood abuse, terrorism, military-related trauma, and mixed trauma and can be used in both outpatient and inpatient settings. The STAIR treatment, with or without the narrative component, provides relief not only from PTSD but also improvement in emotion regulation, interpersonal relationships, perceived social support, and functional status. It should be noted that there is only initial evidence for the effectiveness of STAIR-A and SNT-A at this point. Additional research using larger samples, randomized controlled designs, and replication by independent research groups are needed to enhance the evidence base for this intervention. Of note, two clinical trials of SNT-A are being launched in the United States and in the Netherlands. Despite these limitations, SNT-A and STAIR-A have been used successfully with adolescents exposed to a range of traumatic events who are experiencing a variety of trauma-related difficulties. The intervention has been delivered in group formats in school and inpatient settings, and positive intervention effects have been obtained even when the intervention is flexibly delivered in challenging real-world clinical settings.

References

American Psychological Association (2002) Developing adolescents: a reference for professionals. American Psychological Association, Washington, DC

Breslau N, Wilcox HC, Storr CL et al (2004) Trauma exposure and posttraumatic stress disorder: A study of youths in urban America. J Urban Health 81:530–544

Cantrell PJ, MacIntyre DI, Sharkey KJ et al (1995) Violence in the marital dyad as a predictor of violence in the peer relationships of older adolescents/young adults. Violence Vict 10:35–41

Cicchetti D, Ackerman BP, Izard CE (1995) Emotions and emotion regulation in developmental psychopathology. Dev Psychopathol 7:1–10

Cloitre M, Cohen LR, Koenen KC (2006) Treating the trauma of childhood abuse: psychotherapy for the interrupted life. Guilford, New York

Cloitre M, Farina L, Davis L, Levitt J, Gudiño OG (2014) Skills training in affective and interpersonal regulation for adolescents – revised version (Unpublished manual). National Center for PTSD, Palo Alto

Cloitre M, Jackson C, Schmidt JA (2016) Case Reports: STAIR for Strengthening Social Support and Relationships among Veterans with Military Sexual Trauma and PTSD. Military Medicine 181:e183–e187

Cloitre M, Schmidt JA (2015) STAIR Narrative Therapy. In U. Schnyder, M. Cloitre (eds.), Evidence Based Treatments for Trauma-Related Psychological Disorders: A Practical Guide for Clinicians. Springer International Publishing Switzerland, pp. 277–297. DOI 10.1007/978-3-319-07109-1_14

DeBellis MD, Baum AS, Birmaher B et al (1999) Developmental traumatology part I: biological stress systems. Biol Psychiatry 45(10):1259–1270

Eisenberg N, Cumberland A, Spinrad TL et al (2001) The relations of regulation and emotionality to children's externalizing and internalizing problem behavior. Child Dev 72(4):1112–1134

Gudiño OG, Lau AS, Yeh M et al (2009) Understanding racial/ethnic disparities in youth mental health services: do disparities vary by problem type? J Emot Behav Disord 17(1):3–16

Gudiño OG, Weis JR, Havens JF et al (2014) Group trauma-informed treatment for adolescent psychiatric inpatients: a preliminary uncontrolled trial. J Trauma Stress 27(4):496–500

Gudiño OG, Leonard S, Cloitre M (2016) STAIR for girls: a pilot study of a skills-based group for traumatized youth in an urban school setting. J Child Adolesc Trauma 9(1):67–79. doi:10.1007/s40653-015-0061-0

Havens JF, Gudiño OG, Biggs EA et al (2012) Identification of trauma exposure and PTSD in adolescent psychiatric inpatients: an exploratory study. J Trauma Stress 25:171–178

Kilpatrick DG, Ruggiero KJ, Acierno R et al (2003) Violence and risk of PTSD, major depression, substance abuse/dependence, and comorbidity: results from the National Survey of Adolescents. J Consult Clin Psychol 71(4):692–700

Kim J, Cicchetti D (2010) Longitudinal pathways linking child maltreatment, emotion regulation, peer relations, and psychopathology. J Child Psychol Psychiatry 51(6):706–716

Lansford JE, Dodge KA, Pettit GS et al (2002) A 12-year prospective study of the long-term effects of early child physical maltreatment on psychological, behavioral, and academic problems in adolescence. Arch Pediatr Adolesc Med 156(8):824–830

Layne CM, Greeson JKP, Ostrowski SA et al (2014) Cumulative trauma exposure and high risk behavior in adolescence: findings from the National Child Traumatic Stress Network Core Data Set. Psychol Trauma 6(1):S40–S49

McLaughlin KA, Koenen KC, Hill ED et al (2013) Trauma exposure and posttraumatic stress disorder in a national sample of adolescents. J Am Acad Child Adolesc Psychiatry 52(8):815–830

Mueser KT, Taub JT (2008) Trauma and PTSD among adolescents with severe emotional disorders involved in multiple service systems. Psychiatr Serv 59:627–634

National Research Council (2014) Preventing psychological disorders in service members and their families: an assessment of programs. National Academies Press, Washington, DC

Nooner KB, Linares LO, Batinjane J et al (2012) Factors related to posttraumatic stress disorder in adolescence. Trauma Violence Abuse 13(3):153–166

Shipman K, Zeman J, Fitzgerald M et al (2003) Regulating emotion in parent-child and peer relationships: a comparison of sexually maltreated and nonmaltreated girls. Child Maltreat 8(3):163–172

Eye Movement Desensitization and Reprocessing Therapy (EMDR)

13

Francine Shapiro, Debra Wesselmann, and Liesbeth Mevissen

13.1 Theoretical Underpinnings

Eye movement desensitization and reprocessing (EMDR) is an empirically validated psychotherapy approach used to treat mental health disorders stemming from trauma and other adverse life experiences in children, adolescents, and adults (Shapiro 1995/2001, Shapiro 2014a, b). EMDR therapy involves eight standardized phases to comprehensively address the clinical picture. Treatment includes targeting and implementing the standardized information processing procedures to address (1) the memories of disturbing events that are etiological to emotional, cognitive, and behavioral problems, (2) current situations that trigger dysfunction, and (3) the incorporation of needed skills for future challenges. The case conceptualization, procedures, and protocols are based on the adaptive information processing (AIP) model, which posits that memories of disturbing events may be physiologically stored in unprocessed form, leading to problems in day-to-day functioning.

F. Shapiro, PhD (✉)
Emeritus, Mental Research Institute, Palo Alto, CA, USA
e-mail: fshapiro@mcn.org

D. Wesselmann, MS, LIMHP
The Attachment and Trauma Center of Nebraska, Omaha, NE, USA
e-mail: deb@atcnebraska.com

L. Mevissen, MSc
Department Intellectual Disability and Psychiatry, Mental Health Organization GGZ Friesland, Friesland, Netherlands
e-mail: liesbeth.mevissen@ggzfriesland.nl

13.1.1 The Adaptive Information Processing (AIP) Model

The AIP model serves both as an explanatory framework for the development of personality and psychopathology and, more specifically, as a means of predicting and guiding successful clinical outcomes of EMDR therapy. At the heart of the model is the recognition that the information processing system facilitates the interpretation of current experiences by linking them with previously established memory networks of similar events. For example, the occurrence of falling down a flight of stairs will connect with memory networks from a related earlier accident or perhaps a variety of experiences of physical pain in general. Under normal circumstances the information processing system makes the appropriate physiological connections within the larger context of stored memories. That which is useful is drawn from the event and used to guide future behavior. That which is not is discarded.

Unfortunately, the information processing system does not always function optimally, particularly when confronted with an especially disturbing life experience. The result is a failure to process the event, thereby preventing it from linking up with the memory networks of related previous life experiences that have been adaptively stored. Not only is the adverse event "frozen in time" but so too its associated negative effects, sensations, and beliefs. It has been proposed that the underlying basis for this dysfunction is a failure of episodic memory to be integrated into the semantic memory system (e.g., Stickgold 2002). Such inadequately processed memories can be readily activated by both internal and external stimuli and manifest themselves in the form of clinical symptoms that can include disturbing emotions, beliefs, and behaviors. Unprocessed traumatic events can result in the flashbacks, nightmares, and intrusive thoughts that characterize post-traumatic stress disorder (PTSD) (see Chap. 1). However, even adverse life experiences that do not qualify as "Criterion A" trauma can underlie a variety of psychological problems that include dysfunctional affects, cognitions, and somatic responses (Felitti et al. 1998; Shapiro 1995, 2014a), an observation that was predicted by the AIP model. In fact, nontraumatic stressful life experiences may produce even *more* PTSD symptoms than do the major traumatic events traditionally associated with PTSD (Mol et al. 2005).

In contrast to behavioral models of psychopathology, the AIP model does not view self-characterizations such as "I don't deserve to be loved" as *causes* of emotional dysfunction but rather *symptoms*. Specifically, they are viewed as evidence of unprocessed earlier life experiences and their emotional/perceptual accompaniments. Whereas with cognitive behavioral therapy (CBT), therapeutic change occurs via behavioral, narrative, and cognitive tasks, with EMDR therapy (as guided by the AIP model), it is conceptualized as a consequence of memory processing from the internal associations that are elicited during sets of bilateral stimulation (eye movements, taps, or tones). A recent meta-analysis of 26 randomized controlled trails (RCTs; Lee and Cuijpers 2013) has demonstrated the positive effects of the eye movement component, including declines in negative emotions. It is hypothesized that eye movements (a) place a burden on working memory, (b) stimulate the orienting reflex and associated parasympathetic activity, and (c) elicit the same or similar processes that characterize rapid eye movement (REM) sleep (see Schubert et al. 2011). The EMDR therapy procedures generate and foster an associative process in the brain that connects the maladaptive memory networks with stored adaptive information (Shapiro 2001, 2014a). The processing of the memory transforms the disturbing event into a learning experience and a source of resilience.

As attested by the session transcripts below, EMDR therapy moves rapidly, as each period of bilateral stimulation leads to increased insight, along with shifts in the emotions, sensations, and memories connected with the traumatic event. It is posited that these changes emerge from the links formed between the memory network of the initially unprocessed experience and those of extant, related experiences. This process involves the integration of the disturbing episodic memory within semantic networks (Stickgold 2002; Shapiro 2014a). Thus, treatment by EMDR therapy causes an initially isolated memory to be integrated into a constellation of adaptive networks of previous events. This accelerated learning experience includes a replacement of negative effects and cognitions with positive ones, which in turn provides a foundation of psychological resilience. It has been proposed that the role of the repeated bilateral stimulation in this process is to elicit a prolonged orienting reflex, which in turn activates brain states that accelerate learning (Stickgold 2002). This neural activity is posited to be similar or identical to that occurring during REM sleep. The latter has been shown to facilitate the processing of episodic memories by enhancing insight and understanding of these memories, reducing or eliminating accompanying negative effects, and facilitating the integration of these memories into already-present semantic networks (Stickgold and Walker 2013; Walker and van der Helm 2009).

It has also been proposed that a major outcome of EMDR therapy is the reconsolidation of memory (Shapiro 2014a) in which the memory of the traumatic event is modified and stored. This represents a critical distinction between EMDR and exposure-based trauma-focused cognitive behavioral therapies (TF-CBT) in which it is posited that a new memory is created, while the old one remains unaltered. Support for the distinction between extinction and reconsolidation comes from Suzuki et al. (2004), indicating that the lengthy exposures typical of TF-CBT cause memory extinction, while shorter exposures such as those used in EMDR therapy cause memory reconsolidation. In the words of Craske et al. (2006), ". . . recent work on extinction and reinstatement . . . suggests that extinction does not eliminate or replace previous associations, but rather results in new learning that competes with the old information" (p. 6). One of the major theoretical implications of this difference is that the memory reconsolidation that results from EMDR therapy may be directly responsible for such treatment effects as the elimination of phantom limb pain that are not found with extinction (e.g., De Roos et al. 2010). These outcomes are relevant to a wide number of somatic conditions across the lifespan that appear to be a concomitant of the stored physical sensations experienced when a traumatic event occurred (see Shapiro 2014a).

13.2 How to Do EMDR Therapy

13.2.1 EMDR Therapy Sessions

EMDR with children follows the eight-phase protocol as outlined in Table 13.1 (Shapiro 2001).

The eight phases outlined in the table are customizable to meet the needs of children and their families, as the language and instructions can be adapted to the child's developmental level and preparation phase activities extended as needed. EMDR therapy is recommended for children with single-incident or complex trauma as

Table 13.1 Overview of eight-phase EMDR therapy treatment

Phase	Purpose	Procedures
History taking	Obtain background information. Identify suitability for EMDR treatment. Identify processing targets from events in client's life according to standardized three-pronged protocol	Standard history-taking questionnaires and diagnostic psychometrics. Review of selection criteria. Questions and techniques (e.g., Floatback) to identify (1) past events that have laid the groundwork for the pathology, (2) current triggers, and (3) future needs
Preparation	Prepare appropriate clients for EMDR processing of targets	Education regarding the symptom picture. Metaphors and techniques that foster stabilization and a sense of personal control (e.g., Safe Place)
Assessment	Access the target for EMDR processing by stimulating primary aspects of the memory	Elicit the image, negative belief currently held, desired positive belief, current emotion, and physical sensation and baseline measures
Desensitization	Process experiences toward an adaptive resolution (no distress)	Standardized protocols incorporating eye movements (taps or tones) that allow the spontaneous emergence of insights, emotions, physical sensations, and other memories
Installation	Increase connections to positive cognitive networks	Enhance the validity of the desired positive belief and fully integrate within the memory network
Body scan	Complete processing of any residual disturbance associated with the target	Concentration on and processing of any residual physical sensations
Closure	Ensure client stability at the completion of an EMDR therapy session and between sessions	Use of self-control techniques if needed. Briefing regarding expectations and behavioral reports between sessions
Reassessment	Ensure maintenance of therapeutic outcomes and stability of client	Evaluation of treatment effects. Evaluation of integration within larger social system

Reprinted from Shapiro (2012)

well as for those who have been impacted by adverse events that do not meet the current DSM definition of trauma, such as bullying or being belittled. EMDR processing of past traumas is contraindicated for children who feel unsafe in their present-day environment, for example, one in which violence is a common occurrence.

As indicated in the World Health Organization (WHO 2013) practice guidelines, "EMDR does not involve (a) detailed descriptions of the event, (b) direct challenging of beliefs, (c) extended exposure, or (d) homework" (p. 1). These characteristics can facilitate the use of EMDR therapy with children of all ages and allow effective treatment over a series of days, rather than weekly, an efficient means of dealing with families in crisis. EMDR phases 1 through 8 are commonly provided in 1–3 60-minute sessions for single-incident trauma, which includes only a very brief preparation phase directly following history taking. Children with a history of complex trauma may suffer from problems related to self-awareness and self-regulation that require several preparation sessions involving EMDR self-regulation strategies and other common skill-building activities. The number of sessions needed for the reprocessing phases is dependent upon the number of traumatic experiences and present-day triggers but in the empirical literature has ranged from three to eight sessions. However, EMDR processing of one traumatic event results in generalization of effects to other similar events; therefore, it is not necessary to target each traumatic incident in the child's life.

The decision to keep parents in the session depends upon the wishes of the child and clinical judgment regarding the child's need for parental support. An additional benefit is the increase in the parents' understanding and compassion for their children's experiences. However, when parents' emotional responses threaten to interfere with the provision of emotional support or when children have adequate skills for self-regulation and prefer more independence, EMDR trauma work is implemented without parents in the room. In this case, parents are provided information and guidance so they can be appropriately supportive to the child following the session. Most of the RCT studies involving children (ranging from 6 to 18 years of age) do not mention parent presence. The procedures of one study, however, specify treating children alone unless children request parents to stay, another describes the inclusion of parents for 15 min of the child's session or in a separate meeting, and a third notes the inclusion of four parent guidance sessions. Procedures were the same for treatment and control groups.

Bilateral Dual Attention Stimulation The EMDR therapy standard protocol includes a very specific set of procedures, of which visual, audio, or tactile bilateral dual attention stimulation is one component. As described in the WHO (2013) practice guidelines, "the treatment involves standardized procedures that include focusing simultaneously on (a) spontaneous associations of traumatic images, thoughts, emotions and bodily sensations and (b) bilateral stimulation that is most commonly in the form of repeated eye movements" (p. 1). Most children are able to track the therapist's hand as it moves from side to side at eye level or watch a bright light shifting bilaterally on an electronic eye scan machine. Younger children can be assisted with eye movements by encouraging them to watch as the therapist moves a brightly colored puppet or toy from side to side. Eye movements are the preferred method for processing. However, if the child is unable to perform the eye movements or prefers an alternate method, the therapist may use tactile bilateral stimulation, most commonly applied through gentle, alternating taps on the child's hands or knees or the use of electronic tactile pulsars. Alternating audio stimulation in the form of tones is another option and may be implemented by means of headphones.

13.2.2 Single-Incident Trauma

The following example illustrates the use of the eight phases of treatment with a 9-year-old boy who was referred for EMDR therapy due to post-traumatic stress symptoms from an attack by a neighbor's large dog 6 months prior to the initial session. In this case, the EMDR processing is completed within one session; single-event traumas such as this one are typically brought to closure within one to three sessions.

- *Phase 1. History taking*: The EMDR therapist conceptualizes and treats child the symptoms by addressing the "three prongs" of past, present, and future. She gathers information about the current symptoms and contributing antecedent events by meeting first with Zachary's parents, who describe the attack. They explain that since the attack, Zachary has refused to play outside with neighborhood friends or enter the home of anyone who owns a dog. He is experiencing nightmares and waking frequently at night. Prior to the attack, he exhibited no problems in functioning. Next, the therapist asks to speak with Zachary, who willingly joins her and briefly describes his ordeal with the neighbor's dog. He goes on to say that he wants to get over his fears because he misses being outside with his friends.
- *Phase 2. Preparation*: In the latter part of the session, with his parents present, the therapist prepares Zachary for processing with psychoeducation about EMDR and a Safe Place exercise. She introduces EMDR therapy to Zachary and his parents as a treatment that "helps the different parts of the brain work together to make upset feelings smaller and positive feelings stronger." She shows Zachary how to follow her fingers from side to side with his eyes and demonstrates alternating hand taps.
Next, the Safe Place exercise is conducted to provide Zachary with a technique for self-calming. The therapist initiates the Safe Place exercise by saying, "Zachary, let's see if we can figure out a place where you can go in your imagination to help you feel calm and relaxed. It can be a place you have visited, or it can be a place you invent with your imagination." Zachary decides that he would like to imagine himself in an enormous tree house, and the therapist helps Zachary think about all of the things that he would want there. Zachary prefers closing his eyes as he enjoys thinking of what he might see, touch, smell, or hear in his safe place tree house, and the therapist applies slow, alternating taps on the backs of

his hands to deepen the experience. She encourages Zachary to practice recalling his calm place as he falls asleep at night. Before the session is over, she asks him to draw a "container" to which he can send his upsetting memory for the time being, and he draws and colors a picture of a trunk.

Zachary and his parents return a few days later, and he indicates that he would like his parents to remain present for the trauma work. The therapist explains to his parents, "It might be tempting to jump in with a thought or idea when Zachary is processing, but it will be important for us to stay quiet and allow Zachary's brain to do the work."

- *Phase 3. Assessment*: Formal measures are used during the history-taking phase to assess symptomology when needed. However, a standardized Assessment Phase is used to delineate special aspects of any adverse event targeted for processing. This phase generally takes about 15 minutes. The therapist initiates the Assessment Phase with questions specific to the traumatic memory, identifying the important components of the disturbing memory and obtaining simple baseline measures (see below.) The "worst picture" is identified by asking Zachary, "When you think about the dog attack, what is the most upsetting picture in your mind?" The therapist finds Zachary's negative cognition by asking, "What is the most upsetting thought that goes along with that picture?" The desired positive cognition is found by asking, "What would you rather think instead?" Although Zachary has no difficulty answering questions about his thoughts, some children require assistance with this process. For example, the therapist may tentatively offer some suggestions until a belief is found that resonates for the child.

The validity of the preferred positive cognition (VoC) is found by asking Zachary to point to a number on a visual representation of a 1 (completely false)-to-7 (completely true) scale to "show how true it feels deep down." He rates it as a "4." When asked how he feels when thinking of the incident, Zachary describes his emotion as "scared," and a similar visual representation of a 0–10 scale is used to obtain a subjective unit of distress (SUD) rating of "8." Finally, the therapist asks, "Zachary, where do you feel your upsetting feelings in your body? Before you answer me, take a minute to notice what you're feeling inside your head, your throat, your shoulders and arms, your chest, and your stomach."

The following are the components of Zachary's memory that were identified during the Assessment Phase:

Image (representing the worst part of the experience in the present): "Raino (the dog) digging into my arm with his teeth."
Negative cognition: "I'm going to die."
Positive cognition: "I'm safe."
Validity of positive cognition (VoC) on a scale of 1–7, with 1 being completely false and 7 being completely true: 4
Emotions (currently experienced): Scared
Subjective units of distress scale (SUD) from 0 (no disturbance) to 10 (highest): 8
Body sensations (experienced in the present): Tension in his stomach and arms

Reprocessing Phases Consist of Desensitization, Installation, and Body Scan

Memory processing for an individual target is considered complete when the SUD level is zero (or "ecologically valid"), the VoC is seven, and there is a clear body scan. For an individual trauma, this is usually achieved with children in one or two sessions. As demonstrated below, it is typical for the child to review the experiences of the event only once during the session.

- *Phase 4. Desensitization*: After the Assessment Phase, the therapist commences the Desensitization Phase, which uses standardized procedures to address the entire memory network. In the following transcript, the symbols <<<< represent the therapist prompt, "Go with that," a set of approximately 20–24 repetitions of eye movements, and then the therapist's words, "What are you noticing now?" Depending upon the client's response after a set of eye movements, the therapist guides the next focus of attention.
  The therapist begins by saying: *"Remember, there is no way to do this wrong. Let's see if you can follow my fingers for just a little bit, and then I'll stop and check on what you are thinking or feeling. Then you'll follow my fingers again, and then I'll stop and check in with you again. Does that sound OK?"* (Zachary nods.) *"Do you remember how you can tell me you want to stop?"* (Zachary nods and holds up his hand as a stop sign.) *"Great. OK, now, just let your brain think of Raino's teeth in your arm, the upset thought 'I'm going to die,' and those feelings in your chest. Now follow my fingers with your eyes. There you go, you're doing great."* (The therapist commences approximately 20 repetitions of eye movements.) *"What are you noticing, Zachary?"*

Zachary: *"Raino was growling and snarling. I tried to get away but I couldn't!"*
<<<<
Zachary: *"It hurts! I couldn't get him off me!"* (Tearful now)
<<<<
Zachary: *"Scared. He was really big. He was like a monster!"* (Still tearful)
<<<<
Zachary: *"It felt like a stab."*
<<<<
Zachary: *"Scared. Like a bad dream."*
<<<<<
Zachary: *"Pain – my arm."*
<<<<
Zachary: *"Lots of blood!"*
<<<<
Zachary: *"Pushing and kicking him."*
<<<<
Zachary: *"He was too big, it was scary!"*
<<<<
Zachary: *"Bill came running and screaming at Raino. He yanked him off me."*

<<<<
Zachary: *"My arm was a mess. It hurt!"*
<<<<
Zachary: *"In the car with mom and Bill on the way to the hospital."*
<<<<
Zachary: *"Mom had a towel on my arm."*
<<<<
Zachary: *"They were really nice at the hospital. My dad showed up too."*
<<<<
Zachary: *"Nothing else really."*
Therapist: *"Zachary, take a moment to think of the incident with Raino again. What's there now? Thoughts? Feelings?"*
Zachary: *"Mad!"*
<<<<
Zachary: *"I could kill Raino! Ugly dog!"*
<<<<
Zachary: *"Stupid, stupid dog!"*
<<<<
Zachary: *"He's dead now. Bill had him put down."*
<<<<
Zachary: *"I felt kind of bad for Bill but I don't feel bad for Raino."*
<<<<
Zachary: *"Bill didn't know Raino had dug a hole under the fence."*
<<<<
Zachary: *"He thinks something was wrong with Raino's brain."*
<<<<
Zachary: *"OK, I feel sort of sorry for Raino. Maybe he had a tumor in his head or something."*
<<<<
Zachary: *"Bill got a little dog this time. His name is Pooch."*
Therapist: *"Zachary, when you think of the incident now, what do you notice?"*
Zachary: *"He's dead now, and that's that."*
Therapist: *"Zachary, when you think of the incident with Raino, how upset do you feel now? Look at this scale and point, anywhere from 0 to 10."*
Zachary points to the 0.

- *Phase 5. Installation:* Because the SUD has reached 0, the therapist proceeds with focusing on the positive cognition. The validity of the positive cognition increases spontaneously as a memory is processed during the Desensitization Phase. Alternatively, a more desirable cognition may emerge. During the Installation Phase, its status is assessed and targeted. First, she checks to make sure the preferred thought she and Zachary previously identified is still a good fit for Zachary.
  Therapist: *"Zachary, when you think of what happened, does the thought 'I am safe' still seem like the one you want to have?"* (Zachary nods.)
  "Think about what happened and the words 'I am safe,' and look at

this scale. Point to the number on this scale that shows how true those words feel, anywhere from 1, not true, to 7, completely true." (Zachary points to the 7). Therapist: *"Think of the incident with Raino and the thought, 'I am safe' and follow my fingers."*
(Eye movements)
When the VoC is less than 7, the therapist continues applying sets of eye movements until a 7 is achieved.

- *Phase 6. Body Scan:* The therapist next initiates the Body Scan to determine if there is any residual disturbance felt in the body.

   Therapist: *"Think of the incident and the thought, 'I am safe' and see if you notice any tightness, pressure, or anything in your body anywhere. Notice your head, your neck, your shoulders, your chest, and your stomach."*
   Zachary: *"I can't notice anything."*

   If there had been remaining body sensations, the therapist would have asked him to focus on them and continued sets of eye movements until the sensations were eliminated. Zachary's body scan is clear, so the therapist proceeds to closure, in which she gives some directions to Zachary.

- *Phase 7. Closure*:
   Therapist: *"You did really good work today. How are you feeling?"*
   Zachary: *"Good."*
   Therapist: *"There is no need to think anymore about what we worked on, but if something about it does pop up in your mind, or if you notice any feelings, can you tell your parents so they can write it down for me?"*
   Zachary: *"Yes."*

   If Zachary's session had been incomplete, the therapist would have asked Zachary to place everything they worked on into his container (the trunk.) The therapist would have then asked Zachary to imagine himself inside his safe treehouse in order to establish a calm affect state. Zachary would have been asked to identify the most helpful thought or idea he had learned from the session and to take the thought with him. She would have told Zachary to continue using his container (the trunk) and his safe place (the treehouse) and instructed him to tell his parents if he had any upset feelings or thoughts before the next session.

- *Phase 8. Reevaluation:* During the Reevaluation Phase, the therapist checks to see whether the previous target remains clear. Then she looks for recent triggering situations related to the trauma, which may remain due to second-order conditioning. When Zachary and his parents return, he is asked to bring up the dog attack in his mind and notice his response. Zachary reports no escalation in disturbance related to the memory, and his parents confirm that he is sleeping well and no longer afraid to go outside. However, the day before the appointment, Zachary showed some anxiety around another neighbor's large but friendly dog.

Present-Day or Recent Trigger Phases 3 through 7 are implemented with the recent triggering situation involving the other dog. The event is reprocessed with the standard procedures until Zachary reports no remaining disturbance and rates the positive cognition, "I am safe," with a VoC of 7.

Future Template The future template involves the use of imagination to visualize a positive response to a challenging future situation and reinforcing the positive response with bilateral stimulation. In the latter part of the same session, the therapist and Zachary discuss how he would like to respond to the friendly, big dog in the future. He closes his eyes and imagines staying calm and petting the dog, while the therapist applies alternating taps to the backs of his hands to deepen feelings of confidence.

- *Phase 8. Reevaluation Phase*: In a follow-up phone call, Zachary's parents report that Zachary has been sleeping well and playing outside without anxiety. He had also interacted positively with his uncle's German shepherd.

13.2.3 Complex Trauma

The following is a complex trauma case involving a child (Karen, age 12) who was removed from her biological family due to maltreatment. Children who have experienced multiple adverse experiences within their attachment relationships frequently exhibit extremely challenging behaviors related to their traumatic stress. Families are often stuck in very negative dynamics, and the child's placement may be at risk. In this case, the preparation phase may be longer and involve family therapy work as well as EMDR preparation activities. EMDR resource development involves accessing a positive feeling or trait such as strength or courage through imagery and then deepening it with bilateral stimulation. A customized EMDR resource development activity used with children who lack a secure attachment involves the creation of experiences of closeness in the office and strengthening the child's feelings of security and trust with bilateral stimulation (Wesselmann et al. 2014).

History Taking. Phase 1 During the initial interview with her mother, the therapist learns that Karen had been adopted 2 years earlier. She had been removed from her biological parents by social services at age 7 due to maltreatment. Both biological parents suffered from mental illness and substance addiction, and they had also become involved with a satanic cult, to which Karen had been exposed.

During the interview, Karen's adoptive mother describes her as defiant, dishonest, detached, passive-aggressive, manipulative, angry, impulsive, controlling, and anxious. Karen had been hospitalized and placed in a psychiatric residential treatment facility for 5 months earlier in the year. The mother describes herself as exhausted and defeated, and she states that she does not know if Karen will be able to stay in their home. For this reason, Karen's EMDR therapist decides to collaborate with a trauma-informed family therapist to help interrupt the negative interactional patterns in Karen's family and coach the family in new skills. (See Sect. 13.3 below.)

Preparation. Phase 2 Karen's EMDR therapist begins the Preparation Phase by implementing the Safe Place exercise. From her history and behaviors, it appears that Karen does not have a secure attachment to her adoptive parents, leading the therapist to customize the resource development activity to strengthen attachment security. The therapist first meets individually with Karen's mother to prepare her for the exercise and then invites her into the session. She suggests that the mother and daughter sit together on the sofa if they are comfortable with that position. They comply and Karen's mother places her arm around her daughter's shoulders. Next, the therapist encourages the mother to talk about the qualities that she appreciates in Karen. Karen has chosen tactile bilateral stimulation for the exercise, which the therapist implements, slowly, during her mother's discourse, deepening Karen's feelings of connection with her mother and the positive self-view as seen through her mother's eyes. The therapist next asks Karen's mother to talk about her favorite early memories related to first meeting her daughter, activities she has enjoyed with her, and her future hopes and dreams for their relationship. During each of her mother's responses, the therapist implements the bilateral stimulation to reinforce Karen's feelings of closeness and comfort.

Due to Karen's mistrust of her parents and emotional and behavioral dysregulation, two more EMDR sessions are devoted to additional resource work for strengthening attachment and for increasing a calm affect state together with feelings of maturity. The therapist commences trauma work in the following session. Karen's adoptive mother is invited to provide support for Karen during the session. She is instructed to stay silent but emotionally available during the memory processing, which helps Karen stay present with respect to her emotions and regulated throughout the work. Her mother is also told that the therapist might ask her questions intermittently during EMDR processing to help provide Karen with some needed information or an adult perspective.

Assessment. Phase 3 One of Karen's traumatic memories involves the witnessing of her biological father killing several animals on the kitchen table when she was around 6 years of age. The therapist asks Karen a series of questions to elicit the following basic information and baseline measures.

Image (representing the worst part of the experience in the present): "My dad stabbing the dog."

Negative cognition: "I am not safe."

Positive cognition: "I am safe."

Validity of positive cognition (VoC) on a scale of 1–7, with 1 being completely false, 7 being completely true: 4

Emotions (currently experienced): Scared

Subjective units of distress scale (SUD) from 0 (no disturbance) to 10 (highest): 9

Body Sensations (experienced in the present): Tension in arms, back, and legs

Desensitization. Phase 4 In the following transcript, the symbols <<<< represent the therapist prompt, "Go with that," the eye movements, and "What is there now?"

Therapist:	"Karen, I would like you to sit by your mom so you can feel her supporting you today." (Karen moves over next to her mother who puts an arm around her.) "Then I would like you to pay attention to that upsetting picture, your thought, 'I am not safe,' and the tension in your body. Now just follow my fingers for a bit." (Karen follows the therapist's fingers for about 20 repetitions of eye movements.)
Karen:	"I was so scared I felt frozen. I didn't want to watch, but I couldn't stop myself."
<<<<	
Karen:	"I love animals. I didn't want them to get hurt."
<<<<	
Karen:	(Crying) "It's horrible. I hate it."
Therapist:	"Remember, your feelings won't hurt you. Just notice them."
<<<<	
Karen:	"Scared. Still really tense, all over my body." (Her mother nods at the therapist; she can feel the tension in Karen's body.)
Therapist:	"Remember, it's not happening now. Just notice the tension, Karen."
<<<<	
Karen:	"It's a little less now."
<<<<	
Karen:	(Tearful) "Why would they do this? It makes me sick."
<<<<	
Karen:	"Sad and mad."
Therapist:	"What do you notice in your body?"
Karen:	"I feel tense in my arms."
<<<<	
Karen:	"My younger siblings were too little to know what was going on. I'm kind of jealous of them. They don't have to remember this."
<<<<	
Karen:	"Why did they act like that?"
<<<<	
Karen:	"The drugs made them act scary--and mental illness, too."
<<<<	
Karen:	(Tearful) "I should have stopped him from killing them. I should have saved the animals."

(Children sometimes reach a stuck point during reprocessing due to lack of information that is needed to reach adaptive resolution. In this case, the insertion of a brief question or statement, termed a "cognitive interweave," can help. It is important that it be done in a way that does not interrupt the client's processing. In Karen's case, she is not aware that young children are unable to control adults, so the therapist uses a visual aid to help with a cognitive interweave that provides an adult perspective by pulling a small pair of shoes from her drawer.)

Therapist:	"Mom, would Karen's feet have been about this size?"
Mom:	"Yes, that would be about right."
Therapist:	"Karen, look at these cute little shoes. Could a little girl this size stop a grown-up from doing something he wanted to do?"

Karen: "No, I don't think so."
<<<<
Karen: "Now I feel alone. I didn't have anyone who could help."
<<<<
Karen: "I still feel alone."

(Karen did not feel safe in the past, and she is still not old enough to feel powerful or safe without the protection of a trusted adult in her life. The therapist enlists Karen's mother to provide a cognitive interweave related to her role as protector.)

Therapist: "Mom, if you and Dad could fly back in time and walk into that kitchen, what would you do?"

Mom: "Dad would have stopped your other dad from killing the animals. And I would tell 6-year-old Karen, 'You don't have to be alone anymore.' I would take her to our safe home and hold her and rock her and keep her safe." (Karen leans into her mom, and her mom holds her closer.)
<<<<
Karen: "I'm really not alone."

Therapist: "Can you go back to the incident now and just notice what comes up?"
<<<<
Karen: "There is only a little bit of tension left in my hands."
<<<<
Karen: "My body is more relaxed."

Processing continues until Karen reports that the tension is completely eliminated and Karen reports a SUD of 0.

Installation. Phase 5 The therapist proceeds with installation of the positive cognition, "I am safe," until Karen reports the belief to feel true at a 7 on the 1–7 scale.

Body Scan, Closure, and Reevaluation. Phases 6–8 The therapist asks Karen to scan her body for residual sensations, but Karen reports her body is clear, and the session moves to closure. Reevaluation with Karen during the following session showed that the desensitization effects were maintained.

Karen was discharged following 6 months of treatment consisting of 15 EMDR therapy sessions and 15 family therapy sessions. In family therapy, the parents received guidance, and Karen and her parents practiced new skills, such as strategies for listening and communicating effectively. The EMDR sessions included one history-taking session, three preparation sessions, and six sessions focused on EMDR trauma work (phases 3 through 8) related to five traumatic memories. In the other five EMDR sessions, processing targeted current triggers and the development of future templates for adaptive responses. EMDR therapy resulted in elimination of the disturbance related to Karen's traumatic memories and integration of the memory with adaptive information and a present-day perspective. Karen's emotional reactions to present-day triggers were eliminated and replaced with new emotional and behavioral responses.

At the end of 6 months, Karen's mother reported that Karen was cooperative and helpful at home. She said, "I feel close to her now. She is relaxed, spontaneous, and open with her feelings. She has empathy. We talk and have fun together. I enjoy spending time with her. I even trust her to babysit her younger brothers and sisters." She went on to report that the lying, manipulation, and aggressive outbursts were gone. The therapist followed up with her by phone at 6 months posttreatment, and she reported that all of Karen's gains had been maintained.

13.3 Special Challenges

A variety of obstacles may be encountered when treating children and adolescents. This section will address some of the most common of these, including challenging behaviors related to past abuse and neglect, the death of a parent, intellectual disability, autism, parent issues, and difficulties encountered when working with very young children and adolescents.

13.3.1 Past Abuse and Neglect

Parental abuse or neglect leaves children like Karen in a double bind: The person to whom they wish to run for comfort is at the same time a cause of their emotional pain. Even when their environment becomes safe, they are unable to feel safe or utilize caretakers for comfort due to the presence of stored, unprocessed attachment traumas. Whether children remain with a biological parent or have foster, adoptive, or guardianship homes, an inability to trust can lead to severe emotional and behavioral dysregulation. It is not uncommon for children with a history of maltreatment to exhibit symptoms of aggression, defiance, stealing, lying, and the hoarding of food, all of which may be driven by stored, unprocessed traumatic memories. Parents, in turn, frequently respond with anger and frustration, which intensifies the children's mistrust. For children with severe behaviors, the stuck, negative interactions in the family can become a roadblock to trauma work. Children need to feel safe and supported by their parents in order to access vulnerable emotions and memories, but stuck negative interactions create an unsupportive emotional environment.

An integrative EMDR and family therapy approach provides family intervention in tandem with trauma work (Wesselmann et al. 2012, 2014). The family therapist helps the parents understand the child's problems through the AIP model, while the EMDR therapist commences EMDR resource work for strengthening attachment security. Next, the family therapist teaches and coaches parents and children in skills that promote the family's emotional health and the sense of security and safety for the child during trauma work.

13.3.2 Parent Problems and Concerns

Parents' emotional issues can have a negative impact on the emotional welfare of any child or adolescent, no matter the presenting issue. When the EMDR therapist recognizes that parents' emotional functioning is interfering with therapeutic gains or the child's overall emotional growth, s/he should utilize a compassionate tone and attitude while communicating observations directly, encouraging parents to seek additional support for themselves and participate in their own EMDR therapy as needed. For example, the therapist may say, "You have had and continue to have many stressors in your life, including the stress of meeting your child's needs. Let's talk about how you can get the support you need. I am also going to suggest that you participate in your own EMDR therapy to help you feel better overall and reduce your triggers during interactions with your child." Although the child's therapist can provide EMDR therapy for the parents, a referral to a colleague should be offered as an alternative. Some parents and some children prefer not to "share" their individual therapist with another family member.

13.3.3 Intellectual Disability (ID) and Autism Spectrum Disorder (ASD)

Severe emotional and behavioral problems exhibited by children with intellectual disability (ID) and autism spectrum disorder (ASD) are often attributed to the congenital abnormalities (i.e., the cognitive impairments and the ASD or ID itself) known as "diagnostic overshadowing." When trauma symptoms are recognized in people with ASD, there is often great restraint in offering trauma treatment due to fear of an increase in psychiatric symptoms. Through a reliable and valid interview to assess PTSD in children with mild-to-borderline ID (IQ 50–85) (Mevissen et al. 2014; 2016), it was found that symptoms of PTSD do not differ in type in children with or without mild-to-borderline ID. Children with ID experience adverse life events (e.g., bullying, sexual, emotional and physical abuse, medical problems, surgeries and treatments, parental divorce, and placement outside the home) at a relatively high frequency but are poorly equipped to cope with them.

In view of its nonverbal components and applicability regardless of the client's mental age, EMDR therapy is ideally suited for children with ID (Mevissen et al. 2012). Depending upon the level of client disability, the EMDR therapist may need to be quite directive and use simple language. In the case of very limited verbal and/or cognitive abilities (mental age < 3 years), a storytelling method (Lovett 1999, 2015) can be applied to identify and process target memories. Following history taking and preparation (phases 1 and 2), the therapist, with the help of the child's parents, writes a narrative that begins with positive statements about the child. This is followed by a description of the adverse event, along with the child's emotions and negative beliefs, in order to activate the child's memory networks. The narrative concludes with positive, adaptive information. The written narrative replaces the standard assessment (phase 3) procedures. This entire narrative is read to the child, along with the simultaneous application of bilateral stimulation, which substitutes for the desensitization and reprocessing phases 4 through 7 of the standard protocol. Reevaluation (phase 8) takes place through therapist observation and the parents' report on the child's behaviors in the following session.

ASD occurs in persons with and without intellectual disabilities and refers to persistent deficits in various developmental domains. The EMDR adaptations for children with ASD resemble those used for children with ID, including simplifying instructions, using visual cues, and taking extra time. For children with ASD, the need for such adaptations can vary greatly depending on the child. Some are totally nonverbal, some are over-precise with regard to linguistic usage, some show little emotion, and some exhibit very intense emotions. An apparently trivial incident can be experienced as extremely traumatic, or vice versa.

For example, one boy with ASD had been beaten up by some other children while playing outside. Most non-autistic children would have been able to handle what happened. However, according to his mother, the boy stayed inside the house for about a year and a half. He only went out to go to school by bus, and he became very aggressive toward his brother. After one EMDR therapy session, his pattern of fear was eliminated, and within two sessions, the disturbing memory was completely processed. Subsequently, his behavior returned to what it had been before the distressing event. A therapist who works with children with ASD will customize the EMDR procedures depending on the needs of the child; treatment can take more time due to slow processing of information and long chains of associations filled with details or move incredibly quickly.

Molly was a 6-year-old girl with severe congenital intellectual and physical disabilities. She could not speak, used a wheelchair due to paralysis in her legs, and functioned at a developmental level of an 18-month-old. She was referred for treatment of extreme dental fear, but at intake it was revealed by her mother that she was equally afraid of all physicians. She was also extremely sensitive to touch, especially around the area of her head. Due to her severe physical condition, future medical surgeries and treatments were inevitable.

History Taking. Phase 1 History taking revealed that Molly was tube fed due to a life-threatening illness at the age of 3 months. Her fears had escalated and generalized following a painful surgery by the ear doctor at the age of three. Behavioral interventions had been unsuccessful in reducing her fearfulness. It was hypothesized that Molly's extreme fears were related to her medical traumas. Due to her low level of functioning, it was decided that the EMDR storytelling method as described by Lovett (1999) would be implemented.

Preparation. Phase 2 Two sessions were devoted to educating Molly's parents about trauma and explaining AIP, EMDR therapy, and the storytelling method. In addition, they were asked to identify playful activities that would elicit positive feelings and strengthen attachment bonds in between work with the narrative.

Assessment. Phase 3 The therapist and parents worked together to create stories about Molly's traumatic visits to the ear doctor. These stories included associated emotions and negative thoughts as well as positive, adaptive information.

Storytelling, Desensitization, and Reprocessing. Phases 4–7 The first narrative described an early visit to the ear doctor. While Molly sat in her wheelchair, her mother kindly described lovable baby Molly. Then she went on to describe the memory of being anesthetized. She briefly showed Molly a surgical mask explaining that it "made Molly cry, shout, and lash out. Molly was afraid. Molly couldn't stand it." Molly's father applied bilateral stimulation by tapping her hands. High levels of disturbance were elicited and then faded away. The story was repeated during the session in conjunction with the bilateral stimulation until Molly was able to stay relaxed while looking at the mask, with both parents emphasizing her current strength and safety.

Next, the storytelling procedure was conducted to help Molly reprocess a traumatic doctor visit in which a tube was inserted into her throat. The parent lightly touched Molly's throat to help elicit the dysfunctionally stored memory of the disturbing physical sensations during the storytelling and application of the bilateral stimulation. The storytelling method was also implemented to help Molly reprocess the painful treatment of her ears. Molly's mother held her tightly on her lap (the place where she underwent the treatment) and applied the bilateral stimulation by touching one ear after another during the storytelling.

Closing. Phase 7 A special song was selected as a sign of closure of the session, and Molly was complimented for doing so well. The parents were asked to note any changes or disturbance between sessions.

Reevaluation. Phase 8 Following each session of storytelling, the therapist asked the parents to report any changes they had noted in Molly's functioning before continuing storytelling.

After four sessions of EMDR therapy, which fully processed the three medical memories, the parents reported significant changes in Molly's daily life functioning. They noted increases in her concentration and memory, interest in the environment, attention, and communication. Molly frequently initiated sitting on her parents' laps, and they noticed that she was able to better tolerate loud noises in the environment. Despite these positive signs, her mother was exhausted and no longer felt able to handle Molly's "negative" behaviors.

The therapist invited the mother to participate in her own EMDR therapy session. She told about a recent situation in which Molly had refused to obey. She had become overwhelmed and had yelled at Molly. While processing this event, the mother spontaneously floated back to the memory of giving birth and finding out that Molly was severely handicapped. This memory was targeted along with the negative cognition, "I am bad." The desired positive cognition was, "I am OK." She then described a second memory of "Molly laying in a hospital bed covered with tubes, almost dead, and me standing beside." This memory was reprocessed, along with the negative cognition, "I'm powerless." The desired positive cognition was "I can handle it." It took three sessions to fully process these disturbing memories. Shortly afterward, Molly turned seven. Her mother reported, "For the first time in seven years, I enjoyed her birthday!" She felt relieved and strong and more able to set boundaries when Molly needed them. Molly's therapy was continued by targeting additional memories of dental treatment.

After a total of nine EMDR therapy sessions with Molly and six parent guidance sessions, mother and father reported that Molly was able to undergo dental checkups and medical surgeries without panicking. When it was really painful, she cried, but this passed quickly, and they were able to provide strong support for her. They also reported that Molly now tolerated washing her face, combing her hair, and cleaning her ears. Moreover, positive changes with regard to healthy parent-child bonding were observed: Molly initiated hugging her parents, something she had never done before. She also became inconsolable for a while when separated from them. She showed increased interest and skills in a variety of play materials. It became apparent that processing the traumatic material had allowed her to learn to trust and bond, leading to exploration and the learning of new skills.

13.3.4 Adolescents/High-Risk Behaviors

Adolescents present their own unique challenges. Due to their developing independence and desire for autonomy, they may be resistant to therapy initiated by their parents. Under these circumstances, extra preparation time is needed to develop therapeutic trust. The therapist sidesteps power struggles by avoiding judgments or lectures, instead listening and attuning to the adolescent's emotions and thoughts. Motivation is achieved by involving the adolescent in the EMDR treatment plan and helping him or her identify the most personally troubling problem areas.

Many adolescents in therapy are engaged in high-risk compulsive or addictive activity. These behaviors may have become associated with pleasurable feelings despite creating unpleasant life consequences. Thus, the positive affect is maladaptive under the circumstances, leading to more of the same behaviors and the same negative outcomes. Targeting the compulsive behavior along with the maladaptive positive affect facilitates processing and the natural associative process, bringing the adolescent to a heightened awareness of the negative consequences (Miller 2012). One 13-year-old female who was compulsively stealing small items from the desks and backpacks of her fellow students reported experiencing a feeling of "excitement and happiness" after each act of thievery. She grinned widely the first time she talked about this positive sensation. EMDR therapy was implemented by targeting the compulsive act along with the maladaptive positive affect. As she watched the therapist's fingers, the young girl spontaneously associated to memories of the friends she had lost, the loss of trust from her parents, and the brevity of the positive feelings associated with each new acquisition. The strong positive feeling quickly shifted to sadness and accompanied by the comment, "This doesn't make any sense!"

Another method of reducing compulsive behaviors involves targeting a situation, thought, or feeling that triggers an urge (Popky 2009). While bilateral stimulation is being applied, the youth is instructed to recall the trigger and to notice the associated desire. Processing is continued until the feeling is eliminated, and the procedure is repeated with each successive compulsivity trigger. In all cases the full EMDR therapy protocol that processes past events, current triggers, and future challenges is employed (Shapiro 2001).

13.3.5 Very Young Children

Very young children, typically ages 3–7, may be unable to track bilateral movements easily with their eyes, and their attention span, insight, and vocabulary may be quite limited. The EMDR therapist simplifies the language and protocol as necessary to meet the developmental needs of these children (Adler-Tapia and Settle 2008; Shapiro 2001). For example, the therapist may implement the bilateral stimulation in a child-friendly way using a puppet, wand, or tactile methods such as playful, bilateral hand-clapping games. The therapist may ask the child to hold his hands wide apart or closer together to demonstrate the level of distress the child is experiencing. When implementing EMDR therapy with toddlers and preschoolers, identification of negative and positive beliefs may not be feasible. Younger children who cannot verbalize their traumatic or disturbing experience may be asked to create a drawing or sand tray picture of the event. Alternatively, the parents may be coached to elicit the child's memory of the event by telling a story (prior to the onset of the bilateral stimulation) about what had happened. In addition, simple instructions that elicit imagery and a somatic response can be used to initiate reprocessing. For instance, a 3-year-old had been unable to move past grief after her mother's live-in boyfriend of 2 years, Ted, moved away. She described feeling "sad in my heart." She was instructed to think of Ted, notice "the sad in your heart," and watch a light moving bilaterally on an electronic horizontal bar, about 10–12 repetitions per set. Each time the therapist paused the lights, the little girl talked about happy memories that had come to mind. At one point she remarked, "These lights make pictures go through my brain very, very fast!" After the session, the mother called and stated that her daughter seemed to have made a complete adjustment to the situation.

In summary, the eight phases of EMDR therapy can be customized for children as needed, depending upon their developmental level, functional impairments, complexity of traumatic history, ability to safely experience emotions, and family circumstances. The EMDR child therapist has the option of adapting the language and procedures throughout the eight phases, applying cognitive interweaves, utilizing caregivers for emotional support, and attending to family systems issues as necessary. With the proper modifications tailored to the individual circumstances of each child, EMDR therapy is an efficient and effective approach for resolving emotional and behavioral symptoms, improving the quality of life and fostering posttraumatic growth across the full clinical spectrum.

13.4 Research Review

EMDR therapy and trauma-focused cognitive behavioral therapy (CBT) are the only psychotherapies recommended by the World Health Organization (WHO 2013) for the treatment of post-traumatic stress disorder (PTSD) in children, adolescents, and adults. The efficacy of EMDR therapy with trauma-related disorders has been supported by over 25 RCTs, eight of which specifically evaluated the treatment of children (Ahmad et al. 2007; Chemtob et al. 2002; de Roos et al. 2011; Diehle et al.

2014; Jaberghaderi et al. 2004; Kemp et al. 2010; Soberman et al. 2002; Wanders et al. 2008). Three RCTs assessing the effects of EMDR therapy with civilian adults suffering from single-event trauma have established that approximately 5 hours of treatment results in 84–100 % remission of PTSD (see Shapiro 2014a). These studies have established the baseline expectation for EMDR therapy outcomes in clinical practice across the lifespan. While individual traumas can be effectively treated in 1–3 sessions without homework, the amount of treatment time for multiply traumatized populations depends upon the number of adverse life experiences needing to be processed and the amount of preparation time needed to address affect instability.

As noted above, the efficacy of EMDR therapy with children in the treatment of PTSD symptoms has been supported by eight RCTs. The studies concerned a wide range of adverse events. Six of the studies focused primarily on PTSD symptoms, and of these, three used a wait list control. Kemp et al. (2010) compared EMDR to a wait list control condition with children suffering from persistent PTSD symptoms following a motor vehicle accident. The treatment group showed significant improvement on the Child Post-Traumatic Stress-Reaction Index following four sessions of EMDR, as compared to no improvement for the control condition. This effect was maintained at 3 and 12 months. In another RTC (Ahmad et al. 2007), children suffering from PTSD symptoms related to an explosion received either eight sessions of EMDR or were referred to a wait list. Only the treatment group revealed significant improvement in psychiatric and PTSD symptoms, specifically reexperiencing and avoiding symptoms 2 months posttreatment. A study of children with PTSD 1 year after a natural disaster using a randomized lagged-group design (Chemtob et al. 2002) reported a significant reduction in traumatic stress symptoms on a standardized measure after three sessions of EMDR therapy, an improvement that was maintained at 6 months follow-up. The remaining three published RTCs randomly assigned children to CBT or EMDR. In a study by de Roos et al. (2011), children suffering from PTSD following an explosion were treated with up to four sessions, and parents were provided four parent guidance sessions. Blind evaluators determined that both groups improved significantly on all PTSD and behavioral measures, but the EMDR group required overall fewer sessions. Treatment gains were maintained at 3 months follow-up. In a study by Diehle et al. (2014), children suffering from full or partial PTSD following exposure to at least one traumatic event of varying types received eight sessions of either EMDR or CBT. Both groups exhibited a significant improvement on measures of traumatic stress completed by children and their parents. In another study (Jaberghaderi et al. 2004), sexually abused Iranian girls ages 12–13 were randomly assigned CBT or EMDR therapy. While an equally significant reduction in PTSD and behavioral problems was obtained for the two groups, participants in the EMDR condition achieved this gain in about half the number of sessions as those in the CBT condition and with considerably less homework (i.e., "minimal" vs "about 10–15 hours").

Two other RTCs assessed behavioral issues in children with disturbing memories. In a study by Soberman et al. (2002), boys with conduct problems and traumatic stress symptoms in residential or day treatment were randomly assigned to treatment-as-usual or treatment-as-usual plus three trauma-focused EMDR sessions. The

EMDR group exhibited large and significant reduction in memory-related distress and positive trends toward reduction of traumatic stress symptoms. At 2 months follow-up, the EMDR group showed large and significant improvement in behavioral problems and memory-related distress as compared to only slight improvement for the control group. Finally, in a study by Wanders et al. (2008), children with behavioral and self-esteem problems were randomly assigned to four sessions of either EMDR therapy or CBT that focused on their distressing memories. Parents, mentors, and children completed a wide variety of measures prior to and immediately after four sessions and at 6 months follow-up. Both treatments resulted in significant improvements in behaviors and self-esteem, with the EMDR group showing larger improvements in target behaviors.

A meta-analysis (Rodenburg et al. 2009) reported a substantial reduction in PTSD symptoms in traumatized children ages 4–18 years following EMDR therapy, compared to therapy-as-usual or no-treatment control groups. In the studies that compared CBT with EMDR therapy for children with PTSD, both approaches were effective in reducing symptoms of traumatic stress, although EMDR was determined to add "a small but significant incremental value" (Rodenburg et al. 2009, p. 604).

Thirteen nonrandomized child studies have reported significant positive effects with EMDR therapy. Of particular note are those studies shedding light on efficacy as a function of age, treatment duration, war, and disability. In a naturalistic study (Hensel, 2009), 36 children between 1 and 18 years old with a single trauma were treated with 1–3 sessions of EMDR therapy. Clinical outcomes demonstrated substantial benefits at posttest and follow-up, with very young children showing equal improvement as compared to older children. In a delayed treatment comparison, 17 out of 20 children improved significantly after one session of EMDR therapy following single-incident trauma (Puffer et al. 1997). EMDR therapy was also found effective in treating Iraqi children suffering from PTSD (Wadaa et al. 2010). In case studies, EMDR has been found beneficial in treating PTSD in children and adults with intellectual disabilities (e.g., Mevissen et al. 2011; Mevissen et al. 2012).

Given the potentially dire consequences of childhood trauma worldwide (see Shapiro 2014b), it is important to note that several noncontrolled studies have found significant reductions in reported and observed symptoms of traumatic stress after only one session following a group EMDR therapy protocol with children affected by both man-made and natural disasters (Aduriz et al. 2009; Fernandez 2007; Fernandez et al. 2004; Jarero et al. 2006, 2008). In one nonrandomized trial (Zaghrout-Hodali et al. 2008), Palestinian children experiencing ongoing traumatic events showed substantial treatment effects after four sessions of the EMDR group protocol, including an elimination of PTSD symptoms, reduction in behavioral problems, and increased feelings of security and resilience to subsequent trauma.

Although the majority of child research has focused on the impact of EMDR therapy on PTSD, it has also been widely used to reduce broader symptoms, functional problems, and disorders. Ongoing research indicates that children with a history of abuse and/or foster or orphanage care in out-of-home placements with internalizing and externalizing symptoms experience significant improvement in scores on attachment, traumatic stress, and behavioral measures at 36 weeks with outpatient integrative EMDR and family therapy that includes an EMDR resource development activity (Attachment and Trauma Center of Nebraska 2011). Separate case studies show similar effects with abused and neglected children in out-of-home placements treated with integrative EMDR and family therapy (Wesselmann 2013; Wesselmann and Shapiro 2013; Wesselmann et al. 2012). While EMDR therapy has been validated in the treatment of PTSD across the lifespan, randomized controlled trials are needed to further investigate all these additional areas of interest.

References

Adler-Tapia R, Settle C (2008) EMDR and the art of psychotherapy with children: treatment manual. Springer Publishing, New York

Aduriz ME, Bluthgen C, Knopfler C (2009) Helping child flood victims using group EMDR intervention in Argentina: treatment outcome and gender differences. Int J Stress Manag 16:138–153

Ahmad A, Larsson B, Sundelin-Wahlsten V (2007) EMDR treatment for children with PTSD: results of a randomized controlled trial. Nord J Psychiatry 61:349–354

Attachment and Trauma Center of Nebraska (2011) EMDR integrative team treatment for attachment trauma in children: treatment manual. Attachment and Trauma Center of Nebraska, Omaha

Chemtob CM, Nakashima J, Carlson JG (2002) Brief-treatment for elementary school children with disaster-related PTSD: a field study. J Clin Psychol 58:99–112

Craske M, Herman D, Vansteenwegen D (eds) (2006) Fear and learning: from basic processes to clinical implications. APA Press, Washington, DC

De Roos C, Veenstra A, de Jongh A, den Hollander-Gijsman M, van der Wee N, Zitman F, van Rood Y (2010) Treatment of chronic phantom limb pain using a trauma-focused psychological approach. Pain Res Manag: J Can Pain Soc 15(2):65–71

de Roos C, Greenwald R, den Hollander-Gijsm M, Noorthoorn E, van Buuren S, de Jongh A (2011) A randomized comparison of cognitive behavioural therapy. Eur J Psychotraumatol 2:5694–5704

Diehle J, Opmeer BC, Boer F, Mannarino AP, Lindauer RJ (2014) Trauma-focused cognitive behavioral therapy or eye movement desensitization and reprocessing: What works in children with posttraumatic stress symptoms? A randomized controlled trial. Eur Child Adolesc Psychiatry 24:227–236

Felitti VJ, Anda RF, Nordenberg D, Williamson DF, Spitz AM, Edwards V, Koss MP, Marks JS (1998) Relationship of childhood abuse and household dysfunction to many of the leading causes of death in adults: The Adverse Childhood Experiences (ACE) Study. Am J Prev Med 14:749–379

Fernandez I (2007) EMDR as treatment of post-traumatic reactions: A field study on child victims of an earthquake. Educ Child Psychol. Special Issue: Therapy 24:65–72

Fernandez I, Gallinari E, Lorenzetti A (2004) A school-based EMDR intervention for children who witnessed the Pirelli building airplane crash in Milan, Italy. J Brief Ther 2:129–136

Hensel T (2009). EMDR with children and adolescents after single-incident trauma an intervention study. Journal of EMDR Practice and Research 3:2–9.

Jaberghaderi N, Greenwald R, Rubin A, Dolatabadim S, Zand SO (2004) A comparison of CBT and EMDR for sexually abused Iranian girls. Clin Psychol Psychother 11:358–368

Jarero I, Artigas L, Hartung J (2006) EMDR integrative group treatment protocol: a post-disaster trauma intervention for children and adults. Traumatology 12:121–129

Jarero I, Artigas L, Lopez-Lena M (2008) The EMDR integrative group treatment protocol: application with child victims of mass disaster. J EMDR Pract Res 2:97–105

Kemp M, Drummond P, McDermott B (2010) A wait-list controlled pilot study of eye movement desensitization and reprocessing (EMDR) for children with post-traumatic stress disorder (PTSD) symptoms from motor vehicle accidents. Clin Child Psychol Psychiatry 15:5–25

Lee CW, Cuijpers P (2013) A meta-analysis of the contribution of eye movements in processing emotional memories. J Behav Ther Exp Psychiatry 44:231–239

Lovett J (1999) Small wonders: healing childhood trauma with EMDR. The Free Press, New York

Lovett J (2015) Trauma-attachment tangle: modifying EMDR to help children resolve trauma and develop loving relationships. Routledge, New York

Mevissen L, Reinout L, Seubert A, De Jongh A (2011) Do persons with intellectual disability and limited verbal capacities respond to trauma treatment? Journal of Intellectual & Developmental Disability 36(4):278–283

Mevissen L, Lievegoed R, Seubert A, De Jongh A (2012) PTSD treatment in people with severe intellectual disabilities: a case series. Dev Neurorehabil 15:223–232

Mevissen L, Barnhoorn E, Didden R, Korzilius H, De Jongh A (2014) Clinical assessment of PTSD in children with mild to borderline intellectual disabilities: a pilot study. Dev Neurorehabil 17:16–23

Mevissen L, Didden R, de Jongh A (2016) Assessment and treatment of PTSD in people with intellectual disabilities. In: Martin C, Preedy V, Patel V (eds) Comprehensive guide to post-traumatic stress disorder. Springer International Publishing, Switzerland.

Miller R (2012) Treatment of behavioral addictions utilizing the feeling-state addiction protocol: a multiple baseline study. J EMDR Pract Res 6:159–169

Mol SSL, Arntz A, Metsemakers JFM, Dinant G, Vilters-Van Montfort PAP, Knottnerus A (2005) Symptoms of post-traumatic stress disorder after non-traumatic events: evidence from an open population study. Br J Psychiatry 186:494–499

Popky AJ (2009) The desensitization of triggers and urge reprocessing (DeTUR) protocol. In: Luber M (ed) Eye Movement Desensitization and Reprocessing (EMDR) scripted protocols: special populations. Springer, New York, pp. 489–511

Puffer M, Greenwald R, Elrod D (1997) A single session EMDR study with twenty traumatized children and adolescents. Traumatology-e 3(2):Article 6

Rodenburg R, Benjamin A, de Roos C, Meijer AM, Stams GJ (2009) Efficacy of EMDR in children: a meta-analysis. Clin Psychol Rev 29:599–606

Schubert SJ, Lee CW, Drummond PD (2011) The efficacy and psychophysiological correlates of dual-attention tasks in eye movement desensitization and reprocessing (EMDR). J Anxiety Disord 25:1–11

Shapiro F (1995/2001) Eye movement desensitization and reprocessing: basic principles protocols, and procedures. Guildford Press, New York

Shapiro F (2012) EMDR therapy training manual. EMDR Institute, Watsonville

Shapiro F (2014a) The role of eye movement desensitization & reprocessing (EMDR) therapy in medicine: addressing the psychological and physical symptoms stemming from adverse life experiences. Perm J 18:71–77

Shapiro F (2014b) EMDR therapy humanitarian assistance programs: treating the psychological, physical, and societal effects of adverse experiences worldwide. J EMDR Pract Res 8:181–186

Soberman GB, Greenwald R, Rule DL (2002) A controlled study of eye movement desensitization and reprocessing (EMDR) for boys with conduct problems. J Aggress Maltreat Trauma 6:217–236

Stickgold R (2002) EMDR: a putative neurobiological mechanism of action. J Clin Psychol 58:61–75

Stickgold R, Walker MP (2013) Sleep-dependent memory triage: evolving generalization through selective processing. Nat Neurosci 16(2):139–145

Suzuki A et al (2004) Memory reconsolidation and extinction have distinct temporal and biochemical signatures. J Neurosci 24:4787–4795

Wadaa NN, Zaharim NM, Alqashan HF (2010) The use of EMDR in treatment of traumatized Iraqi children. DOMES 19:26–36

Walker MP, van der Helm E (2009) Overnight therapy? The role of sleep in emotional brain processing. Psychol Bull 135(5):731–748

Wanders F, Serra M, de Jongh A (2008) EMDR versus CBT for children with self-esteem and behavioral problems: a randomized controlled trial. J EMDR Pract Res 2:180–189

Wesselmann D (2013) Healing trauma and creating secure attachment through EMDR. In: Solomon M, Siegel DS (eds) Healing moments in psychotherapy: mindful awareness, neural integration, and therapeutic presence. Norton, New York

Wesselmann D, Shapiro F (2013) Eye movement desensitization and reprocessing. In: Ford J, Courtois C (eds) Treating complex traumatic stress disorders in children and adolescents. Guilford Press, New York, pp. 213–224

Wesselmann D, Davidson M, Armstrong S, Schweitzer C, Bruckner D, Potter A (2012) EMDR as a treatment for improving attachment status in adults and children. Eur Rev Appl Psychol 62:223–230

Wesselmann D, Schweitzer C, Armstrong S (2014) Integrative team treatment for attachment trauma in children: family therapy and EMDR. Norton, New York

World Health Organization (2013) Guidelines for the management of conditions that are specifically related to stress. WHO, Geneva

Zaghrout-Hodali M, Alissa F, Dodgson P (2008) Building resilience and dismantling fear: EMDR group protocol with children in an area of ongoing trauma. J EMDR Pract Res 2:106–113

Attachment, Self-Regulation, and Competency (ARC)

14

Margaret E. Blaustein and Kristine M. Kinniburgh

14.1 Attachment, Self-Regulation, and Competency (ARC)

14.1.1 Theoretical Underpinnings

A substantial percentage of youth exposed to trauma experience multiple or prolonged adversity (Copeland et al. 2007; Finkelhor et al. 2009; Spinazzola et al. 2005a), often resulting in a complex array of symptoms and functional impairments that include but go beyond PTSD. These behavioral, emotional, and functional challenges may result in placement in and services from a wide range of systems. As compared with nonexposed youth, youth impacted by multiple traumas are overrepresented in juvenile justice, residential, and other acute treatment systems (see Chaps. 20 and 21), are at risk for involvement with the child welfare system and disruption from multiple out-of-home placements, have a higher likelihood of eligibility for special education services, and seek medical care at higher rates (Abram et al. 2004; Annerback et al. 2012; Dube et al. 2003; Kisiel et al. 2009; Zelechoski and Beserra 2013). This high service utilization across settings suggests the need for trauma-focused treatment for this complex population that incorporates, but goes beyond, traditional therapy approaches.

The Attachment, Regulation, and Competency (ARC; Blaustein and Kinniburgh 2010; Kinniburgh and Blaustein 2005) treatment framework was developed to address the complicated needs of the population of children and

M.E. Blaustein, PhD (✉)
Trauma Training and Education, The Trauma Center at Justice Resource Institute,
Brookline, MA, USA
e-mail: mblaustein@jri.org

K.M. Kinniburgh, LCSW
Justice Resource Institute Connecticut Division, National trauma trainer and consultant,
The Trauma Center at Justice Resource Institute, Brookline, MA, USA
e-mail: kkinniburgh@jri.org

families defined by exposure to multiple, chronic, and often ongoing adversity. ARC is a core component intervention designed to be translatable across systems and explicitly incorporates the range of caregivers (primary, resource, milieu, etc.). ARC identifies three *core domains* and eight primary *treatment targets*. Theoretical underpinnings and rationale for primary domains targeted in ARC are briefly described here.

The *attachment* domain focuses on strengthening the system surrounding children by enhancing supports, skills, and relational resources for adult caregivers. Caregiver functioning has a significant impact on mental health outcomes for trauma-impacted children, and the presence of inadequate caregiving and/or stressed adult systems impacts both placement stability and risk for further victimization. Because complex childhood trauma by definition takes place within a relational context, the caregivers of these children are often themselves recovering from traumatic exposures.

The *regulation* domain addresses a core factor in negative outcomes among youth who have experienced complex trauma, namely, dysregulation of emotion, physiology, and behavior. A substantial body of research emphasizes the impact of traumatic stress on both physiological underpinnings of regulation and on the emotional and behavioral expression of this dysregulation, and both existing trauma-related diagnoses and newer proposed diagnostic categories attend to markers of dysregulation such as hyperarousal, behavioral reactivity, shifting mood states, and constriction/avoidance of affect.

The *competency* domain addresses key factors associated with resilience in stress-impacted populations. Research on risk and resilience stresses protective factors, including internal resources and external supports, in predicting long-term positive outcomes. A goal of ARC intervention is to go beyond pathology reduction to enhance resilience among youth receiving intervention; as such, the framework actively targets specific skills linked with resilient outcomes.

14.1.2 How To Do ARC

14.1.2.1 Structure of ARC

Each core domain described above has specific targets that are addressed in treatment; in turn, each target has identified subskills. These are described in Table 14.1. In addition, attention is paid to three crosscutting factors: (1) building mastery and safety through the use of *routines and structures*; (2) attention to *engagement* by exploring and identifying stake of the child, caregiver, and/or system for all goals; and (3) providing *psychoeducation* to build empowerment, understanding, and client/system stake.

In the service of trauma experience integration, all ARC targets are intended to be woven into treatment throughout the process, with providers identifying goals specific to the client and family system. Treatment moves in a staged process that mirrors classic phase-oriented models of treatment, emphasizing initial engagement and formulation; support for regulation, distress tolerance, and relational safety; building capacity for caregiver reflection (attunement) as well as youth self-understanding;

14 Attachment, Self-Regulation, and Competency (ARC)

enhancing strengths; and gradually shifting and transforming the impacts of traumatic experience. Given the complexity of the population typically treated with this framework, providers are encouraged to think of phases as "dynamic," in which the present state of the child/caregiver may shift the specific application of skills in the moment. For instance, the presence of stressors, trauma reminders, and/or ongoing

Table 14.1 ARC broad domains, core targets, and key subskills

Broad domain	Core targets	Key subskills
Attachment	Caregiver affect management	Trauma education, normalization, validation
		Identify challenging situations
		Build self-monitoring skills
		Enhance self-care and support
	Attunement	Parallel attunement to caregivers
		Support active curiosity
		Use reflection to mirror child experience
		Integrate attunement skills into support for youth regulation
		Support fluidity/pleasure in dyadic engagement
	Effective response	Proactively identify target behaviors
		Use attunement to identify behavior patterns
		Use "go-to" strategies (meet needs, support regulation) to reduce and address identified behaviors
		Identify, experiment with, and enhance behavioral response strategies that increase youth and environmental safety
Regulation	Identification	Language for emotions and arousal
		Connection of emotions, body sensations, behavior, and cognition
		Contextualization of emotions/arousal to internal and external experience
		Accurately reading others' emotional expression
	Modulation	Understanding of degrees of energy and feeling
		Understanding comfortable and effective states
		Explore arousal states and develop agency over tools
		Support and facilitate strategies which successfully lead to state change
	Expression	Explore goals of expression; build comfort and safety in relationship
		Identify/establish resources for safe expression
		Build skills to support effective use of resources
		Facilitate self-expression

(continued)

Table 14.1 (continued)

Broad domain	Core targets	Key subskills
Competency	Executive functions	Active recognition of capacity to make choices
		Age-appropriate active evaluation of situations
		Capacity to inhibit response
		Ability to generate and evaluate potential solutions
	Self and identity	Identify personal attributes
		Build internal resources and identification of positive aspects of self
		Build a sense of self which integrates past and present experiences, and incorporates multiple aspects of self
		Capacity to imagine and work toward future goals/outcomes
Trauma experience integration	Work with children to actively explore, process, and integrate historical experiences into a coherent and comprehensive understanding of self in order to enhance capacity to effectively engage in present life	

exposure to instability or trauma may lead to unanticipated shifts in child or family functioning within and across intervention sessions. As a result, the attunement of the provider is crucial to support appropriate use of ARC skills. Sequential application of skills with a child/family system is described in the case that follows.

14.1.2.2 The Case of Leo

As noted above, the ARC model may be applied in a range of settings, incorporating clinical intervention as well as organizational strategies such as staff training, system policies, and milieu practices. For the purposes of this chapter, an outpatient clinical application is described via the case of "Leo." Note that throughout the case description, key ARC targets underlying the intervention will occasionally be noted in **bold** to assist the reader in identifying them. The fluid stages of treatment will be denoted by subheadings in *italics*.

Leo is a 9-year-old Caucasian boy of Italian-American background who had recently moved into a kinship home. He was referred for treatment by his pediatrician due to aggressive and oppositional behaviors. Leo's caregivers, his biological father's cousin Jim and his wife, Lisa, were described as feeling burnt out. Leo's case was assigned to outpatient clinician "John."

Initial Engagement and Formulation: Caregivers

During the initial stage of treatment (typically two to four sessions each with child and caregiver), emphasis is placed on engagement and gathering information to inform formulation and treatment planning. Caregiver engagement practices include conversations about the ARC treatment approach, the role of the caregiver, and treatment "match." They also include identifying treatment goals, aligning both with the family's goals as well as core ARC targets, providing an early frame linking life stressors with current challenges, establishing a frame of transparency and psychoeducation, and enacting attunement by taking a curious, reflective stance about strengths and challenges in the child and family system. Embedded within provider attunement is the goal of developing a strong formulation of the child and family system in order to match treatment goals with identified needs.

The clinician, John, met with Jim and Lisa first. Jim described his relationship with Leo's father as distant and noted that he had little contact with Leo prior to placement. They have one older child, a daughter in her first year of college and living out of the home. Jim described Leo's father Lenny as "troubled":

> He was always a hard kid, always had a temper and seemed kind of off. I remember he got in some trouble when he was in high school, drinking, hanging out with bad kids. I saw him once when I came by to visit our grandmother, and he was high as a kite. We didn't see each other much after that.

Jim reported that he had few details about Leo's early life. He knew that Leo's parents met in high school, and Leo was born when his mother Janine was 19. Both parents were described as drug users, and multiple reports of neglect and physical abuse were made by neighbors and by the school. Leo and his younger brother Matty, now 5, were removed when Leo was 7, after he was seen in the emergency room with a broken arm. Although initially placed together, Leo's challenging behaviors (stealing, lying, aggression, and withdrawal) led to several disruptions. Ultimately, Matty entered a pre-adoptive home and Leo briefly entered a group home before moving in with Jim. Jim described himself as, "The kid's last hope. We weren't exactly looking to do this all over again, but they called and said it was either us or an institution. He's my blood, even if his father's a jerk." When asked what their long-term plan is, Jim and Lisa look at each other and then away. "Hard to say," Jim finally answers.

Behaviorally, Lisa and Jim describe Leo as "a challenge." Lisa reports, "He's a sweet kid when he wants to be, but just gets so stuck. The littlest things can set him off, like, 'Did you do your homework?' Sometimes he just loses it, yelling, throwing things. Then he shuts down, and you can't get him to talk to you." They report that Leo has extra supports in school, where he likes his counselor but has a hard time with friends and academics. "He always thinks that kids are picking on him when they're not, and then gets in fights or blows out of class." When asked what they want, they say that they want their days to be more peaceful; for Leo to be less reactive, and to feel more confident that they're doing the right thing.

John talks with them about the treatment process, including the important role of caregivers. Jim asks whether their participation will give Leo "enough time to work his own stuff out," and John responds, "That's a great question, and one we'll want to figure out. Given what you've described to me, though, it sounds like at least part of what's hard is the interactions among you two and Leo. Those challenges make sense, because Leo has had so many hard things happen to him in his family and because this is all new to you. So at least some of our work is going to be to help you all help each other and help him."

Initial Engagement and Formulation: Child

Early meetings with a child or adolescent client emphasize engagement, information gathering, and laying a foundation for reasonable therapeutic safety. This process includes establishing interest in the whole child, rather than just the presenting problem(s), engaging around child-specific goals, co-creating session routines, establishing a frame of transparency, incorporating psychoeducation, and linking trauma and targeted skills.

Leo is brought in for his first session by Jim, and the clinician initially meets with them together. Leo is silent and makes little eye contact but appears to be scanning the room. He is restless, digging his toes into the ground and playing with his fingers. The clinician asks Leo what he knows about coming in, and when Leo shrugs, John describes himself as, "Someone who works with kids who have been through really hard things in their lives, like I understand you have." John reports that he has already met with Jim and Lisa and learned a bit from them, but, "I obviously don't know you at all yet. I know your Uncle Jim and Aunt Lisa are worried about the ways things feel hard sometimes at home, and want ideas on how to help everyone get along better and help you feel better. I'm not sure yet what *you* want, but that's something I'm hoping to learn as I get to know you."

With Leo's permission, Jim leaves the room after several minutes. John shares with Leo information about himself (where he went to school, how long he's been working at the center), and begins to gather information about Leo. John begins psychoeducation by sharing "the trauma frame," which normalizes the child's emotional experience and behavioral strategies:

> Your aunt and uncle told me some of the things that happened in your family, but there's a lot they don't know. One of the things I do know is that when kids go through really hard experiences, like being hurt by parents or living in a lot of different homes, they can have big feelings that can be hard to deal with. They may get in fights, or just want to be left alone. I'm guessing some of that happens to you sometimes, and part of our work will be learning why these things make sense, and how to help with your feelings. But to do that, we'll need to get to know each other. So how about we take some time today to start learning about each other? You don't have to tell me anything you don't want to, and you can ask me whatever you'd like.

The remainder of the session is spent exploring normative aspects of identity (child interests); talking about typical components of therapy (i.e., talking, checking in, practicing activities, time for "child choice"); and allowing Leo to ask questions.

Support for Regulation, Distress Tolerance, and Relational Safety Caregivers

A primary goal of ARC is to enhance caregiver capacities. Key targets – supporting adult emotional safety, building rhythm in relationship by enhancing curiosity and effective response, and supporting trauma-informed behavioral response strategies may be targeted in primary caregivers, in collaterals, in systems, and by the clinical provider. In early stages of work, emphasis is placed on stabilization and support, with the assumption that a stressed system will struggle with supporting the child.

14 Attachment, Self-Regulation, and Competency (ARC)

At the start of treatment, John worked out a contact structure with Jim and Lisa. This included several initial meetings held separately from child meetings, involvement during portions of Leo's sessions, and – in the beginning – weekly brief phone check-ins (15 min). This work had a two-part goal: to support Jim and Lisa and to help them begin to build an attuned understanding of Leo's behaviors. In each of these meetings, John provided the caregivers with psychoeducation about trauma and attachment and particularly about the link between trauma triggers and hyperarousal.

Caregiver Affect Management John worked with both Jim and Lisa to identify which of Leo's behaviors they found hardest, to reflect on their own responses, and to develop coping strategies which might reduce their feelings of helplessness. The clinician emphasized in-the-pocket tools (taking a deep breath when upset, repeating a phrase in their head, "He's not doing this on purpose," taking a break if they felt frustrated) as well as ongoing self-care. A key stressor was their feeling of isolation: both reported a more active social life prior to taking Leo in, and felt like they had lost contact with friends and each other. John helped them develop a plan to reconnect, including identifying friends to reach out to, shifting their social plans (i.e., meeting for coffee versus going out at night), identifying and challenging fears about where they could reengage (i.e., how might they handle things if Leo misbehaved in church?), and brainstorming ways to achieve a bi-weekly "date night."

Routines and Structures John targeted routines to further support family regulation. First, he engaged Lisa, Jim, and Leo in doing a "walk-through" of a typical day, attending to what felt like did and didn't work. All three members of the system had similar identified "trouble spots," though different perspectives. For instance, Lisa identified bedtime as "a nightmare, he drags his heels and when I think he's in bed I hear him walking around." She viewed this as oppositional and reported feeling exhausted at the end of the day. Leo also felt frustrated, saying, "It's not that I don't want to, I can't. I'm just red *[referring to the color codes he and John used in modulation work; see below]* and I can't get to green!" John was able to support the family in identifying Leo's hyperarousal as a factor that interfered with falling asleep, and which Leo had learned to cope with by expending energy. Leo's difficulties with bedtime were representative of his challenges regulating throughout the day, and particularly the afternoons, which Lisa described as "a chaotic mess."

Together, the family co-created a new routine which included emphasis on matching activity to Leo's modulation needs as well as key family functions (i.e., dinner time). This included building in downregulation strategies after school (quiet time in his room, listening to music), a plan for reconnection that minimized social demand (i.e., completing homework in a location near Lisa, but without an expectation that he engage in conversation), free time to expend energy and transition to dinner, a set time after dinner for family connection, and then transition time to settle down for bed.

As part of this work, John asked the family to identify a list of activities they all enjoyed, thinking in particular about activities that could be accomplished in "15 min or less." The trio reported surprise at how many things they were able to identify, including listening to favorite songs, taking a walk around the block and playing games. To support development of positive relationship, the family was asked to commit to engaging in an activity at least two times per week after dinner, with a goal of building to once daily.

Child
Early stages of work with a child also focus on establishing a foundation of safety, particularly when the presentation is marked by instability. This may include co-creating and adjusting session routines, exploring the child's modulation needs; and building language for emotional and physiological experience. The work is anchored in exploration of identity, with an emphasis on engaging strengths.

Identification, Modulation During the first few months of treatment, Leo and John developed a session routine that included a check-in, modulation practice, "Leo's choice" (activity of Leo's choosing), "John's choice" (targeted goal activity), and "family time" or time in the session held jointly with Jim and/or Lisa.

John noticed that Leo felt most comfortable when he had something to do with his hands, so he introduced a basket of sensory objects (balls, clay). Leo was usually silent as they walked down the hall, but after fidgeting with objects for a few moments appeared able to engage in conversation. Each session began by checking in about the week. Because of Leo's observed guardedness, John kept early check-ins event focused, asking Leo about "anything good" and "anything hard" this week, as well as his actions ("What did you do when that happened?" "Was there anything you wish you could have done but didn't?"). As Leo grew more comfortable, John began to incorporate emotion labels ("How did it feel when…?") as well as daily emotion and energy checks ("How are you feeling today?").

Exploration of energy and arousal provides the foundation for modulation work. A key part of this psychoeducation is the linkage between feelings and energy states and particularly the link between the trauma response and surges or freezing of arousal. Importantly, the clinician emphasizes that neither "high" nor "low" energy is necessarily better or worse but that different kinds of energy can feel more or less *comfortable* in our bodies and can be more or less *effective* for the situation we are in.

John introduced the concept of degrees of energy by tuning into Leo's observable rhythms during a check-in:

> One of the things I talk with kids a lot about is the way they manage their body's energy. Let me ask, have you ever felt like people keep telling you to calm down? (Leo laughs and nods.) The thing is, we all have different levels of energy in our body – sometimes we're relaxed, and sometimes we're revving. I'm noticing that you're tapping your fingers and wiggling around a lot today, so I'm guessing you have a fair amount of energy in you. What do you think – if you take a look at this scale, which goes from really shut down, like feeling nothing at all, up to bursting-out-of-your-body energy, where do you think you'd be right now?

As Leo grew comfortable with the concept, John began asking Leo to regularly tune into and rate his energy, his comfort level, and whether he felt in a good space for meeting or not. Leo initially struggled with using numerical anchors (i.e., a 0–10 scale) but liked color anchors for effectiveness (green = can handle things/yellow = struggling/red = really can't handle this) as well as sensory anchors for comfort (audio: "quiet and clear" up to "way too much noise, like a stereo blasting"). Using Leo's anchors, they created an individualized check-in using a color scale, along with a physical dial built out of layered pieces of construction paper. After they checked in, they experimented with different activities (tossing a ball, jumping on a trampoline, doing a puzzle) to see whether and how the activity shifted Leo's energy and helped him feel more or less comfortable and in control of his body.

John also began to link reported experiences to energy and to verbally observe and link Leo's energy changes to coping strategies. For instance, when Leo came into the meeting one day very shut down, John said, "I can see you're looking quiet today. I can't tell if your energy is feeling shut down, or if it's high but just hiding." When Leo shrugged, John replied, "It's ok if you don't want to talk. I know that sometimes when your energy is kind of low, it helps for us to do something quiet. Would you like to do a puzzle together before we check in?" Leo agreed, and after working quietly for a few minutes, Leo was able to describe a negative interaction with a teacher in which he felt singled out unfairly. During this initial stage of treatment, John's response remained primarily on present-focused strategies which stayed attuned with and validated Leo's experience. "I'm sorry you had such a tough day. It sounds like your teacher said something that felt hurtful to you." Leo agreed, saying strongly, "It's not fair! Everyone is always picking on me."

During these early months, themes of injustice and shame arose frequently in Leo's conversation, and John utilized attunement skills to mirror Leo's perceived experience (that injustice exists, and feels hard); and to identify potential coping strategies ("It sounds like when things feel unfair, you start to feel lousy and alone. I'm wondering what we can figure out to help with that.") In part, this involved experimentation with a range of activities in session (deep breathing, muscle stretches, yoga poses). These strategies were largely practiced in less aroused moments, to help Leo build a felt sense of control over body sensations. To support in-the-moment coping, emphasis was placed on linking specific strategies to identified "hard times" and on engaging caregiver supports. For instance, they identified different places where Leo might feel upset (i.e., school vs. home), available tools and resources (i.e., his counselor, his music player), different things influencing use of tools (i.e., did he want anyone to know he was trying to manage feelings or not), and clues that might tell him it was time to try a tool. Identified adults (his teacher, his counselor, Jim, and Lisa) were engaged in supporting Leo, and specific plans were made for each setting.

Building Attunement and Self-Understanding: Child and Caregiver

As treatment progresses and both child and caregiving system are able to better recognize and respond to overwhelming distress, increasing attention is paid to building adults' ability to reflect upon and understand child behaviors, needs, and emotions and the child's own awareness of emotional and behavioral patterns.

Attunement, Effective Response, Identification, and Modulation Challenging behaviors are one of the primary reasons for referral for trauma-impacted youth, and addressing these behaviors is typically an important goal in treatment. In ARC, caregivers are supported in *identifying patterns* (understanding the triggers, function, and need addressed by the child's behavior), using *core behavior response strategies* (meeting child needs, supporting regulation), and *using selective behavior response strategies* (such as targeted praise and reinforcement, limit setting, and problem-solving) based on child patterns, caregiver capacities, and environmental context. Response plans are characterized as experiments.

John explored Lisa and Jim's own history of being parented and the way they had parented their daughter Livvy. Both parents reported growing up in "less than perfect" homes; Jim described his parents as emotionally distant, while Lisa reported the opposite: "My mom was pretty out there, you know? Everything was always drama, and always about her." Both described order as important to them, and acknowledged discomfort with strong emotion. They described their daughter as having been, "a really easy kid. If you said stop, she stopped, if you said go, she went. She never really gave us any trouble."

Leo was described as "the exact opposite – he'll argue if you tell him the sky is blue!" They acknowledged this as one of their primary challenges, with Jim saying, "Honestly, it felt so easy with Livvy. Sure, she was tough sometimes, but it wasn't the crazy we have now." Lisa and John reported particular frustration with Leo's oppositionality, which felt "personal," along with his rapid escalation when upset.

John normalized the challenge of parenting someone for whom none of your "tried-and-true" strategies feel effective and brought in psychoeducation about the ways that the danger response shift behaviors and behavioral compliance, so that "can't" becomes a better interpretation than "won't."

> We've talked about the ways Leo seems like he's always ready for a fight, right? And how that fight response is sometimes a really good sign that his danger brain has kicked in, and that when the danger brain is on, his thinking brain gets out of the way and action takes over. I'm wondering if we can start to figure out what gets him there and how to help get his thinking brain back online, and also how to keep you sane in the process.

John began by asking them to track times when Leo refused to comply with or became easily upset by a demand, noticing situation, their own reactions, and what they tried in the moment. Early tracking indicated frequent power struggles: for instance, on one occasion Lisa asked Leo to clean up his homework; after being ignored several times, she turned off the show he was watching and repeated the request. Leo got upset and threw a book. In response, Jim became angry and yelled, and Leo shut down and refused to talk for the rest of the evening.

John engaged Lisa and Jim in exploring these patterns, focusing on understanding what led to escalation (the triggers), whether these seem related to Leo's previous experiences (for instance, verbal abuse by his father), their own identified push buttons (intense emotion and loss of order), Leo's needs in the moment ("What do you think he is trying to do with his behaviors?"), and their own needs in the moment (to feel in control, to regain a sense of order).

During this time, both joint and individual meetings were held. Meetings with Leo continued to explore regulation strategies and patterns of response. Meetings with the caregivers followed a similar strand but also incorporated more vulnerable parenting content (i.e., the parents' triggers and responses to Leo's behaviors). In joint meetings, the family talked about core values ("What matters to all of us?") and core rules ("We try to talk to each other in ways that feel respectful") and began to troubleshoot ways to be successful in meeting these.

Subsequent behavior response plans, developed with Leo's input, placed a heavy emphasis on "regulation breaks," in which any family member could call a "time out." Language developed by Leo during previous modulation work was built in, and in session Leo and his guardians practiced respectful cues ("I'm so red! I need a break!" "Ok, everyone's dial just went way up – we need to take a break to dial it back") and ways to support each other in using their developed "regulation toolbox." Joint time in sessions shifted to an emphasis on "the week in review" or reflection upon the family's interactions during the week. More challenging interactions were used as "learning opportunities" to support increasingly effective regulation and response in the future.

As treatment progressed, family relationships stabilized, and Leo appeared to have a more extensive language for awareness of internal experience; John began to support Leo in linking his reactions not just to *current* events but also to historical experiences including trauma exposures. For instance, when Leo angrily described a teacher's "unfair" response in school, John stated:

> So I'm curious about something – you know how we've been talking about how we all have things that kick up bigger feelings in us, because they remind us of something that happened before? One of the clues we talked about was having your feelings or energy start to go into the red, or go really high or low on the dial. It sounds like that's where you were, so I wonder if this might be one of those push-buttons.

When Leo acknowledged that this might be possible, John said, "So that means this is a really good chance for us to start collecting clues – like how we know your buttons are being pushed, what kinds of things push them, and what makes you feel better or worse." A "Clue book" was created in which they began to log patterns of behavior, starting with more concrete data (How I know when I'm upset) and slowly weaving in more vulnerable data (What might this remind me of?).

Enhancing Child and Family Strengths

An important part of enhancing safety and building a foundation for developmental competency is exploration and support for positive experiences, connection, and reflective capacities that go beyond simply "surviving" a moment. This work becomes increasingly feasible as youth and their surrounding systems become more stable, able to acknowledge and manage both day-to-day and more intense moments of arousal, and begin to develop a shared common language for and understanding of experience.

Expression, Executive Functions, Self, and Identity As the work progressed, Lisa and Jim appeared better able to tolerate and put language to Leo's distress and support him in calming down. They were also able to remain aware of and manage their own responses to anger or disconnection. In turn, Leo's distressed moments began to happen less often, and he was better able to use Jim and Lisa for support.

This growing ability to handle challenges was supported through continued focus on enhancing the family system. During the "family time" portion of session, John worked with Jim, Lisa, and Leo to develop and practice routines for communicating. With John's support, "family figure-it-out meetings" were held in session incorporating structured, predictable elements each week. These included identifying a hard moment from the previous week; allowing each family member to share something they were thinking or feeling during the interaction; concrete listing on a white board of the sequence of events ("Leo said X, then Jim said Y, then Leo left the room and Lisa followed"); a chance for each family member to share what they were proud of and/or what they wish would have happened; and then a search for "clues" to help understand what got in the way, what might have helped everyone respond in a different manner, and what they might want to do the next time. Incorporated in this work was reference to a growing list which included each family member's "push button" and coping tools.

John also worked with the family to increase their focus on the positive. In session, they incorporated an "I'm proud of…" routine, in which family time each week began with each person naming one thing they were proud of in him- or herself and in another family member that week. This was initially hard for Jim, who acknowledged, "You know, growing up, we didn't do this kind of thing. Doing the right thing, it's what you're supposed to do, isn't it? Not get a trophy for it." With practice, however, he became more adept at it, identifying subtle strengths both in himself ("I was feeling really frustrated, but I held it together") and in Leo ("I could tell he was steamed, but instead of flipping his lid, he talked to Lisa and used that clay stuff to relax.") This attunement to the positive became increasingly part of the family repertoire; Leo reported to John one day, "Guess what? We started doing that 'I'm proud' thing at dinner! Pretty cool, huh?"

Managing the Inevitable Crisis Moments

When working with youth and families who have and who continue to experience multiple adversities, it is almost inevitable that periods of stabilization, growth, and positive functioning can derail during periods of increased stress or transition. Although these cycles are expected and make sense in the context of the clients' lives, when moments of crisis occur after times of relative safety, they can feel particularly overwhelming to families and to provider systems, as the sudden resurgence of turmoil can bring with it feelings of "failure." An important part of building the core ARC competencies is using crisis as an opportunity to observe, reflect upon, and practice emergent and solidifying skills. In these moments, the attuned, affect-managed response of the provider is crucial.

Leo had been living with Jim and Lisa for nearly a year and in treatment for 7 months when contact with his biological mother was reinitiated. Having recently

14 Attachment, Self-Regulation, and Competency (ARC)

completed a substance abuse treatment program, she petitioned for and was granted visitation with her sons. Janine was inconsistent in her follow-through, and Jim reported that she "does her usual chaotic thing," not calling when scheduled or calling at inappropriate times. Over the course of the next month, Leo's behavior deteriorated, with periods of constriction alternating with surges of reactivity. Although Jim and Lisa tried to be supportive, both felt demoralized and overwhelmed. Jim said to John, "How are we supposed to keep putting in the energy to do this right when the courts just mess everything up again?"

Lisa received a call from school one day that Leo had been in a fight; Lisa was asked to pick him up and told he would be suspended for several days. Because this was not Leo's first suspension, the principal told Lisa that he would need to be reviewed for alternative placement. Jim asked John for an emergency meeting, stating, "I'm just not sure we can keep doing this. Maybe we're not the right people to help him work out his issues."

When the family arrived for session, the affect in the room was palpable; Leo was constricted and sat with his arms folded and eyes down; Jim sat clenching and unclenching his fists, and Lisa appeared tired and drawn. John began their meeting by sticking to established routines and supporting in-the-moment awareness of energy and use of strategies: "I know everyone is upset, and that this isn't our usual day to meet. But we've found a rhythm that works pretty well for us, so I'd like to stick to at least some of it. I can see a lot of different reactions happening here – can I ask everyone to do a quick check of yourselves and see where your energy is at, so that we can figure out what we might need to do to have a helpful conversation?"

As each family member checked in, provider attunement was an important vehicle for mirroring and putting language to each family member's experience. For instance, with Leo, John named and reflected his current perceived experience ("It sounds like you got so upset you felt like you didn't have any other choice but to fight. I'm so sorry you had such a hard day."). With Jim and Lisa, John reflected and validated their frustrations and fears ("I know you've both been working hard, and things have been getting better. It's especially hard to have things feel like they're going south when you feel like you've made progress") while simultaneously integrating psychoeducation ("I know it doesn't feel like it, but I can tell you from my experience working with families, that a hard day, a hard week, even a hard month doesn't mean that everything is falling apart. You've built a lot of skill up this past year, and I'm guessing that with supports you all can handle even this kind of very hard day.")

Building on previous "family figure-it-out meetings," John pulled out a list of identified triggers and reactions:

> Leo, I don't really know much about what happened today, but something we've talked a lot about is that behavior makes sense. If you hit someone, then I'm guessing it means that something pushed your buttons and your energy went into the red. I'm thinking maybe if we sort through what happened, your Uncle Jim and Aunt Lisa can help you figure out what button might have been pushed, and what you might have been trying to accomplish by fighting.

John had multiple goals in integrating Jim and Lisa into the conversation: to support them in engaging reflective process, rather than just reactive/emotional (a reminder that "we know how to handle this"), and to reduce Leo's felt isolation in this moment, by reconnecting him to his established safe resource.

While engaging the family in exploring and identifying Leo's triggers, which unfolded to include a moment of shame ("You're so stupid!") and a feeling of being unwanted ("Jim and Lisa are probably going to let my mom have me back, they never wanted me anyway,"), John supported them in engaging in-the-moment modulation strategies: "Jim, I'm noticing that when you talk to Leo about his mom, he's kind of shutting down. Leo, I wonder if it might help for you and your uncle to toss a ball while you talk. What do you think?"

By the end of the meeting, the affect and arousal levels had shifted. Jim spontaneously hugged Leo, saying, "Listen, you know fighting's not ok, right? But it's been a lousy hard few weeks, and it's hard for me to blame you when I'm on edge myself. We'll figure it out, all right?" John highlighted the work the family did in session, stating, "I know that figuring out the puzzle pieces doesn't necessarily solve what happened today, but it's really important to understand that when Leo fights, it happens for a reason. I'm so impressed with all of you for doing the hard work to try to figure that out, and we can take some time together to think about how we can help Leo to keep working on making different choices."

Shifting and Transforming Traumatic Experience
Therapeutic work with children and families who have experienced complex trauma may continue to address safety and stabilization for lengthy periods of time, particularly when surrounding life continues to be chaotic or dangerous. With greater safety, however, there is increasing space to build toward shifting the experience of the child and family system from a focus on survival toward increasingly empowered present engagement. One vehicle for supporting this is development of a life narrative that allows the youth a broader understanding of self in context that includes vulnerabilities, strengths, resources, and challenges.

Leo and John had been working on supporting self and identity throughout the treatment process by incorporating various self-activities into the "John's choice" portion of session. These grew from an early focus on broader attributes (exploring and identifying favorites, opinions, and interests) to deeper exploration of Leo's experiences and ways they shaped him. Initially, Leo focused primarily on positive memories (his room when he lived with his parents; a memory of sitting on his mother's lap) and denied having any hard memories. However, as he started to feel safer with Jim and Lisa, Leo was able to acknowledge the links between "hard feelings" in the present and things he was reminded about.

Salient memories included a time his father hit him, the day his dog disappeared, and the day he left his parents' home. Memory work was organized through use of a concrete timeline, on which John and Leo mapped out details of Leo's life. Specific details such as where Leo had lived were written directly onto the timeline; other memories were labeled with numbers, recorded on separate sheets of paper, and put away into a separate "memory box" to support containment and to allow for gradual unfolding of Leo's story. Layered onto the challenging memories of Leo's time with his parents were other, more positive memories (for instance, a teacher he liked in first grade), and these memories were incorporated into Leo's "story of me" as well.

Leo slowly became able to share some of his memories with Jim and Lisa, who added what they knew to Leo's story. With support from John, as they continued to feel a great deal of anger themselves, Jim and Lisa were able to tolerate and reinforce Leo's mixed feelings of love and anger toward his parents.

Although there is certainly utility for shorter-term work in complex trauma, therapeutic work with youth who have experienced complicated relational trauma may best be thought of as a longer-term process, and Leo and his family's work with John progressed over a period of 18 months. During that time, the early crisis and overwhelm that each family member was experiencing stabilized, only to be derailed when the court process around parental rights and visitation reemerged. Several months after Leo's mother regained visitation, she abruptly disappeared and 2 months later, the child welfare system petitioned for and achieved termination of parental rights. After much discussion, Jim and Lisa began the process of finalizing Leo's adoption. Treatment reduced initially to bi-weekly sessions and eventually terminated. During the termination process, emphasis was placed on anticipating and troubleshooting future challenges, identifying and making explicit the skill set and routines the family had developed to manage those moments, and actively identifying the range of internal and external resources available for this next stage of the family's journey together.

14.1.3 Special Challenges

Treatment of the short and long-term effects of complex trauma is challenging for many reasons, not the least of which is the complicated presentation and surrounding environment that are by definition inherent to this population. The case of Leo, presented above, is in many ways on the less complicated end of the spectrum of what a provider might face: Leo has difficult but not extreme behaviors, is living in a reasonably safe albeit distressed caregiving system, is separated from biological parents but remains connected to his larger family system, and is "in placement," but despite several early transitions, he has remained relatively stable over the course of a year, with increasingly invested caregivers who have been able to commit to the treatment process. The family is resourced enough to access services (has transportation, low-middle SES but adequate to meet basic needs); is a member of a cultural majority (Caucasian, English-speaking); and is living in a reasonably safe neighborhood. The greatest complications in this case lie in Leo's significant history of abuse and neglect; in his ongoing involvement with the court system; and in the continued uncertainty of his placement.

However, Leo's case does serve to illustrate a number of common challenges in this work, and some of the ways that ARC treatment incorporates and addresses these challenges. These include the following:

14.1.3.1 Issues of Engagement

Engagement in the therapeutic process is hard for many families impacted by trauma, for a myriad of reasons that includes logistical and relational barriers and those barriers attributable to complicated mental health symptoms. Many families are experiencing not just historical but current stressors which may fluctuate and influence functioning and treatment continuity.

Although the process of engagement has not been specifically researched within ARC treatment, significant attention has been paid to the available literature on engagement in therapy, particularly for complicated populations. Drawing from that literature, ARC training emphasizes the importance of the provider addressing engagement from the first contact and continuously throughout treatment. Emphasis is placed on identifying and addressing perceived barriers, identifying both caregiver and child stake in all treatment goals, establishing transparency around goals and process, and building a relational context that allows honest and collaborative evaluation of the treatment experience. Provider attunement to the family system is identified as a core subskill within the attachment domain, and training emphasizes the role of the provider's embodiment of attachment processes (such as being affectively managed, building an accurate and empathic understanding of client behaviors, maintaining consistency in therapeutic routines/rhythms) in building a therapeutic relationship that provides a foundation for the change process.

14.1.3.2 Complexity of Youth Presentation

One of the challenges of establishing effective treatments for the most complicated clients exposed to trauma is the current practice of evaluating treatment effectiveness for particular diagnostic presentations (in the case of trauma, PTSD), and ruling more complicated individuals out of treatment studies (Spinazzola et al. 2005b). A primary vulnerability of this practice is that for many trauma-exposed children, PTSD is a portion but not the entirety of the clinical presentation (D'Andrea et al. 2012).

Although resolution of trauma-related affect and support for present engagement is a primary goal of ARC treatment, ARC was specifically developed to address the range of challenges often present in youth who have experienced developmental trauma. As such, aggression, self-injurious behaviors, parent-child conflict, substance use, and other presenting issues which might otherwise be cause for referral for adjunctive services or delay of trauma-focused intervention are seen within ARC as manifestation of underlying developmental challenges and alternative adaptations, and therefore important fodder for application of targeted skills. Development of effective caregiving practices, for instance, is embedded within psychoeducation on trauma, development of attunement, identification and understanding of youth triggers and responses, and support for caregivers' regulatory capacity, rather than approached as purely behavioral skill development.

14.1.3.3 Complexity of Caregiving Systems

One of the natural challenges in working with children and adolescents is the reality that providers are treating not just individuals, but individuals embedded within larger systems. Historic approaches to child treatment emphasized intervention as held within the provider-child dyad, with parents or other caregivers viewed as adjunctive at best. Greater attention to the role of the attachment system has shifted an understanding of the role of caregivers in treatment, particularly for trauma-focused intervention. However, caregivers are often viewed as primarily in a "support role": their job is to facilitate/support (or at least not detract) from the work that the child is doing in treatment. Complicated caregivers – those who are most at risk of derailing intervention efforts – are often not addressed.

In ARC, intervention with and support of the caregiving system is viewed as a primary therapeutic task, and emphasis is placed on applying skills matched with current level of functioning. With highly distressed caregivers, for instance, emphasis may be on provider parallel attunement, supporting caregivers in coping with their own intense affect, and identification of a range of supports and resources; more stable caregivers may be better able to engage in reflective intervention about their own and their child's experience. Training emphasizes the importance of tuning in to "relative success": for one caregiver, success may be as basic – and monumental – as being able to disconnect and walk away from a charged situation with their teen, or being able to remain connected to a provider even while experiencing crisis. Importantly, ARC does not emphasize the need for an individual provider to address all of a caregiver's challenges – for instance, in many instances, significant complications suggest the need for a team approach, engagement of alternative resources, etc. – but does emphasize that understanding and addressing caregiver functioning is a core goal of treatment.

An additional note in this area: in both writings about ARC as well as in training, significant care is taken to utilize the language of "caregivers" rather than "parents"; this is due to a recognition and acknowledgment that for many of the young people with whom we work, there are not stable caregivers available who are willing, able, or identifiable as treatment participants. In this case, the provider's own embodiment of attachment principles becomes particularly important, along with attention to the development of a surrounding support team.

14.1.3.4 The Crisis of the Moment

The "weekly crisis" has long been bemoaned as the derailer of effective intervention, and a driver of that is certainly the reality that the content of family crisis has strong potential to take over a given session as the point of focus, delaying the process of change ("I know we're working on how to manage relationships, but I'm so upset about my housing/e-mail I got from my brother/call I got from the school today/the bill for my auto repair that I can't talk about anything else!"). In ARC, a distinction is made between engaging in the *content* of the crisis ("Housing issue? Let me pull out a list of housing advocates/help you think of places you can go, etc.") and the application of *skill set* to the crisis. In the example provided above of Leo, Jim, and Lisa, Leo's crisis at school (one of many faced by this family over the course of treatment) provided a rich opportunity to apply skills that were already a focus of intervention. By the provider remaining aware of choice points (for instance, is this a good opportunity to address identification, support modulation, engage in reflective problem-solving, build attunement), the moments of crisis – which are certainly of interest to the client and therefore an important source of stake and engagement – become the primary vehicles in which to build client skills. Training therefore emphasizes the importance of not avoiding the routine challenges that are so often present in the lives of our clients, but rather utilizing these effectively, while maintaining the rhythms of intervention.

14.1.3.5 Ongoing Exposure to Violence and Chaos

A common tenet of many training approaches is that "trauma treatment" cannot be undertaken until a client is "safe"; any intervention prior to establishment of safety may be viewed as essentially adjunctive or supportive. The dilemma this raises is the reality that so many of the youth and families we work with are not safe and yet are desperately in need of support: these individuals remain embedded in unsafe neighborhoods and communities; experience ongoing chaos in their family systems; are living in a state of impermanency; have primary caregivers who struggle with substance use, mental health issues, or numerous other stressors that impact their functioning and yet remain "good enough" for the child to remain in the home; and have developmental vulnerabilities such as relational neediness or poor judgment that leave them vulnerable to ongoing risk for acute traumatization. Our understanding of trauma has shifted from one in which there is perceived to be a clear "before" and "after," and a clear event or sequence of events to be processed, to a recognition that for many youth and families, their entire life has been embedded – often across generations – in traumatic context. An expanded definition of "trauma treatment" is therefore crucial.

This expanded view holds that trauma encompasses a range of adversities that are often layered and ongoing and that trauma treatment includes but goes beyond the development and integration of the trauma narrative. Trauma treatment highlights attention to the range of factors that support the achievement of safety and resilience, rather than just recovery from "posttraumatic" pathology. As such, trauma treatment includes attention to core developmental capacities that allow for thoughtful decision-making; support for development of caregiver skill sets and capacities that increase the likelihood of adequate safety in surrounding systems; and acknowledgment of the crucial role of context in clients' application of learned skill sets. For instance, for many youth it makes sense to approach the world *as if* it is dangerous – because it largely still is. Rather than challenging that perspective, treatment may need to explore and validate it and examine ways to survive current context, achieve safety in moments, and build toward a shifted future.

14.1.4 Research

The ARC framework has an emerging evidence base that provides preliminary support for its use in a range of settings and with various subpopulations. Data from several outpatient evaluations is available; this data comes primarily from pre-/post evaluation of community-based samples with comparison to the client's own baseline scores or to treatment non-completers. In pre-/post evaluation of adoptive children ages 6–12 ($n = 481$) completing a 16-week ARC-based treatment including individual child/family sessions along with both child and caregiver skills groups, pre-/post analyses using HLM multilevel regression indicated significant decrease in child PTSD symptoms, reduction in broad behavioral symptoms according to both self-report and maternal report, and increase in maternal-reported adaptive skills. Both mothers and fathers demonstrated reduced parenting distress (Hodgdon et al. 2016).

Positive results have also been seen in child-welfare-involved children and families. In a sample of young (0–12) child-welfare-involved youth in Alaska, 54 % of children enrolled in treatment had both baseline and follow-up or discharge data available; of these, 52 % ($n = 21$) were considered treatment completers. Reasons for premature ending included relocation out of the region (26 %), treatment dropout (14 %), and lost to follow-up (8 %). Treatment completers exhibited a drop in overall behavior problems which was significantly greater than that of children who ended treatment prematurely. Importantly, 92 % of completers had achieved permanency in placement by treatment cessation (adoptive, pre-adoptive, or biological family reunification), a favorable rate as compared with a 40 % permanency rate after 1 year for the state as a whole (Arvidson et al. 2011). Similar results appear to be emerging in preliminary data from a statewide initiative targeting children in child-welfare-involved families ($n = 52$) in Illinois; in this sample, significant reduction has been seen across time points in clinician-rated child trauma symptoms (grief, reexperiencing, avoidance, numbing, dissociation, adjustment to trauma) as well as in a range of emotional and behavioral needs (i.e., anxiety, anger control, somatization) (Kisiel et al. 2013).

These findings are supported by data from examination of the pool of children served by sites within the US National Child Traumatic Stress Network (NCTSN). In the final report of the Cross-Site Evaluation of NCTSN activities and services between 2005 and 2009 (ICF Macro 2010, December), analysis of baseline and 3-month and 6-month client measures indicated that children receiving ARC-based treatment services demonstrated significant reductions in behavioral problems and posttraumatic stress symptoms; this evaluation report indicates that these reductions did not differ from those observed in children receiving TF-CBT (Cohen et al. 2006), a well-established gold standard treatment for childhood PTSD.

Preliminary evidence also exists for positive outcomes in residential settings. In two residential programs serving adolescent girls implementing systemic integration of ARC (including individual and group treatment, staff training, and milieu components), a subsample of adolescent girls (ages 12–19, $M = 16$ years; $N = 126$) served during the evaluation time period for whom data was available demonstrated significant reductions in behavior problems and PTSD symptoms. In addition, significant reductions were demonstrated in use of physical restraint by staff over the course of the intervention period (Hodgdon et al. 2013).

Preliminary support also exists for the integration of ARC concepts into a comprehensive systems approach in early intervention. In a Head Start program serving high-risk youth and families, ARC concepts were systematically utilized as a primary training approach for all staff, parents, and extended family; this training was integrated with provision of TF-CBT (Cohen et al. 2006) for students referred and found eligible for more intense services. For those youth receiving intensive services ($N = 81$; ages 3–5 years), teachers reported significant reduction in attention problems, externalizing, and oppositional defiant behaviors, while parents reported reductions in attentional and internalizing problems. Ratings of emotional climate and organization in all participating classrooms (including non-referred youth) suggested positive movement on all scales over the project period, though these were not able to be statistically analyzed. Although the mechanism for change cannot be definitively identified within this multipronged approach, data suggests that ARC may be an effective part of an overall organizational change process in early childhood programs (Holmes et al. 2015).

To date, the research base largely centers on effectiveness of ARC in real-world applications, including naturalistic and reference group comparison designs. Further research is needed to establish efficacy. The positive results seen to date, however, for youth across the developmental span and served within a range of systems and for caregivers including primary, educational, and mental health staff, support the utility of ARC as an intervention approach for youth and families who have experienced complex trauma.

References

Abram KM, Teplin LA, Charles DR, Longworth SL, McClellan GM, Dulcan MK (2004) Posttraumatic stress disorder and trauma in youth in juvenile detention. Arch Gen Psychiatry 61:403–410

Annerback EM, Sahlqvist L, Svedin CG, Wingren G, Jimtaffson PA (2012) Child physical abuse and concurrence of other types of child abuse in Sweden – Associations with health and risk behaviors. Child Abuse Negl 36:585–595

Arvidson J, Kinniburgh K, Howard K, Spinazzola J, Strothers H, Evans M, Andres B, Cohen C, Blaustein M (2011) Treatment of complex trauma in young children: developmental and cultural considerations in applications of the ARC intervention model. J Child Adol Trauma 4:34–51

Blaustein M, Kinniburgh K (2010) Treating traumatic stress in children and adolescents: how to foster resilience through attachment, self-regulation, and competency. Guilford Press, New York

Cohen J, Mannarino A, Deblinger E (2006) Treating trauma and traumatic grief in children and adolescents. Guilford Press, New York

Copeland WE, Keeler G, Angold A, Costello EJ (2007) Traumatic events and posttraumatic stress in childhood. Arch Gen Psychiatry 64(5):577–584

D'Andrea W, Ford J, Stolbach B, Spinazzola J, van der Kolk B (2012). Understanding interpersonal trauma in children: Why we need a developmentally appropriate trauma diagnosis. J Am Orthopsychi, 82(2):187–20.

Dube S, Felitti V, Dong M, Giles W, Anda R (2003) The impact of adverse childhood experiences on health problems: evidence from four birth cohorts dating back to 1900. Prev Med 37:268–277

Finkelhor D, Turner H, Ormrod R, Hamby S (2009) Violence, abuse, and crime exposure in a national sample of children and youth. Pediatrics 124(5):1411–1423

Hodgdon H, Kinniburgh K, Gabowitz D, Blaustein M, Spinazzola J (2013) Development and implementation of trauma-informed programming in residential schools using the ARC framework. J Fam Violence 28:679–692

Hodgdon HB, Blaustein M, Kinniburgh K, Peterson ML, Spinazzola J (2016) Application of the ARC model with adopted children: supporting resiliency and family well being. J Child Adol Trauma 9(3):43–53

Holmes C, Levy M, Smith A, Pinne S, Neese P (2015) A model for creating a supportive trauma-informed culture for children in preschool settings. J Child Fam Stud 24(6):1650–1659

ICF International (2010) Evaluation of the national child traumatic stress initiative: FY 2010 annual progress report, executive summary. Calverton, MD

Kinniburgh K, Blaustein M (2005) Attachment, self-regulation, and competency: a comprehensive framework for intervention with complexly traumatized youth. A treatment manual. Author, Boston

Kisiel CL, Fehrenbach T, Small L, Lyons J (2009) Assessment of complex trauma exposure, responses and service needs among children and adolescents in child welfare. J Child Adol Trauma 2:143–160

Kisiel C, Torgersen E, Villa C (2013) Understanding complex trauma in children and adolescents: advances in clinical, research, and diagnostic issues. The 27th Annual San Diego International Conference on Child and Family Maltreatment, San Diego

Spinazzola J, Ford JD, Zucker M, van der Kolk BA, Silva S, Smith SF, Blaustein M (2005a) Survey evaluates complex trauma exposure, outcome, and intervention among children and adolescents. Psychiatr Ann 35(5):433–439

Spinazzola J, Blaustein M, van der Kolk B (2005b) Posttraumatic stress disorder treatment outcome research: the study of unrepresentative samples? J Trauma Stress 18(5):425–436

Zelechoski AD, Sharma R, Beserra K, Miguel JL, DeMarco M, Spinazzola J (2013) Traumatized youth in residential treatment settings: prevalence, clinical presentation, treatment and policy implications. J Fam Violence 28(7):639–652

Child-Parent Psychotherapy: An Evidence-Based Treatment for Infants and Young Children

Vilma Reyes, Barclay Jane Stone, Miriam Hernandez Dimmler, and Alicia F. Lieberman

15.1 Theoretical Underpinnings

Child-parent psychotherapy (CPP) is an intervention for children from birth to five who have experienced or witnessed a traumatic event and are exhibiting attachment, behavioral, or emotional difficulties as a result. The primary goal is to strengthen the relationship between the child and his or her primary caregiver as a vehicle to restore their sense of trust and safety, regulate affect, and return to a healthy developmental trajectory. CPP normalizes the trauma-related response, supports the parent in recognizing and contextualizing their children's behavior, and joins the dyad in co-constructing a developmentally appropriate trauma narrative to help organize and integrate their experience (Lieberman and Van Horn 2005).

CPP objectives include (a) promoting the child's development by encouraging play, affection, and language; (b) providing reflective, culturally congruent developmental guidance; (c) highlighting parent's protective behavior when it occurs and modeling an appropriate protective response to threat when needed; (d) providing trauma-informed potential meaning behind behavior; and (e) offering case management, advocacy, and crisis intervention as needed (Lieberman and Van Horn 2005).

CPP clinicians encourage parents to reflect on the ways their own childhood experiences can serve as traumatic reminders with the risk of intergenerational transmission, referred to as "ghosts in the nursery" (Fraiberg et al. 1975). CPP clinicians also encourage parents to recall moments in which they felt safe and protected in their own childhood, hoping to increase their capacity to draw upon these experiences when parenting their own children. These moments are referred to as "angels in the nursery" (Lieberman et al. 2005b).

There are several resources which describe CPP more (e.g., Lieberman and Van Horn 2005, 2008; Lieberman et al. 2016). For the purposes of this chapter, a brief summary of CPP will be presented, along with research outcomes and a case example to illustrate the theoretical concepts.

15.2 How to Do Child-Parent Psychotherapy

CPP is usually conceptualized, as a year-long intervention (including the foundational phase and the termination phase), consisting of weekly hour-long parent-child sessions that may be supplemented by collateral meetings with the caregiver as needed. This duration may be modified to better suit individual circumstances, for example, a younger child who routinely cleans up all the toys and goes and stands at the door after 30 min, indicating that this is the appropriate session length for him or her (Lieberman and Van Horn 2005, p. 32). Child-parent psychotherapy is a flexible model that responds to the family's needs. Thus, the play therapy sessions may take place at the clinic, at the child's school, at a community agency where the family feels comfortable and connected, or in the family's home. Each of these settings provides its own advantages and disadvantages. For example, home visiting may make the intervention accessible to caregivers who do not have the resources to travel to the clinic, but it may mean a loss of privacy if neighbors see the clinician arrive or other family members come in and out of the home during therapy. If home visiting is an option, it is important for the CPP clinician to be thoughtful and collaborative about factors related to safety (his or hers and the family's), privacy, and culture and about how to balance the dual roles of being a guest in the family's home and a helping professional there to focus on a clinical goal (Lieberman and Van Horn 2005).

15.2.1 Foundational Phase

CPP clinicians meet with the caregiver alone on a weekly basis for an average of five times. Depending on the caregiver's ability to come in consistently, this foundational phase before introducing the child into the sessions can take from one up to three months. This period is critical for building a strong alliance and thoroughly assessing the caregiver and child's trauma history and the caregiver's understanding of how these experiences impacted the child's functioning and their relationship. The assessment includes several evidence-based instruments to assess trauma and other symptoms and behaviors. CPP clinicians help the caregiver understand the importance of holding their own trauma history in mind so that they can offer support if the caregiver experiences traumatic triggers from their own history.

The CPP clinician is prepared to intervene with crisis intervention or case management. For example, if the dyad is still unsafe, they may need referrals to a confidential domestic violence shelter, or help obtaining a restraining order. The clinician may need to advocate with the client to prevent an eviction, to consult with the child's school if he/she risks expulsion for challenging behaviors, or to help the client connect with agencies that can offer help with housing, legal issues, or enrolling other children in school or daycare. These interventions are crucial to help the family achieve increased safety and stability as well as building the therapeutic alliance (Lieberman and Van Horn 2005).

The foundational stage serves as the anchor for subsequent sessions by preparing the caregiver for the dyadic portion of treatment. During this stage, CPP clinicians support the caregiver in making the connection between the child's trauma history and his/her behavioral and emotional presentation by contextualizing and exploring the meaning behind the behavior that concerns the caregiver. The CPP clinician provides psychoeducation about traumatic reminders and works together with the caregiver to anticipate and prepare for potential traumatic reminders for the child and the parent. The therapist also prepares the caregiver by helping him/her understand that play is the predominant vehicle for communication with young children. Additionally, the caregiver is invited to join in play as much as they are comfortable to explore and respond to the child's internal world. Cultural values and experiences with play are explored as necessary and a set of toys are jointly selected. Toys that can be used to represent the child's traumatic experience as well as toys to help self-regulate and take normative breaks from trauma processing are encouraged.

Finally, the CPP clinician and caregiver meet for a feedback session where all the results from the screening instruments are summarized in the context of the family's history. This session is a unique opportunity to offer a strength-based integrative narrative about the caregiver's story, their resilience, and their hopes for treatment. In this session, the CPP clinician and caregiver explore how the caregiver wants his/her child to understand the traumatic event that occurred and how the caregiver would prefer to present treatment to the child. While it is important to respect the caregiver's perspective, CPP is contraindicated if a caregiver denies that a traumatic event occurred or blames the child. The risk of the child feeling invalidated or blamed for their experience by the caregiver takes priority over the potential for the caregiver to shift his/her perspective. In these situations, it would be more appropriate to extend the foundational phase with caregiver only hoping that once their perspective is acknowledged, they can create room for their child's experience. If the family is still not a good fit for CPP, the CPP clinician can refer them to individual treatment or other supportive services, as needed.

The CPP clinician encourages the caregiver to prepare his/her child for the first dyadic session but also repeats this introduction upon meeting the child. This introduction includes an acknowledgement of what the child experienced, how he/she may have felt, and his/her current struggles as a result. It is important to highlight the caregiver's commitment to keep him/her safe now (assuming this is the case) and the desire to bring him/her to treatment to support his/her healing process.

15.2.2 Treatment Phase

Ports of entry or clinical opportunities for interventions are selected by the CPP clinician as moments arise. Therapists conducting the interventions should hold in mind the intervention's potential impact on the child, the caregiver, and ultimately their relationship; the overarching goal of strengthening the dyadic relationship should be prioritized. Ports of entry can be the child or caregiver's behavior, the interactions between them, the mental representations and attributions of each other, the child's play, and the relationship to the CPP clinician. Systemic ports of entry include continuing to offer concrete assistance with problems of daily living by providing ongoing consultation and a bridge to community resources, such as legal aid services.

CPP does not determine a specific order of interventions, although CPP clinicians are encouraged to start with simple and direct interventions, such as offering developmental guidance, highlighting the importance of physical and emotional safety, and normalizing the traumatic response. CPP clinicians highlight moments of attunement in the caregiver-child relationship and foster the caregiver's attempts at restoring themselves as a protective shield. All interventions should hold in mind that it is the caregiver's rightful place to guide the child through their healing process. The overarching goal is to promote their ability and readiness to take on this role. All interventions also have the common goal of promoting hope, safety, and competence in both the caregiver and child.

Play and physical contact serve as vehicles to explore themes of danger and safety, celebrate joy and mutual enjoyment, and co-construct a trauma narrative. Play is the most natural language for children and it's the main medium used. The categories of toys provided should include toys that can be used to play traumatic themes (family of dolls that match the client's race, police car, ambulance, playhouse), toys that promote nurturing (doctors kit, kitchen toys), and art supplies. The caregiver should be given a "toy tour" in the feedback session, and a joint decision should be made about which toys to present to the child in the first dyadic session. Caregivers are encouraged to join the child in play as a way to build their understanding of the child's worldview as exhibited in the play and to enhance their capacity for spontaneous connection and pleasure in being together. CPP clinicians may build on what the child is playing to bring narrative coherence to their experience, address relevant themes in the caregiver-child relationship, or expand insight and make connections. For example, if a child has been playing out a theme of a baby in danger, the CPP clinician may stay in the play and comment on the baby needing help and encourage the caregiver to be engaged in the play rescue, or he/she may connect the play to the child's story. If a CPP clinician chooses to connect the play to their story, it is important to normalize the traumatic response, highlight what the caregiver was and is doing to keep them safe now, and encourage hope. For example, "you are showing us how you felt when you heard fighting and loud noises outside your house. You might have been scared and confused. Your mommy is here to protect you (Lieberman and Van Horn 2008)."

As the therapeutic relationship builds, clinicians can test more complex interventions such as addressing the generational transmission of trauma and challenging negative attributions about the child (Lieberman and Van Horn 2005). As trust deepens in the therapeutic relationship, new ports of entry may open up. CPP clinicians must be able to balance important concerns while remaining aware of the caregiver and the child's pace, as well as their ability to make use of the interventions. Well-timed and tactful interpretations can bring unconscious repetition of past dynamics into awareness and can cause powerful changes in understanding situations. For example, young children tend to blame themselves for traumatic events that have occurred in their life. CPP clinicians may give the caregiver this developmental guidance and create an opportunity for the caregiver to correct this common distortion in the child.

Many parents who present to treatment for their children have also experienced traumatic events themselves (Ghosh Ippen et al. 2011). The CPP clinician needs to attend to the child and the parent's traumatic reminders, attributions, and affect dysregulation. This creates one of the most significant challenges in CPP, but also sets the stage for the greatest potential for deep, long-lasting transformation in two or more generations. Many events traumatize both the caregiver and child at the same time, but each one may encode the multiple moments in the event in a different way or from a different perspective. Traumatic reminders may include certain sounds, smells, tone of voice, and/or facial expressions. Intense negative affect or relational closeness may become traumatic reminders in either caregiver or child, or both. CPP clinicians help caregivers identify, predict, and minimize traumatic reminders. For example, a caregiver may be encouraged to notice when she becomes triggered by her son's aggressive play (or neutral play that is perceived as aggressive due to caregiver's history) prompting her to withdraw. Furthermore, the CPP clinician may highlight that the caregiver's withdrawal, in turn, is a traumatic reminder for the child, prompting him to become more emotionally dysregulated and escalating his aggressive behavior.

Most importantly, CPP clinicians must communicate emotional availability, hope, and nonjudgment for any intervention to be effective. Trauma assaults people's self-worth and can cause or exacerbate feelings of guilt and shame. Parenting under the best circumstances tests the individual's resources and can lead to self-doubt and sensitivity to judgment. Conditions such as poverty, institutionalized racism, implicit bias, and discrimination lead to feelings of powerlessness, anger, and distrust. CPP clinicians need to consider what they represent to the caregiver as a person in a position of power. One should be very cautious not to collude with oppressive systems and instead should embody a tone that is respectful and empowers the caregiver as the rightful guide to their child's healing.

15.2.3 Termination Phase

Loss can be a significant traumatic reminder for caregivers and children. The termination phase in CPP is an integral part of the treatment, and it should be carefully planned out with the caregiver over the course of on average of 6 weeks. Ideally, the timing is mutually determined and occurs once the caregiver feels capable to continue guiding the child through their healing process independently. CPP clinicians highlight a sense of hope, summarize the strengths the dyad have shown in the process, and help the caregiver anticipate and prepare for traumatic reminders in the future. Once the caregiver and CPP clinician have decided on the timing, they prepare the child by explaining the reasoning for ending, highlighting the caregiver's strengths in continuing the process independently and normalizing their reactions to the goodbye. CPP clinicians may create a project such as a calendar for child to decorate and mark the weeks left to instill predictability to the goodbye or create a picture the family can take with them as a tangible reminder of their journey in therapy.

A Case Example
A local agency that provides phone support to distressed caregivers referred this dyad to the Child Trauma Research Program (CTRP), emphasizing how awful the trauma was, how symptomatic the dyad was, and how urgent it was that we take the referral. The identified trauma was that the child's father had tried to kill his 3.10-year-old son by injecting him with drugs, resulting in several weeks of hospitalization for the child. The family dog was found dead at the scene. At the time of the referral, the mother reported that the child was angry, aggressive, fearful about being separated from her, defiant, frequently asked for his father, and was "needy" at school with his peers.

Foundational Phase
The mother, "Autumn," was 24, of Southeast Asian descent, and born and raised in the San Francisco Bay Area; the father "Rick" was White and a number of years older than his wife. The mother worked to support the family, while the father had been the primary caregiver. She had recently left the father and moved to a neighboring city as a result of domestic violence and had not been able to explain to the child why they moved or why he was not regularly seeing his father. The attempted murder happened when the child was visiting his father for an afternoon.

The clinician was a White postdoctoral fellow with the Child Trauma Research Program (CTRP), serving families who met clinic criteria at a family services agency. Autumn was already receiving help with housing at the agency, and so it was decided that the postdoc, a third-year trainee with CTRP, would see the dyad at the agency.

When they met to begin the foundational phase, the young mother was terrified and overwhelmed. She had been told at the emergency room that her little boy was very hurt and that he might not wake up. During his several weeks of hospitalization, he had to relearn how to breathe, eat, and walk. With help, she had been able to give the child, then 4 years old, a wonderful explanation of the referring trauma:

"Your dad gave you bad medicine. You got hurt and mom had to call the ambulance. That is why you went to the hospital." The child would ask why daddy gave him the bad medicine, and Autumn would answer "daddy was not thinking properly." She threw up her hands. She didn't think this was adequate but didn't know what else to tell him. She had not told him the dog was dead, thinking this would be too much for the 4 year old, so every time he asked for the dog, she told him the pet was at his paternal grandmother's house.

Though the child—"Janu"—complained of aches and pain and showed some one-sided weakness, the neurologist's report was remarkably positive. The recommendation was for psychotherapy for the child's trauma symptoms and behavioral problems, continued occupational and physical therapy, and a follow-up visit with the neurologist in 1 year.

As the clinician and the mother filled out the child symptom checklists, it became clear that Janu's aggressive behavior was changing Autumn's attributions of the child, creating problems in the mother-child relationship. Autumn said that Janu really missed his father and asked "where's daddy?" about five times a day. She answered by appropriately explaining that it was not okay for dad to give him bad medicine and so dad was in jail, where he was getting help. Janu would respond angrily "when my daddy gets out he'll push you against the wall!" (which he had witnessed several times). He was quick to anger and to criticize her, blaming her for "taking him away from his father" and his beloved pet dog. Autumn felt very hurt and rejected by the child and fearful that his aggression meant that he would become violent like his father. She struggled with her own PTSD from the domestic violence and the horror of thinking her child could have died. She also felt overwhelmed by suddenly becoming the primary caregiver to a very traumatized child in a new city with little money or familial support.

As they talked about the changes in the child's behavior and how they made Autumn feel, the clinician used psychoeducation about trauma reactions in young children to increase the mother's understanding of and empathy for her son's aggressive reactions. The clinician shared that children discharge the bulk of their anger with the person with whom they spend the most time and feel the safest with. Autumn responded positively to psychoeducation and started shifting the meaning she made out of Janu's aggressive behavior. Autumn was also responsive to the clinician's highlighting what Autumn was already doing to increase Janu's sense of security, such as giving Janu one of her necklaces to take to school for moments when he missed her.

Understandably, Autumn's feelings were so overwhelming that she needed to push them away. She referred to the attempted murder as "the incident," brought in lists of the child's behaviors that worried her, and handed over copies of reports from hospitals, neurologists, and occupational therapists. The supervisor helped the clinician see the function of this defense in protecting her from the pain of being attuned to Janu's experience. At the end of one assessment session, at the door, Autumn asked for reassurance "Does this treatment *really* work? Does it really work for PTSD in young children?" The clinician began quoting data about the efficacy of child-parent psychotherapy. The supervisor recommended not reassuring Autumn, but instead allowing her to explore her fears.

In one of the assessment sessions, Autumn described the trauma—coming into the house and finding her son pale, not breathing, with needle sticks all over his body and a syringe lying on his chest and the dead dog nearby. As if pressured to evacuate the terrible memory, she quickly took out her phone and pulled up the photo she had taken of the scene. The clinician had no time to slow her down and discuss the meaning of this. Autumn was holding out the phone, waiting for the clinician to take it. She thought "if I refuse to see the photo it may send the message that I can't handle what happened to them… she might feel alone and rejected." The clinician examined the photo, noting that the child's color was abnormal and that he looked dead. Autumn commented that the child frequently asked to see "the bad medicine picture." The clinician did not know how to respond. After this session, she began to have heartburn and intrusive images of the photo (as discussed in Sect. 15.3). The safe and reflective space provided by her supervisor allowed the clinician to help Autumn gently explore and tolerate her difficult feelings, instead of the clinician taking those feelings on herself.

After five assessment sessions, Autumn and therapist met for the feedback session: to review the results of the measures and plan for treatment. Autumn reported that Janu was already rapidly improving. The child was no longer threatening mom with future violence from dad, he was separating easily to go to preschool, and he was again doing some of the sweet gestures she was accustomed to from her little boy. Additionally, the occupational therapist and the physical therapists both discharged him.

"What is helping?" the clinician asked. "I give him choices like which shirt to put on or who goes down the stairs first. But he knows I'm in charge," Autumn responded. She also shared that she felt reassured by psychoeducation about trauma reactions in children "I know he's traumatized but he's not ruined. These are normal behaviors given the situation." Autumn described how she had softened her responses to his outbursts or aggression, reassuring him and helping him feel safe. The clinician underlined this, explicitly crediting the mother's ability to see the fear beneath Janu's aggression and to respond to her son's fear in a way that made him feel secure. Janu was then able to calm down and express his feelings instead of being aggressive, which made Autumn feel more confident both in her parenting and in her child's future. She was returning to some of the soothing rituals they shared before they moved, like inventing bedtime stories that starred a little boy named Janu.

Together the mother and the clinician developed the introduction to treatment—a "triangle" linking the traumatic events, feelings, and behaviors. They wondered together what the child might want to play and how the mother thought she would respond.

Treatment Phase

At the first dyadic play therapy session, Janu was 4 years and 4 months. When mother and child entered the playroom, Janu immediately began inspecting the emergency vehicles. He seemed calm and alert, comfortable in the new setting. The clinician asked Autumn what she had told him about today's visit. "I told him, 'we are coming to talk and play with a lady who is a doctor but not the kind of doctor who gives shots.'" Janu looked at the clinician and asked "do you give shots?" The clinician answered no. She asked Autumn if she would like to present the reason for treatment now, and as many caregivers do, she asked the clinician to tell him.

The clinician told Janu, "Your mommy has been coming to talk to me, and she told me that some really scary things have happened to your family. You saw your daddy push your mommy up against the wall. Then you didn't live with daddy anymore and you missed him a lot." "Yeah," Janu said. He was looking at the rug, rolling the cars around. She continued, "Then your mommy told me your dad gave you bad medicine, and it hurt you." "Yeah," he said again. Then he rolled the police car away, making siren sounds. The clinician wondered if this was too much for him. When he turned back toward her, she continued, "Janu, all those things can make kids as little as you really scared and sad. Your mommy told me that now you cry a lot and you miss your daddy; that it's hard to listen to mommy, and that you choke mommy and your cousin. This is a safe place where we can play and talk about what happened. You can ask your mommy questions if you are confused. And we will also just play and have fun." He was inspecting the emergency vehicles as she talked and not seeming to pay much attention.

The clinician watched Janu carefully, interested in what he would do after hearing "the triangle." Another child had left a baby figure in the back of the ambulance, and Janu took the baby out, asking "is the baby hurt or dead?" The clinician asked Janu what he thought. "I don't know," he answered.

Then he found two small figures seated in a police car. He said "that one is police and that one is the bad guy." The clinician was watching and casually narrating his actions. The child took out the bad guy and threw him on the floor, saying "He's dead." The clinician asked him, "What does it mean when someone is dead?" "It means they're hurt," he said. "That's important for us to know," the clinician commented to Autumn.

Janu spent some time driving the police car around the room, exploring, and then invited the mother and the clinician to be police with him. He said "we are looking for bad guys" and requested a jail. He put the figure in jail and said "he's *never* getting out." He spent some time putting "bad guys" (only animals) in the jail. Then he announced that he was a firefighter, though he continued putting nonhuman toys in jail. The clinician hypothesized to herself that the distance—incarcerating bad snakes, not people—made this play tolerable for the child.

He said that his mother could be the ambulance driver. This brought his attention back to the baby in the back of the ambulance. "The baby is dead," he told us, and the clinician responded, "It is so sad the baby is dead. It is so scary and sad when a kid gets hurt." Janu responded that he was going to take the baby to the hospital, and asked his mom to drive the ambulance to the hospital. But first he had to load some more "people" onto the ambulance, pieces of furniture from the dollhouse. He announced that he was the doctor and put on the stethoscope. He listened to the baby's heart and then got out the syringe and asked if the "people" needed shots. Autumn said yes, and he carefully gave each one a shot. He directed the rest of the medical care to the baby, checking "her," and then asking mom if she needed a Band-Aid. Mom said yes. He covered the baby with a giant Band-Aid and he said that she was all better. In fact, all of the people were all better now and they were going home. Autumn looked happy and told him what a good doctor he was and helped him take the "people" back to the dollhouse.

When they arrived for the second session, Autumn said Janu had been eagerly waiting to come back all week. He immediately began playing the same sequence putting the figures in jail and saying emphatically "they will never get out!" (though they did). Mom said, "He wants to be police so he can let his dad out and put the other police in jail"; Janu got noisy and began moving around the room. The clinician wondered if this explicit link to his history had been too much for him.

Janu introduced a new game announcing, "Now we're going to play that we are firefighters. I'll be the fire truck, Mommy you are the ambulance, and Doctor B you are police." He rushed off to the dollhouse with the fire truck, making siren noises, saying, "The house is on fire. Somebody died." He told mom to take the baby to the hospital and be the doctor. Autumn quickly checked the baby, giving the baby "medicine" with a syringe and putting a Band-Aid on it. Janu said, "The baby is okay now, I'm going to take her home." He played this several times in exactly the same way, illustrating the driven, repetitive nature of traumatic play. As he took the baby doll home from the hospital for the third time, the clinician added, "I am so glad the baby is okay! It is so scary when a baby gets hurt." Janu paused and looked at her and added, "It is scary. Even an… an old baby." The clinician agreed, "It is scary even when an older baby gets hurt."

With his mother and the clinician to witness his experience, Janu continued to elaborate on his story. He initiated a game where he was a "bad guy" in a tiny race car and mom and the clinician were police and had to chase him but could never catch him. He giggled a lot as mom chased him around—the clinician was wondering if some of it was nervous energy, if even playing at being bad was too anxiety provoking—but the mother was laughing too and the clinician pointed out, "You are laughing so much! Mommy is laughing so much! I think you guys are having fun playing together!" (as generally the dyad did seem to have fun playing). At this, the mother scooped him up and hugged him—he smiled and leaned his head into her shoulder for a second—and then she released him to keep playing. They both seemed lifted by this attachment-promoting intervention, as they would during the entire treatment.

In the following session, he initiated the firefighter game as usual—"the baby is dead!"—racing his firetruck over, urging mom to drive the ambulance to the dollhouse too. He ran to the bin of bad guys and pointed out the same figure as last time, saying "this bad guy did it! He put fire in the house!" The clinician raced her police car over and captured the bad guy, saying, "You put fire in the house! The baby got hurt! That was bad!" (Then she thought to herself that "bad" was not the language she wanted to be using and decided to use the "safe" language used at the child's preschool). Child answered, "Yeah the baby already has fire on him!" The clinician said, "Oh no poor baby! That is not safe! It is so scary when babies get hurt!" "Yeah!" Janu added loudly. This is an example of the healing power of play, not only as a vehicle to express Janu's internal world but also as a restorative agent in itself.

Autumn was able to tolerate Janu's three repeated play themes, remaining engaged and initiating attachment-promoting games when she sensed he needed a break. For example, she asked "Do you want to be a flatbread?" He said yes and she said "I'm going to knead you... (kneading his body) and roll you out... (rolling him on the floor) and cook you... and eat you up!" She pretended to take bites of him while he giggled. The clinician asked if this was something they played at home and she said yes, they took turns being the flatbread. The clinician acknowledged the importance of this game that regulated the emotions he held in his body, restored safe loving touch, and strengthened their attachment.

As he felt safer, slowly Janu was able to get closer to his own story through the play, moving a step closer, and then regulating himself through cooperative play with blocks, Play-Doh, or pretend food. In the fifth session, Janu said "I was on fire in the house and I died." This was followed by food play to help him regulate. He continued expanding his traumatic play and trying on different roles. With his mother's help, he sorted animals into bad and good ones, he played with the scary bad snakes, and then he had them flee to the dollhouse, where Janu said "*I* put fire on them and then they died." By becoming the perpetrator in his play, Janu was perhaps experimenting with the feeling of being the powerful one, perhaps trying on a revenge fantasy, perhaps addressing his fear of being bad (the clinician watched his play for signs that he thought daddy gave him bad medicine because he was a bad child), and perhaps trying to connect with his absent father by imitating him.

Feeling safer at home and working through his trauma in play helped Janu become less symptomatic—less aggressive and defiant and less anxious and clingy. His mother then felt less overwhelmed and more confident in her skills. Seeing him improve so quickly helped her grow even more into her role as a loving but firm primary caregiver. When Autumn identified the ways that Janu was improving, the clinician asked "how do you understand that?" and Autumn responded "he became himself again once he felt safe."

When Janu cried for his father, Autumn felt "helpless and heartbroken," but reassured him "I'm here. I'll take care of you." Showing him photos of his father made him "happy," but was triggering for his mother. She had made bedtime their special time to talk about anything Janu wanted, and he seemed less sad at bedtime than before. The mother also said she was helped by understanding the bedtime neediness as a loss reminder—this created more sympathy for him, which let her be more patient. Before she was worried that he was "just doing it to get attention" and she didn't want to reinforce that kind of behavior. Now she just cuddled him. The clinician helped her think about reassuring bedtime routines and ways Janu could access a photo of his father in a way that didn't trigger Autumn.

To enhance safety, the clinician, with mom's collaboration, discussed the domestic violence when Janu brought it up. For example, he stated "yesterday daddy pushed mommy against the wall." The clinician responded, "your mommy told me about that and that can be scary for kids as little as you." He said, "it wasn't scary for me. I said 'no no no no no no.'" Recognizing her error in labeling the child's feeling for him, the clinician just repeated his statement. He added, "and then I said 'don't push my mommy!'" The clinician repeated this, saying, "it wasn't good for anybody that daddy pushed mommy. It wasn't good for daddy, or you, or mommy...," Janu talked over the clinician, and she knew this likely meant he was flooded and she followed his lead to transition to another topic. Autumn and the clinician knew that young children's tolerance for strong affect is brief and respected Janu's titration of his narrative.

By session #12 mother reported that Janu was doing much better getting along with peers, following rules, and not doing dangerous things. She also added that he wanted to call his dad. "*That* was a surprise." She said, "So this morning we called his dad on the pretend phone." Janu chimed in, "Dr. B, I want *you* to call my dad." The clinician felt how the mother likely felt—nervous and caught off guard. "Okay. What do you want me to say to him?" "*I* don't know," Janu answered nervously. The clinician picked up the pretend phone, made a ringing noise, and started talking to dad. "Rick? I'm Dr. B. I'm here with Janu and his mom. They are coming to see me because it was so so scary for everyone when you gave him bad medicine." Janu was fidgeting nervously with Play-Doh. "Should I keep talking?" the clinician stage-whispered to the child. He nodded yes. "Janu also really misses you a lot. He is sad at bedtime because you used to put him to bed. He misses playing with you. He is sad and he is scared and he doesn't know why you gave him the bad medicine. And mom is scared too and she is working so hard to keep her Janu safe. And they are both doing really well. Okay I will talk to you later." She hung up. Janu had his mom put his pretend phone away and the clinician joined them at Play-Doh.

The clinician wondered if she needed to be making more explicit links to his history. His mother said that he seemed to have no memory of "the incident" and frequently asked to see "the bad medicine picture" or asked mother to tell him everything that happened after she hugged him goodbye that day, leaving him to visit with his father. This made sense, since the drugs given to the child cause retrograde amnesia. The supervisor suggested that the clinician try to find out what those drugs might feel like in the body, as they couldn't find another way to understand the child's prominent fire play "I had fire on me and I died." The mother was baffled as well "he's never seen a house fire or anything...." The clinician and the supervisor imagined that his "memories" could be scattered sensory experiences, and the clinician wondered if she should be doing more to help him integrate these bodily memories into a verbal, conscious trauma narrative.

The clinician decided to try to put words to the sensations he expressed in his play. Janu began his firefighter game as usual. "Oh no the house is on fire! Somebody died!" and all three raced over with their emergency vehicles. As Autumn was taking the baby to the hospital, Janu stopped and stroked the fire truck and said "My fire engine has fire all over it and I died." The clinician said "When your dad gave you the bad medicine maybe it burned in your body." He said "No" and immediately wanted to switch to playing with Play-Doh. This explicit link to his history flooded him, signaling to the clinician to stay within the language of play.

In a collateral meeting, the clinician said to mom, "I have been wondering about this fire play for a while and I know you have too. I was wondering if heroin burns when it enters the body, and I even did some research about it." Autumn said, "it does. I know it does." She said she sometimes had pain from a childhood injury and one day her husband offered to inject her with a synthetic narcotic. "It felt like my whole vein was on fire," she said. "I could feel it burning up to my heart, and my heart was burning and contracting. I really regretted it because I was nauseous the whole day. I never tried it again." Hearing "heart burning," the clinician got the chills, remembering the heartburn she had when she began working with this family, reflecting again on how powerfully the child held his experience in his body. She also reflected silently on how satisfying and rewarding this case now was and how much she looked forward to the weekly sessions. Autumn mused, "you know, Janu tells me sometimes that his heart hurts. I thought he said it when he was sad, but now I wonder if he has that same sensation."

As she often did, mother began the next dyadic session by reporting their most recent trauma-related conversations. "Janu told me that when he grows up, he's going to be a good daddy and not push people." Janu added, "My daddy pushed my mommy against the wall." The clinician, delighted at this opportunity, continued "when your daddy was little, he didn't learn how to use his words when he was upset. He didn't learn not to push people. No one is born knowing not to hurt. Everybody has to learn that. And you are learning it too! Your mom told me that you used to choke her and your cousin. Now you don't do that anymore. Your mom is teaching you that, and she is going to teach you everything you need to know to be a good daddy." This was a relatively long speech to make to a 4-year-old, but he kept listening, transfixed.

Autumn had a remarkable capacity to put aside her terror of her husband to help Janu hold onto the positive memories of his father, both in and out of session. She helped him name and expand on favorite activities and memories with dad. The clinician supported Autumn's efforts, adding "children know to some extent that they are part mommy and part daddy. When little boys think or hear that their fathers are all bad, they think that they are condemned to be all bad too. He needs some positive parts of his father to identify with as he grows into a man. You do such a beautiful job of helping him with this."

As Janu continued to feel safer, he began sharing even more painful worries. Due to their cognitive egocentricity, children his age often think that bad things are their fault, and they frequently worry that they are bad. The clinician always wondered who really was the bad guy in the "bad guy game"—was it dad, was it Janu, or was it both? One day, mom stopped by to share that Janu asked "Do you know why daddy gave me the bad medicine?" Autumn said she could tell it was a rhetorical question. "Why?" she asked her son. "Because I was being a bad bad bad boy, that's why daddy gave me the bad medicine." Mom told him "that's not what happens when you are a bad boy. When you are a bad boy you get a time out or I take your iPad." The clinician, imagining how painful this could be for her, said, "Janu must feel incredibly safe with you to be able to bring up such a scary thought. You have really helped him feel safe again. I know it must be hard for you, but talking about it with him the way you do is a huge part of that." Autumn visibly relaxed.

Termination Phase
Organically, the mother and the clinician began talking about when they might end treatment. After 40 dyadic sessions, Janu's symptoms were almost gone, and the concerns that mom brought up were developmentally normal, such as "he wants to

win all the games we play and he makes up his own rules." The mother's increased capacity to be protective and stand firmly on the side of safety was certainly a factor. At this point she was telling Janu things like "I'll do whatever it takes to protect you, even when you don't like it." When the child talked about his father getting out of jail in 20 years—which he often spoke about as a longed-for event—mother would tell him "I won't let him hurt you again."

Autumn and the therapist met to plan for termination. With 4 weeks left, they introduced the topic to the child. Janu got out the emergency vehicles and, just as he used to, assigned the ambulance to his mother; the fire truck to himself, and the police car to the clinician "but we only need you if there's a bad guy." He selected a baby and, for the first time, a mother doll, and put the baby in the house, saying "The mom left! The baby is dead!" (The dolls' skin color was close to theirs.) Autumn repeated "the mom left?"; Janu had his mother take the baby to the hospital and "fix" it. Then he called the mother doll—who was somehow back at the dollhouse—and told her to come get the baby and take it home. He had the mom doll walk in and kiss the baby. The clinician said "The mommy didn't know that something would happen to the baby or she never would have left! She thought everything was safe."

Then Janu selected a white man doll and had him shoot the baby with a tiny toy gun. He commanded the clinician, who was still holding the police car, "Get him!" The clinician-police stage-whispered to Janu "Okay, now what should I do?" He guided her to take away the man's gun and put him in jail, and the clinician added passionately "It's not okay to hurt a baby no matter what!!" Then Janu had the man come out of jail and apologize to the mother doll and the baby doll. Then he briskly cleaned up all the toys.

At the very last session, Janu seemed anxious—shrieking, spinning, and avoiding eye contact. The clinician interpreted this to him and mother; "we are saying goodbye today, and you are spinning and being loud. Sometimes kids feel sad or mad and they feel yucky in their bodies and want to move around a lot." Janu did not want to talk about termination or take photos together, though he did eat his celebratory cupcake. The clinician thought to herself that the "real" last session had been when Janu had the white man doll apologized to the brown mother and child for hurting and frightening them. She was confident that Janu's mother would continue their work—the real goal of child-parent psychotherapy is to make the clinician obsolete.

She and Autumn met two more times to complete a posttreatment assessment and then compare the results to the pretreatment assessment. At intake, the child symptom checklists had been so elevated that they were flagged as invalid. Now, a year and a half later, there were no elevations whatsoever on the child symptom checklists or on the measure of parental stress. Autumn's depression and PTSD symptoms were half of what they were, and the clinician emphasized to mom, "look how you were able to help your little boy even though you were struggling with some of the same feelings!" Then Autumn spontaneously asked if she could retroactively consent to share their data for research. At intake she was too frightened to consider it and couldn't take in the clinician's careful explanations of how their confidentiality would be protected.

Another goal of child-parent psychotherapy is to create a positive feedback loop in which caregiver and child continue to improve after treatment is over. About 6 months after ending therapy, the clinician had an opportunity to see how Autumn and Janu had continued to heal. In keeping with the collaborative nature of CPP, the clinician asked Autumn's permission to write their story for this chapter. Autumn enthusiastically agreed and participated in changing details of the case to disguise their identity. They agreed to meet so that Autumn could review the draft and suggest changes. Coincidentally, Rick was to be sentenced for the attempted murder the week prior.

Autumn welcomed the clinician to her office with a warm hug, and they sat down to debrief about the sentencing. The clinician thought she looked happy and grounded. Autumn said with pride "My body was shaking beforehand, but I got up in front of the judge and read my statement about how Rick's actions impacted Janu. And I didn't cry! He even smirked at me at one point, but I looked him in the eyes. I thought to myself, 'we're safe from you now. All of these people here will keep us safe." Autumn went on to say that she had also, for the first time, revisited the house she, Rick, and Janu had shared and taken Janu to see his paternal grandparents. "It's over… I can do whatever I want with my life now. I feel like I can breathe again, and I didn't even know I was holding my breath."

15.3 Special Challenges

Vicarious Trauma
Vicarious traumatization refers to the psychological phenomenon that can occur when helpers who are exposed to hearing about traumatic events develop symptoms that mimic posttraumatic stress disorder. In contrast to burnout, vicarious trauma can happen suddenly, and it can include reexperiencing, avoidance, and changes in arousal, as well as harmful alterations in cognitions about self, others, and the world (Saakvitne and Pearlman 1996). Working with traumatized people can evoke strong reactions in the provider and perhaps even more so when working with traumatized young children who hold the trauma and related emotions in less conscious and less modulated ways. Reflective supervision—a safe and confidential space that preserves room for an examination of the clinician's experience and feelings—is a necessary part of CPP, not just for trainees, but for clinicians of all levels (Lieberman and Van Horn 2005).

In the case example above, the clinician, a postdoctoral fellow, experienced symptoms of vicarious trauma during the foundational phase, due to a combination of the clinical content, the mother's defensive style, and the clinician's wish—common in newer therapists—to help or save the family. During the foundational phase, the mother presented as overwhelmed and needing to distance herself from her own and her child's fear. After the mother showed the clinician a photograph of the trauma in which the child looked dead, the clinician had intrusive images of the photograph. Additionally, and unusually for her, she had heartburn and could barely eat. The heartburn and the intrusive images continued for several days, and the clinician reflected that she had only had heartburn one other time in her life, at a time when she was taking responsibility for things that she had no control over. She sat down, lit a candle, and reminded herself, "Responsibilities? My only responsibilities in this case are to show up to the sessions and be present with the family, write my process notes, and go to supervision. I am not responsible for 'saving' or 'fixing' anyone." The heartburn vanished immediately.

The clinician was able to share all of this with her primary supervisor, highlighting the importance of reflective supervision when doing trauma-focused CPP. The supervisor supported the clinician in changing the sessions to earlier in the week, right before the supervision hour, and provided a safe place for the clinician to share all of her own feelings about the case. She also supported the clinician in continuing her nightly ritual of lighting a candle and reminding herself what her "responsibilities" truly were in this work.

Not only did the symptoms of vicarious trauma not reoccur with this family, but the clinician left her training program feeling well-equipped to continue offering trauma-focused therapy. Vicarious trauma is a construct that considers the interaction between the person of the helper, the work, and the work environment (Saakvitne and Pearlman 1996). Reflecting the agency's commitment to managing vicarious trauma, they offered trainings about vicarious trauma in addition to plentiful reflective supervision, manageable caseloads, support for personal psychotherapy, and sufficient vacation time (Saakvitne and Pearlman 1996, p.43).

The trainee learned to notice and address symptoms of vicarious trauma and to consider how her own culture, history, and personality style interacted with clinical material. She began learning how to transform those symptoms into the rewards and growth inherent in offering trauma-focused therapy. Hernández et al. (2007) posit that there is a specific resiliency that develops when working with trauma survivors "vicarious resilience." Their study elucidated a number of elements that contribute to positive growth for therapists: "…witnessing and reflecting on human beings' immense capacity to heal; reassessing the significance of the therapists' own problems; incorporating spirituality as a valuable dimension in treatment; developing hope and commitment; articulating personal and professional positions regarding political violence; articulating frameworks for healing; developing tolerance to frustration; developing time, setting, and intervention boundaries that fit therapeutic interventions in context; using community interventions; and developing the use of self in therapy" (p. 2). Addressing and transforming the symptoms of vicarious trauma and cultivating vicarious resilience needs to be a lifelong personal and professional journey. Saakvitne and Pearlman's (1996) workbook "Transforming the Pain: A workbook on vicarious traumatization" is an invaluable resource for therapists and other helping professionals. Sustaining trauma-focused work requires deep self-awareness and a commitment to ongoing individual and systemic prevention of burnout and vicarious trauma.

Losing the Caregiver as a Result of the Trauma
Not just in traumatic bereavement cases, but in other cases as well, the trauma can result in the child losing one of their primary caregivers. Domestic violence

may lead to the parent's separation or divorce, or to the perpetrator's incarceration or deportation. The child and the caregiver may struggle with conflicting feelings about the perpetrator—love, longing, anger, fear, or relief. Inevitably there are moments when the two are "on different pages": the caregiver expressing righteous anger about the abuse while the child feels sadness and longing for that parent; the child using animals to angrily act out the violence at a moment when the caregiver is feeling calm and stable; or the caregiver reminiscing about the positive moments of the relationship while the child is experiencing fear or anger. The CPP clinician often intervenes by reflecting (and thus legitimizing) the differing feelings: "Sometimes you miss daddy and sometimes you are angry at daddy. Sometimes mommy misses daddy and sometimes mommy is angry at daddy. Right now you miss daddy and mommy is angry at daddy and that is hard for both of you." It helps to empathize with how hard it can be to be on different pages and encourage the dyad to find ways to together grieve, remember positives, and talk about how the violence was not okay, at moments when both can tolerate it.

Due to their cognitive egocentricity, children 0–5 often blame themselves for events. The child may think the violence and/or the caregiver's disappearance was his or her fault. The CPP clinician and the parent need to carefully assess for this kind of misunderstanding. Directly asking "are you worried that it is your fault that daddy left?" could suggest this possibility to a child who had not been considering it! The child's play usually provides clues about this pathogenic belief. In one case, a little boy who had been sent to stay with his grandparents in Central America when he was a toddler played repeatedly that a little boy doll was arrested, put in a police car, driven to the airport, and put on the plane by police. The treatment must help the child change this attribution about the self and come to an accurate, developmentally appropriate view of events.

In cases where the perpetrating parent still has legal custody of the child, that parent should be informed about treatment. He or she has the right to forbid or terminate treatment if he or she is not in agreement, which is much more likely if he/she has not been told about it. If dyadic treatment sessions have already begun and the parent suddenly finds out the child is being taken to therapy without his or her assent and pulls the child from treatment, the sudden end to the therapy is another loss and probably a traumatic reminder. Getting the other parent's permission for treatment must be done during the foundational phase.

Understandably, many survivors of domestic violence may be hesitant or fearful about talking to their former partner, or a restraining order may prohibit contact. If the client is not able or willing to broach the topic of treatment, the clinician can volunteer to contact him or her. It is helpful to reassure the client that the other parent has a legal right only to information about the child and that confidentiality prevents the clinician from sharing information about the client with his or her ex. The clinician asks the offending parent if he or she has any concerns about the child, what he or she observes when the child is with him or her, and what goals he or she might have for the child's treatment. When appropriate, the clinician asks for his or her perspective on the violence and/or separation and they think together about ways to talk to the child that feel acceptable "your mommy and your mama had grown-up problems and they fought too much and that wasn't good for anybody. They decided to live in different houses but they both love you so much and will always be your mommy and your mama."

15.4 Research

CPP's efficacy has been empirically documented in five randomized controlled trials. The samples include high-risk toddlers and preschoolers exposed to interpersonal violence and/or abuse and depressed mothers with chronic trauma histories.

The randomized trial at San Francisco General Hospital consisted of a sample of 75 multiethnic preschooler-mother dyads from a range of socioeconomic backgrounds (Lieberman et al. 2005a). All of the preschoolers had been exposed to domestic violence. Additionally, 49 % had experienced abuse themselves, 46.7 % had been exposed to community violence, and 14.4 % had suffered sexual abuse. Dyads were randomly assigned to either weekly CPP treatment for 1 year or case management plus a referral for individual therapy in local community agencies. The mothers and toddlers were assessed for emotional and behavioral challenges and posttraumatic stress symptoms. Analysis of variance supported CPP's efficacy with a reduction on children's total behavioral problems, traumatic stress symptoms, and diagnostic status and improvements on cognitive functioning. Findings also support more positive caregiver attributions toward their children, reduction in mother's avoidance symptoms, overall PTSD symptoms, and parental distress. Six months after treatment had ended, the dyads were reassessed, and symptom reduction for children's total behavior problems and mothers' general distress was sustained (Lieberman et al. 2006). A reanalysis of these data showed that the children with four or more traumatic or stressful life events showed significantly greater improvements in PTSD and depression symptoms, PTSD diagnosis, number of co-occurring diagnoses, and behavior problems. The mothers of these same children also showed greater reductions in symptoms of PTSD and depression (Ghosh Ippen et al. 2011).

Toth et al. (2002) studied the efficacy of CPP in altering preschoolers' representations of their mothers and themselves. These mental representations or internal working models set a template for children's future relationship expectations. Mental representations were assessed with Bretherton et al. (1990) MacArthur Story Stem Battery (MSSB). The study included 112 maltreated preschoolers of whom 76.2% were reportedly ethnic minorities. Abuse types included physical abuse, sexual abuse, emotional maltreatment, and neglect, with 60% of children experiencing more than one form of maltreatment. Groups were randomly assigned to either CPP, psychoeducation home visitation (PHV), or community standard (CS). There was also a normative comparison group (NC). Multiple findings suggest that the CPP intervention was effective in improving preschoolers' representations of self and their mothers: the CPP group exhibited significantly greater reductions in negative self-representation compared to children in the other three groups, significantly greater reductions in maladaptive maternal attributions compared to the children in the NC group, and significantly greater improvements in relationship expectations compared with children in the NC group with a trend for greater improvement than the PHV group.

Cicchetti et al. (2006) compared a relationship-based versus a parental psychoeducation intervention in changing infants' attachment classification. Participants included 137 12-month-old infants and their mothers recruited by reviewing child welfare records. Of the mothers, 74.1% were reported to be ethnic minorities. 64.4% of the infants had directly experienced neglect or abuse, while 33.6% were living in families where their siblings had experienced abuse or neglect. At intake 0% of the infants randomly assigned to the CPP group were classified as securely attached; at post, 60.7% of those infants were now classified as securely attached, significantly greater than the community standard group.

In addition, four published studies provide support for the efficacy of relationship-based models with at risk samples, including anxiously attached dyads (Lieberman et al. 1991) and toddlers of depressed mothers (Cicchetti et al. 1999, 2000; Toth et al. 2006).

Cicchetti and colleagues examined the effects of CPP on toddlers' attachment security (1999), toddlers' cognitive development (2000), and reorganizing attachment (2006). Similar procedures were used in all studies, and Cicchetti et al. (1999) and Cicchetti et al. (2000) are subsamples of the Toth et al. (2006) study. The mothers were mostly Caucasian (92.9%), and all had met DSM-III-R criteria for major depressive disorder during the child's lifetime. CPP was proven to significantly improve attachment security, significantly improve the child's cognitive scores, and reorganize the toddlers' attachment—at intake, few children of depressed mothers were found to be securely attached (CPP group = 16.7%), while at post, 67.4% of the toddlers who had participated in CPP were now securely attached.

The Lieberman et al. (1991) study involved a sample of low-income Spanish-speaking immigrant women and their babies aged 11–14 months. Trauma histories were not specified, but mothers averaged 11.34 stressful events on Cochrane and Robertson's (1973) Life Events Inventory (LSE). Anxiously attached dyads were randomly assigned to the CPP intervention ($n = 34$) or the comparison group ($n = 25$). Securely attached dyads ($n = 34$) formed a second control group. The outcomes were measured by coding free play interactions before and after treatment. At post, CPP toddlers scored lower than comparison group toddlers in avoidance, resistance, and anger and scored higher in partnership with mother; mothers had higher scores in empathy and interactiveness with children; and the CPP group did not differ from the securely attached comparison group on any outcome measures.

References

Bretherton I, Oppenheim D Buchsbaum HK, Emde RN, The MacArthur Narrative Group (1990) MacArthur story stem battery, unpublished manuscript

Cicchetti D, Toth SL, Rogosch FA (1999) The efficacy of toddler-parent psychotherapy to increase attachment security in offspring of depressed mothers. Attach Hum Dev 1:34–66

Cicchetti D, Rogosch FA, Toth SL (2000) The efficacy of toddler-parent Psychotherapy for fostering cognitive development in offspring. J Abnorm Child Psychol 28:135–148

Cicchetti D, Rogosch FA, Toth SL (2006) Fostering secure attachment in infant in maltreating families through preventive interventions. Dev Psychopathol 18:623–650

Cochrane R, Robertson A (1973) The life events inventory: a measure of the relative severity of psycho-social stressors. J Psychosom Res 17(2):135–139

Fraiberg S, Adelson E, Shapiro V (1975) Ghosts in the nursery: a psychoanalytic approach to the problems of impaired infant-mother relationships. J Am Acad Child Adolesc Psychiatry 14(3):385–559

Ghosh Ippen C, Harris WW, Van Horn P, Lieberman AF (2011) Traumatic and stressful events in early childhood: can treatment help those at highest risk? Child Abuse Negl 35:504–513

Hernández P, Gangsei D, Engstrom D (2007) Vicarious resilience: a new concept in work with those who survive trauma. Fam Process 46:229–241

Lieberman AF, Weston DR, Pawl JH (1991) Preventive intervention and outcome with anxiously attached dyads. Child Development 62(1):199–209

Lieberman AF, Van Horn P (2005) "Don't Hit my mommy!": a manual for child-parent psychotherapy with young witnesses of family violence. Zero to Three Press, Washington, DC

Lieberman AF, Van Horn P (2008) Psychotherapy with infants and young children: repairing the effects of stress and trauma on early attachment. Guilford Press, New York

Lieberman AF, Van Horn P, Ghosh Ippen C (2005a) Towards evidence-based treatment: child-parent psychotherapy with preschoolers exposed to marital violence. J Am Acad Child Adolesc Psychiatry 44:1241–1248

Lieberman AF, Padron E, Van Horn P, Harris W (2005b) Angels in the nursery: the intergenerational transmission of benevolent parental influences. Infant Mental Health J 26(6):504–520

Lieberman AF, Ghosh Ippen C, Van Horn P (2006) Child- parent psychotherapy: 6 month follow up of a randomized controlled trial. J Am Acad Child Adolesc Psychiatry 45(8):913–918

Lieberman AF, Ghosh Ippen C, Van Horn P (2016) Dont hit my mommy: a manual for child-parent psychotherapy with young children exposed to violence and other trauma, 2nd edn. Zero to Three Press, Washington, DC

Saakvitne KW, Pearlman LA (1996) Transforming the pain: a workbook on vicarious traumatization. W.W. Norton & Company, New York

Toth SL, Maughan A, Manly JT, Spagnola M, Cicchetti D (2002) The relative efficacy of two interventions in altering maltreated preschool children's representational models: implications for attachment theory. Dev Psychopathol 14:877–908

Toth SL, Rogosch FA, Cicchetti D (2006) The efficacy of toddler-parent psychotherapy to reorganize attachment in the young offspring of mothers with major depressive disorder: a randomized preventive trial. J Consult Clin Psychol

Parent-Child Interaction Therapy

Robin H. Gurwitch, Erica Pearl Messer, and Beverly W. Funderburk

16.1 Introduction

Parent-child interaction therapy (PCIT), a program for young children and their families, is a strong evidence-based treatment that repeatedly receives the highest rankings possible in reviews of such treatments (e.g., California Evidence-Based Clearinghouse for Child Welfare, 2015; nrepp.samhsa.gov). PCIT was originally developed for use with young children (2–7 years of age) with disruptive behavior problems (McNeil and Hembree-Kigin 2010; Zisser and Eyberg 2010). As PCIT continued to show significant positive outcomes including improved child behaviors, reduced parenting stress, and improved parent-child relationships (Brinkmeyer and Eyberg 2003; Eyberg and Robinson 1982), the application of PCIT to children at risk or exposed to trauma seemed a logical step.

When PCIT was initially developed circa 1974 (Funderburk and Eyberg 2011), the diagnosis of PTSD did not exist, and recognition of child abuse was only just dawning. However, parents and caregivers of many children presenting with behavior problems reported a history of child trauma. Over the years, PCIT has been specifically applied to this population. Results are positive for children with such histories and for children in the foster care system (McNeil et al. 2005; Pearl et al. 2012; Timmer et al. 2006). PCIT is endorsed by the National Child Traumatic Stress Network as an appropriate treatment for young children (see www.nctsn.org) and the Kaufman Best Practices Project final report (2004) lists PCIT as one of the three best practices for working with children with a history of maltreatment.

R.H. Gurwitch, PhD (✉)
Duke University Medical Center, Durham, NC, USA
e-mail: robin.gurwitch@duke.edu

E.P. Messer, PsyD
Cincinnati Children's Hospital Medical Center, Cincinnati, OH, USA

B.W. Funderburk, PhD
University of Oklahoma Health Sciences Center, Oklahoma City, OK, USA

16.2 Theoretical Underpinnings

Sheila Eyberg, the developer of PCIT, was influenced by Baumrind's parenting models (Baumrind 1966, 1967), Hanf's two-phase model (1969), play therapy (Axline 1947; Funderburk and Eyberg 2011), Patterson's behavioral parent training being conducted at the University of Oregon (Patterson 1976), and attachment theory (Ainsworth 1979). Baumrind (1967) identified unique parenting styles: permissive (high warmth, low control), authoritarian (low warmth, high control), and authoritative (high warmth, high control). Authoritative parenting, associated with positive outcomes of long-term social-emotional well-being, combines children's need for nurturance with their need for limits, creating positive parenting and positive parent-child interactions.

PCIT, like other evidence-based behavioral parenting models developed in that time (e.g., defiant children (Barkley 1987), helping the non-compliant child (Forehand and McMahon 1981), incredible years (Webster-Stratton 2011, Webster-Stratton and Reid 2003)), is based on a two-stage operant model (Hanf 1969). Operant conditioning posits that learning is guided by the consequences of behaviors. Ideally, attention is given for appropriate positive behaviors (reinforcement), while inappropriate behaviors are ignored or receive negative consequences (punishment).

Traditional play therapy, emphasizing the development of a warm and safe therapeutic relationship in which change can occur (Funderburk and Eyberg 2011), also influenced PCIT. The child's play is followed with undivided attention, which includes describing the child's play, imitating the play, and reflecting and expanding on the child's verbalizations. Eyberg noted that "play is the primary medium through which children develop problem-solving skills and work through developmental problems (Eyberg 1988, p. 38)." While children and therapists appeared to enjoy their interactions, little improvement in the child's behavior was actually noted. Furthermore, the bond that developed was between the child and the therapist, not the child and his/her parent.

A third influence on PCIT came from Patterson's coercive cycle of parenting (Forgatch et al. 2004; Patterson 1982). Here, a child's behavior problems are inadvertently developed and maintained by their interactions with the parent. Power struggles arise as parents try to control or stop behavior through negative, coercive tactics. The cycle increases the child's disruptive behaviors and maintains the parent's inconsistent discipline. For example, if a child cries for candy at the check-out counter in the store, the parent seeks to stop this. Yelling may ensue from both the parent and the child, and the parent may threaten punishment. Facing escalation by the child, the parent may "give in" and offer the child the candy, thus stopping the child's negative behavior and reinforcing "giving in." However, the child has been reinforced to yell when he wants candy at the store. The cycle can also be set if the parent is aggressive (spanking, hitting, threatening). The child may temporarily stop a behavior, so the parent is reinforced to continue this harsh response to a child's unwanted behavior. Through parental modeling, aggressive behaviors on the child's part are reinforced. Furthermore, the unwanted behaviors tend to return or increase in multiple settings.

Patterson's coercive cycle was influenced by Bandura's social learning theory (1977). The parent-child relationship is bi-directional (each influences and is influenced by the other). Negative behaviors are shaped and maintained through dysfunctional patterns of interactions. The coercive cycle can ultimately result in a hostile parent-child relationship that, in addition to harsh, inconsistent discipline, is characterized by a lack of recognition or unresponsiveness to appropriate behaviors exhibited by children. Unresponsiveness to appropriate child behavior or needs, deteriorated relationship quality, and withdrawn or weak parent-child attachments form a relational context for physical abuse and neglect (Stith et al. 2009).

Attachment theory (Ainsworth 1979) describes different relationships between infants/young children and their parents: secure, anxious-avoidant, anxious-resistant, and disorganized. The latter three types are insecure attachments and have been associated with child aggression, poor coping skills, lower self-esteem, and more maladaptive relationships with others (Greenberg et al. 2001; Hildyard and Wolfe 2002). Increased parental stress and increased risk for child maltreatment also exist with an insecure attachment (Venet et al. 2007). With secure attachment, parents serve as a consistent base from which a child can explore. The parent is warm and responsive to a child's physical and emotional needs. Emotional and behavioral regulation in the child results from this type of attachment.

Integrating all of these influencing theories and ideas, Eyberg developed PCIT. PCIT, a strength-based, supportive therapy, includes the Hanf-influenced two phases of treatment: Child-Directed Interaction (CDI) and Parent-Directed Interaction (PDI). PCIT focuses not on specific behavior problems, but in changing the pattern of the parent-child interactions in which these problems occur. These two phases parallel an overall authoritative parenting style. The first phase, CDI, is heavily influenced by attachment theory and play therapy concepts. However, rather than the traditional play therapy approach of a therapist working directly with the child, the parent becomes the "expert therapist" of their child's play, coached in vivo by the therapist. Live coaching and feedback are unique features of PCIT, highlighting findings that practice with feedback improves outcomes of treatment (Kaminski et al. 2008). Using play therapy techniques, the parent shapes appropriate child behaviors through praise of positive child behaviors while ignoring negative behaviors. This new pattern of interaction conveys warmth and acceptance of the child, creating a more secure attachment.

With heavy influence from Patterson's coercive cycle, the PDI phase of treatment involves a predictable, positive discipline program, which the parent can effectively implement across all settings. PDI disrupts the coercive cycle and establishes consistent and appropriate contingencies for child behavior. PCIT teaches the parent ways to avoid escalating coercive interactions with the child while reinforcing compliance in the child's behavior. Consistent with attachment theory, the parent becomes a more predictable partner for the child, offering clear limits and supporting the child's developing emotional and behavioral regulation.

As a whole, Eyberg combined concepts from the best parenting style, attachment and social learning theories, and behavior modification ideas to create a unique and effective therapy, PCIT, to work with young children and their parents to achieve significant improvements in both positive child behaviors and the parent-child relationship. This robust evidence-based intervention continues to grow and make lasting, positive differences in the families receiving the services, including children at risk or with a history of trauma and/or maltreatment.

16.3 How to Do PCIT

16.3.1 Therapy Structure and Format

As with any evidence-based therapy, PCIT begins with an assessment of the presenting problem via clinical interview and appropriate standardized measures. In addition, PCIT includes an observational assessment. The parent and child are observed in three different 5-min situations. In the first, the child is in control of the play, and the parent is simply instructed to follow the child's lead (low-demand situation). Next, the parent is told to set the rules of the play, getting the child to follow the parent's lead (moderate-demand situation). Finally, the parent is instructed to have the child clean up all toys and return these to their appropriate places, without help from the parent (high-demand situation). All interactions are coded using an empirically validated coding system, the Dyadic Parent-Child Interaction Coding System-IV (DPICS-IV) (Eyberg et al. 2013) These observations add important information to that collected during the interview and serves as the baseline for parent skills, child compliance, and the quality of the parent-child interaction.

As noted, PCIT consists of two phases (i.e., the Child-Directed Interaction (CDI) and Parent-Directed Interaction (PDI)). Each phase begins with a "teaching" session where the parents[1] meet with the therapist (typically without the child) and phase-specific skills are introduced, modeled, and role-played with the parent(s). These teaching sessions are followed by "coaching" sessions where the therapist communicates with the parent from an observation room via a wireless earphone while the parent interacts with the child one-on-one. Although live parent-child skill practice approaches are more labor intensive than group didactic delivery modes, it has been demonstrated that program delivery via direct skill practice with the parent's own child is one of the most powerful predictors of larger effect sizes across both parent and child outcomes (Kaminski et al. 2008). This may be particularly important for child welfare clients where significant behavior changes are important goals. The peak ages for child maltreatment are in the preschool and early school-age years (Children's Bureau 2005), which corresponds well with the age range targeted by PCIT.

Coaching sessions each have a specific protocol with an integrity checklist for the therapist to use to assure treatment integrity (Eyberg and Funderburk 2011). At each coaching session, the parent completes a brief rating of the child's behavior since the

---

[1] In PCIT, the parent is defined by the family. The parent is the primary adult caregiver(s) of the child. This could include biological parents, kinship parents, foster parents, etc. For this chapter, the term parent(s) will be used to describe the parent(s)/caregiver(s).

last session (Eyberg Child Behavior Inventory (ECBI), Eyberg and Pincus 1999). The therapist then reviews the week and homework assignments for 5–10 min. The majority of the session (30–40 min) is spent with the parent and child playing in one room while the therapist observes and coaches skills. This begins with the therapist coding a 5-min behavioral observation using the DPICS-IV to assess skills and set coaching goals. The therapist then coaches the parent toward skills mastery for approximately 30 min. Coaching time is divided if two parents are present, with each parent observing the other's time playing with the child, allowing for vicarious learning to occur. As PCIT is an extremely transparent intervention with the therapist and parent working as a team to achieve the treatment goals, the session concludes with the therapist re-entering the treatment room for 5–10 min to review session progress, skills, and assigned homework. This includes review of summary sheets of skills, ECBI scores, and homework completion to gauge progress.

PCIT is typically conducted with the parent and child in weekly, 1-h sessions. The average length of the PCIT intervention is 12–14 sessions, although reports from community samples average approximately 20 sessions. The primary goal of the first phase of PCIT (the Child-Directed Interaction (CDI) phase) is to develop and strengthen positive parent-child relationships and to strengthen the child's prosocial behaviors. Other goals of this phase include improved anger and frustration tolerance and increased attention, concentration, and impulse control. A decrease in negative behaviors and acceptance of limits begins to occur during CDI. In this phase, parents learn to implement techniques described as *behavioral play therapy*, which includes differential social attention. Parents learn how to attend to appropriate child behaviors (e.g., sharing, using manners, playing nicely) while actively ignoring attention-seeking, inappropriate child behaviors that do not cause any safety concerns (e.g., whining, playing roughly with toys, temper tantrums, disrespectful behaviors). To accomplish the goals of CDI, parents learn and utilize a specific set of skills known as the "PRIDE" skills to enhance the parent-child relationship, to reward children's appropriate behaviors, and to increase the frequency of those behaviors through: (a) Labeled *Praise:* recognizing and encouraging specific prosocial behaviors. (b) *R*eflection: utilizing active listening skills to enhance verbal communication. (c) *I*mitation: doing what the child is doing to promote positive behaviors and improve warmth. (d) *D*escription: pointing out what the child is doing to sustain interest in positive behaviors and increase attention and focus. (e) *E*njoyment: playing warmly, genuinely, and enthusiastically

The basic rule for parents in the CDI phase is to follow the *child's lead*. As such, parents learn to avoid behaviors that can direct the play or can negatively impact the budding positive parent-child interaction (e.g., questions, commands, criticisms). In addition to weekly sessions, parents practice CDI skills during 5 min of daily "Special Time" with their child. PCIT is an assessment-driven, mastery-based intervention; therefore, before progressing to the second phase of the PCIT intervention (Parent-Directed Interaction, PDI), parents must meet CDI mastery criteria by demonstrating at least ten labeled praises, ten behavioral descriptions, ten reflective statements, and no more than a total of three questions, commands, or criticisms to the child during a 5-min observation period. These quantitative skills serve as proxy measures for enhanced warmth and engagement in the parent-child interaction and a more secure attachment. Once mastery is met, the parent and child transition to the next phase of treatment.

The essence of the second phase of PCIT, the Parent-Directed Interaction (PDI) phase, is to teach parents to give effective commands, set consistent and fair limits, follow through with commands in a predictable manner, and provide reasonable, age-appropriate consequences for misbehavior within the context of a positive parent-child relationship. Like with CDI, the parents attend the PDI teach session to learn the skills associated with this phase and then resume coaching sessions with the child. Emphasis continues on the CDI skills in clinic sessions and home practice even as the PDI skills are added. During the PDI phase, parents learn to utilize a specialized time-out procedure in a calm, neutral manner for child noncompliance and severe misbehavior.

Following the PDI session protocols, therapists coach the parent through PDI while assuring that CDI skills are maintained. Through the PDI phase, increased emphasis is placed on the generalization of PCIT skills outside the clinic environment (e.g., home setting throughout the day, shopping mall, grocery store, restaurants, other outings) to facilitate real-world mastery of PCIT skills. Similar to the CDI phase, the PDI phase requires specific behaviors to reach mastery criteria. For the PDI phase, within a 5-min observation period, parents must demonstrate (a) giving at least 75 % "effective" or properly stated commands that are developmentally appropriate, direct, positively stated, and specific and (b) showing at least 75 % correct follow-through (i.e., labeled praise for compliance, appropriate utilization of the time-out warning/procedures for noncompliance). Parents learn specific words to use with the time-out sequence to increase predictability for the child and to reduce stress and increase consistency in the parent.

Successful completion of the entire PCIT intervention requires that three criteria are met: (a) parents demonstrate mastery criteria of both CDI and PDI skills; (b) the child's behavior, as rated on the ECBI, has moved to within ½ standard deviation of the normative mean (i.e., <114); and (c) the parents express confidence in their abilities to appropriately manage their child's behaviors on their own. PCIT ends as it began, with the three-situation observation assessment of the parent and child. Results and progress are reviewed with the parent and management of future problems, discussed. The parent is instructed to continue to implement learned skills well into the future in order to maintain the gains made in therapy. The parent and child are congratulated on the work they have completed and praised for their positive changes. As they graduate from treatment, both the parent and the child generally receive a certificate for their success in PCIT.

16.3.2 Case Example

"Jake" was a 4-year-old Caucasian boy who had recently lost both parents to suicide. He and his maternal grandmother, "Ms. Adams," were referred to psychological services of a large children's hospital by Jake's pediatrician because of increased crying, temper tantrums that included screaming and hitting his grandmother, frequent nightmares, and noncompliance.

PCIT Assessment
The PCIT assessment was completed over two sessions.

Clinical interview During a 1-h clinical interview with grandmother, Ms. Adams reported that Jake witnessed drug abuse by both parents. Grandmother reported Jake had been displaying internalizing behaviors, such as hypervigilance and avoiding conversations related to his parents. Early developmental, medical, social, and psychological histories were obtained from grandmother. Jake had a normal birth history and no major medical problems were noted. He reached developmental milestones within the normal range and was attending Head Start. Grandmother reported that Jake appeared to be functioning at his age level, but she was concerned that he was somewhat behind his peers in identifying colors and letters. Jake reportedly got along well with peers, but he could be shy at times. When asked about discipline strategies, grandmother stated that while Jake's parents used corporal punishment, she did not use this, except in rare situations. She had tried time-out with Jake (i.e., standing in the corner until he is ready to apologize), but that was woefully ineffective. Grandmother reported Jake is well behaved at school with no concerns voiced by his teachers. Given circumstances associated with the referral (loss due to suicide, exposure to substance abuse, change of placement), time was also spent with Ms. Adams to discuss the impact of traumatic events on child development and behavior. The therapist also discussed Ms. Adams' coping and support systems because these events were difficult for her as well.

Measures obtained At the clinical interview, grandmother completed measures.

- *Eyberg Child Behavior Inventory* (ECBI; Eyberg and Pincus 1999). The ECBI is used in all PCIT cases. Although ideally used at every session, it should be used at a minimum at pretreatment, mid-treatment, and posttreatment. Grandmother's ECBI was 198 (T score of 79), which indicated that Jake's disruptive behavior was in the clinically significant range (Raw score > 133; T-score > 70).
- *Parenting Stress Index-Short Form* (PSI-SF, Abidin 1990). Though not required in PCIT, the PSI-SF provides a measure of parenting stress; it is administered pre- and posttreatment. At the pretreatment assessment, she endorsed items in the clinically significant range (above 80 %) on the subscales of parental distress, parent-child dysfunctional interaction, difficult child, and total stress.
- *Trauma Symptom Checklist for Young Children* (TSCYC, Briere et al. 2001). Given Jake's history, grandmother completed the TSCYC to assess trauma symptoms. The following subscales were elevated (T-score > 70): depression, anger/aggression, posttraumatic stress intrusion, posttraumatic stress avoidance, posttraumatic stress arousal, and posttraumatic stress total.
- *Dyadic Parent-Child Interaction Coding System* (DPICS-IV, Eyberg et al. 2013). For the second assessment session, grandmother brought Jake for the observational

assessment of their interactions. The DPICS-IV is used in PCIT for the observational baseline assessment described above and throughout treatment to assess progress in parent skills, child behaviors, and their interactions. The structured observations with Jake and his grandmother took approximately 20 min. Ms. Adams was noted to be warm and attentive during the observations. She interacted primarily by asking questions, and when she was asked to lead the play, she offered many corrections (e.g., "No, that's not how it goes") and avoid direct requests by making a challenge of tasks ("I bet you can't get those toys in the box."). Afterward, the therapist gathered information from Ms. Adams about how typical these were. Grandmother noted that Jake was better behaved during the observation than he is at home. For example, she reported that he usually was easily frustrated during play involving building activities, but not during this observation. She was surprised that he willingly agreed to play with her choice of toy in the parent-led play situation. Finally, she stated that he normally refused to clean up toys at home, yet he did so during the session. The therapist placed these differences in context, explaining that children may behave more appropriately in new situations and with new toys. The therapist assured grandmother that the behaviors she reported were believed and, together, they would work to improve these and help Jake to reach his potential.

At the conclusion of the two assessment sessions, it was determined that Jake met diagnostic criteria for *adjustment disorder with mixed disturbance of emotions and conduct*. Treatment goals were developed to enhance the parent/child relationship, to increase Jake's positive behaviors, to teach grandmother strategies to be more consistent in discipline, and to improve Jake's compliance to directions.

Child-Directed Interaction (CDI) Teach Session
One week following the DPICS observation session, Ms. Adams returned for a 1-h didactic on the CDI phase of PCIT; Jake did not attend this session. During this session, the therapist provided an overview of PCIT and expectations of treatment. She taught each of the PRIDE skills (do skills) and avoid skills to be mastered in CDI, described when and how to ignore negative attention-seeking behavior, and instructed Ms. Adams on how to handle dangerous and/or destructive behaviors. "Special Time" for a structured 5 min each day with Jake to practice the PRIDE skills at home was explained. The therapist helped the grandmother determine appropriate toys they had for Special Time as well as the "when" and "where" for this daily practice. The therapist role-played all of the skills with the grandmother. Finally, several handouts pertaining to CDI and PRIDE skills were given to Ms. Adams.

Child-Directed Interaction (CDI) Coaching Sessions
Ms. Adams and Jake attended six weekly 1-h CDI coaching sessions. At the beginning of each CDI coaching session, the therapist briefly checked in with the family and reviewed homework (5–10 min). Together, they problem-solved any homework or treatment concerns. Ms. Adams also completed an ECBI measure at each session.

The grandmother and Jake began to play while the therapist went behind the one-way mirror. Next, the therapist used the DPICS-IV to code the play interaction between Ms. Adams and Jake for 5 min as this mirrored Special Time in the home. Based on the coding data, the therapist identified specific coaching goal of the session (e.g., a PRIDE skill for the primary focus of the coaching). The therapist then coached Ms. Adams for approximately 30 min each session using a bug-in-ear microphone device as grandmother and Jake played together. Coaching involved prompts ("what can you praise him for?"), direct line-feeds on occasion (say, "you're drawing a horse"), and observations ("he's loving this time with you"). Gentle corrections ("oops, was that a question?") were used sparingly based on research suggesting that parents tended to drop out of treatment when therapists used more criticism than praise (Fernandez and Eyberg 2009). Coaching in PCIT is focused on the positive to help increase rapport and comfort with the therapist, with live coaching, and to build the parent's confidence. During the last 5–10 min of the session, the therapist reviewed the PRIDE skill progress, the ECBI score graph, and the assigned homework for the week. (Note: In PCIT, the skill summary sheets and ECBI score graph are shared with the parent throughout treatment to bolster engagement, motivation, and praise for progress or problem-solve for challenges.) Relevant handouts were given for any skill(s) that needed refining. Ms. Adams met mastery criteria for CDI skills at the sixth CDI coaching session.

Teaching Parent-Directed Interaction (PDI) Discipline Skills
After mastering the CDI skills, Ms. Adams attended a 1-h PDI teaching session to learn skills for further improving behaviors and to implement a positive discipline procedure. Her ECBI graph of weekly scores was reviewed to update treatment goals for the PDI portion of treatment. Ms. Adams was taught several important components of PDI including how to give good commands, determining compliance vs. noncompliance, and how to implement an effective time-out procedure to handle noncompliant behaviors. Time-out was introduced with care, answering all concerns she had about this procedure. The therapist highlighted differences between this procedure and how time-out had been tried in the past. The time-out discussion included (1) how to give time-out warnings, (2) type of chair to use, (3) placement of the time-out chair, (4) appropriate length of time for time-out (3 min + 5 s of quiet), (5) parent behavior during time-out, (6) managing escape from the time-out chair, (7) ending time-out, and (8) what to do immediately following time-out. Ms. Adams role-played the time-out procedure with the therapist. The therapist stressed the importance of continued Special Time for the next week and of *not* practicing the time-out procedure at home until Ms. Adams practiced the sequence with therapist coaching and support. Ms. Adams reported an eagerness to try this new approach.

Coaching Parent-Directed Interaction (PDI) Discipline Skills
Ms. Adams and Jake attended six PDI coaching sessions. The structure of the initial PDI coaching sessions was similar to the CDI sessions; however, simple commands and minding/listening exercises were integrated into the play. At the

beginning of each PDI coaching session, CDI homework (and PDI homework when relevant) was reviewed for about 5–10 min. Following these discussions, the therapist went behind the one-way mirror and coded CDI skills for 5 min. Based on the coding data, if any skills had dropped below mastery, the therapist would coach Ms. Adams for a few minutes on these. By the third PDI session, the therapist also coded Ms. Adams' PDI skills for 5 min. The therapist then coached Ms. Adams for 30–40 min in parent-directed play. Coaching in PDI was initially very directive, with the therapist telling Ms. Adams the exact commands to use until Ms. Adams was able to generate appropriate commands on her own. For example, Ms. Adams was instructed to give play commands such as, "Your potato head cannot see. Please give him some eyes" and to point to where the piece was to be placed. As sessions progressed, commands increased in difficulty, moving from very simple play commands to "real-life" commands that simulated issues Jake faced outside of the clinic setting. These included having Jake transition from preferred to less-preferred activities, compliance with academic-type tasks, and commands related to cleaning up after his play. If Jake required a warning or timeout, the therapist coached Ms. Adams with the exact words and actions to use so that the procedure went as smoothly as possible and became predictable and consistent for both Jake and his grandmother. Following compliance, she was instructed to respond only to compliance (e.g., "Thank you for doing what I told you to do so quickly.") while ignoring any negative attitude. Grandmother then returned to use of CDI skills with Jake to underscore their positive relationship. Coaching also involved helping Ms. Adams ignore attention-seeking behavior when Jake was in the time-out chair. The coach kept her apprised of the amount of time remaining of his time-out and provided support (e.g., "Take a deep breath. You are doing a great job of staying calm while he is yelling."). Following timeout, Jake was required to comply with the original command or return to the chair. After compliance, Ms. Adams was coached to acknowledge his behavior and immediately give a second similar command. Jake showed learning with compliance to the second command, which was followed by a praise from his grandmother and a return to PRIDE skills.

As PDI sessions progressed, more advanced concepts were introduced, such as "real-life" directions in the home setting (e.g., getting Jake to bring his dishes to the sink), applying the discipline skills throughout the day, establishing house rules (standing consequences for dangerous or aggressive behaviors), and using PDI skills in public. For the latter, the therapist and grandmother problem-solved and role-played (a) expected behaviors in public, (b) how to do time-out in public, and (c) how to address bystanders and grandmother's potential embarrassment. Corresponding homework assignments were given. To help ensure that Ms. Adams did not overuse the time-out procedure, she came to one session to review other discipline tools to utilize for managing future behaviors.

Posttreatment and Follow-Up Assessment
Using the standard PCIT termination criteria, the family graduated from PCIT when Ms. Adams had achieved mastery criteria on CDI and PDI skills, ECBI intensity

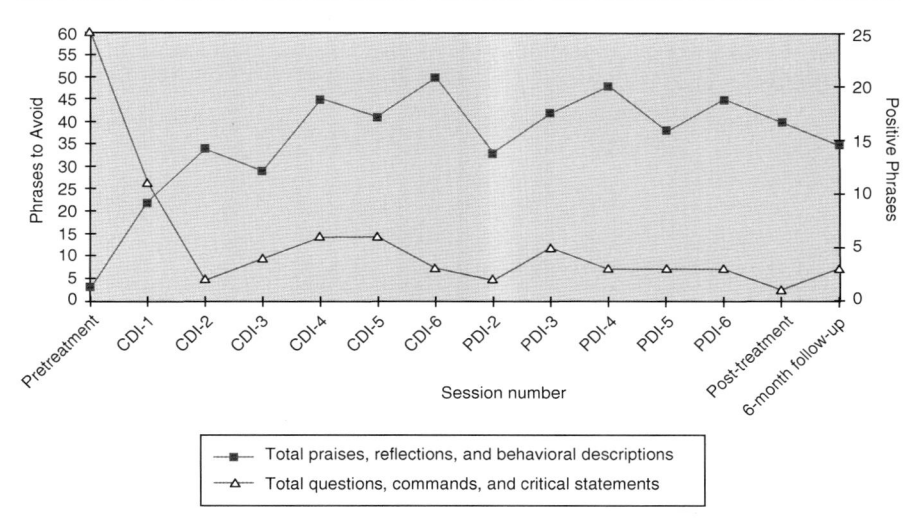

Fig. 16.1 Total number of CDI positive phrases and total number of CDI avoid phases coded during 5-min DPICS observations. *CDI* child directed interaction, *PDI* parent directed interaction

raw score was 114 or below (i.e., within ½ standard deviation of the normative mean), and Ms. Adams reported comfort in applying the skills on her own and was observed generalizing the skills outside of the session. Once these were met, Ms. Adams and Jake were again assessed in the three situations (e.g., pre- and post-assessments). A review of her skill acquisition over the course of treatment was shared. Ms. Adams and Jake were congratulated on their progress and accomplishments; a certificate was given to each of them. Ms. Adams and Jake were assessed again at a booster session approximately 6 months after termination and feedback, provided.

Ms. Adams' skills showed significant improvements over the course of treatment. For the 5-min observations, her CDI positive phase skills went from a total of <5 pretreatment to >40 at posttreatment and maintaining at 6 months. The goal is approximately 30 total statements. The phrases to avoid began at 60, falling to 1 at posttreatment and <5 at follow-up; the goal is <3 of these statements (Fig. 16.1).

Jake's improvement in various behaviors was also assessed throughout the course of treatment. ECBI intensity scores are presented in Fig. 16.2 for Jake. At initial assessment, Jake's ECBI intensity score was 198 (T-score of 79), with a problem score of 30 (T-score of 80). These scores reflect significant concerns associated with disruptive behavior, falling in the conduct problem range. At posttreatment and follow-up, the ECBI intensity was more than one standard deviation below the clinical cutoff (108 and 113, respectively, with T-scores below 70), and the problem score was in the normal range (8 and 6, respectively, with T-scores below 70).

Figure 16.3 outlines the Parenting Stress Index-Short Form (PSI/SF) percentiles obtained for pretreatment, posttreatment, and follow-up. The PSI/SF yields a total

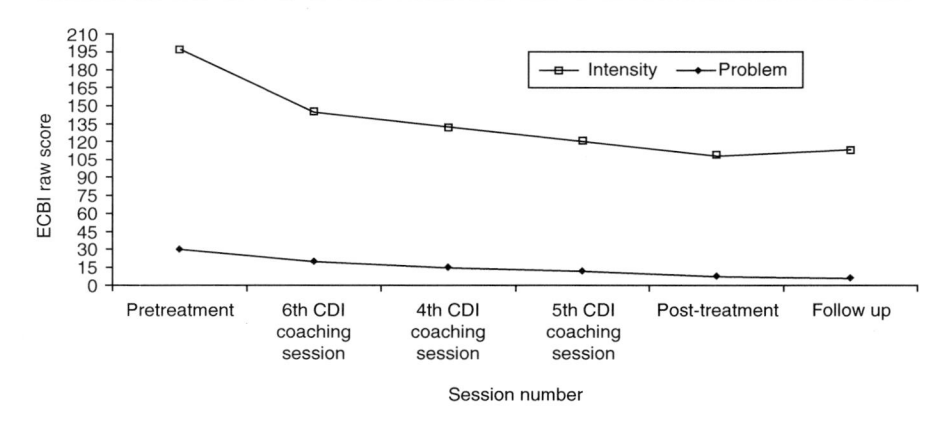

Fig. 16.2 Changes in Eyberg Child Behavior Inventory (ECBI raw scores)

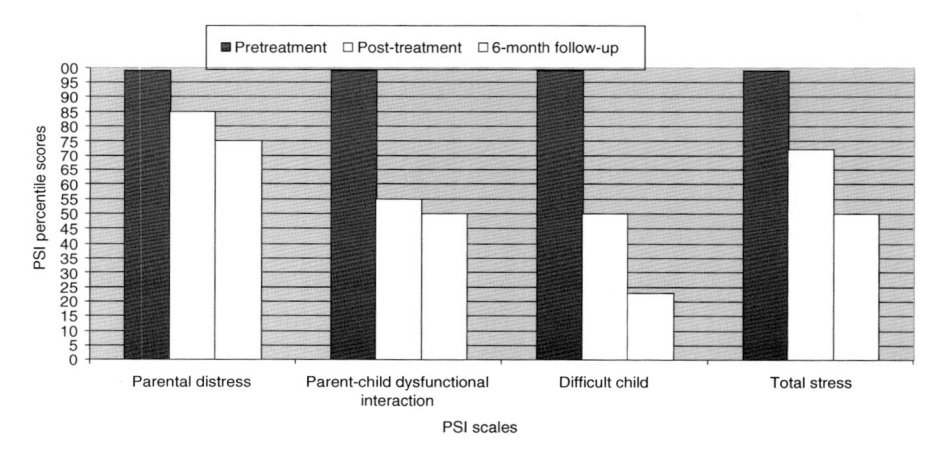

Fig. 16.3 Percentile scores for each subscale of the PSI at pretreatment, posttreatment, and 6-month follow-up

stress score from three scales: parental distress, parent-child dysfunctional interaction, and difficult child. The normal range is between the 15th and 80th percentile rank, with the higher percentile reflecting a higher degree of stress. Percentiles ranging from the 85th to 99th percentile and higher indicate clinically significant levels of parental stress. At the pretreatment assessment, Ms. Adams endorsed items in relation to Jake in the "clinically significant" range on the subscales of parental distress, parent-child dysfunctional interaction, difficult child and total stress. During the posttreatment and the 6-month follow-up assessment, the parent-child dysfunctional interaction and difficult child subscales and total stress fell within the normal range.

Figure 16.4 outlines the Trauma Symptom Checklist for Young Children (TSCYC) scores obtained for Jake at pretreatment, posttreatment, and follow-up.

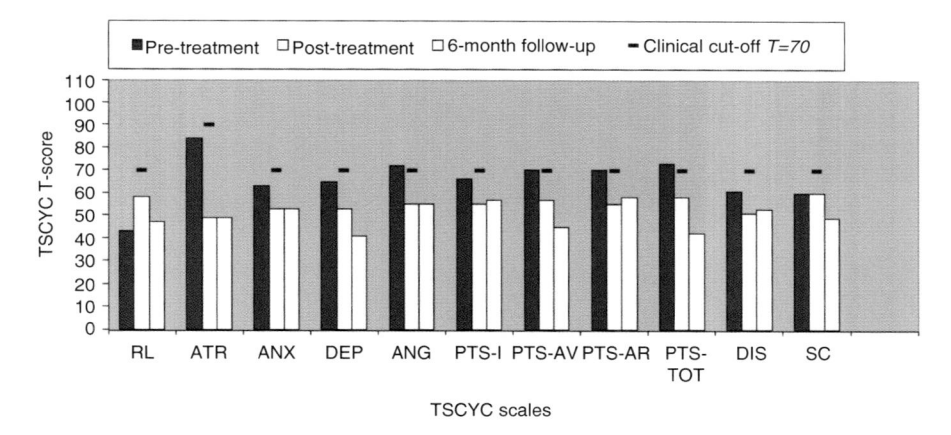

Fig. 16.4 T-scores for the Trauma Symptom Checklist for Young Children (TSCYC) subscales at pretreatment, posttreatment, and 6-month follow-up

On the TSCYC, T-scores have a mean of 50, and T-scores that fall between 65 and 70 suggest "possible concerns." Scores that are greater than 70 are considered "clinically significant." The TSCYC has two validity scales: (a) one that taps the parent's tendency to deny symptoms (i.e., RL) and (b) one that indexes a tendency to overreport symptom items (i.e., ATR). The cutoff score for the ATR is higher (90 T) than the other cutoff scores as parents of children in mental health settings tend to endorse more unusual TSCYC symptoms, for valid reasons, than parents in the general population. During pretreatment, Jake had four subscales (i.e., anger/aggression, posttraumatic stress avoidance, posttraumatic stress arousal, and posttraumatic stress total) falling in the clinically significant range. At posttreatment and follow-up, Jake did not have any subscales in the clinically significant range.

At the conclusion of PCIT treatment, Ms. Adams noted she was pleased with the progress Jake had made. The therapist advised Ms. Adams to continue doing Special Time daily so that treatment gains would be maintained over time. She also recommended Ms. Adams seek an evidence-based individual trauma therapy for Jake in the future should Jake's anxiety symptoms related to his parents' death return and/or if he began to express difficulties related to his parents' deaths (e.g., sleep disturbances or an increase in repetitive talk or play that had death-related themes that interfered with daily functioning). No further problems were reported.

16.4 Special Challenges

PCIT treatment is highly rewarding to families and clinicians because strong positive changes are achieved in a relatively short time. Providing PCIT to children exposed to trauma, however, is not without challenges. To increase effectiveness with this population, clinicians need to (a) understand and respond to trauma symptoms displayed in the course of treatment, (b) address barriers to parent participation in treatment, including motivation, and (c) adapt, when needed, PCIT for children outside of the 2–7 year age range.

When using PCIT with children in the traditional PCIT age range of 2–7 who have a trauma history, treatment modification is more tailoring than a systemic adaptation of core treatment elements, requiring sensitivity on the part of the clinician. In the case example, the therapist's intake incorporated an exploration of the grandmother's own coping methods and support systems as she dealt with the recent loss of loved ones and sudden new demands as a parent. The therapist monitored Ms. Adams' coping throughout the course of treatment, as is standard PCIT practice. Although Ms. Adams was experiencing the grief and guilt feelings associated with the suicide of family members, she reported that Jake's disruptive behavior increased her day-to-day stress and decreased her ability to connect with her support network such as church and social activities. Furthermore, tailoring with this population often includes measures of trauma symptoms, such as the TSCYC (Briere et al. 2001), as was done with Jake. Teach sessions and coaching incorporate trauma education, placing behaviors and PCIT skills in this context. For Jake's grandmother, information on young children's developmental understanding of loss and links between trauma and behavior were woven into every aspect of treatment. The therapist works with the parent to help the child move toward emotion regulation when trauma talk and/or play is observed, adding an emphasis on validating and helping label the child's emotions when coaching the CDI skills. For example, when Jake's play incorporated baby animals being orphaned when the parent animals were killed, Ms. Adams was coached to validate the sadness of the baby and model the arrival of alternative strong animals to care for the baby animal. When Jake volunteered that he missed playing with his Daddy, Ms. Adams initially froze the then tried to change the subject. The therapist coached her to reflect Jake's feelings ("You miss playing with your Daddy"), to validate his feelings ("I'm glad you told me how you are feeling. I know you miss them and I miss your Mommy and Daddy too."), and then to provide assurance of safety ("We miss them very much, but I am here to take care of you and I'm happy that we get to play together and build this big zoo.") At that point Jake easily returned to the play, and Ms. Adams was coached to resume more "standard" CDI skills. In feedback after coaching, Ms. Adams and the therapist problem-solved and briefly practiced how Ms. Adams might respond to Jake's comments at home in a similar way. The therapist also briefly discussed how these statements about the loss affected Ms. Adams, and, together, they problem-solved her coping strategies. Finally, in cases where a trauma history is present, if symptoms remain elevated following improvements in the parent-child relationship and reduction in negative behaviors, a referral to a trauma-specific treatment is recommended (e.g., trauma-focused cognitive behavioral therapy, Cohen et al. 2006, 2012). Trauma-specific therapy is often not initially feasible because disruptive behaviors make it extremely challenging for the child and parent to effectively engage in the treatment. In Jake's case, his disruptive behaviors and significant attention problems would have made success of other treatment modalities extremely difficult. With PCIT, all goals, including reduction of trauma symptoms, were met, so no further referrals were indicated.

While much research supports the utility of PCIT for children with externalizing behavior problems, children with a history of maltreatment and/or trauma exposure may also experience internalizing behavioral concerns. Growing evidence points to PCIT benefits in internalizing problem domains (e.g. depression, anxiety, PTSD symptoms) (Eyberg and Chase 2008; Lenze et al. 2011; Thomas and Zimmer-Gembeck 2011, 2012). Findings from uncontrolled trials of PCIT *without* any significant adaptions have reported specific reductions in trauma-related symptoms (Pearl et al. 2012); an adapted version of PCIT found significant reductions in anxiety symptoms (Puliafico et al. 2012).

Parents with a history of maltreatment may have problems with self-control, insensitivity, negative attributions, and inappropriate expression of anger. Tailoring of traditional PCIT coaching in the RCT research conducted by Chaffin and colleagues with this population (Chaffin et al. 2004, 2009, 2011) implemented additional supportive actions during PDI coaching, especially during implementation of the time-out procedure. These included help with self-monitoring and deep breathing. CDI coaching was tailored toward selectively reinforcing parental self-control or sensitivity toward the child when appropriate. These actions are considered minor modifications as PCIT coaching should always be geared to the unique presentation and needs of the parent and child. Greater emphasis was placed on educating parents about developmentally normal child challenges and expectations, and the use of role-plays was expanded. As noted below, RCT of tailoring and adaptations of PCIT for child maltreatment demonstrated significant positive outcomes (Chaffin et al. 2004, 2011); these results have been supported by other research in this area (Timmer et al. 2005; Timmer and Urquiza 2014). Parents, particularly those who have been victimized by domestic violence or those who have not been in a parenting role, may have trouble with the assertiveness needed to set clear limits with a disruptive child. Standard PCIT practice offers emotional support of the parent as they learn, through coaching, that within the context of a nurturing relationship, it is possible for a parent to set and enforce clear limits without "damaging" the parent-child attachment. Ms. Adams was supported as she began to impose limits that promoted Jake's safety and well-being (e.g., rules to wear safety belt, to refrain from hitting peers, to conform to an appropriate bedtime) without worrying that Jake should be protected from every frustration since he had already suffered great loss.

There is debate outside of the PCIT community regarding PCIT's role as a treatment for children with attachment disorders, with concern about the discipline procedures used in PDI. As PCIT is *grounded* in attachment theory, PCIT advocates contend that the dual focus on strengthening parent-child relationships and providing safe, predictable limits offered in PCIT can be ideal for children who have experienced disrupted attachments (Troutman 2015; Allen et al. 2014.). To date, arguments pro and con have been largely theoretical because few good measures of attachment exist for children older than toddlers, and well-controlled research has yet to be conducted.

Attachment is often a concern in cases that involve the child welfare system and mandated treatment. To address challenges for PCIT with this coerced population, adaptations were made in a series of RCTs (see below). The first and primary adaptation was the inclusion of a pretreatment motivational intervention (Campbell et al. 2014). An additional adaptation to standard PCIT was an extension of the age range to include children between 7 and 12 years of age. However, this was for families presenting with abusive or neglectful parenting practices. The modifications made for the older child focus on taking into account the child's perception of treatment in both phases of PCIT. The CDI skills and PDI consequences were adjusted to match developmental expectations and developmental maturity. CDI incorporates age-appropriate activities and language, including using drills to "prime" skills to help parents master skills with a more age-appropriate interaction. The emphasis in PDI is changed from absolute compliance expected from preschoolers to acceptance of reasonable consequences in the older child. These adaptations drew from elements of the Defiant Children's program (Barkley 1987) and the Common Sense Parenting program (Burke et al. 2006). While the older children in the studies had a range of behavioral difficulties, the children did not receive diagnostic evaluations because the parent was the presenting client. The adaptation has not been evaluated with children in the 7–12 age range who have a primary referral for disruptive behavior problems. Future research is needed to evaluate efficacy before PCIT is implemented with this referral population.

Adaptations in PCIT may also be required for parents who have limited opportunities to practice skills or complete homework because their children are in out of home placement. These adaptations include using role-plays, practicing CDI during scheduled visits, or practicing with other children in the home. To be successful, PCIT requires that parents have adequate access to the child to practice the skills. PCIT is *not* recommended with the biological parent in cases where the child in foster care is unlikely to ever return home or if return may be delayed until well after PCIT is completed, because delays have been found to be associated with loss of treatment benefit (Chaffin et al. 2011). If reunification is imminent, PCIT is recommended only when the parent has ready access to interact with the child and practice skills at least three times per week in addition to the PCIT treatment session.

Children who have experienced sexual abuse may also benefit from PCIT when treatment is provided with a non-offending caregiver. PCIT is not recommended as a treatment for perpetrators of sexual abuse because the treatment goals of enhancing the parent-child relationship and increasing the child's compliance with adult requests may be contraindicated.

16.5 Research

It is often stated that PCIT was developed for children with disruptive behavior disorders and later adapted for children with a history of maltreatment, but, in reality, PCIT always treated children exposed to adverse life experiences. In the late 1970s to early 1980s when the initial effectiveness studies of PCIT were being conducted, the nascent field of child maltreatment focused on descriptive studies rather than interventions. Post-traumatic stress disorder did not appear in the DSM until 1980 and then primarily as a diagnosis for war veterans. Recognition of trauma-related anxiety and depression in young children came several years later. The initial PCIT randomized controlled trials (RCT) included only children with clinically significant levels of disruptive behavior, likely attributable to a variety of antecedents, including ineffective parenting practices, child maltreatment, developmental concerns such as prenatal substance exposure, or conditions such as autism spectrum disorders. Later studies evaluating PCIT as a treatment for parents at risk for child maltreatment eliminated the requirement for documented disruptive behavior disorders on the grounds that the treatment targeted presumed deficits in parenting rather than behavior problems in the child. In summary, diagnostic and screening conventions for children seen in PCIT have evolved over time, but the heterogeneous mix of children treated with PCIT has been relatively constant.

A series of randomized controlled trials established the effectiveness of PCIT for parents with a history of physically maltreating and/or neglecting their child (Chaffin et al. 2004, 2009, 2011). These studies demonstrated that when PCIT is combined with techniques to enhance motivation to change parenting practices, parents with a history of child maltreatment are much more likely to complete treatment and to evidence benefits in the form of significantly reduced future child welfare reports (e.g., less than 20 % at 2 years posttreatment). PCIT alone was shown to be more effective than PCIT combined with an ad hoc array of additional services, family preservation services, or standard parenting classes (Chaffin et al. 2004). It appears clear that motivational enhancement is important to address when providing PCIT to parents referred through the child welfare system because without motivational intervention, they tend to have very low treatment completion rates (Thomas and Simmer-Gemback 2012; Timmer et al. 2005; Lanier et al. 2014).

It is less clear whether the description of PCIT as a mastery-based treatment is essential to outcome. Thomas and Zimmer-Gembeck (2007) reviewed PCIT RCT's for 8 cohorts and found that 9 of 13 published studies represented time-limited PCIT rather than mastery-based. Thomas and Zimmer-Gembeck (2012) assessed participants after 12 sessions of PCIT and again at full mastery, finding marginal additional gains when treatment was extended, notable reductions in child internalizing symptoms, and increases in parents' emotional sensitivity.

PCIT has a wide body of research, with over 300 published articles documenting its effectiveness with externalizing behaviors (see PCIT.org for bibliography). PCIT gains generalize to untreated siblings (Brestan et al. 1997) and to the school setting (Funderburk et al. 1998), with PCIT treatment gains lasting upward of 6 years (Hood and Eyberg 2003). Format changes have also been implemented, yielding positive results; these include in-home treatment (Masse and McNeil 2008; Galanter et al. 2012), intensive or shortened treatment (Graziano et al. 2014), and group PCIT (Bertrand 2009; Niec et al. 2005). Effectiveness has been demonstrated for children with disorders of development (Bagner and Eyberg 2007; Bertrand 2009; Ginn et al. 2015). It has been applied successfully to various populations and cultural groups in the United States (Bigfoot and Funderburk 2011; McCabe and Yeh 2009; Gurwitch et al. 2013). PCIT has been used around the world with similar results; countries with PCIT implementation include Australia, China, Germany, Hong Kong, India, Japan, Norway, the Netherlands, New Zealand, South Korea, and Taiwan.

PCIT is a robust evidence-based treatment, which appears effective across a variety of settings, formats, and populations. Over the past decade, children specifically with a history of trauma and/or maltreatment have become a strong focus of PCIT practice and research. PCIT shows significant promise not only to reduce trauma symptoms and improve overall behaviors and relationships but also to find a significant reduction in recidivism in a population which continues to challenge the child welfare and family and drug court systems.

As PCIT is being disseminated across the United States and around the world, efforts have been made to maintain the fidelity and integrity of this treatment. In 2009, PCIT International incorporated as a governing body helps assure these goals are met as the treatment expands its reach. Agency readiness and therapist training guidelines were developed, a uniform treatment protocol was adopted, and a certification process for PCIT therapists and trainers was established to assure the sustainability and high standards of this strong evidence-based intervention.

References

Abidin RR (1990) Parenting stress index manual. Pediatric Psychology Press, Charlottesville

Ainsworth MS (1979) Infant-mother attachment. Am Psychol 34:932–937

Allen B, Timmer SG, Urquiza AJ (2014) Parent–child interaction therapy as an attachment-based intervention: theoretical rationale and pilot data with adopted children. Child Youth Serv Rev 47:334–341. doi:10.1016/j.childyouth.2014.10.009

Axline V (1947) Play therapy. Houghton Mifflin, Boston

Bagner DM, Eyberg SM (2007) Parent–child interaction therapy for disruptive behavior in children with mental retardation: a randomized controlled trial. J Clin Child Adolesc Psychol 36(3):418–429

Bandura A (1977) Social learning theory. Prentice Hall, Englewood Cliffs

Barkley RA (1987) Defiant children: a clinician's manual for parent training. Guilford Press, New York

Baumrind D (1966) Effects of authoritative parental control on child behavior. Child Dev 37:887–907

Baumrind D (1967) Child care practices anteceding three patterns of preschool behavior. Genet Psychol Monogr 75:43–88

Bertrand J, [On behalf of the Interventions for Children with Fetal Alcohol Spectrum Disorders Research Consortium] (2009) Interventions for children with fetal alcohol spectrum disorders (FASDs): overview of findings for five innovative research projects. Res Dev Disabil 30(5):986–1006

BigFoot D, Funderburk B (2011) Honoring children, making relatives: the cultural translation of parent-child interaction therapy for American Indian and Alaska Native families. J Psychoactive Drugs 43(4):309–318

Briere J, Johnson K, Bissada A, Damon L, Crouch J, Gil E, Hanson R, Ernst V (2001) The Trauma Symptom Checklist for Young Children (TSCYC): reliability and association with abuse exposure in a multi-site study. Child Abuse Negl 25:1001–1014

Brinkmeyer M, Eyberg SM (2003) Parent-child interaction therapy for oppositional children. In: Kazdin AE, Weisz JR (eds) Evidence-based psychotherapies for children and adolescents. Guilford, New York, pp 204–223

Burke R, Herron R, Barnes BA (2006) Common sense parenting®, 3rd edn. Father Flanagan's Boys' Home, Boys Town

Campbell C, Chaffin M, Funderburk B (2014) Parent-child interaction therapy (PCIT) in child maltreatment cases. In: Reece R, Sargent J, Hanson R (eds) Handbook of child abuse treatment, 2nd edn. Johns Hopkins University Press, Baltimore

Chaffin M, Silovsky J, Funderburk B, Valle LA, Brestan EV, Balachova T, Jackson S, Lensgraf J, Bonner BL (2004) Parent-child interaction therapy with physically abusive parents: efficacy for reducing future abuse reports. J Consult Clin Psychol 72:500–510

Chaffin M, Valle LA, Funderburk B, Gurwitch R, Silovsky J, Bard D et al (2009) A motivational intervention can improve retention in PCIT for low-motivation child welfare clients. Child Maltreat 14(4):356–368

Chaffin M, Funderburk B, Bard D, Valle L, Gurwitch R (2011) A combined motivation and parent-child interaction therapy package reduces child welfare recidivism in a randomized dismantling field trial. J Consult Clin Psychol 79(1):84–95. doi:10.1037/a0021227

Chase R, Eyberg S (2008) Clinical presentation and treatment outcome for children with comorbid externalizing and internalizing symptoms. J Anxiety Disord 22(2):273–282

Children's Bureau (2005) Child welfare outcomes 2002-2005. Administration on Children, Youth and Families, Department of Health and Human Services. Retrieved from http://archive.acf.hhs.gov/programs/cb/pubs/cwo05/cwo05.pdf

Cohen JA, Mannarino AP, Deblinger E (2006) Treating trauma and traumatic grief in children and adolescents. Guilford, New York/London

Cohen JA, Mannarino AP, Deblinger E (2012) Trauma-focused CBT for children and adolescents: treatment applications. Guilford, New York/London

Eyberg SM (1988) Parent-child interaction therapy: integration of traditional and behavioral concerns. Child Fam Behav Ther 10(1):33–46

Eyberg SM, Funderburk B (2011) Parent-child interaction therapy protocol. Copyright 2011 PCIT International, Inc.

Eyberg SM, Pincus D (1999) Eyberg child behavior inventory and Sutter-Eyberg student behavior inventory-revised: professional manual. Psychological Assessment Resources, Odessa

Eyberg SM, Robinson EA (1982) Parent-child interaction training: effects on family functioning. J Clin Child Psychol 11:130–137

Eyberg S.M, Nelson MM, Ginn NC, Bhuiyan N, Boggs SR (2013) Dyadic Parent-Child Interaction Coding System (DPICS): comprehensive manual for research and training, 4th ed. Copyright 2013 PCIT International, Inc.

Fernandez MA, Eyberg SM (2009) Predicting treatment and follow-up attrition in parent-child interaction therapy. J Abnorm Child Psychol 37(3):431–441. doi:10.1007/s10802-008-9281-1

Forehand RT, McMahon RJ (1981) Helping the noncompliant child. The Guilford Press, New York

Forgatch MS, Bullock BM, Patterson GR (2004) From theory to practice: increasing effective parenting through role-play. The Oregon Model of Parent Management Training (PMTO). In: Steiner H (ed) Handbook of mental health interventions in children and adolescents: an integrated developmental approach. Jossey-Bass, San Francisco, pp 782–814

Funderburk BW, Eyberg S (2011) Psychotherapy research centers and groups. In: Norcross JC, Vandenbos GR, Freedheim DK (eds) History of psychotherapy: continuity and change, 2nd edn. American Psychological Association, Washington, DC, pp 415–420. ISBN: 978-1-4338-0762-6

Funderburk BW, Eyberg SM, Newcomb K, McNeil C, Hembree-Kigin T, Capage L (1998) Parent-child interaction therapy with behavior problem children: maintenance of treatment effects in the school setting. Child Fam Behav Ther 20:17–38

Galanter R, Self-Brown S, Valente JR, Dorsey S, Whitaker DJ, Bertuglia-Haley M, Prieto M (2012) Effectiveness of parent-child interaction therapy delivered to at-risk families in the home setting. Child Fam Behav Ther 34(3):177–196

Ginn NC, Clionsky LN, Eyberg SM, Warner-Metzger CM, Abner JP (2015) Child-directed interaction training for young children with autism spectrum disorders: parent and child outcomes. J Clin Child Adolesc Psychol. 1–9. doi:10.1080/15374416.2015.1015135

Graziano PA, Bagner DM, Slavec J, Hungerford G, Kent K, Babinski D, Derefinko K, Pasalich D (2014) Feasibility of intensive parent–child interaction therapy (I-PCIT): results from an open trial. J Psychopathol Behav Assess:1–12. doi:10.1007/s10862-014-9435-0

Greenberg MT, Speltz ML, DeKlyen M, Jones K (2001) Correlates of clinic referral for early conduct problems: variable- and person-oriented approaches. Dev Psychopathol 13:255–276

Gurwitch RH, Fernandez S, Pearl E, Chung G (2013) Utilizing parent-child interaction therapy to help improve the outcome of military families. Children, Youth, and Families Newsletter.

http://www.apa.org/pi/families/resources/newsletter/2013/01/parent-child-interaction.aspx. Accessed 6 Mar 2015

Hanf M (1969) A two stage program for modifying maternal controlling during mother-child (M-C) interaction. Paper presented at the meeting of the Western Psychological Association, Vancouver

Hildyard KL, Wolfe DA (2002) Child neglect: developmental issues and outcomes. Child Abuse Negl 26:679–695

Hood KK, Eyberg SM (2003) Outcomes of parent–child interaction therapy: mothers' reports of maintenance three to six years after treatment. J Clin Child Adolesc Psychol 32(3):419–429. doi:10.1207/S15374424JCCP3203_10

Kaminski JW, Valle LA, Filene JH, Boyle CL (2008) A meta-analytic review of components associated with parent training program effectiveness. J Abnorm Child Psychol 36:567–589. doi:10.1007/s10802-007-9201-9

Kaufman Best Practices Project (2004) Kaufman best practices project final report: closing the quality chasm in child abuse treatment; identifying and disseminating best practices. http://www.chadwickcenter.org/Documents/Kaufman%20Report/ChildHosp-NCTAbrochure.pdf. Accessed 1 Feb 2015

Lanier P, Kohl PL, Benz J, Swinger D, Drake B (2014) Preventing maltreatment with a community-based implementation of parent–child interaction therapy. J Child Fam Stud 23:449–460. doi:10.1007/s10826-012-9708-8

Lenze SN, Pautsch J, Luby J (2011) Parent-child interaction therapy emotion development: a novel treatment for depression in preschool children. Depress Anxiety 28:153–159. doi:10.1002/da.20770

Masse JJ, McNeil CB (2008) In-home parent-child interaction therapy: clinical considerations. Fam Behav Ther 30(2):127–135

McCabe K, Yeh M (2009) Parent–child interaction therapy for Mexican Americans: a randomized clinical trial. J Clin Child Adolesc Psychol 38(5):753–759

McNeil CB, Hembree-Kigin TL (2010) Parent-child interaction therapy. Springer, New York

McNeil C, Herschell AD, Gurwitch R, Clemens-Mowrer LC (2005) Training foster parents in parent-child interaction therapy. Educ Treat Child 28(2):182–196

Niec LN, Hemme JM, Yopp JM, Brestan EV (2005) Parent-child interaction therapy: the rewards and challenges of a group format. Cogn Behav Pract 12(1):113–125. http://www.sciencedirect.com/science/article/pii/S107772290580046X

Patterson GR (1976) The aggressive child: victim and architect of a coercive system. In: Mash EJ, Hamerlynck LA, Handy LC (eds) Behavior modification and families. Brunner/Mazel, New York, pp 267–316

Patterson GR (1982) The early developmental of coercive family process. In: JB

Pearl E, Thieken L, Olafson E, Boat B, Connelly L, Barnes J, Putnam F (2012) Effectiveness of community dissemination of parent-child interaction therapy. Psychol Trauma Theory Res Pract Policy 4(2):204–213

Puliafico AC, Comer JS, Pincus DB (2012) Adapting parent-child interaction therapy to treat anxiety disorders in young children. Child Adolesc Psychiatr Clin N Am 21(3):607–619. doi:10.1016/j.chc.2012.05.005

Reid JB, Patterson GR, Snyder J (eds) (2002) Antisocial behavior in children and adolescents: developmental theories and models for intervention. American Psychological Association, Washington, DC, pp. 25–44

Stith SM, Liu T, Davies LC, Boykin E, Meagan C, Harris JM, Som A, McPherson M, Dees JEEG (2009) Risk factors in child maltreatment: a meta-analytic review of the literature. Aggress Violent Behav 14:13–29

Thomas R, Zimmer-Gembeck MJ (2007) Behavioral outcomes of parent-child interaction therapy and triple P-positive parenting program: a review and meta-analysis. J Abnorm Child Psychol 35(3):475–495

Thomas R, Zimmer-Gembeck MJ (2011) Accumulating evidence for parent–child interaction therapy in the prevention of child maltreatment. Child Dev 82(1):177–192. doi:10.1111/j.1467-8624.2010.01548.x

Thomas R, Zimmer-Gembeck MJ (2012) Parent child interaction therapy: an evidence based treatment for child maltreatment. Child Maltreat 17(3):253–266. doi:10.1177/1077559512459555

Timmer SG, Urquiza AJ (2014) Parent-child interaction therapy for maltreated children. In: Timmer S, Urquiza A (eds) Evidence-based approaches for the treatment of maltreated children. Springer, New York

Timmer SG, Urquiza AJ, Zebell N, McGrath NM (2005) Parent-child interaction therapy: application to maltreating parent-child dyads. Child Abuse Negl 29(7):825–842. doi:10.1016/j.chiabu.2005.01.003

Timmer SG, Urquiza AJ, Zebell N (2006) Challenging foster caregiver-maltreated child relationships: the effectiveness of parent-child interaction therapy. Child Youth Serv Rev 28(1):1–19. doi:10.1016/j.childyouth.2005.01.006

Venet M, Bureau J, Gosselin C, Capuano F (2007) Attachment representations in a sample of neglected preschool-age children. Sch Psychol Int 28:264–293

Webster-Stratton C (2011) The incredible years parents, teachers, and children's training series: program content, methods, research and dissemination 1980-2011. Incredible Years, Inc., Seattle

Webster-Stratton C, Reid MJ (2003) Treating conduct problems and strengthening social and emotional competence in young children: the Dina Dinosaur Treatment Program. J Emot Behav Disord 11(3):130–143

Zisser A, Eyberg S (2010) Parent-child interaction therapy and the treatment of disruptive behavior disorders. In: Weisz JR, Kazdin AE (eds) Evidence-based psychotherapies for children and adolescents, 2nd edn. Guilford Press, New York, pp 179–193

Trauma Systems Therapy for Children and Adolescents

17

Adam Brown, Christina Laitner, and Glenn Saxe

17.1 Theoretical Underpinnings

Understanding child traumatic stress requires an appreciation of complexity. Effective treatment of child traumatic stress requires the ability to translate understandings of this complexity into a set of specific therapeutic actions that will help for the defined traumatic stress problem. Trauma systems therapy (TST) is designed to help providers to do this. What are the origins of this complexity? The traumatized child is comprised of a complex biological system – developing over time – and embedded in complex social systems including family, peer group, school, neighborhood, and culture. The traumatic event, itself, is complex and involves many factors such as duration, frequency, developmental period, and trauma type. Out of this complexity, what determines the child's response to trauma and how treatment should address these determinants? This notion has critical practical applications. TST addresses not only a traumatized child's difficulty regulating survival states but also the role that the child's social environment plays in either helping the child to cope or in triggering and/or perpetuating these survival states. This

---

A. Brown (✉)
Department of Child and Adolescent Psychiatry, The Atlas Project NYU Child Study Center, New York, NY, USA
e-mail: adam.brown2@nyumc.org

C. Laitner
Department of Child and Adolescent Psychiatry, Center for Stress, Trauma, and Resilience NYU Child Study Center, New York, NY, USA
e-mail: Christina.Laitner@nyumc.org

G. Saxe
Department of Child and Adolescent Psychiatry,
The Child Study Center at NYU Langone Medical Center, New York, NY, USA
e-mail: glenn.saxe@nyumc.org

© Springer International Publishing Switzerland 2017
M.A. Landolt et al. (eds.), *Evidence-Based Treatments for Trauma Related Disorders in Children and Adolescents*, DOI 10.1007/978-3-319-46138-0_17

interactive duality of internal and external factors forms the core approach to understanding and treating child traumatic stress within TST. Thus, TST focuses on the critical systemic factors that can contribute to a youth experiencing traumatic stress by understanding the fit between the child's strengths and vulnerabilities and their social context.

In our experience many children with traumatic stress have problem lists that may be exceedingly long. TST begins with an assessment process that considers all possible determiners of the child's problems and concludes with an understanding of the most important ones to address in treatment. How does TST do this?

1. We understand that biological systems related to trauma have evolved to promote survival in the face of threat. Accordingly, our first pass at understanding the child's emotional or behavioral responses to trauma is to consider how these responses relate to survival preservation.
2. We understand that the child's social environment following trauma is, usually, no longer threatening, but children will respond to their environments – as if it is threatening – in certain situations. In cases where the child's environment is actually threatening, treatment is fully dedicated to preserving safety.
3. The child's emotional, behavioral, and cognitive shift to respond to their current environment as if it were threatening is the defining feature of traumatic stress responses. We call this response a *survival state*, defined as follows: "An individual's experience of the present environment as threatening to his or her survival with corresponding thoughts, emotions, behaviors, and neurochemical, and neurophysiological responses" (Saxe et al. 2016, p.10).
4. We understand that *survival states* do not occur randomly, but are in response to environmental signals that the child perceives (consciously or unconsciously) as threatening. Usually these signals have some knowable connection to the child's experience of trauma: but such connection may not be readily apparent and is understood through the process of assessment.
5. The occurrence of the child's *survival states* in the context of specific threat signals usually defines the episodes for which the child needs treatment. These signals may be very subtle (e.g., a type of glance or tone of voice). Accordingly, a key part of the assessment process is to identify patterns by which threat signals lead to *survival states*.
6. Threat signals may come from any area of the child's social environment (e.g., home, school, peer group). TST will focus on areas of the social environment in proportion to the degree that threat signals are found.
7. It is the identification of these patterns of links between threat signals and *survival states* that defines the clinical problems to be addressed in TST treatment. This will usually result in a small number of high-value problems that become the focus of treatment: out of the great many possible problems that could have been the focus of treatment.

These ideas enable clinicians and clinical teams to consider child traumatic stress in all its complexity and to translate the complexity into the specific therapeutic actions that will help a child given their needs. Theoretically this is a systems process (hence the name trauma *systems* therapy). We define the trauma system as (Saxe et al. 2005):

> A traumatized child who experiences survival states in specific definable moments; and,
> A social environment and/or system of care that is not able to help the child to regulate these survival states.

As previously stated, this conceptual framework is what sets TST apart from other child trauma models. This interactive duality of internal and external factors forms the core approach to understanding and treating child traumatic stress within TST.

TST began in the outpatient clinic of a large, urban medical center in Boston (Boston Medical Center) in which the initial developers of TST had been providing interventions for children with complex trauma histories in the "usual and customary" way, that is, in a clinic, in individual sessions, and with a primary focus on the child. Although this approach at the time was in line with evidence-based, individual child treatments (Wethington et al. 2008), two major challenges were faced. First, there was not a sufficient recognition that the children referred to the clinic were coming from unstable home environments typically mired in poverty and affected by racism/discrimination, inadequate schools, and community violence. As such, these complex environmental and social factors were directly contributing to the children's presenting problems and suggested the need for intervention to reach beyond the individual. Second, there was a lack of clarity about whether the work was having a positive impact on the children and their families. This uncertainty was reinforced when some of the children and families did not truly engage in treatment – a situation typically reflected by treatment dropout. Such attrition is especially prevalent in ethnic minority youth and with children and adolescents who have histories of child maltreatment (Lau and Weisz 2003). The team thus embarked on a mission to develop a different and better way to help the children and families.

As we set out to change the way we practiced, we followed four guiding principles: (1) treatment must be developmentally informed, (2) treatment must directly address the social environment/ecology, (3) treatment must be compatible with systems of care, and (4) treatment must be "disseminate-able." Affective (or emotional) dysregulation has been found to be one of the major problems experienced by children exposed to complex trauma (Cicchetti and Toth 1995). For such children, problems in emotion regulation (ER) can be understood as a core feature of traumatic stress associated with biological systems that help the individual survive in the face of threat (Frewen and Lanius 2006; Hopper et al. 2007). When confronted with reminders of past trauma or actual threats, children who have been traumatized respond with hyper- or hypo-arousal and other forms of emotional lability. We therefore chose to specify ER, which we refer to as survival in the moment states, as a crucial focus of TST. This approach is consistent with other treatment approaches described in this book.

The important work of Urie Bronfenbrenner (1979), with its emphasis on understanding the developing child in the context of her/his social ecology and the transactions that occur between that child and the various layers of her/his social environment, was a catalyst that focused TST on the social ecology/environment of the traumatized child. Bronfenbrenner's framework is particularly appropriate to these children due to the many threats and dangers that are in their environment and the absence of support or protection that may also be part of the environment. For instance, a child subjected to parental physical abuse who is also exposed to community violence may have difficulty recovering from symptoms due to the ongoing threat in the community. The treatment team decided to focus TST on addressing aspects of the social environment that directly relate to a child's survival states. This focus will be explained in detail below.

Although comprehensive approaches have been developed to coordinate and deliver an array of mental health services from multiple agencies (e.g., systems of care; Pumariega and Winters 2003), our experience indicated that multi-provider approaches tend to be fragmented, uncoordinated, and thus not very effective. Consequently, we decided to devise an intervention approach that literally "brings to the table" each provider across all systems of care in a multispecialty clinical team. The TST team is typically comprised of home-based clinicians, a psychopharmacologist, psychotherapists, a legal advocate, and a supervising clinician with trauma treatment expertise. The intent was for TST to provide a team approach involving all systems of care with which a traumatized child is involved. These providers, in turn, were engaged with the various parts of the child's social environment (i.e., home, neighborhood/community, school, etc.). We thus set about to develop not only an effective treatment model but also one that could be successfully disseminated across a variety of "real-world" settings.

One critical strategy that we used in the creation of TST was to create a model that is "disseminate-able" and that incorporates services that are available in most regions of the United States. TST is provided via a traditional multidisciplinary team that also possesses two unique members (i.e., home-based clinician and legal advocate). A second feature of TST that improves its successful adoption and implementation is that the model is fully operationalized in a published manual (Saxe et al. 2016), which is in line with other empirically supported, manualized, social-ecological models (e.g., multisystemic therapy; Henggeler et al. 2002). Another feature of the TST model is the development of a treatment adherence approach to help ensure that treatment is delivered with sufficient fidelity. Specifically, fidelity is guided by adherence to a well-articulated approach to assessment, treatment planning, child and family engagement, and intervention centered around three phases of treatment and is consistent with the notion of "flexibility within fidelity" to lead to a child-centered, individualized treatment approach (Kendall et al. 2008).

TST provides a central organizing structure that brings together different service systems that are involved in a child's care. In order to provide TST, a service system must be able to provide four types of services/skills:

- Individual skills-based, trauma-informed psychotherapy (emotional regulation and then cognitive/trauma processing skills)
- Home or community-based care
- Legal advocacy
- Psychopharmacology

The configuration of a team providing these services differs by community and is typically *built out of existing resources* by surveying services already provided by a given agency that can be integrated or that are already provided by other agencies in a region and can be integrated through interagency agreement. TST also places a strong emphasis on engaging families in treatment utilizing specific strategies to develop the treatment alliance and troubleshooting practical barriers to treatment engagement. A critical element of treatment engagement is the *families' culture-based understanding* of emotion, mental health, and mental health intervention.

17.2 How to Do Trauma Systems Therapy

TST is both a clinical model for the effective and efficient treatment of child traumatic stress and an organizational model to help a program that works with traumatized youth embed the model within their practices, procedures, and organizational culture. All TST materials and details can be in found in the TST manual (Saxe et al. 2016). We do not train individual clinicians in TST, but rather plan with an organization to train a team of providers to implement the model. TST thus begins by helping an organization to create a TST leadership team. This team engages in a process of TST organizational planning designed to elicit an understanding of the most important priorities from the perspectives of the various members of the leadership team, which usually includes administrators and program leaders. The organizational planning process is also designed to understand what gets in the way of accomplishing these important priorities. A plan is then created to determine how TST can best help to address these concerns and help the organization to achieve these goals. This planning process also includes a detailed understanding of what is necessary in order to successfully implement TST. For instance, if the organization does not provide all the service elements necessary for TST, a plan for creating interagency agreements will be developed. This plan also spells out the mechanism for identifying which youth will be a part of the TST program, how many youth can be served at a given time, and how progress toward organizational goals will be tracked.

TST is delivered by a multidisciplinary team of providers who work in a tightly coordinated way. These providers represent the four core service elements of TST: skills-based psychotherapy, psychopharmacology, home- and community-based interventions, and legal advocacy. Each of these core elements is represented at the weekly TST treatment team meetings.

TST is delivered within a defined sequence of activities beginning with an *assessment process* to gather needed information, a *treatment planning process* to decide how to organize treatment based on the assessment information, a *treatment engagement process* to reach a good-enough agreement with the child and family on the treatment plan, and a *treatment implementation process* that delivers the treatment as defined within the agreed upon treatment plan. It is beyond the scope of this chapter to detail all aspects of this sequence. In the next sections, we provide an overview of these activities. All details are provided in the TST manual (Saxe et al. 2016).

17.2.1 Assessment

The TST assessment process seeks to gather all relevant information to make decisions about the focus of treatment. In this section, we will describe two categories of information that are perhaps most important for making these decisions: (1) the way a child shifts to *survival state* and (2) the characteristics of the child's *trauma system*. As defined in Sect. 17.1, there are often a great many plausible problems that might be addressed in treatment, given the complexity of children's responses to trauma. Which ones are most important? As will be detailed, we define the most important problems to address as those that lead to a child's shift to survival state (also called survival-in-the-moment state). Once assessed, it is often possible to determine specific environmental signals that the child and others may not even be aware of that repeatedly lead to survival states. As the child's survival state – by definition – involves the expression of extreme emotion and/or behavior related to survival, the ability to intervene to prevent these states will be among the most important components of intervention. What modalities of intervention will be effective to prevent survival states? This involves understanding the trauma system that – by definition – involves the interface between the child's shift to survival state and the capacity of those around the child to help and support them given their specific vulnerability. As will be described, the interventions chosen will depend on the specific interface between these two domains.

17.2.1.1 Assessing the Child's Shift to Survival State
Providers are trained to identify episodes of dysregulation. These are the moments when a child has lost control over their emotional and/or behavioral state. For a child with traumatic stress, what drives this loss of control are signals in the environment that are reminiscent of the past trauma experiences and lead to survival-laden emotion and defensive behavior to manage threat. Of note, these signals can be very subtle (e.g., an odor, a type of glance, a tone of voice) such that the child and others may not even be aware that the child's reactions are related to specific signals. Not all episodes of extreme emotion and/or behavior are related to survival or even a part of a dysregulation process. This must be assessed. The primary way this process is assessed within TST is with a method that we (and others) have called a *moment-by-moment assessment*.

A moment-by-moment assessment is conducted by focusing on the sequence of events surrounding an identified episode when the child was not in control of emotion and/or behavior. What was going on before the child was not in control of emotion and/or behavior? What was the child doing and feeling? What was the child aware of? What happened next? How did the child's state of emotion, behavior, and awareness shift? What notable stimuli were present in the child's environment immediately preceding this shift? This assessment is not only conducted with the child. Providers are trained to gather information from any observer of the episode. Providers are also trained to gather the facts around the episode without any presumptions about what might have led to the shift in emotion, behavior, and awareness. A TST provider is trained to solve a mystery: Why did this particular child lose control over emotion and/or behavior in this particular moment? We approach the solving of this mystery with the gathering of clues using the moment-by-moment assessment and train providers to resist all temptations to make assumptions without first gathering these clues or facts. Since the provider was (in most cases) not at the episode and was not at the traumatic event or events, we cannot presume knowledge of the signal that may have led to the survival state. We generate this knowledge by gathering the facts. A complete discussion of the moment-by-moment assessment and the tools used to conduct it is detailed in the TST manual (Saxe et al. 2016). This outline was provided in the service of communicating the basic logic of this assessment. Once the facts are gathered – in this way – about a specific episode, it may be possible to see patterns among specific signals and shift in emotional/behavioral state between episodes. As will be detailed in the treatment planning section, these patterns define the priority problems to be addressed in treatment.

17.2.1.2 Assessing the Child's Trauma System

Once we have knowledge about the child's pattern of shifting to survival state, we are in position to define the child's trauma system. As will be detailed in the treatment planning section, it is the knowledge of the trauma system that determines the modalities of intervention that will be needed. The trauma system is defined as the interface between two domains: (i) the child's tendency to shift to survival state and (ii) the capacity of those in the child's environment to help them with this tendency to shift to survival state. Each of these domains is assessed in three categories. These will be described next:

(a) *The child's survival state*: In rating the child's survival state, two questions are asked: Does the child shift to survival state at all? If the child shifts to survival state, does the child engage in dangerous or risky behavior in the survival state? The answer to these two questions places the child in one of the following three categories:
   (i) No survival states
   (ii) Survival states
   (iii) Dangerous survival states
(b) *The capacity of the social environment*: Two qualities of the social environment are rated: *help and protect. Help* connotes the capacity of those around the child to help the child manage emotion. It is based on the degree to which these individuals are attuned to the child's emotional state and able to help the child

maintain states of regulation. *Protect* connotes the capacity of those around the child to identify the specific signals that lead to survival state for the child and minimize the likelihood of exposure to these signals within the bounds of reality (and unless exposure to these signals is clinically indicated as part of the defined treatment plan). *Protect* not only connotes the protection of the child from signals that are reminiscent of past trauma experiences (but will not actually cause harm in the present), it also connotes the protection of the child from actual threats of harm. This distinction is extremely important for treatment planning/treatment implementation purposes, and TST providers are trained to carefully make this distinction. Thus, this assessment places the child's social environment in one of three categories:

(i) Helpful and protective
(ii) Insufficiently helpful and protective
(iii) Harmful (child can be exposed to actual threats)

Again, details of how these ratings are made are provided in the TST manual. In this section on TST assessment, we have focused on the two most important areas of assessment. TST assessment also includes other domains such as the child and family's priorities and goals, strengths, and plausible barriers to treatment engagement. Although each of these domains is very important for treatment planning, space considerations precluded their inclusion in this chapter.

17.2.2 Treatment Planning

Within TST, the defined treatment planning process is dedicated to making decisions about how the treatment will be implemented, based on the information gathered in the assessment process. In this chapter, we focus on two of the most important treatment planning decisions that are based on the assessment information gathered in the previous section. These decisions concern the phase of treatment that will be offered to the child and family and the priority problem or problems that will be addressed in that defined treatment phase. As will be detailed, TST treatment implementation is organized via three sequential treatment phases that fully define the interventions that are delivered. Accordingly, it is very important to accurately determine the child's phase of treatment.

17.2.2.1 Determining the TST Treatment Phase

The child's treatment phase is fully determined by the information assessed about the child's trauma system described in the previous section. The rating about the trauma system as recorded in a two-dimensional grid called the *TST Treatment Planning Grid*. This grid is shown in Fig.17.1. As can be seen the ratings of the child's shift to survival state and the environment's capacity to help and protect directly translate to a determination to one of three treatment phases. This should make intuitive sense as a child who shifts into dangerous survival states and lives in a harmful environment would be expected to need quite different intervention

	The Environment's Help and Protection		
TST Treatment Planning Grid	Helpful and Protective	Insufficiently Helpful and Protective	Harmful
The Child's Survival States — No Survival States	Beyond trauma	Beyond trauma	Safety-focused
Survival States	Regulation-focused	Regulation-focused	Safety-focused
Dangerous Survival States	Regulation-focused	Safety-focused	Safety-focused

Fig. 17.1 The TST treatment planning grid

modalities than a child who shifts to (non-dangerous) survival states but lives in a helpful and protective environment. The three phases of treatment will be detailed in the treatment implementation section. Briefly, they are:

(a) Safety-Focused Phase: focuses on creating safe and stable environments
(b) Regulation-Focused Phase: focuses on building emotional regulation skills
(c) Beyond Trauma Phase: focuses on gaining perspective about the trauma and living beyond it

17.2.2.2 Determining the TST Priority Problems

TST *priority problems* will become the primary targets of the treatment interventions and are based on the understanding gained via the assessment process about how and why a child will tend to shift to a survival state. Often these episodes of survival state are the reason the child is brought to treatment, but these episodes may be considered as completely disconnected events. The information gathered about these episodes through moment-by-moment assessments enables the possibility of seeing how they may be connected. Thus, we arrive at the definition of a TST priority problem: "patterns of links between a traumatized child's perception of threat in the present environment and the child's transition to a survival state" (Saxe et al. 2016, p. 192). The TST providers and their teams are trained to examine at least three episodes with moment-by-moment assessments and aim to determine patterns of perceived threat and consequential shift to survival states between these episodes. These patterns are then used to define the TST priority problem (or problems). In order to help providers see these patterns, we have created a worksheet called the *TST Priority Problem Form* to record information about the episodes of dysregulation and to abstract the themes that may then define a given priority problem (see Fig. 17.2). The details of completing this complex form are given in the manual (Saxe et al. 2016); the following outline how the form is used. We will provide an example of the use of this form later in this chapter.

TST Priority Problem Form

Environment-Present Threat (from *E-Present Revving*)

Survival-in-the-Moment response (from 3A's Re-experiencing)

Episode 1 | Information about Environment-Past that may inform response to Environment-Present | Episode 1

Episode 2 | Theme of E-Present Threat | Theme of Survival-in-the-Moment response | Episode 2

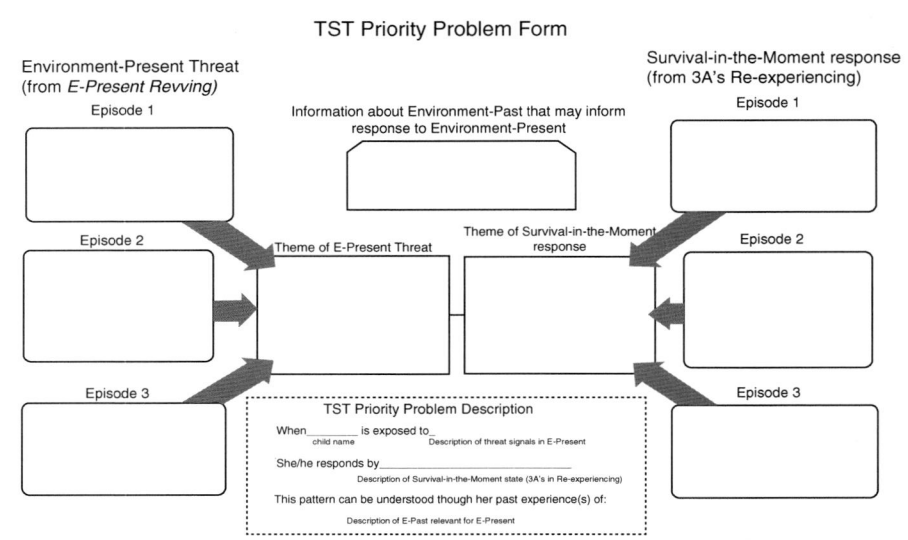

Episode 3 | Episode 3

TST Priority Problem Description
When_____ is exposed to_____
   child name   Description of threat signals in E-Present
She/he responds by_____
                    Description of Survival-in-the-Moment state (3A's in Re-experiencing)
This pattern can be understood though her past experience(s) of:
                    Description of E-Past relevant for E-Present

TST Priority Problems: Patterns of links between the thaumatized child,s perception of threat in the present environment and the child's transition to a Survival-in-the-Moment state.

Fig. 17.2 TST priority problem form

(a) The three boxes on the left (labeled Environment Present Threat) are meant to record information from each of three moment-by-moment assessments of the environmental information that directly preceded the shift in survival state.
(b) The three boxes on the right (labeled Survival-in-the-Moment state) are meant to record information about the child's emotional/behavior when this shift in state occurred for each of those moment-by-moment assessments.
(c) The two middle boxes (labeled Theme of E-Present and Theme of Survival-in-the-Moment) are meant to record possible common environmental and emotional/behavioral themes, respectively, from the three identified episodes. As detailed, it is the abstraction of these themes that will define the priority problem.
(d) The box at the top ("Information about Environment Past") is to examine the child's history of trauma and to infer what about that history may have primed the child to shift to survival state in the face of the environmental stimuli identified. In TST we call this trauma inference.
(e) The box at the bottom (TST Priority Problem Description) enables providers and teams to have a common way of describing the TST priority problems defined through this process.

Once the treatment phase and priority problems are defined through the treatment planning process, providers and teams are about ready to begin to implement treatment. They have, however, one last process to insert before they are ready to go. We define this process as Ready Set Go, and it describes how children and families are engaged in treatment.

17.2.3 Treatment Engagement (Ready Set Go)

Throughout the assessment process, the team is gathering information to understand the child and caregivers in order to understand them from the perspective of their motivations, priorities, strengths, frustrations, and fears. It is only through developing a genuine sense of caring and understanding that the team can gain the trust and partnership necessary to engage youth and families in treatment. This is accomplished by understanding what is most important to them from their perspective, what are their biggest *sources of pain*, and developing an agreement about how working together can address these concerns. Ready Set Go process is captured in the *treatment agreement* letter (Saxe et al. 2016, p. 435). More information about this can be found in the next section.

17.2.4 Phase-Based Intervention

Each of the three phases of treatment has a distinct focus and is accompanied by two guides which anchor and organize the work of the TST team:

(a) Safety-Focused Treatment: The goals of this phase are to ensure the youth is in an adequately safe environment and to diminish the likelihood a child will shift into a dangerous survival state by improving his or her ability to recognize and manage their reactions, and/or by improving the caregiver's capacity to be helpful and protective, or help get the child to an environment that has the capacity to provide sufficient help and protection for a child with dangerous survival states. Service advocacy is often a main focus of intervention in the safety-focused phase. Safety-focused treatment is typically provided in the home and/or community. Two guides are used in this phase: the safety-focused guide to organize and coordinate the work of the team and the HELPers guide to be used directly with the caregiver to help them build skills and get support to manage their own needs (Saxe et al. 2016, p. 441–455).

(b) Regulation-Focused Treatment: The focus of this phase is on building children's skills regulating emotion so that they don't switch to survival states when a threat signal is perceived – or if a survival state begins, they are able to use skills or accept help to switch back again to a regulated state. A child in this phase is not at risk of engaging in dangerous behavior if triggered, and the environment is not harmful to the child. Regulation-focused treatment is centered on psycho-education about trauma and trauma reactions and the building of skills to recognize and manage survival states. These skills are taught to the child, and the child's plan for using these skills is shared with key adults in that child's life who are in a position to help that child to cope. Regulation-focused treatment is typically provided in an office, as home-based stabilization is no longer required. Engaging caregiver in regulation-focused treatment is critical. Two guides are used in this phase: the regulation-focused guide, which helps to coordinate the work of the team around choosing appropriate skills and planning to share these coping strategies with others, and the managing emotions guide (MEG) which helps a child learn to understand that there is a pattern to their survival state reactions, which they can learn to recognize. The MEG is organized around the three As and the four Rs and helps a child learn to recognize and manage their changes in state. Both guides can be found in the TST manual (Saxe et al. 2016, p. 456–466).

(c) Beyond Trauma Treatment: A child in the beyond trauma phase no longer experiences survival states and lives in an environment that is helpful, protective, nurturing, and safe. This does not mean, however, that there is no longer a need for intervention. The child may still be impacted by their prior experiences of both traumatic events and survival in the moment states. Children may be plagued by negative views of themselves, others, and their future. Similarly, caregivers may harbor beliefs that their child is damaged or may never have a normal life. The primary goals of beyond trauma treatment are to help a child and their caregivers move forward from the trauma, so that it does not define the child's sense of self and others and so that the child does not feel limited by or held back by their past. This phase also addresses how the child and family can achieve lasting meaning from the experience of trauma, which can help to develop a positive and hopeful sense of future that does not require the ongoing involvement of a treatment team.

Treatment is provided by experienced mental health clinicians with training in these trauma-specific interventions and who can facilitate gradual exposure via a trauma narrative (which is specifically designed to address both single incident and chronic trauma) and provide cognitive restructuring skills. Caregivers are an integral part of treatment in this phase, which is conducted in the office. There are two guides used on beyond trauma treatment: the Beyond Trauma Guide (Saxe et al. 2016, p.479), which organizes the treatment and includes a template for the trauma narrative, and the Cognitive Awareness Log (Saxe et al. 2016, p. 491), which is a tool for helping children to recognize and change maladaptive cognitions.

17.2.5 Case Example Emily

Identifying Information and Referral Concern

Emily is a 10-year-old girl who lives with a foster family. She recently disclosed to a teacher that she had been repeatedly sexually abused by her mother's boyfriend (Jerry), while her mother was at home. A child protective services (CPS) investigation was initiated, and Emily was removed from her home as her mother was found to have failed to protect her. Charges were filed against Jerry. At the time of the referral for mental health services, the legal proceedings were ongoing including a court-ordered forensic evaluation and an order of protection against Jerry. Emily's foster mother requested that Emily receive mental health support following several incidents in which Emily banged her head against a wall and made statements about wanting to die. Emily's foster parents appear to genuinely care for Emily, but at times, they seem overwhelmed by her behavior. The team has some concerns about the potential for placement disruption if Emily's behavioral dyscontrol is not able to be reduced.

Emily is in the fourth grade and receives special education services. Although Emily's problematic behavior tends to occur outside of school, her teachers worry that Emily often seems withdrawn or distracted. Emily appears to want to establish friendships but has difficulties maintaining relationships. Both Emily's foster parents and her teachers describe her as smart and artistically and athletically talented.

Assessment and Treatment Planning
The child welfare agency which placed Emily in a home has a trauma systems therapy program where both the child welfare and mental health staff use the model to guide their interventions. The TST team, which consists of caseworkers, social work clinicians, a community-based psychiatrist, and a team leader, reviewed the referral and determined that given Emily's trauma history and her problems regulating her emotional and behavioral states (which appear plausibly related to her trauma history), she was a good fit for inclusion in the TST program.

During the assessment process, the team focused on gathering information about Emily's episodes of problematic behavior (using the moment-by-moment assessment process), the impact of this problematic behavior on Emily and others in her social environment, and the ability of others around Emily to help and to protect her when she shifts into dangerous survival states. During the assessment process, the team also evaluated whether there are additional needs that may be impacting Emily and her family. There is a shared understanding between the team and the family of what the problem is (head banging, passive suicidal ideation statements, maladaptive beliefs that Emily "destroyed her family"), so the task of the team is to systematically gather data about what may have led to shifts in Emily's behavior in specific moments. The goal is to connect the dots between episodes or moments of problematic behavior to identify a pattern between Emily's perception of threat in her environment and her shift into a dangerous survival state.

The clinician worked with Emily and her foster family using the MMA process to form the TST priority problem (see Fig.17.3). The team identified three instances of problematic behavior and gathered information from Emily and her foster parents about what Emily was doing, feeling, and focused on just prior to the shift in her behavior and what was happening in the environment that may have provoked the shift in Emily's behavior. The team also gathered information about what factors in the environment may have helped to maintain her shift into a dangerous survival state. Through this process, the team discovered that Emily bangs her head or punches herself and expresses passive wishes to die after she is exposed to situations in which she feels disloyal to her biological family for disclosing being sexually abused. This pattern can be understood through Emily's past experiences of sexual assault from her mother's boyfriend, subsequent removal from her home following disclosure, and being told by her mother that she "ruined" their family.

TST Priority Problem Worksheet

Perceived Threat in Present Environment	Past Trauma Environment	Shift to Survival State
Episode 1: During a phone call with her biological mother, Emily's mother said, "How can you be so sure that Jerry did it? He's been so nice to you."	Repeated Sexual abuse by mother,s boyfriend, while mom was in the apartment. After Emily disclosed the abuse to a teacher and was subsequently removed by Child Protective Services, Emily's mother told her that she "destroyed their family"	**Episode 1**: Emily banged her head against her bedroom wall and stated that she wants to die.
Episode 2: Emily was interviewed by the police and a forensic psychologist about her sexual abuse allegation.	**Pattern of Perceived Threat**: Situations in which Emily Feels disloyal to her family for disclosing sexual abuse.	**Pattern of Survival-in-the-Moment**: Feeling like she needs to be punished. Emily bangs her head and punches herself. Emily also expresses wishes to die (passive suicidal ideation).	**Episode 2**: Emily banged her head against the car window on the way home from the interview.
Episode 3: Emily was watching a movie on TV in which the main character expressed the importance of family loyalty, "Families first, no matter what".		**Episode 3**: Emily started sobbing, ran into her bedroom where she punched herself and stated that she "just wants to die."

TST Priority Problem Statement

When ____Emily____ is exposed to __Situations where she feels disloyal to her family for disclosing sexual abuse__,
          Child,s name   Description of perceived threat

She/he responds by __Feeling like she needs to be punished and die, She bangs her head and punches herself__.
                                  Description of Survival State

This pattern can be understood through past experience(s) of:
Sexual abuse by mother,s boyfriend, disclosure of abuse and removal from home, told by mother that she "destroyed" their family.
Description of past trauma to inform related to Survival State

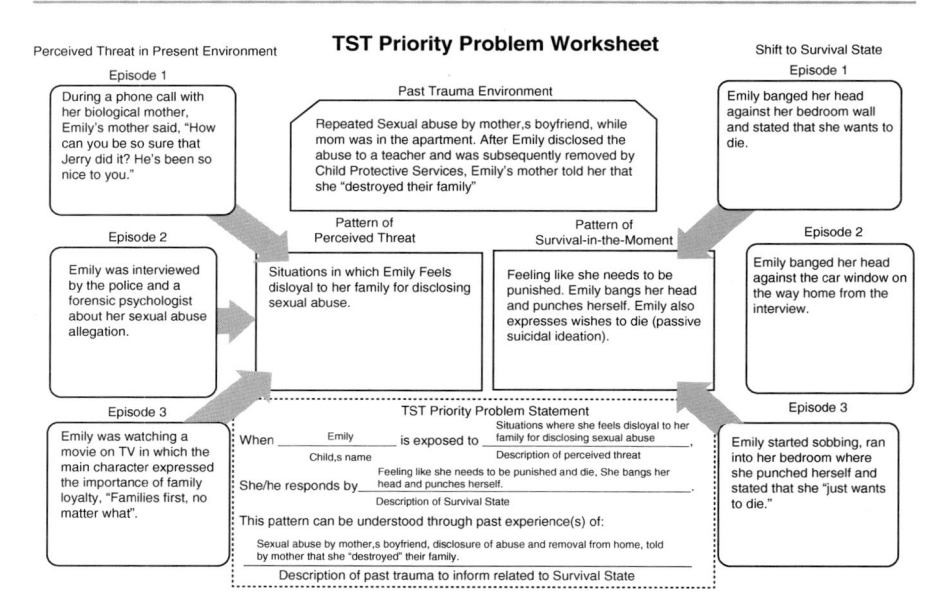

Fig. 17.3 Emily's priority problem worksheet

Although not the highest priority to address, the team also identified other problems to address during treatment including maladaptive beliefs and cognitions (e.g., "If I hadn't told anyone, everything would have been ok"), social difficulties, and withdrawal and distractibility at school.

After the team also categorized the trauma system, Emily's vulnerability to shift to survival states was rated as "dangerous" given that when she perceived threat in her present environment, she experienced shifts in emotional/behavioral state that included dangerous behaviors (head banging). The team rated the social environment as insufficiently helpful and protective. The team considered the multiple social environments in which Emily routinely interacts and rated the environment based on the most problematic setting. Emily continued to be exposed to upsetting stimuli including communications of blame from her biological mother. In addition, although Emily's foster parents were committed to getting support for Emily, at the time of the assessment process, they did not have the requisite skills to help Emily regulate her behavior. Using the TST Treatment Planning Grid (Fig.17.4), the team determined that Emily will initiate treatment in the *safety-focused phase* of treatment.

Prior to initiating the safety-focused interventions, the TST team shared their treatment strategy with Emily and her foster family in the form of a treatment agreement letter to ensure that there is shared agreement and documented accountability of what everyone, including the TST team, will do as part of treatment.

Phase-Based Interventions

Emily began treatment in the *safety-focused (SF)* phase of treatment. During this phase, the majority of treatment was provided by home-based care providers

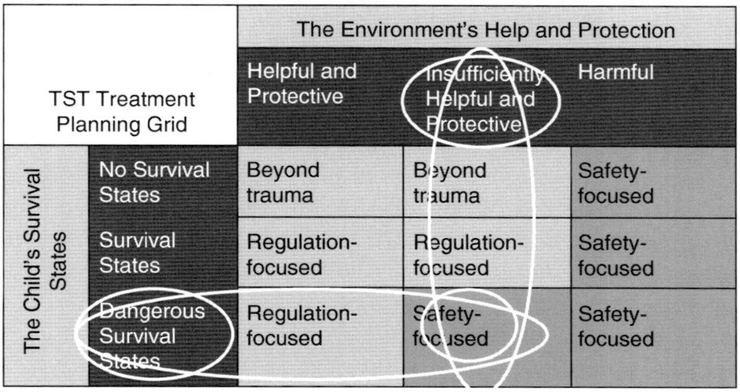

17 Trauma Systems Therapy for Children and Adolescents

TST Treatment Planning Grid		The Environment's Help and Protection		
		Helpful and Protective	Insufficiently Helpful and Protective	Harmful
The Child's Survival States	No Survival States	Beyond trauma	Beyond trauma	Safety-focused
	Survival States	Regulation-focused	Regulation-focused	Safety-focused
	Dangerous Survival States	Regulation-focused	Safety-focused	Safety-focused

Fig. 17.4 *The TST treatment planning grid* for Emily, indicating her current treatment phase

(caseworker) with close involvement from mental health clinicians on the TST team. The emphasis of treatment during this phase was twofold. The first was to protect Emily from situations where she is made to feel that she has "destroyed" her family (i.e., improve the environment so that it is no longer harmful). This component of treatment was accomplished by identifying the types of situations that lead to survival state (i.e., situations in which Emily perceives that she has been disloyal to her family) and helping the foster parents to reduce Emily's exposure to these situations and to teach the parents concrete strategies to help Emily when exposure to these situations is unavoidable. The team worked with the Department of Social Services to monitor and limit contact with Emily's biological mother. The team also worked with the TST legal advocate to ensure that Emily was only interviewed when absolutely necessary as part of the forensic proceedings. The second emphasis during SF treatment was on helping Emily and her foster parents learn skills to bolster their ability to help Emily improve her regulation capacity. As Emily's head banging was of significant concern, the team and specifically the home-based provider worked with Emily to teach replacement behaviors including throwing a bean bag against a wall, pacing back and forth in the hallway, and drinking ice water. The home-based care providers completed the *HELPers guide* with the foster parents to plan for dangerous survival states, learn strategies to handle difficult moments, and teach concrete coping skills to help regulate their own emotional reactions. The home-based providers taught Emily's foster parents strategies of what they can do and whom they can reach out if and when Emily engages in dysregulated and dangerous behavior. Through using the *HELPers guide*, Emily's foster parents were able to gain skills to help Emily reduce dangerous behaviors and to protect Emily from perceived threats in the environment. Importantly, as Emily was no longer exhibiting dangerous survival states, her foster parents became much more hopeful about their ability to safely maintain Emily in their home, and they were much more able to focus on Emily's positive behaviors. The work in SF treatment lasted about 2 months, at which time Emily's behavior was sufficiently regulated and her environment was sufficiently helpful and protective to transition to regulation-focused treatment. During SF treatment, the TST home-based provider met with Emily and her foster mother in their home twice per week.

Emily transitioned to the *regulation-focused (RF)* phase of treatment once her social environment became adequately helpful and protective, and Emily no longer exhibited dangerous survival states. In addition to Emily's foster parents gaining skills to help and protect Emily, the forensic interviews had been completed, and thus Emily was no longer exposed to traumatic reminders inherent in the interview process. In order to maintain the social environmental safety achieved during SF treatment and to provide an opportunity to build Emily's emotional regulation skills, communication with Emily's biological mother was limited during regulation-focused treatment. During the SF treatment, Emily's biological mother did not exhibit willingness to modify her behavior related to communicating to Emily that she has harmed her family for reporting Jerry's abuse. The team also suspected that Emily's biological mother had ongoing contact with Jerry. Emily continued to display survival states but no longer engaged in dangerous behavior.

While the TST home-based team continued to supervise contact between Emily and her birth mother, the majority of the TST phase-based interventions took place at the clinic. Emily began to meet with a clinician for individual sessions, and the same clinician also met regularly with Emily's foster parents. The TST clinician anchored her work with Emily on building emotional regulation skills when Emily is reminded of her sexual abuse, particularly in instances where she feels disloyal to her family for disclosing the abuse. As reflected in the priority problem, in those instances, Emily can feel that she has "destroyed" her family or origin and she is vulnerable to shifting to a dangerous survival states. The TST clinician used the *Managing Emotion Guide* to help Emily and her foster parents understand exactly how Emily switches to survival states and how to use that understanding to increase regulation and then to share that knowledge among all relevant caregivers. The clinician helped Emily and her foster parents learn how to promote regulation and use skills to help Emily become re-regulated in times when she notices herself become dysregulated. Throughout this phase, the clinician engaged Emily and her foster parents in the MMA process to continue to hone the understanding of how and why Emily experiences these shifts. As a result of this ongoing work, the clinician was able to help the family identify which emotional regulation skills helped to maintain Emily's regulatory states and what skills helped to transition Emily back to a regulated state. For example, if Emily was becoming dysregulated, she could color a mandala, do the "being a noodle" muscle relaxation exercise, or dance around her room to her favorite playlist. Similarly, the clinician worked with the foster parents and Emily to come up with what they can help Emily do when she was revved including reminding her to try the "being a noodle" activity, allowing her to play music in her room, and validating her conflicted feelings regarding disclosing the abuse.

Emily was able to move to the *beyond trauma (BT)* phase of treatment once she and her foster parents developed the requisite RF skills such that Emily no longer shifted into survival states. The RF phase lasted approximately 2 months, during which time the TST team was also able to help the foster parents continue to maintain stability and safety within Emily's social environment. The majority of the BT interventions took place at the clinic with Emily's primary clinician who continued to work with Emily and her foster parents. During BT, the clinician first worked to strengthen Emily's cognitive skills. Through the MMA and TST assessment process, the team was able to identify a number of maladaptive beliefs that Emily held about her trauma and herself (e.g., "I destroyed my family by telling on Jerry"; "If I hadn't told anyone, everything would have been ok"; "I am broken."). These cognitions were unhelpful to her and caused her to feel sad and to withdraw. While these worries no longer lead to survival states, Emily continued to feel very sad and sometimes withdrew from activities when she felt this way. The team also perceived that these beliefs were interfering with Emily's social relationships. The team worked with Emily to help her learn to notice when she had thoughts that were unhelpful or inaccurate and helped her develop alternative ways of thinking that were more helpful. The team continued to work with the foster parents around how best to help Emily when she felt sad and began to withdraw.

Once Emily learned to recognize unhelpful thoughts and how to replace them with more helpful thoughts, the clinician worked with Emily to develop a single-incident trauma narrative. The clinician determined that Emily and her foster parents had developed the requisite emotional regulation skills during RF in order to prepare Emily to engage in the gradual exposure work. Although Emily was subjected to multiple incidents of sexual abuse, they occurred within a defined period of time, and thus the clinician determined that a single-incident approach was more appropriate than a chronic trauma narrative. At this point, individual psychotherapy sessions focused on helping Emily to tell the story of her traumatic experience, using the Beyond Trauma Guide to help shape the development of her narrative (this guide provides a template for creating the narrative, with specific chapter headings and guidelines). As Emily completed the trauma narrative and processing work with her therapist, the therapist concurrently worked with Emily's foster parent to prepare them for Emily to ultimately share her narrative with them. Although actively engaged and genuinely wanting to help Emily, the foster parents expressed some discomfort with the idea of hearing the narrative and wondered if it would be best if "she could just forget what happened." The clinician met separately with the foster parents for several meetings to prepare them to hear the narrative and on ways to best support Emily during the process. As Emily completed the narrative work, she decided that she would like to make a comic book to help other kids who have "had horrible stuff happen to them too" and share what she learned as part of TST. Through the process of making the comic book, Emily was able to make meaning out of what happened to her and move towards living a life that is not defined by her traumatic experiences.

The team determined that given the biological mother's ongoing blame and disbelief in the value of talking about the sexual abuse with Emily, it would be more clinically appropriate for Emily to share the narrative with her foster parents. The team referred Emily's biological mother for her own mental health treatment to address her ongoing unresolved feelings and reactions to Emily's sexual abuse. Although Emily's biological mother was unable to fully participate in the narrative work, with the support of the team, she entered her own individual mental health treatment. The child welfare agency continued to work with Emily's mother to reinstate more frequently supervised visits and eventually worked up to unsupervised overnight weekend visits. The team continues to plan for Emily's eventual return to her biological mother, and in the interim Emily has developed a close and safe relationship with her foster family, which helps her to experience signals of care and to avoid survival states while the plan is being carried out.

Figure 17.3 shows Emily's priority problem based on 3 moment-by-moment assessments, and Fig. 17.4 shows her initial phase at the beginning of TST treatment.

17.3 Special Challenges

One of the biggest challenges to effective implementation of any model is creating a balance between maintaining model fidelity, while encouraging adaptations designed to meet the needs of specific populations and the various settings where services are delivered. The TST development team has addressed this important need by creating a process of collaborative innovation. Based on the concept of lead user innovation (von Hippel 2005), we believe that adaptations to our treatment approach are best conceived of by the people implementing that model in real-world settings.

We have developed a "community of innovators," who, through collaboration with the development team, have developed a number of TST adaptations. At the time of this writing, TST has been disseminated and is being currently implemented in twelve US states, the District of Columbia, and the country of Singapore. Adaptations have been developed for specialized population including refugee children and families, traumatized youth with comorbid substance abuse, and unaccompanied alien minors. TST has been adapted for various service settings as well, including child welfare, residential treatment centers, hospitals, outpatient clinics, shelters, community-based prevention programs, and school-based mental health programs. Each adaptation adheres to key features of TST, while making crucial changes necessary to meet the individualized needs of the population and setting, demonstrating the concept of "flexibility within fidelity" (Kendall and Beidas 2007). For more information about TST adaptations, please see our manual (Saxe et al. 2016) and our website (www.traumasystemstherapy.com).

Another challenge commonly encountered when implementing treatment for childhood trauma is lack of commitment and follow-through with the treatment process on the part of both children and caregivers. It is common to attribute this to qualities of the youth and families. While this may be true in some cases, it is equally important to consider whether there has been a failure on the part of the clinician to adequately engage these children and their caregivers in the treatment process. To address this, TST includes a specific engagement strategy, which we call *Ready Set Go* (RSG). This begins during the assessment process and includes gathering detailed information from both the child and caregiver about their goals and priorities. In order to engage someone in a meaningful way, it is imperative to know what is most important to them and what gets in the way of achieving what is most important. We refer to this as the person's "major source of pain." If the child and caregiver come to believe that working with the team will help to alleviate their source of pain and achieve their goal, they are much more likely to trust the team, keep commitments, and engage fully in the process. True treatment engagement in TST is achieved when there is a mutually agreed upon understanding of the problem and the way in which the team will work together to solve the problem. This agreement is captured in writing on a form called the *TST treatment agreement letter*. This is a document which is initially created by the team as a draft, based on their work with the family. It is then shared at a meeting with the child and caregivers, where it is reviewed. If anyone has objections or suggestions, changes are made. Once there is full agreement, all team members sign the letter, and it becomes the guide for the rest of the work.

Another important challenge we have encountered involves the specific context in which youth exposed to abuse and neglect most commonly come into contact with child-serving professionals: the child welfare system. Children and families involved with the child welfare system have almost by definition experienced trauma, both because of the maltreatment that brings them into contact with the system and the invasive nature of system involvement itself. The child welfare system is particularly challenging in that it is not, as the name might imply, a well-defined system with clearly articulated processes and mechanisms for meeting the needs of the youth in its care. Typically, children who receive services in the child welfare system come into contact with multiple providers from different aspects of the system, including child protection, family court, social services, and private agencies that are contracted by the child welfare system to provide mental health, preventive services, and foster care. Treatment and service approaches are provided within and between organizations that have their own needs and mandates. Over time, organizations develop cultures related to the conduct of their work. The public mandate of the child welfare system – a compulsory system – is quite different than the mental health system – a voluntary system; accordingly, providers within these systems will prioritize different aspects of the work and have different relationships with families. Additionally, when public agencies contract for services, the fit between a given treatment or service and the way services are financed, supported, and sustained within an organization is pivotal; inadequate fit between a treatment or service approach and the way the organization finances and provides services makes desired outcomes unlikely.

Addressing trauma-related mental health needs of children in the child welfare system requires effective approaches to integrating the two systems. Additionally, addressing the trauma-related needs of children is not solely about linking them with appropriate treatment services. Rather, many different child welfare practices and activities exist, from preparing and supporting foster parents to working with other stakeholders such as the judicial system, that must also be informed by the impact of trauma. Given the different mandates and workplace cultures between child welfare and mental health, successful approaches must also be able to "speak both languages" and provide value to the needs of both child welfare and mental health professionals and the organizations for which they work.

TST uniquely addresses these needs by creating a structure for integrating the various service system providers to facilitate them working together as an integrated team.

TST provides a common language for understanding the needs of child welfare involved youth and families and requires that they all participate in the TST treatment team meetings, with team members from various parts of the system each providing a specified role in addressing the TST priority problem. In addition, we have developed specific tools to train case workers and foster parents to use the TST approach to understand and meaningfully impact the children in their care (Saxe et al. 2011).

The specific nature of service provision within TST presents several unique challenges. These include the provision of home-based as well as office-based services, as well as the creation of a closely integrated multidisciplinary team. These elements are required for TST and are funded via leveraging existing resources, so as not to require grant funding, which is typically not sustainable. The provision of multiple services is often accomplished via creating interagency agreements.

17.4 Research and Evidence

The first study that initially demonstrated TST's efficacy was an open trial conducted at two sites: a child psychiatry outpatient clinic of a large, urban general hospital and a joint program of countywide departments of mental health and social services in rural upstate New York (Saxe et al. 2005). Each site had a team trained in TST, which was implementing prior to the study. One hundred and ten children aged 5 to 20 years old ($M = 11.2$, $SD = 3.6$) and their families were enrolled in treatment. The Child and Adolescent Needs and Strengths-Trauma Exposure and Adaptation Version (CANS-TEA; Kisiel et al. 2009) was used as the primary treatment outcome measure after TST had been delivered for 3 months. For those children who remained in treatment (82, 72 % of the enrolled sample), improvement was found in PTSD symptoms, emotion regulation, behavior regulation, caregiver's physical and mental health, caregiver psychosocial support and stability, and social environmental stability. Positive changes in children's functioning were also strongly and positively correlated with changes in those dimensions that are specifically targeted by TST (e.g., ER and stability of the social environment). Moreover, 58 % of the children transitioned from more to less intensive phases of treatment during the 3 months of the study.

The aforementioned joint program in upstate New York was the end result of the first successful TST dissemination effort (Hansen et al. 2009). The adoption and implementation of TST came to fruition after the program's realization that:

1. The primary reason for referral was "environmental/family dysregulation" as opposed to more isolated psychiatric disorders in the child being referred for services (e.g., oppositional defiant disorder, conduct disorder, PTSD)
2. The majority of referred cases had histories of trauma, including abuse, neglect, and extreme poverty
3. The clinical model used at the time had proven to be ineffective at providing services to these families, who presented as stressed, unable to organize themselves, and unable to keep members safe
4. Resource barriers for the families (e.g., lack of childcare and/or transportation) and a general mistrust of the system that resulted in poor engagement in therapy.

As a consequence, the program decided to incorporate TST into its overall treatment framework, which also includes aspects of play therapy and cognitive behavior therapy. Recent evaluation data provide empirical support for the program's clinical as well as cost effectiveness (Ellis et al. 2011). Across a 15-month period, 124 children between 3 and 20 years old who had experienced three to nine potentially traumatic events received TST. Measures of clinical course (hospitalization, need for intensive vs. office-based services) and children's psychiatric and psychosocial functioning and social-environmental stability were taken at intake, 4–6 months (early treatment), and 12–15 months (late treatment). Cost savings were evaluated through a comparison of pre- and post-implementation hospitalization rates and lengths of stay for all children under the care of the county mental health department. Emotion regulation, social environmental stability, and child functioning/strengths improved significantly over the course of treatment. Early treatment improvement in child functioning/strengths and social environmental stability were associated with overall improvement in emotion regulation across the duration of the intervention. Children who were able to transition from crisis stabilization to office-based services during early treatment tended to stay in treatment and improve through late treatment. For the 72 % of youth who completed treatment, the need for crisis stabilization services at 15 months was reduced by over 50 %. Compared to children served prior to the implementation of TST, hospitalization rates were 36 % lower and the average length of stay was 23 % lower.

Such short- and long-term gains cannot be attained unless children and families are actively engaged early in treatment. Initial findings indicate that *Ready Set Go!*, the engagement approach used in TST, is associated with high levels of treatment retention (Saxe et al. 2011). In a small, randomized controlled trial of traumatized youth ($N = 20$), 90 % of TST participants were still in treatment, whereas only 10 % of "treatment-as-usual" participants remained at the 3-month assessment (Saxe et al. 2011). While preliminary evidence for the effectiveness of TST is promising, the initial RCT could not be completed since 90 % of the treatment as usual sample did not complete treatment. Although the results of this study were encouraging about treatment engagement, no conclusions can be drawn about outcomes. Currently a new randomized trial of TST is under way, and a large independent evaluation of TST for foster care – using a quasi-experimental design – has recently been completed, and preliminary results look very promising.

References

Bronfenbrenner U (1979) The ecology of human development. Harvard University Press, Cambridge, MA

Cicchetti D, Toth SL (1995) A developmental psychopathology perspective on child abuse and neglect. J Am Acad Child Adolesc Psychiatry 34(5):541–565

Ellis BH, Fogler J, Hansen S, Beckman M, Forbes P, Navalta CP (2011)Trauma systems therapy: 15-month outcomes and the importance of effecting environmental change. Psychol Trauma Theory Res Pract Policy Adv online publication. doi: 10.1037/a0025192

Frewen PA, Lanius RA (2006) Toward a psychobiology of posttraumatic self-dysregulation: reexperiencing, hyperarousal, dissociation, and emotional numbing. In: Yehuda R, Yehuda R (eds) Psychobiology of posttraumaticstress disorders: a decade of progress, vol 1071. Blackwell Publishing, Malden, pp. 110–124

Hansen S, Saxe G, Drewes AA (2009) Trauma systems therapy: a replication of the model, integrating cognitive behavioral play therapy into child and family treatment. In: Blending play therapy with cognitive behavioral therapy: evidence-based and other effective treatments and techniques. Wiley, Hoboken, pp. 139–164

Henggeler SW, Schoenwald SK, Rowland MD, Cunningham PB (2002) Serious emotional disturbance in children and adolescents: multisystemictherapy

Hopper JW, Frewen PA, van der Kolk BA, Lanius RA (2007) Neural correlates of reexperiencing, avoidance, and dissociation in PTSD: symptom dimensions and emotion dysregulation in responses to script-driven trauma imagery. J Traumatic Stress 20(5):713–25

Kendall PC, Beidas RS (2007) Smoothing the trail for dissemination of evidence-based practices for youth: flexibility within fidelity. Professional Psychology: Research and Practice 38(1):13–20

Kendall PC, Gosch E, Furr JM, Sood E (2008) Flexibility within fidelity. J Am Acad Child Adolesc Psychiatry 47(9):987–993

Kisiel C, Blaustein ME, Fogler J, Ellis BH, Saxe GN (2009) Treating children with traumatic experiences: understanding and assessing needs and strengths. Rep Emot Behav Disord Youth 9(1):13–19(17)

Lau A, Weisz J (2003) Reported maltreatment among clinic-referred children: implications for presenting problems, treatment attrition, and long-term outcomes. J Am Acad Child Adolesc Psychiatry 42:1327–1334

Pumariega AJ, Winters NC (2003) Handbook of child and adolescent systems of care: the new community psychiatry. Jossey-Bass, San Francisco

Saxe GN, Ellis BH, Fogler J, Hansen S, Sorkin B (2005) Comprehensive care for traumatized children. Psychiatric Annals 35(5):443–48

Saxe GN, Ellis BH, Fogler J, Navalta CP (2012) Preliminary evidence for effective family engagement in treatment for child traumatic stress: Trauma systems therapy approach to preventing dropout. Child Adolesc Mental Health 17(1):58–61. doi:10.1111/j.1475–3588.2011.00626.x

Saxe GN, Ellis BH, Brown AB (2016) Trauma systems therapy for children and teens, 2nd edn. Guilford Press, New York

von Hippel EA (2005) Democratizing innovation. MIT Press, Cambridge

Wethington HR, Hahn RA, Fuqua-Whitley DS, Sipe TA, Crosby AE, Johnson RL, Chattopadhyay SK (2008) The effectiveness of interventions to reduce psychological harm from traumatic events among children and adolescents: a systematic review. Am J Prev Med 35:287–313

Pharmacological Treatment for Children and Adolescents with Trauma-Related Disorders

18

Julia Huemer, Michael Greenberg, and Hans Steiner

18.1 Theoretical Underpinnings and Evidence

Across the scope of treatment for pediatric PTSD, the limited research examining the efficacy of pharmacotherapy has focused on interventions within four classifications: second-generation antipsychotics, mood stabilizers, selective serotonin reuptake inhibitors, and antiadrenergic medications. While each classification varied in its depth of research and significance in open or randomized controlled trials (RCTs), the overall evidence to substantiate pharmacological interventions is often weak and often more dependent on results obtained from adult populations. The following section outlines the most common pharmacological interventions used in children and adolescents with PTSD, along with the research done to validate usage.

18.1.1 Selective Serotonin Reuptake Inhibitors (SSRIs)

Despite being one of the first lines of treatment for treating pediatric PTSD, research on the effectiveness of SSRIs is mixed. Based on evidence for their efficacy in adults, SSRIs were theorized to be beneficial in the treatment of children with PTSD (Tareen

---

[$]Equal contribution as first authors.

J. Huemer, MD (✉)
Department of Child and Adolescent Psychiatry, Medical University of Vienna,
Währinger Gürtel 18-20, 1090 Vienna, Austria
e-mail: julia.huemer@meduniwien.ac.at

M. Greenberg, MA
The Wright Institute, 2728 Durant Ave, Berkeley, CA 94704, USA

H. Steiner, MD
Department of Psychiatry and Behavioral Sciences, Stanford University School of Medicine,
401 Quarry Road, 94305 Stanford, CA, USA

© Springer International Publishing Switzerland 2017
M.A. Landolt et al. (eds.), *Evidence-Based Treatments for Trauma Related Disorders in Children and Adolescents*, DOI 10.1007/978-3-319-46138-0_18

et al. 2007). In the overall context of pediatric pharmacotherapy, 95 % of child psychiatrists use SSRIs and alpha-adrenergic agonists in the treatment of PTSD (Cohen et al. 2001). SSRIs are typically recommended for treating a broad range of symptoms (anxiety and depression) and for improving social and occupational functioning (Donnelly 2003). SSRIs are used to target the reexperiencing, avoidance, and numbing symptoms that are characteristic of PTSD (Cohen et al. 2001). Despite their prevalent use in pediatric pharmacology, 20–30 % of patients (children and adolescents) show little to no benefit from SSRI treatment (Rapp et al. 2013). The most typical SSRIs used to treat pediatric PTSD are sertraline, fluoxetine, and citalopram.

The SSRI sertraline for pediatric PTSD has been tested in two RCTs, both of which failed to demonstrate a significant effect; additionally, sertraline was used in a secondary preventive approach in a third RCT (Stoddard et al. 2011). The first RCT with sertraline compared a flexibly dosed (50–200 mg daily) plus trauma-focused CBT treatment group to a placebo and trauma-focused CBT group of 24 children and adolescents (Cohen et al. 2007). Following 12 weeks of treatment, no single group demonstrated a significant effect over the other. The other RCTs by Robb et al. (2008) examined the results of placebo versus sertraline treatment in 131 children and adolescents with PTSD symptoms. After 10 weeks of treatment, no significant difference in the primary outcome measure (UCLA PTSD-I Score) was found between the two groups. Despite the fact that sertraline has demonstrated efficacy in both adult and pediatric populations with regard to obsessive-compulsive disorder (OCD) (March and Curry 1998), generalized anxiety disorder (Rynn et al. 2001), depression (Wagner et al. 2003), separation anxiety (Walkup et al. 2008), and social phobia (Walkup et al. 2008), currently no evidence exists to demonstrate efficacy in the treatment of child/adolescent PTSD.

Aside from sertraline, the only other SSRI that has been evaluated in an RCT is fluoxetine. In a 1-week trial (Robert et al. 2008), fluoxetine and imipramine were compared to a placebo in a population of children being treated for acute stress disorder from thermal burns. The results showed no difference between the three treatment groups; however, with such a brief treatment period, a clinical result might have been unlikely.

Unlike sertraline and fluoxetine, citalopram has yet to be evaluated in an RCT, but initial exploration has demonstrated positive results in case studies and open-label trials. In the first open-label trial by Seedat (Seedat et al. 2001), patients' measures on the Clinician-Administered PTSD Scale – Child/Adolescent Version (CAPS-CA) showed a 38 % reduction, yet citalopram did not improve self-reported depressive symptoms. In another open-label trial (Seedat et al. 2002), the efficacy of citalopram was evaluated in 24 children and adolescents, with results demonstrating a reduction in CAPS total scores, Clinical Global Impression (CGI) ratings, and symptom cluster scores.

18.1.2 Antipsychotics

Antipsychotics have been utilized in the treatment of PTSD for correcting major dysfunctions in dopaminergic neurotransmission. Despite the extensive research of second-generation antipsychotics (SGAs) in the adult PTSD population (Strawn et al.

2010), limited research has assessed their effectiveness in children and adolescents. Furthermore, while generally safer than the classic antipsychotics, SGAs still carry the risk of extrapyramidal side effects, along with weight gain, dyslipidemia, increase blood glucose, hyperprolactinemia, and increased QTc intervals (Strawn et al. 2010).

While no RCTs have been conducted with risperidone in the child and adolescent population, two open-label trials and one case study have demonstrated notable symptomatic improvements (Horrigan and Barnhill 1999; Keeshin and Strawn 2009; Meighen et al. 2007). The first open-label study (Horrigan and Barnhill 1999) found a remission of PTSD symptoms in 13 out of 18 youths. In a case study by Keeshin and Strawn (2009), significant improvements were noted with a 13-year-old boy receiving risperidone adjunctive to divalproex sodium and clonidine for PTSD symptoms related to sexual abuse and neglect. Finally, the study by Meighen et al. (2007) found that risperidone treatment alleviated PTSD-related symptoms in pediatric patients suffering from acute stress disorder.

Like risperidone, quetiapine has yet to undergo an RCT with a pediatric population, but it does show some promise within open-label trials. In a study by Stathis et al. (2005), six adolescents between the ages of 15 and 17 received flexibly dosed quetiapine (50–200 mg/day) for a period of 12 weeks. At the conclusion of each case study, all the participants demonstrated significant improvements on their traumatic symptom checklists.

18.1.3 Mood Stabilizers

Approaching the treatment of PTSD through the lens of anticonvulsants, mood stabilizers modify the GABAergic and glutamatergic neurotransmission within the brain, targeting the symptoms of aggression, anger, and impulsivity often associated with PTSD. While extensive open-label and RCT research has been done among adults with mixed to moderate effects, very little research has explored these medications in the pediatric population (Strawn et al. 2010). The two studies assessing the efficacy of mood stabilizers in children and adolescents have focused on carbamazepine and divalproex sodium.

In a study by Looff et al. (1995), 28 children and adolescents with sexual abuse-related PTSD were administered with carbamazepine at varying dosages of 300–1200 mg daily. At the conclusion of the treatment, 22 participants were symptom free, with the other 6 showing improvements in functioning. A double-blinded, 7-week randomized controlled trial of divalproex sodium by Steiner et al. (2007) compared the effects of a low or high dosage of divalproex sodium in a population of 71 adolescents with conduct disorders and 12 with comorbid PTSD. Those who received a higher dosage demonstrated improvements in CGI scores over the course of the trial.

18.1.4 Antiadrenergic Agents

Antiadrenergic medication has drawn focus due to its ability to reduce noradrenergic hyperactivity (Cohen et al. 2001), which has been implicated in the development and presentation of PTSD symptoms. Theorized as an effective treatment against the hyperarousal symptom clusters, a variety of antiadrenergic agents have been explored for their effectiveness in treating pediatric PTSD. The most common medications used in this category are guanfacine, clonidine, prazosin, and propranolol.

Guanfacine and clonidine are alpha-2 agonists that have demonstrated positive results in open-label trials for their ability to mediate symptoms of hyperarousal in both children and adults with PTSD (Donnelly 2003). In an 8-week open-label study by Connor et al. (2013), extended-release guanfacine was given to 19 child and adolescent patients, which concluded with 71 % of the participants classified as responding to guanfacine, with a decrease in severity from all three symptom clusters (reexperiencing, hyperarousal, and avoidance). Although limited and dated, a study by Harmon and Riggs (1996) found that clonidine was effective in reducing symptoms of aggression, hyperarousal, and sleep difficulties in a population of seven school children.

Prazosin is an alpha-1 antagonist that has been used specifically to treat nightmares and intrusive symptoms associated with PTSD. In several case studies (Strawn et al. 2009; Fraleigh et al. 2009), prazosin demonstrated marked effectiveness as both a mono and adjunctive treatment for four adolescent patients suffering from frequent and intrusive nightmare symptoms. After reaching dosage levels between 1 and 3 mg daily, all the case studies demonstrated significant improvements in sleep. Unfortunately, while RCTs and open-label studies have found prazosin to be effective in treating PTSD in the adult population, only case studies have been conducted in pediatric populations (Oluwabusi et al. 2012).

Unlike other antiadrenergic medications, propranolol is a beta-antagonist that has been designed to work as a preventive, rather than a reactive, measure toward pediatric PTSD. While an initial study by Famularo et al. (1988) observed significantly fewer symptoms in 11 cases of children who had experienced childhood trauma, the only propranolol study conducted in the pediatric population failed to demonstrate significant findings (Nugent et al. 2010; Sharp et al. 2010).

18.2 How to Administer Pharmacological Treatment

18.2.1 Ethical and Legal Considerations

Pharmacotherapy is challenging since an increase in prescriptions is in conflict with uncertainties of safety and efficacy topics. Due to the lack of clinical trials in child and adolescent psychiatry, drugs are most frequently used off-label, entailing a non-age-specific use. Of particular importance in this respect is the fact that youth displays developmentally dependent metabolic conditions and a high vulnerability for adverse medication reactions. Given these facts and the evidence for psychotherapy as first line therapy for youth with PTSD, it is of great importance to provide adequate education and make sure that children and adolescents and their caregivers provide informed consent when medication is intended as a treatment option for PTSD.

Table 18.1 Indications for pharmacotherapy for pediatric trauma-related disorders

Psychotherapy is unavailable
Patient presents with comorbidity
Patient presents with treatment-resistant PTSD
Age of the child

18.2.2 Indication for Pharmacotherapy

When working in the context of PTSD and trauma within the pediatric population, it is important to approach treatment from several levels, including psychotherapy and pharmacotherapy. The first line of treatment for trauma-related disorders in children and adolescents is psychotherapy. While medication can function to decrease the symptoms of hyperarousal, depression, and anxiety (Cohen et al. 2001; Strawn et al. 2009), trauma-focused psychotherapy, in addition to improving post-traumatic symptomatology, serves to address the deficits in interpersonal functioning, self-esteem, and fear mastery.

PTSD guidelines published by the UK's National Institute for Health and Clinical Excellence (NICE) in 2005 and the Australian National Health and Medical Research Council in 2013 state that pharmacotherapy should not be routinely prescribed to children or adolescents (National Institute for Health and Care Excellence 2005; Phoenix Australia – Centre for Posttraumatic Mental Health 2013). PTSD guidelines published by the American Academy of Child and Adolescent Psychiatry in 2010 state that while trauma-focused psychotherapies are the first-line treatments, pharmacotherapy can be considered (AACAP Official Action 2010). However, medication should not be used without psychotherapy.

In some examples, pharmacotherapy may be indicated instead of psychotherapy (Table 18.1). This would be the case if no psychotherapy was available or if relevant comorbidity hinders the implementation of psychotherapy.

Despite the lack of controlled research on the use of pharmacotherapies for pediatric PTSD, SSRIs serve as the primary method of treatment by child psychiatrists due to their ability to treat a broad range of both anxiety and depressive symptoms (Cohen et al. 2001). Sertraline is an SSRI approved for the treatment of pain disorder, depression, and obsessive-compulsive disorder and is often a first-line treatment recommendation for pediatric PTSD as a way to mitigate the reexperiencing, numbing, and avoidance symptoms typical of the disorder (Cohen et al. 2001). While other types of medication, such as the alpha-1 and alpha-2 agonists prazosin, guanfacine, and clonidine, have demonstrated some limited success with treating hyperarousal symptoms in children with PTSD (Strawn et al. 2009; Connor et al. 2013; Harmon and Riggs 1996), there is not enough evidence yet to substantiate their off label use in the treatment of children with PTSD.

18.3 Special Challenges and Case Studies

18.3.1 Case 1: PTSD with Comorbid Bulimia Nervosa

Lilly, a 15-year-old adolescent, is brought into your office by her concerned mother. The mother articulates that her daughter has been caught purging her meals in the restroom, waking up the entire house due to screaming fits and night terrors, and failing all of her classes at school. Lilly's mother reports that the behavioral problems began 6 months earlier after she left Lilly to stay at her father's place for a month, while she had gone abroad for vacation. Upon returning to her mother's house, Lilly began presenting with symptoms of extreme mood irritability, anxiety, nightmares, and impulsivity. When questioning her mood changes, Lilly would only remark that her mother would not be able to understand. As the weeks went on, Lilly began to engage less with her mother and stepfather, spending time isolated alone in her room while fixating on her image on social media websites. Eventually, Lilly was caught purging in the bathroom and was given the ultimatum of seeing a psychiatrist. After a few family sessions reviewing her binging and purging behaviors, Lilly asks to meet with you 1:1. It is during this private session that she suddenly breaks down in tears and reports that her father had sexually molested her on several occasions.

Symptom Presentation When a client presents with a comorbid case of PTSD and bulimia nervosa, it is important to understand the shared symptom profile of these two disorders and how they relate to the patient's emotionally dysregulated state. The common symptoms of PTSD, such as hyperarousal, anger, emotional numbing, and avoidance, along with the characteristic binging and purging in bulimia nervosa, communicate a patient's unsuccessful attempts at regulating negative affect. Another hallmark characteristic of both bulimia and PTSD is alexithymia, or difficulty in identifying and describing one's emotions along with deficits in interoceptive awareness. In the case presented above, Lilly presents with symptoms of nightmares, reexperiencing of the traumatic sexual abuse, isolation, impulsivity, aggression, and the binging and purging of her meals in an attempt to facilitate control over her dysregulated emotional state.

Special Challenges There are several inherent challenges when working with children and adolescents with this symptom profile due to the often vulnerable context of their environment and family relations. First, while this is not an inherently psychopharmacological consideration, it is of primary importance to make sure that the patient is not being continuously exposed to whatever traumatic event precipitated their symptoms in the first place. In the case presented above, Lilly's mother was not aware of the sexual molestation that took place between Lilly and her father. As Lilly is a minor, a CPS (Child Protective Services) report would need to be promptly made upon the discovery of this alleged abuse, along with safeguards set in place to ensure no further contact between Lilly and her father. In cases like these, the patient might still be living with their abuser while being routinely violated and re-traumatized.

Another important challenge to consider when working with comorbid PTSD presentations is the presence of side effects. With a typical PTSD presentation, SSRIs are usually the first line of pharmacological treatment (adjunctive to psychotherapy) due to their application toward a broad range of symptoms (Donnelly 2003). However, when dealing with comorbid presentations, the use of atypical antipsychotics and anticonvulsants might be warranted to treat the symptoms of mood instability, impulsivity, or psychosis that would otherwise remain untreated by the typical SSRI application. The additional challenge posed by antipsychotics/anticonvulsants is the often severe and difficult side effect profile that can come with them. Extrapyramidal side effects such as weight gain, dyslipidemia, increased blood glucose, and hyperprolactinemia are just a few of the side effects caused by SGAs and can be especially difficult for children/adolescents to deal with in their already vulnerable states. Furthermore, when working with medications that can elicit strong side effect reactions, it is important to discuss proper medication compliance, especially when a significant duration of time has elapsed with no notable symptom improvement. It is important to consider that PTSD symptoms will often persist beyond 12 weeks and that medication adjustment might be necessary.

Treatment Recommendations As noted above, the first-line treatment is always psychotherapy, such as individual CBT for the patient and family therapy. When working with a patient who is suffering from a comorbid presentation of PTSD and bulimia nervosa, it is important to provide them with the means of helping them to regulate their internal states. The first-line recommended psychopharmacological interventions for PTSD are SSRIs, such as sertraline and fluoxetine, as recommended by Marshall (Marshall et al. 2001) and Brady (Brady et al. 2000). In this specific case of comorbid bulimia nervosa with PTSD, the medication fluoxetine would be recommended over sertraline, because it is licensed for the treatment of bulimia (SPC 2011). Given the comorbid presentation, an additional psychopharmacological intervention besides psychotherapy is warranted.

One final area of consideration with comorbid presentations is any medical complications that might arise from chemical imbalances or illicit drug interactions. In the case of bulimia, there can be severe medical complications, like electrolyte imbalance, depending on how much purging is going on. Thus, a consultation with a pediatrician should routinely be performed.

18.3.2 Case 2: Atypical Presentation

You receive a patient referral for a 6-year-old male who has been diagnosed with attention deficit hyperactivity disorder (ADHD). After a few pharmacological regimens of methylphenidate, the patient does not seem to be benefiting in any way from the medication. He continues to present with symptoms of inattentiveness and impulsivity, resulting in impaired functioning at school and difficulties socializing with peers. During one of your consultations with the patient's mother, she mentions that her child was doing seemingly well in school until the accident. After inquiring further, the parent articulates that her son was in a traumatic car accident with his father 2 years prior, but she cannot understand how such an old event could be related to her child's ADHD, especially because her son did not exhibit any symptoms until 6 months posttrauma. Since the incident, however, her son seems to "zone out" during car rides, does not engage with his peers or play as frequently as he used to, and is often irritable. As a result of his mood and social withdrawal, the mother has had difficulties finding play dates for her son and has resigned herself to trying to get her son to do anything but play alone with his toys and video games. After giving you the case history and circumstances, the mother wants you to prescribe her child a new medication to ameliorate his behavioral problems.

Symptom Presentation In children age 6 and below, the Diagnostic and Statistical Manual (5th ed.; DSM–5; American Psychiatric Association [APA] 2013) criteria for PTSD preface the expression of negative alterations in mood through the emergence of irritability and tantrums. Due to a young child's limitations in cognition and labeling, symptoms of mood negativity more often present as aggression and agitation (APA 2013). Unfortunately, many behavioral problems can mirror symptoms of ADHD, including inattentiveness and difficulties with concentration (APA 2013). In the case described above, the child presents with symptoms of irritable behavior, diminished interest in play, dissociative reactions, problems with concentration, and significant impairment in functioning both socially and at school. Furthermore, this patient's symptom presentation did not appear until 6 months after the traumatic car crash. Given the time disparity between the traumatic event and the emergence of symptoms, it is very easy to see why the patient's parents might have misinterpreted their child's symptoms to be related to poor behavioral adaptation or ADHD.

Special Challenges The challenges associated with this case are giving an appropriate differential diagnosis and utilizing a treatment that would be safe and effective for a child of this young age. With a clear and thorough history, a health care practitioner would not have trouble differentiating a PTSD diagnosis. However, given the loose association of events and the parents' focus on finding an appropriate medication for their child, a clinician might struggle to conceptualize this case appropriately. If only presented with the behavioral problems, inattentiveness, and poor concentration, a clinician might settle for a different diagnosis that would continue to ignore the patient's underlying trauma.

In consideration of this child's age, a major question is how appropriate are pharmacological interventions to the safety and well-being of this child. Notwithstanding the scarcity of research and support toward the efficacy of medication in the treatment of pediatric PTSD, any form of drug treatment given to this child runs the risk of precipitating potential damage to his neurobiological development. With a patient at the height of his vulnerability and without the evidence to support the efficacy of the treatment, psychopharmacology would be potentially disadvantageous to the patient.

Treatment Recommendations Taking into consideration the patient's young age and presenting problems, the treatment recommendations for this case would be to use trauma-focused cognitive behavioral therapy (TF-CBT) as a first-line treatment (see Chap. 8).

18.3.3 Case 3: Treatment-Resistant Presentation of PTSD

Alex is a 14-year-old male who was brought in by the police to an adolescent inpatient unit at a behavioral hospital. During his intake, his father articulates that his son has been progressively escalating in symptom severity over the past year. A year prior, Alex had stumbled upon his mother's lifeless body after she had overdosed on prescription medication. Initially, Alex responded in a way that seemed appropriate to the circumstances, presenting as deeply depressed and isolative. However, as time progressed, Alex's mood and behavior grew increasingly dysregulated. Starting with acts of impulsivity, such as minor shoplifting and marijuana abuse, Alex then started to present as increasingly aggressive and unpredictable toward his family and peers. Alex would become explosive and violent when he wouldn't get his way, punching holes in the wall and breaking plates. Eventually, he started to have fits of rage, during which he was seemingly inconsolable until his anger was exhausted. Sometimes his behavior was unsolicited, throwing furniture, screaming, and striking at his father until restrained. During his most recent incident, Alex was reportedly being shamed by a fellow peer when he suddenly snapped into a violent rage. According to the police report, Alex grabbed the nearest rock and proceeded to bludgeon his peer into unconsciousness. When the police arrived on the scene, Alex was still exhibiting violent and disassociated behavior.

Symptom Presentation Alex's primary symptom presentation of aggression, emotional reactivity, impulsivity, and reexperiencing is representative of an atypical PTSD presentation. In Alex's case, the emotional dysregulation precipitated by PTSD is expressed through behavioral impulsivity and aggression. With his emotional reactivity compounded by the shame and disconnection he experiences with his peers and family, Alex has demonstrated very little tolerance for stress and triggering situations. Given the use of illicit substances, it can also be presumed that there is some attempt on his part to self-medicate or emotionally withdraw from the severe dysregulation he experiences.

Special Challenges There are several challenges inherent in a case with this level of acuity. Challenges such as discerning an appropriate diagnosis and treatment compliance can hinder the overall treatment success with a case of this severity.

Due to this patient's symptom profile exhibiting several characteristics that are atypical of PTSD, a clinician must be careful to establish an appropriate differential diagnosis that supports the etiology of the symptoms. Cases of childhood PTSD will typically present with the core symptom clusters of the disorder; however, they also can present with a broad range of additional symptoms that are not typical in an adult case. Symptoms such as regression, reckless behavior, hyperactivity, distractibility, and psychosomatic complaints can often complicate or distort the clinical picture (Kaminer et al. 2005). With regard to the dissociative and violent incidents exhibited by Alex, it would be important to explore the nature of these episodes in relation to psychosis and drug abuse. Through the acquisition of a clear and cohesive history, the patient can be treated for the correct diagnosis accordingly.

Once an appropriate diagnosis has been made (in the described example, this would be a complex PTSD presentation, see also Chap. 1), the clinician must work carefully with the patient to ensure proper treatment compliance. With a difficult case like Alex, a clinician must not only work to build a trusting relationship with the patient but also destigmatize the concept of medication while reinforcing the importance of adhering to a strict medication regimen. With factors such as being held involuntarily and a history of mistrust and aggression, a patient like Alex can be very averse to following treatment recommendations. Once a patient has agreed to take medication, the ongoing challenge of medication compliance can become an issue. If a patient has been taking a medication for several months with no evident changes in symptom presentation, it may be the case that they are not taking their medication as prescribed. Another point of consideration is the fact that the literature has yet to demonstrate significant evidence for large effect sizes in the use of SSRIs and SGAs in children and adolescents (Rapp et al. 2013) (Strawn et al. 2010).

The importance of establishing trust and close observation cannot be emphasized enough, as this sometimes makes the difference between a patient's recovery and deterioration.

Treatment Recommendations When approaching a case like the one described above, it is important to consider a treatment for the most problematic of the presenting symptoms. In Alex's case, his violent episodes impair the safety of himself and others, while his mood dysregulation and impulsivity prevent him from successfully regulating his emotions and behavior. In addition to psychotherapy, the typical first line of pharmacological treatment for adolescents with PTSD is SSRIs (Tareen et al. 2007), but in this case, given Alex's extreme aggression and violence, SGAs might be considered as an adjunctive approach to treatment. The two SGAs risperidone and quetiapine have both demonstrated some promise in open-label trials with the adolescent population (Strawn et al. 2010). Once a patient's aggressive and psychotic symptoms are under control, the treatment can proceed into the processing of trauma and the development of skills that will facilitate the management of emotional dysregulation.

18.3.4 Case 4: Acute Medication

A 16-year-old girl is admitted to an inpatient unit presenting with symptoms of extreme anxiety, panic, and inconsolable crying. The attending resident is notified by the child's parents that the patient was playing a game of house harmlessly with her brother, when suddenly she began to cry uncontrollably. The parents, worried about this sudden symptom presentation, rushed her to the hospital only to be told that she was presenting with extreme bouts of panic and anxiety. In order to calm the patient down, the resident prescribes midazolam to help the patient relax. Shortly after being administered with benzodiazepine, the patient begins to react "paradoxically" to the medication, with presenting symptoms of agitation and disinhibition. The patient starts to kick and scream uncontrollably and needs to be quickly restrained so as to not put the other patients in danger. The resident consults with the child's parents about her presenting symptomatology and finds out that the patient had a history of repetitive, traumatic rape at the hands of her biological father. Following the acute medication reaction, the patient begins to present with the primary symptoms of frequent and debilitating nightmares. The nightmares are so intense that the patient is only managing to sleep 3–4 h per night, has developed a strong aversion to the dark, and will do anything she can to avoid going to sleep.

Symptom Presentation The initial symptom presentation of this patient was overt anxiety and panic, triggered by an unknown or seemingly benign event. When administered with benzodiazepine midazolam, the patient began to exhibit paradoxical symptoms, including violent behavior and disinhibition. Following the paradoxical reaction, the patient's PTSD symptoms emerge as severe anxiety and debilitating nightmares. The complexity of this case arises from both the presence of a paradoxical reaction and the prevalent reexperiencing features of the night terrors. In order to treat this patient effectively, the etiology and timeline of the symptoms need to be carefully explored to avoid misdiagnosis or ineffective medication protocols.

Special Challenges In this acute medication case, the special challenges are centered around the paradoxical reaction to the medication and the utilization of off-label and less researched treatment approaches. The attending resident in this case sought to remedy the patient's overt anxiety with the benzodiazepine midazolam. Not making a careful differential, the resident was unaware of this patient's underlying trauma history and prescribed a medication that even without the precipitation of the paradoxical effects would have been ultimately ineffective in treating her psychological disorder (Strawn et al. 2009). While the risk of patients experiencing paradoxical reactions to benzodiazepines is very low, younger children are at a greater risk than adults (Mancuso et al. 2004). Without a quick and effective way to moderate the paradoxical reaction, the patient's underlying PTSD symptoms will be left untreated. Therefore, it is of utmost importance to manage the paradoxical reaction in the quickest and most efficacious method possible. This requires the health care professional to take a multilayered approach to managing each set of symptoms with the appropriate pharmacology. A response to this case might utilize antipsychotics to first treat the paradoxical effects in case those can't be managed by waiting until the substance has been cleared from the body, which would be the preferred course of action, and then transition to psychotherapy, combined with the antiadrenergic medication prazosin to manage the nightmares. The problem then arises with the risk of off-label use and the broad range of side effects that can quickly put a patient at great risk. Extrapyramidal symptoms, along with weight gain and heavy sedation, are just a few of the possible concerns that must be closely monitored in a situation where a younger patient is subject to such a heavy load of pharmaceutical treatments. Furthermore, while research has demonstrated some effectiveness with antiadrenergic medications (Strawn et al. 2009; Fraleigh et al. 2009; Seedat et al. 2001), the evidence is still insufficient to confidently endorse their use in the treatment of pediatric PTSD symptoms.

Treatment Recommendations The steps toward effectively treating a case like the one described above need to include a quick and effective management of the paradoxical reaction and then a transition to the treatment and care of the primary PTSD impairment. To deal with the violent behavior and disinhibition that resulted from the benzodiazepines, the clinician could administer a very low dosage of the antipsychotic olanzapine, in case the symptoms can't be controlled. It is important to again reiterate the myriad of problems associated with the use of SGAs and that the clinician must make both the patient and caretakers aware of the risks brought forth by side effects. Once the patient has returned to an appropriate baseline and the SGAs have been safely discontinued, the treatment will need to move into the next phase, which will focus primarily on psychotherapy and the antiadrenergic medication prazosin to remedy the impairment caused by the patient's nightmares. SSRIs are the most utilized method of treating PTSD symptoms (Cohen et al. 2001) as they can be used to target a wide variety of both anxiety and depressive criteria. Prazosin, while not as well researched as SSRIs, has shown some significant effectiveness in the treatment of intrusive nightmares associated with traumatic PTSD events (Strawn et al. 2009; Fraleigh et al. 2009). Given the primary symptoms expressed in this case, an adjunctive therapy approach with prazosin might serve as an effective complement to psychotherapy, the first-line treatment.

18.3.5 Case 5: Psychopharmacological Side Effects

A 15-year-old female patient is referred to your practice, articulating symptoms of depression and insomnia. After a few sessions, she brings up several traumatic incidents of sexual abuse at the hands of her previous boyfriends. As she continues to describe her ongoing difficulties with nightmares, how she avoids activities associated

18 Pharmacological Treatment for Trauma-Related Disorders

with her previous partners, and how she has been so impacted by her ongoing symptoms that she is unable to perform well in school or socialize with others, you conclude that her symptom profile fits that of PTSD. In addition to organizing a psychotherapeutic setting for her, you give her a prescription for sertraline and slowly titrate the dosage to therapeutic levels. During the patient's next visit, her mood and affect seem more agitated and aggressive, which seem a stark contrast to her typical restricted and low presentation. Throughout the session, the patient raises several red flags, articulating how fed up she is with her family and how she has been thinking about taking all of the sleeping pills her mother hides in the medicine cabinet.

Symptom Presentation In the case described above, the patient initially presented with symptoms of depression and insomnia. As the patient's history unfolds, it becomes apparent that the depression and sleep troubles are a result of a long history of abuse and sexual trauma. With the recent changes made to the diagnostic criteria of PTSD in the DSM-5, Criteria D has been added to include negative alterations in mood that resulted from a traumatic event. Alongside the patient's mood symptoms, she also presents with intrusive symptoms of nightmares, avoidance of stimuli that reminds her of the trauma, and arousal symptoms in the form of sleep disturbances. Together, her symptom profile communicates a clear diagnosis of PTSD. Once medicated with the SSRI, the patient begins to exhibit signs of agitation and suicidal ideation. While research has demonstrated a strong correlation between suicide risk and PTSD diagnosis (Tarrier and Gregg 2004), the abrupt and sudden appearance of suicidal ideation in this case can be connected to the prescribed SSRI (Olfson et al. 2006).

Special Challenges When a health care professional is tasked with treating a patient with any pharmacological intervention, the risks and side effects of the designated treatment are always a concern that needs to remain paramount. The challenge of this specific case is to ensure the patient's continued safety while effectively transitioning her to a different medication regimen. In comparison to the earlier used tricyclic antidepressants, the side effects associated with SSRIs are much less severe (Strawn et al. 2010), which is one of the primary reasons that 95 % of child psychiatrists utilize them in the treatment of pediatric PTSD (Cohen et al. 2001). Despite their effectiveness and relatively benign side effects, in 2004 the FDA recognized potential risks of suicidal ideation associated with SSRI use in children and adolescents (Olfson 2006). While this side effect seems limited to a small subset of adolescents, it is absolutely critical that any health care provider monitors their patients closely for any signs and symptoms of suicidality when utilizing SSRIs. In the case described above, the patient's adverse reaction to this medication challenges the clinician to utilize a different method of treatment that might be less favorable than the relative safety of SSRIs. With the presence of the aggression and inhibition, the provider might switch to a second-generation antipsychotic such as quetiapine, in order to help downregulate the patient's most concerning symptoms. Similar to the newer SSRIs, SGAs are generally safer than the first-generation antipsychotics. However, SGAs still carry a risk of dangerous side effects that include dyslipidemia, weight gain, hyperprolactinemia, and increased QTc intervals and blood glucose levels (Strawn et al. 2010).

Treatment Recommendations Due to the obvious danger of continuing to treat this patient with SSRIs, the appropriate treatment approach to this case would be to safely titrate the patient off of the antidepressants, ensure her safety with regard to her suicidal ideations, and carefully acclimate her to SGAs. In the present case, the patient could benefit from an admission to an inpatient ward in order to establish the discontinuation of the SSRI and the titration to an alternative medication. A different approach to this problem would be to monitor the patient closely and see if the side effect of the prescribed SSRI is only temporarily affecting the patient. SSRIs can lead to a deterioration of mood symptoms at the beginning of their administration, and it is up to the clinician to responsibly consider continuing the SSRI despite potentially temporary side effects. In this case, again, it is of utmost importance to guarantee safety for the patient and therefore consider a potential admission to an inpatient ward.

Conclusions

According to all current guidelines, psychotherapy is the first-line treatment for trauma-related disorders. In some cases, it may be appropriate to use pharmacotherapy as an adjunctive treatment. However, as demonstrated by the limited and contextual research conducted on the most prevalent pharmacotherapies for pediatric PTSD, there is a clear gap between how the medications are used and prescribed and what evidence exists for their efficacy.

Notwithstanding the lack of efficacy demonstrated in the research, SSRIs function as the first line of pharmacological treatment for trauma-exposed children and adolescents suffering from PTSD, due to their demonstrated effectiveness in the adult population, relative tolerability, minimal side effects, and broad application to a variety of mood and anxiety symptoms (Donnelly 2003; Huemer et al. 2010). While certain medications within the antipsychotic, antiadrenergic, and anticonvulsant classifications have demonstrated positive results in open-label trials, these medications have yet to stand up to the rigors of randomly controlled trials and, as such, should be targeted for future exploration. Without further evidence to support the use of the most widely utilized pharmacotherapies in the trauma-exposed population—including a better understanding of the neurobiological differences between adults and children—clinicians run the risk of providing a less than effective treatment for youth suffering from PTSD.

Treating PTSD with psychopharmacology is complex, particularly considering the off-label use of most of the medication described in this chapter. In order to determine the best course of action, the clinician must take into consideration the age of the patient, the presentation, and the specific symptoms. Therefore, pharmacotherapy must be individually targeted. As such, the case vignettes presented in this chapter are by no means binding treatment rules, but rather represent a few possible examples of how to address childhood PTSD by means of medication.

References

AACAP Official Action (2010) Practice parameter for the assessment and treatment of children and adolescents with posttraumatic stress disorder. J Am Acad Child Adolesc Psychiatry 49(4):414–430

American Psychiatric Association (2013) Diagnostic and statistical manual of mental disorders, 5th edn. Arlington: American Psychiatric Publishing

Brady K, Pearlstein T, Asnis GM et al (2000) Efficacy and safety of sertraline treatment of posttraumatic stress disorder: a randomized controlled trial. JAMA 283(14):1837–1844. doi:10.1001/jama.283.14.1837

Cohen JA, Mannarino AP, Rogal S (2001) Treatment practices for childhood posttraumatic stress disorder. Child Abuse Negl 25(1):123–135. doi:10.1016/S0145-2134(00)00226-X

Cohen JA, Mannarino AP, Perel JM, Staron V (2007) A pilot randomized controlled trial of combined trauma focused CBT and sertraline for childhood PTSD symptoms. J Am Acad Child Adolesc Psychiatry 46:811–819. http://dx.doi.org/10.1097/chi.0b013e3180547105

Connor DF, Grasso DJ, Slivinsky MD et al (2013) An open-label study of guanfacine extended release for traumatic stress related symptoms in children and adolescents. J Child Adolesc Psychopharmacol 23(4):244–251. doi:10.1089/cap.2012.0119

Donnelly CL (2003) Pharmacologic treatment approaches for children and adolescents with posttraumatic stress disorder. Child Adolesc Psychiatr Clin N Am 12(2):251–269. doi:10.1016/S1056-4993(02)00102-5

Famularo R, Kinscherff R, Fenton T (1988) Propranolol treatment for childhood posttraumatic stress disorder, acute type. A pilot study. Am J Dis Child 142(11):1244–1247. doi:10.1001/archpedi.1988.02150110122036

Fraleigh LA, Hendratta VD, Ford JD et al (2009) Prazosin for the treatment of posttraumatic stress disorder-related nightmares in an adolescent male. J Child Adolesc Psychopharmacol 19(4):475–476. doi:10.1089/cap.2009.0002

Harmon RJ, Riggs PD (1996) Clonidine for posttraumatic stress disorder in preschool children. J Am Acad Child Adolesc Psychiatry 35(9):1247–1249. doi:10.1097/00004583-199609000-00022

Horrigan JP, Barnhill LJ (1999) Guanfacine and secondary mania in children. J Affect Disord 54(3):309–314. http://dx.doi.org/10.1016/S0165-0327(98)00183-9

Huemer J, Erhart F, Steiner H (2010) Posttraumatic stress disorder in children and adolescents: a review of psychopharmacological treatment. Child Psychiatry Hum Dev 41(6):624–640. doi:10.1007/s10578-010-0192-3

Kaminer D, Seedat S, Stein DJ (2005) Post-traumatic stress disorder in children. World Psychiatry 4(2):121–125

Keeshin BR, Strawn JR (2009) Risperidone treatment of an adolescent with severe posttraumatic stress disorder. Ann Pharmaco 43(7):1374. doi:10.1345/aph.1M219

Looff D, Grimley P, Kuller F et al (1995) Carbamazepine for PTSD. J Am Acad Child Adolesc Psychiatry 34(6):703–704. doi:10.1097/00004583-199506000-00008

Mancuso CE, Tanzi MG, Gabay M (2004) Paradoxical reactions to benzodiazepines: literature review and treatment options. Pharmacotherapy 24(9):1177–1185. doi:10.1592/phco.24.13.1177.38089

March JS, Curry JF (1998) Predicting the outcome of treatment. J Abnorm Child Psychol 26(1):39–51. doi:10.1023/A:1022682723027

Marshall RD, Beebe KL, Oldham M et al (2001) Efficacy and safety of paroxetine treatment for chronic PTSD: a fixed-dose, placebo-controlled study. Am J Psychiatry 158(12):1982–1988. doi:10.1176/appi.ajp.158.12.1982

Meighen KG, Hines LA, Lagges AM (2007) Risperidone treatment of preschool children with thermal burns and acute stress disorder. J Child Adolesc Psychopharmacol 17(2):223–232. doi:10.1089/cap.2007.0121

National Institute for Health and Care Excellence (2005) Post-traumatic stress disorder: management. NICE Guidelines [CG26]. Retrieved from https://www.nice.org.uk/guidance/CG26/chapter/About-this-guideline

Nugent NR, Christopher NC, Crow JP et al (2010) The efficacy of early propranolol administration at reducing PTSD symptoms in pediatric injury patients: a pilot study. J Trauma Stress 23(2):282–287. doi:10.1002/jts.20517

Olfson M, Marcus SC, Shaffer D (2006) Antidepressant drug therapy and suicide in severely depressed children and adults. JAMA 63(8):865–872. doi:10.1001/archpsyc.63.8.865

Oluwabusi OO, Sedky K, Bennett DS (2012) Prazosin treatment of nightmares and sleep disturbances associated with posttraumatic stress disorder: two adolescent cases. J Child Adolesc Psychopharmacol 22(5):399–402. doi:10.1089/cap.2012.0035

Phoenix Australia – Centre for Posttraumatic Mental Health (2013) Australian guidelines for the treatment of acute stress disorder and posttraumatic stress disorder. Australian Government National Health and Medical Research Council. Retrieved from https://www.clinicalguidelines.gov.au/portal/australian-guidelines-treatment-acute-stress-disorder-and-posttraumatic-stress-disorder

Rapp A, Dodds A, Walkup JT et al (2013) Treatment of pediatric anxiety disorders. Ann N Y Acad Sci 1304(1):52–61. doi:10.1111/nyas.12318

Robb AS, Cueva JE, Sporn J et al (2008) Efficacy of sertraline in childhood PTSD. Paper presented at the 55th annual meeting of the American Academy of Child and Adolescent Psychiatry Meeting, Chicago, Oct 28–Nov 2, 2008

Robert R, Tcheung WJ, Rosenberg L et al (2008) Treating thermally injured children suffering symptoms of acute stress with imipramine and fluoxetine: a randomized, double-blind study. Burns 34(7):919–928. doi:10.1016/j.burns.2008.04.009

Rynn MA, Siqueland L, Rickels K (2001) Placebo-controlled trial of sertraline in the treatment of children with generalized anxiety disorder. Am J Psychiatry 158(12):2008–2014. doi:10.1176/appi.ajp.158.12.2008

Seedat S, Lockhat R, Kaminer D et al (2001) An open trial of citalopram in adolescents with posttraumatic stress disorder. Int Clin Psychopharmacol 16(1):21–25

Seedat S, Stein DJ, Ziervogel C et al (2002) Comparison of response to a selective serotonin reuptake inhibitor in children, adolescents, and adults with posttraumatic stress disorder. J Child Adolesc Psychopharmacol 12(1):37–46. doi:10.1089/10445460252943551

Sharp S, Thomas C, Rosenberg L et al (2010) Propranolol does not reduce risk for acute stress disorder in pediatric burn trauma. J Trauma Acute Care Surg 68(1):193–197. doi:10.1097/TA.0b013e3181a8b326

Specific Product Characteristics (SPC) Fluoxetine® (2011, July 12) Retrieved 9 Nov 2015, from http://www.medicines.org.uk/emc/medicine/13431

Stathis S, Martin G, McKenna JG (2005) A preliminary case series on the use of quetiapine for posttraumatic stress disorder in juveniles within a youth detention center. J Clin Psychopharmacol 25(6):539–544

Steiner H, Saxena KS, Carrion V et al (2007) Divalproex sodium for the treatment of PTSD and conduct disordered youth: a pilot randomized controlled clinical trial. Child Psychiatry Hum Dev 38(3):183–193. doi:10.1007/s10578-007-0055-8

Stoddard FJ, Luthra R, Sorrentino EA et al (2011) A randomized controlled trial of sertraline to prevent posttraumatic stress disorder in burned children. J Child Adolesc Psychopharmacol 21(5):469–477. doi:10.1089/cap.2010.0133

Strawn JR, Delbello MP, Geracioti TD (2009) Prazosin treatment of an adolescent with posttraumatic stress disorder. J Child Adolesc Psychopharmacol 19(5):599–600. doi:10.1089/cap.2009.0043

Strawn JR, Keeshin BR, DelBello MP et al (2010) Psychopharmacologic treatment of posttraumatic stress disorder in children and adolescents: a review. J Clin Psychiatry 71(7):932–941. doi:10.4088/JCP.09r05446blu

Tareen A, Elena Garralda M, Hodes M (2007) Post-traumatic stress disorder in childhood. Archives of Disease in Childhood – Education and Practice Edition 92(1):ep1–6. doi: 10.1136/adc.2006.100305

Tarrier N, Gregg L (2004) Suicide risk in civilian PTSD patients: predictors of suicidal ideation, planning, and attempts. Soc Psychiatry Psychiatr Epidemiol 39:655–661. doi:10.1007/s00127-004-0799-4

Wagner KD, Ambrosini P, Rynn M et al (2003) Efficacy of sertraline in the treatment of children and adolescents with major depressive disorder: two randomized controlled trials. JAMA 290(8):1033–1041. doi:10.1001/jama.290.8.1033

Walkup JT, Albano AM, Piacentini J et al (2008) Cognitive behavioral therapy, sertraline, or a combination in childhood anxiety. N Engl J Med 359(26):2753–2766. doi:10.1056/NEJMoa0804633

Part III

Settings

Interventions in Medical Settings

Meghan L. Marsac, Aimee K. Hildenbrand, and Nancy Kassam-Adams

Injury, illness, and associated medical care are among the most frequent potentially traumatic events (PTEs) experienced by children (Murray and Lopez 1996). While most children are resilient and display transient distress after PTEs, a notable subset demonstrates adverse psychological reactions that often include (but can extend beyond) posttraumatic stress symptoms (PTSS; Kahana et al. 2006; Kassam-Adams et al. 2013; Price et al. 2016). *Medical traumatic stress* is defined as PTSS and other emotional reactions that develop because of injury, illness, or their treatment in children and families (Kazak et al. 2006). A meta-analysis revealed that nearly 20 % of injured and 10 % of ill children develop persistent and impairing PTSS; similar rates are reported for parents (Kahana et al. 2006; Landolt et al. 2003). A recent systematic review suggests that roughly 30 % of ill and injured children and their parents experience subthreshold yet clinically significant PTSS (Price et al. 2016). PTSS can be especially problematic in medically involved children, as they are associated with poorer adherence, health-related quality of life, and health outcomes (e.g., mental health, functional impairment, pain perception, general health; Landolt

---

M.L. Marsac (✉) • N. Kassam-Adams
Perelman School of Medicine, University of Pennsylvania,
Children's Hospital of Philadelphia, Philadelphia, PA, USA
e-mail: marsac@email.chop.edu; nlkaphd@mail.med.upenn.edu

A.K. Hildenbrand
Department of Psychology, Drexel University, Center for Injury Research and Prevention,
The Children's Hospital of Philadelphia, Philadelphia, PA, USA
e-mail: hildenbranda@email.chop.edu

© Springer International Publishing Switzerland 2017
M.A. Landolt et al. (eds.), *Evidence-Based Treatments for Trauma Related Disorders in Children and Adolescents*, DOI 10.1007/978-3-319-46138-0_19

et al. 2009; Zatzick et al. 2008). In addition, as described in Chaps. 2 and 3, millions of children have encountered other PTEs such as witnessing violence or natural disasters (Copeland et al. 2007). After PTE exposure, many children interact with healthcare networks, with most families visiting their primary care provider first if they need help managing reactions (Schappert and Rechsteiner 2008). Thus, medical settings can be an ideal setting to identify PTSS and intervene.

Pediatric healthcare settings provide direct access to children recently exposed to potentially traumatic medical events (PTMEs), and medical providers play an important role in facilitating child development. As such, pediatric healthcare networks are an ideal setting for the implementation of "trauma-informed care" (Marsac et al. 2015a, b). The US Substance Abuse and Mental Health Services (2015) has defined a trauma-informed approach as encompassing four key elements: (1) realizing the widespread impact of trauma; (2) recognizing how trauma may affect children, families, and staff; (3) responding by applying trauma knowledge into practice; and (4) preventing re-traumatization. Applying this definition to healthcare, a trauma-informed approach requires that staff understand how PTE exposure affects patients and families as well as healthcare staff and incorporate this understanding into interactions with patients and families throughout healthcare delivery. This includes recognizing and addressing any PTSS associated with pediatric injury or illness and minimizing potential trauma during medical care, as well as recognizing how preexisting trauma may impact a child's reactions to medical care (Marsac et al. 2015a). See Marsac, Kassam-Adams et al. (2015a) for an overview of guiding principles related to implementation of a trauma-informed approach in pediatric healthcare settings.

19.1 Theoretical Underpinnings

Etiological models of child PTSS that have been applied to medical trauma include social cognitive theory, information-processing theories, models of emotion regulation, and models of the interplay between neurobiological processes, emotions, and coping (see Chap. 5 for more on these theories; Kassam-Adams 2014). Perhaps the most comprehensive conceptual framework for understanding psychological reactions and adjustment across various pediatric injury and illness populations is Kazak et al. (2006) integrative model of pediatric medical traumatic stress (PMTS). Five assumptions underlie the model: (1) there are common dimensions across illnesses and injuries related to PTEs and risk/protective factors; (2) there are a range of normative reactions to PTMEs; (3) children and families' preexisting psychological functioning influence risk for PMTS; (4) a developmental lens is essential for understanding responses to medical trauma; and (5) a social ecological or contextual approach is optimal to guide intervention (Kazak et al. 2006).

These models highlight a number of empirically supported risk factors for PTSS across pediatric illness and injury populations (Kassam-Adams 2014; Price et al. 2016). See Table 19.1 for a summary of these risk factors. As noted by Kassam-Adams (2014), those designing interventions to prevent or reduce PTSS should select methods that are likely to change specific etiological processes; thus many of the risk factors in Table 19.1 represent potential targets for intervention.

19 Interventions in Medical Settings

Table 19.1 Risk factors for persistent PTSS related to injury, illness, and/or medical treatment[a]

	Children/Patients	Parents
History of behavioral, emotional, or other mental health problems (Trickey et al. 2012)	√	√
History of past trauma (Copeland et al. 2007)	√	√
Perceived of threat (medical event/condition or world view) (Trickey et al. 2012)	√	√
Elevated heart rate at first medical exam (Alisic et al. 2011)	√	
Child early PTSS (Alisic et al. 2011; Cox et al. 2008)	√	
More severe pain (Hildenbrand et al. 2015)	√	
Specific frightening aspects of treatment experiences (Kazak et al. 1996	√	
Separation from caregivers during/after trauma (Winston et al. 2003)	√	
Low social support (Trickey et al. 2012)	√	√
Parent early PTSS (Alisic et al. 2011)	√	√
Other life stressors or disruptions associated with the index trauma (Trickey et al. 2012)		√

[a]Adapted with permission from the Center for Pediatric Traumatic Stress (2015)

Regardless of the underlying theoretical model, several crosscutting issues are relevant to the design of interventions for children exposed to PTMEs. One key issue is the timing of intervention (Kassam-Adams 2014). Price et al. (2016) updated the integrative model of PMTS, now referred to as the integrative *trajectory* model of PMTS. The updated model emphasizes that phases of PMTS progress according to the course and timing of medical events and treatment. In this model, child and family adjustment are described across three consecutive phases: *peri-trauma, acute medical care, and ongoing care or discharge from care*. Phase I, peri-trauma, includes the initial PTME as well as surrounding events (e.g., emergency transport, invasive procedures, diagnosis). Phase II, acute medical care, is characterized by active treatment and related physical demands of ongoing illness or injury. Phase III, ongoing care or discharge from care, refers to the time beyond active acute medical care when children may have completed care for the index medical event, or may be engaged in long-term care for an illness or for the longer-term sequelae of an injury. The revised model, informed by longitudinal research, also adds several possible trajectories of PMTS, labeled as resilient, recovery, chronic, and escalating PMTS. Most children and families demonstrate a resilient trajectory marked by minimal initial distress that resolves over time, whereas a smaller proportion exhibits a recovery pathway (i.e., high initial PTSS that remits within several months). The smallest subset exhibits chronic or escalating trajectories, characterized by consistently elevated or increasing PTSS (Price et al. 2016). Across all phases of the timeline, children may present for medical care with PTSS related to exposure to PTEs outside the medical setting; this is of particular relevance to primary care providers. Trauma exposure (regardless of whether it is related to medical events or other experiences) can impact medical care (e.g., the child's response to medical procedures or interventions) and child health outcomes (Marsac et al. 2015a).

While the integrative trajectory model of PMTS underlines core features across pediatric populations with regard to psychological adaptation to medical trauma, it also notes that significant variability in PMTS is possible based on child, family, injury/illness, and treatment factors (Price et al. 2016). This suggests that the appropriate level and type of intervention will vary across children and families within each phase. The intensity and target(s) of trauma-informed interventions in medical settings must be matched to risk status and level of need (Kassam-Adams 2014; Kassam-Adams et al. 2013). *Universal interventions* are appropriate for all children exposed to PTMEs, *targeted interventions* are appropriate for those with known increased risk, and *indicated interventions* are for children with more severe and persistent distress requiring formal treatment. *Stepped care models* systematically combine universal, targeted, and indicated interventions, with individuals progressing through these levels of care as warranted. Many universal and targeted interventions can be delivered directly by pediatric healthcare providers, while most indicated interventions must be delivered by mental health (MH) providers (Kassam-Adams 2014). See Table 19.2 for an overview of key interventions across phases of PTMEs.

Table 19.2 Interventions based on level of need and timeline

		Peri-trauma	*Acute medical care*	*Ongoing (post-acute) care or discharge from medical care*
		PTMEs and immediate treatment	*Active medical treatment and ongoing acute illness/injury*	*Time beyond active acute medical care*
Universal	*All children and families presenting for medical care*	Minimize traumatic aspects of medical care Support family in providing effective support to child (e.g., calming child, distract child during stressful procedure) Consider possibility that prior trauma exposure (even if not known to healthcare team) may impact child/family responses Screen for indicators of higher risk	Provide information that supports adaptive coping with injury, illness, acute treatment Consider potential impact of prior medical or other trauma exposure on child's response to medical care and to ongoing stressors related to injury or illness Periodic screening, especially at critical junctures, for indicators of distress/higher risk	Provide information on long-term impact of child's illness/injury/treatment Provide information on common ongoing child/family psychological responses and coping strategies Provide children and families with tools for ongoing self-screening for indicators of distress

(continued)

Table 19.2 (continued)

Targeted	Children with known risk for greater than normal distress or where distress may have more severe consequences	Initiate "watchful waiting" with ongoing screening Address specific mechanisms related to known risk factors Implement strategies to reduce distress/promote coping (e.g., psychological preparation for procedure, extra attention to pain management, possible sedation)	Continue "watchful waiting" Anticipatory guidance and evidence-based self-help resources Address specific mechanisms related to known risk factors Continue strategies to reduce distress or promote coping and plan for use of these strategies during future events and procedures	Screen periodically for indicators of distress; arrange for more thorough mental health assessment if needed Assist with self-assessment of lasting impact of child/family's ongoing needs and strengths Specific suggestions and support for adaptive coping/effective self-help
Indicated	Children with known risk for severe distress or with current severe response	Initiate clinical mental health intervention for severe PTSS and other acute distress Provide more intensive psychological support during current events and treatment	Conduct more thorough assessment Provide trauma-focused treatment for severe acute distress that interferes with functioning/medical care/adherence Plan for provision of more intensive support (psychological and/or medical/sedation) during future events/procedures	Conduct more thorough assessment Trauma-focused mental health treatment

19.2 How to Implement Interventions in Medical Settings

As MH providers, our involvement in supporting psychosocial interventions in medical settings allows us to extend our reach to those who may not otherwise come in contact with MH services. There are various ways in which MH providers become involved with children in healthcare settings. MH clinicians may be integrated as key members of interdisciplinary healthcare teams, may be "co-located" (i.e., delivering MH services within the same facility), or may be external resources who serve as consultants to healthcare teams. Regardless of their role within the healthcare setting, all MH practitioners can serve as partners and advocates for routine MH screening and for the delivery of medical care using a trauma-informed approach. The appropriate type and intensity of intervention is determined based on timing and severity of child or family trauma reactions (see Table 19.2). Each phase of care is described in more detail below. Two core elements should continue throughout all phases of medical care and at all levels of need: implementing trauma-informed pediatric medical care and screening for risk and distress (Marsac et al. 2015a; Price et al. 2016). In acute medical settings (particularly those in which the child or family does not have a long-term relationship with the medical team), MH providers may face additional challenges in systematic implementation of trauma-informed care and screening. MH providers can work with teams to identify how to integrate trauma-informed medical care into their standard practice such that it does not result in additional time. Similarly, assessment tools that are easy to administer and score can be selected; administering screenings electronically that can be directly tied to the medical record may be helpful. Finally, in acute care settings, providers need easy access to referral information.

Trauma-Informed Pediatric Medical Care
MH providers can serve as leaders in medical settings in promoting a trauma-informed approach to care, with the goal of preventing trauma reactions in the early aftermath of PTEs. The DEF Protocol for Pediatric Healthcare Providers (see HealthCareToolBox.org) can be a useful framework for conceptualizing trauma-informed care actions (Center for Pediatric Traumatic Stress 2009). The DEF protocol was developed based on evidence on the etiology of PTSS and preventive techniques. This protocol encourages medical providers to address physical health (i.e., airway-breathing-circulation or the A-B-Cs) while remembering emotional health using D-E-F: reduce *D*istress, promote *E*motional support, and remember the *F*amily. The DEF protocol can be used in primary care, specialty care, and hospital-based care settings. Mutually respectful partnerships among MH providers, physicians, and nurses can enhance the provision of skilled and sensitive trauma-informed care.

In addition to supporting patients exposed to PTEs, a trauma-informed approach recognizes the challenges of providing medical care and takes into consideration self-care for medical staff. Medical providers care deeply about their patients' well-being, which may make them vulnerable to trauma reactions (e.g., burnout, compassion fatigue) related to witnessing children's suffering (Robins et al. 2009). When medical providers experience compassion fatigue or burnout, work performance and patient care can suffer (e.g., providers display less empathy; Najjar et al. 2009). To promote the best possible care for children and well-being of providers, MH practitioners can partner with medical teams to minimize compassion fatigue and burnout (Marsac et al. 2015a).

Screening for Risk and Distress
It is important to distinguish two common uses of the term "screening," each of which has an important role within a comprehensive response to children's trauma

reactions. The first is predictive screening to identify children and families who are likely to be at greater risk for ongoing distress or impairment. The second is concurrent screening to identify children and families who have current psychological distress that may warrant ongoing monitoring or immediate clinical attention. Some screening tools can serve both purposes; predictive screening in the peri-trauma or acute phases may include brief assessment of current psychological symptoms as well as other markers of risk for persistent distress. Both predictive and concurrent screening provide valuable information to healthcare teams in determining how to allocate scarce resources or supportive services based on which children and families have the highest need. In medical settings, plans for screening must take into account that some children have preexisting trauma exposure as well as trauma exposure related to current medical treatment. Screening measures vary in their coverage of preexisting and current risk markers and/or symptoms, and this may be a factor in selecting the most appropriate instrument for a specific patient population (Kassam-Adams et al. 2015a, b; Kazak et al. 2015).

To be valid, screening for future risk requires empirical evidence regarding specific factors that can be assessed at the time of screening and that are associated with later symptoms or psychosocial problems. A number of biological, psychological, and social factors contribute to a child's risk for experiencing significant distress and/or impairment in functioning (Alisic et al. 2014; Cox et al. 2008; Kahana et al. 2006; Trickey et al. 2012). See Table 19.1 for a summary of these evidence-based risk factors, some of which represent potentially malleable mechanisms and targets for prevention efforts.

The state of the art in predictive screening is still evolving, but a number of tools have been developed that assess some combination of these risk factors (Kassam-Adams et al. 2015a, b). In clinical practice, the presence of any of these risk factors may warrant continued assessment of child and family member symptoms, coping, and emotional recovery over time. See Fig. 19.1 for a list of questions to consider

---

1) Is my primary purpose to detect current distress or to predict ongoing needs/ distress?
2) What primary symptoms am I concerned about?
3) Has the measure been validated in my population and for the purpose for which I concerned for the use it?
4) How much time is needed to administer, score, and review results?
5) Who is qualified to administer and interpret results?
6) What is the cost of the measure?
7) Are there critical items on the measure that need to be addressed immediately if endorsed, and do we have staff to manage this?
8) How can we integrate the screening into standard patient care?

Fig. 19.1 Questions to consider in selecting assessment measures for use of with children in medical settings

when selecting screening tools or broader assessment measures. The answers to these questions vary widely depending on the type of medical setting (e.g., primary care, ED, inpatient hospital, specialty centers). Careful consideration of these issues will help MH providers tailor screening and assessment to maximize efficiency, while providing the most relevant and useful information to the healthcare team.

19.2.1 Interventions in the Peri-trauma Phase

During the peri-trauma phase, youth are in the midst of initial PTE exposure (e.g., injury event, new diagnosis), and many are experiencing multiple new PTEs (e.g., challenging medical procedures). Nearly all children and families experience some level of distress and challenges in coping with frightening or painful medical events and procedures. This phase is an optimal time to begin prevention of PTSS or other negative emotional outcomes through the application of trauma-informed care and screening (Marsac et al. 2014). The nature of prevention efforts will vary based on children's initial distress and other risk factors (see Table 19.2).

Universal A key role for MH providers is to facilitate the delivery of trauma-informed pediatric medical care, providing consultation, training, and/or direct services that promote medical teams' knowledge, confidence, and use of specific trauma-informed practices during initial diagnosis and treatment (Marsac et al. 2015a). Trauma-informed care in this phase includes actions by the healthcare team that minimize potentially traumatic aspects of diagnostic and treatment procedures, optimize pain management, attend to emotional distress, promote family presence and emotional support during challenging procedures, and encourage consistent communication between the medical team and the child and family. Regular assessment of the child's pain and optimizing pain management based on the child's perception (rather than assumptions about what the procedure or injury "should feel like") is an essential element of medical care that may also be helpful in preventing PTSS.

In their role as a consultant and trainer for the healthcare team, MH practitioners may find it useful to build on existing skills in patient- and family-centered care and to frame specific skills and practices for trauma-informed care using the DEF protocol (Marsac et al. 2015a; Center for Pediatric Traumatic Stress 2009). Collaboration with medical teams will often help to determine trauma-informed actions for their specific patient population and setting. For example, for children with an acute physical event with anticipation of full physical recovery, a key goal of both medical and psychosocial care is to promote return to normal functioning. For these children, universal trauma-informed care in the peri-trauma phase may include providing psychoeducation about normative physical and emotional recovery, providing a rationale for approaching rather than avoiding situations that may remind the child of the precipitating medical event, and helping parents encourage the child to return to normal activities that are safe (Kassam-Adams et al. 2013). For children with a new diagnosis of a chronic condition, a key goal (for both treatment adherence and PTSS prevention) is to increase child and family perception of safety and control. Thus, universal preventive interventions in the peri-trauma phase might include setting achievable individual goals that promote a sense of efficacy (e.g., help plan age-appropriate ways for the child to be in charge of his/her medication schedule, plan family activities in which the child can participate; Kazak et al. 2007). Primary care centers may want to consider routine screenings at well visits to help identify children with ongoing or new MH needs. A child may be at any phase of a PTE exposure when presenting for a well visit, which routine screening can help determine (Husky et al. 2011).

Targeted While many children will adapt well over time by using their existing coping strategies and social support networks, a significant number develop ongoing PTSS or other psychological distress (Kahana et al. 2006). When initial distress or risk factors are identified, ongoing screening and follow-up (a "watchful waiting" approach) is warranted, possibly supplemented by targeted prevention efforts (Kassam-Adams 2014; Price et al. 2016). At this point, these interventions are not conceptualized as clinical treatment of symptoms or disorder, although ongoing monitoring may reveal the need to offer indicated treatment.

Ideally, targeted prevention efforts in the peri-trauma phase are designed to address specific mechanisms that may lead to ongoing PTSS and other psychological sequelae (Kassam-Adams 2014). When a child has a known history of trauma exposure, medical teams can modify care delivery to reduce the potential for care (even routine procedures) to be re-traumatizing. For example, a child with a history of sexual abuse could be given the choice of whether s/he is awakened before a nurse checks vital signs overnight. Children (and their family members) with prior PTSS or anxiety may appraise new situations as threatening, beyond the realistic threat posed by specific medical event(s) and treatment. Attending to these perceptions and providing specific age-appropriate explanations and information on the duration, severity, or projected outcomes of treatment can be useful in the peri-trauma phase. In children with known PTSS risk factors, MH providers may become more involved in preparation for procedures, conducting thorough assessments of pain and coping and working with the medical team to facilitate effective pain management.

In some cases, the nature of medical event means that the peri-trauma phase also involves preparation for end-of-life care. Palliative care teams have a role here in promoting child and family sense of control and in providing more intensive support to help manage emotional experiences from the initiation of palliative care (e.g., assisting the family in discussing death, their beliefs, and wishes and creating memories through tangible mementos; Kazak et al. 2007).

Indicated Clinical MH treatment is "indicated" in the peri-trauma phase when a child (or family members) experiences severe or impairing psychological distress. In some cases, severe distress may interfere with the child or family's ability to communicate effectively with the healthcare team or to participate in medical care.

Children and families in significant distress may benefit from a psychosocial provider to help them navigate treatment and the healthcare system and from a MH practitioner to initiate trauma-focused interventions to address severe acute PTSS. MH providers who are trained in trauma-focused treatment for children, but who are not familiar with medical settings and medical trauma, may benefit from a review of specific issues relevant to pediatric injury and illness (Center for Pediatric Traumatic Stress 2015). It is likely that children with an indicated need for clinical MH treatment during the peri-trauma phase will continue to need this care in later phases and outside of the medical setting. While the identification of MH problems is increasing in primary care settings, many children are not receiving the treatment that they need for their emotional reactions, particularly those with internalizing symptoms (Chavira et al. 2004). Thus, MH providers can partner with primary care centers to help with referrals or to provide co-located services (Cluxton-Keller et al. 2015).

19.2.2 Interventions in Acute Medical Care Phase

As children and families transition from the peri-trauma to the acute medical care phase, they are still involved in active medical treatment and often face many demands and stressors related to the injury or illness itself. However, the initial shock of the medical event or diagnosis may be wearing off. Often child and family distress begins to decrease as they adapt to this new situation. In this phase, which may last from several days to many months, a medical plan is put into place to address physical health needs, and the family is either still in the hospital or still in regular contact with the medical team. Care may be transitioned to the child's primary care provider at this point. For some children and families, the nature of the acute medical treatment or the seriousness of the diagnosis may continue to pose new or ongoing challenges. The acute medical care phase thus offers opportunities for medical teams and MH providers to implement psychosocial interventions.

Rates of significant PTSS during the acute medical care phase vary depending on the type of medical event and treatment, ranging from 4–16 % of children and 11–50 % of parents (Price et al. 2016). In this phase, the child and parents' PTSS trajectory emerges. It may be too early to determine whether a specific child will ultimately follow a resilient, recovery, chronic, or escalating trajectory; evidence suggests that more than two thirds will follow resilient or recovery trajectories, and a minority will have chronic or escalating PTSS (Price et al. 2016).

Universal The need for trauma-informed medical care for all ill and injured children continues through the acute medical care phase (Marsac et al. 2015a). The same basic principles apply – minimizing potentially traumatic aspects of treatment, attending to pain management, and using the DEF protocol as a guide for specific trauma-informed practices (Center for Pediatric Traumatic Stress 2009). Although the need for trauma-informed care is universal, MH providers can work with medical teams to identify aspects of trauma-informed care that are of particular relevance to their patient population. For example, for children newly diagnosed with a chronic illness, the acute medical care phase often involves efforts to introduce and promote long-term adherence to medical regimens (e.g., medication, diet, restrictions in activities). Knowing that these regimens can potentially trigger traumatic stress reactions, MH providers can help guide the ways in which ongoing treatment regimens are introduced to children and parents (Shemesh et al. 2000). When palliative care is warranted, if support has not already begun during the peri-trauma phase, it should be initiated now.

Information and basic psychoeducation are a key part of universal prevention efforts during the acute medical care phase. MH providers can work with medical providers to ensure that all families receive education about what to expect in regard to medical treatment and normative emotional and psychological responses and to support families' existing adaptive coping strategies and social support systems (Kassam-Adams et al. 2013). Continued periodic screening, especially at critical junctures (e.g., major change in prognosis or treatment plan, discharge), can help to identify children and families that need a higher level of care now and possibly in the future.

It can be very helpful for MH and medical providers to understand not only the child's physical health needs but also the child and family's subjective perceptions of the child's condition and treatment and their beliefs about prognosis and future treatment plans. Research consistently shows that subjective appraisals are key for emotional recovery, much more so than the objective nature or severity of illness, injury, or medical treatment (Price et al. 2016). Trauma-informed medical providers listen carefully to understand the child's and family's understanding of the situation, inquire "What worries you the most?," and provide age-appropriate information about the child's medical condition, procedures, and treatment plan.

Targeted Universal screening during the acute medical phase may identify children and families with distress warranting additional attention. MH providers can support the medical team's readiness to provide additional anticipatory guidance regarding PTSS and expected reactions and to systematically include attention to child distress and emotional support in care plans (during inpatient admission). Based on screening results, MH providers may choose to conduct a more thorough assessment of child symptoms and functional impairment to help target prevention efforts and to determine if a higher level of care is needed. Targeted prevention efforts in this phase should be designed to address specific, malleable risk factors that may lead to ongoing PTSS and other psychological sequelae (Kassam-Adams 2014). Promising targets for prevention during acute medical care include parent responses and children's early maladaptive appraisals and coping strategies (Kassam-Adams 2014).

Preventive interventions appropriate for this phase include evidence-based, self-directed programs for children or parents. The example programs presented here were each designed as a universal preventive intervention, but because research suggests they are particularly useful for children or families at higher risk for persistent PTSS, we include them as targeted interventions. An injured child may benefit from psychoeducational programs such as an informational booklet or website (e.g., "Kids and Accidents"; Cox and Kenardy 2010; Kenardy et al. 2008)); parents of injured children may also benefit from web-based resources (e.g., AfterTheInjury.org; kidtrauma.org; Landolt 2016; Marsac et al. 2013). Programs are under development that teach cognitive restructuring and adaptive coping (e.g., Coping Coach) for children with acute medical events (Kassam-Adams et al. 2015; Marsac et al. 2015b). Children with chronic illnesses can benefit from programs that teach them how to manage disease symptoms, treatment, and associated feelings (e.g., Cellie Coping Kit; Marsac et al. 2012, 2014). Moving beyond evidence-based self-help resources, if a MH provider is available, programs that help families recognize and reframe maladaptive beliefs and work together to face the challenges of life-threatening illness may be beneficial (e.g., Surviving Cancer Competently Intervention Program-Newly Diagnosed; Kazak et al. 2005).

Indicated If children or families' psychological symptoms are creating significant distress, interfering with medical care, and/or interfering with daily functioning, clinical MH services are warranted. Depending on their role within the hospital or healthcare organization, MH providers may initiate and deliver treatment within the medical setting (if co-located or integrated team members), provide treatment in an external setting, or support the child and family in identifying a knowledgeable provider. Effective treatments for child PTSS (e.g., trauma-focused CBT, reviewed in Chap. 8) are relevant for children in the acute medical care phase but may sometimes require adaptation to address medical issues and triggers (Center for Pediatric Traumatic Stress 2015).

19.2.3 Interventions During Ongoing (Post-acute) Care or After Discharge from Care

A small but significant proportion of children demonstrate persistently elevated or delayed onset PTSS, making long-term follow-up care a critical window of opportunity for the provision of trauma-informed assessments and interventions. Primary care providers have a unique opportunity to follow-up on children that have been discharged from specialty care and, with routine screening, may be able to identify children whose symptoms were delayed. In addition to those with chronic or delayed symptom trajectories, some children may require additional monitoring and support for the late effects or complications associated with their injury, illness, and/or medical treatment. After acute medical care has ended, some children and families experience changes in risk and protective factors (e.g., available support systems) and/or exposure to additional PTEs that impact adjustment and/or recovery. Thus, despite the practical emphasis on prevention and intervention efforts in the peri-trauma and acute medical care phases, a comprehensive response to pediatric medical traumatic stress must incorporate the *entire* lifecycle of a medical event, including this longer-term phase after discharge or when acute medical care has transitioned to ongoing care (Price et al. 2016).

Universal Universal interventions for PTSS include continued screening for PTSS during routine follow-up visits and ongoing provision of support, education, and resources targeted toward later stages of PTMEs. For instance, healthcare providers can continue to implement the basic principles of the DEF protocol (Center for Pediatric Traumatic Stress 2009) as a standard part of medical visits. Specifically, providers should screen for current child distress related to either the medical event or its longer-term consequences or complications (e.g., pain, restrictions in activities, missed school, bullying), assess availability of emotional support to cope with distress, and inquire about new or ongoing needs of family members that impact the child's recovery. Partnerships between pediatric healthcare teams and relevant community-based organizations can offer additional opportunities for universal assessment and supports for children in the months and years after a PTE (Kazak et al. 2007).

Universal trauma-informed support includes providing families with psychoeducational resources targeted toward issues relevant to this later phase. For instance, HealthCareToolBox.org offers developmentally appropriate tip sheets for youth and parents regarding adjustment after hospital discharge, dealing with ongoing pain, and fears or worries (Center for Pediatric Traumatic Stress 2009). Several web-based interventions designed for the early weeks after acute medical events (described above) also offer guidance, strategies, and resources for concerns that can emerge in this later stage of recovery (Cox and Kenardy 2010; Marsac et al. 2013).

Targeted Targeted interventions promote recovery and resilience for children at risk for continued or new onset traumatic stress reactions. During routine follow-up visits, medical providers who are concerned about psychological sequelae of medical events should coordinate with MH clinicians to provide more targeted assessment and intervention services. Specifically, clinicians should assess the lasting psychosocial impact of the medical event as well as the child and family's ongoing needs and strengths. Based on this assessment, MH providers can make suggestions and provide support for adaptive coping strategies. Providers should consider ways to enhance social support for children with problematic yet subclinical reactions by connecting them to resources and supports at the healthcare, school, and community levels. For children who are at risk for persistent and impairing symptoms, referrals should be made for more comprehensive, formal assessment to determine whether MH treatment is needed. MH providers in primary care settings are particularly well positioned to provide these targeted assessment and intervention services during the longer-term post-trauma phase, as primary care providers often have the greatest continuity with and exposure to this patient population.

Indicated Children demonstrating significant and impairing PTSS that persist beyond the early weeks and months after medical trauma require referrals to a MH clinician trained in trauma-focused treatments. These interventions are described in detail in section B of this book. MH providers in medical settings can facilitate the referral process by identifying appropriate treatment providers in the healthcare network and/or the community, preparing patients for treatment by providing basic psychoeducation about evidence-based therapies, enhancing motivation to seek treatment, addressing anticipated barriers, and following-up with patients over time to monitor needs. In addition to facilitating referrals to formal treatment services, providers in medical settings should pay particular attention to the impact of symptoms on adherence to medical regimens and health outcomes (e.g., avoidance of hospital, anxiety around medications or procedures).

19.2.4 Stepped Care Models

Stepped care models systematically incorporate universal screening of PTSS, targeted services for those at risk, and provision of indicated trauma-focused psychological interventions to youth with persistent PTSS (Kassam-Adams et al. 2011). These models provide intervention using a stepped approach: only those at risk for significant and persistent symptoms progress to more intensive levels of care (Salloum et al. 2014). For instance, Kassam-Adams et al. (2011) screened injured children for risk factors and subsequently assigned them to either a low-risk or an at-risk group. Those at risk were randomized to usual care or intervention, which included psychoeducation and brief assessments to identify additional needs. Children with identified needs were then offered additional services (e.g., care coordination, assistance with medical adherence, brief intervention to improve communication and coping, evaluation by MH provider, and/or TF-CBT). Similarly, Kenardy et al. (2010)) developed a stepped care intervention for injured children involving a two-stage screening (2 and 6 weeks after injury), followed by child- or family-focused CBT if indicated. Applying stepped care to young children, Salloum et al. (2014) developed a systematic intervention program that begins with an initial assessment, followed by three therapist-led TF-CBT sessions, a parent-child workbook, weekly phone meetings, and provision of a web-based informational resource. Children who demonstrate sufficient clinical improvement terminate active treatment and enter a maintenance phase, comprised of parent-led weekly meetings and continue practicing and using skills learned in the first phase of treatment. Those who did not respond to the first step receive up to nine additional therapist-led TF-CBT sessions. A posttreatment assessment then facilitates decisions around terminating or continuing treatment. While stepped care programs for pediatric traumatic stress are few in number and evidence is preliminary, these models hold promise for providing more efficient, accessible, and cost-effective services relative to standard treatment delivery systems (Salloum et al. 2014).

19.3 Special Challenges

A number of challenges emerge when working to support children and families' emotional health in medical settings. Limited resources can prevent implementing MH interventions on a large scale, particularly those requiring a MH provider. Recent efforts have been made to try to extend our reach of interventions, particularly universal and targeted, while minimizing costs. These include creating programs that do not depend on implementation by a MH provider and developing eHealth applications. These programs require funding for development, evaluation, and sustainability, but can often be disseminated at a low cost.

Evaluation of treatments in medical settings is costly and time consuming. Given that specific populations (e.g., children with cystic fibrosis) are often small in a single setting and agreement to participate in studies can be low with competing medical demands, multi-site studies are often necessary. This can be very costly and challenging, particularly when evaluating a particular type of intervention (requiring consistent implementation by MH providers). Thus, while promising evidence of effectiveness of trauma interventions in medical settings exists, a gold standard of care has yet to be determined.

Another challenge is lack of awareness or training in trauma-informed care for medical providers (Banh, Saxe, Mangione, & Horton, 2008). Most medical providers have limited training in MH and no training in trauma-informed care, resulting in an underestimation of MH symptoms and lack of awareness of available screening tools (Banh et al. 2008). With the heavy demands on medical teams to care for increasing numbers of patients at lower costs, integrating another concept of delivering medical care via a trauma-informed care approach may be overwhelming. However, MH providers can help address this by integrating trauma-informed practices as part of standard care.

Finally, the child and family may want to focus exclusively on the child's physical health. Families may be unaware of how medical events can affect MH, fear stigmas associated with MH treatment, or unable to dedicate time or money to care that extends beyond physical health. If children's emotional health is integrated into their standard medical care to a greater degree, we may be able to overcome or minimize these pervasive stigmas.

19.4 Empirical Support for Interventions in Medical Settings

Evidence on the effectiveness of interventions in medical settings is beginning to grow, but much more research is needed to best support children's emotional health and recovery (Kassam-Adams et al. 2013; Kazak et al. 2007). While trauma-informed care has a strong theoretical background and is solidly anchored in medical traumatic stress and child trauma research, we do not yet know how implementing trauma-informed care directly affects child emotional or physical health outcomes.

As discussed above, screening needs persist across all phases of trauma exposure and can serve two purposes: identifying current distress or predicting future distress.

For children with acute medical trauma (e.g., injuries with expected recovery, sudden, brief illnesses such as appendicitis), a number of screeners have been successfully developed and implemented in medical settings (e.g., Kassam-Adams et al. 2015; Kramer et al. 2013; van Meijel et al. 2015). However, efforts to identify short screeners that can be easily integrated into routine medical care are still underway (Kassam-Adams and Marsac in press). Screening for those with chronic or ongoing medical conditions can be more challenging as the course of medical treatment (thus additional trauma exposure) is often unpredictable. Tools such as the Psychosocial Assessment Tool have had some success in predicting psychosocial service utilization and PTSS in parents of children with cancer (Alderfer et al. 2009). The use of PTSS checklists can be useful in providing information on current distress (Landolt et al. 2003). However, we are in need of validated, brief screeners that can be integrated into medical care to assess and predict child PTSS over the course of chronic illness. Thus, while we can fairly easily determine those children and families who need more attention immediately and suggest who will need to be followed over time, more research is necessary to be able to determine which children will need a high-level intensity of services over time. As our predictive ability improves, we may be able to intervene earlier with these children and better allocate resources to those most in need (given limited funding for MH treatment).

Turning directly to interventions, careful attention is needed in developing and evaluating interventions across phases of medical care. Even the most well-intentioned interventions can have adverse effects, so it is essential that treatments are based in evidence and evaluated as they are developed (Roberts et al. 2009). To date, no clear evidence is available supporting the routine implementation of a specific universal preventive intervention for those exposed to trauma (Roberts et al. 2009). However, some interventions have shown promising results. An example of a promising universal intervention that was initiated during peri-trauma (and continued through later phases) is Stoddard et al. (2011) pharmacological intervention (i.e., 24-week course of sertraline initiated during burn hospitalization); this intervention reduced PTSS in children by parent report (but not by child report). Initiating an intervention during the acute trauma phase, Kenardy et al. (2008) provided children with an informational booklet following an injury. They found a reduction in anxiety (but not PTSS) for the intervention group. Providing this information to children online and with a booklet to parents replicated the same effect (i.e., reduced anxiety in children; Cox and Kenardy 2010). Also during the early acute phase, Zehnder et al. (2010) had success in reducing depression (but not PTSS) in preteens following an injury using a single-session intervention (a therapist met with parents and children together to provide psychoeducation and facilitate reconstruction of the injury event). Finally, during the ongoing/discharge phase, results from the Surviving Cancer Competently Intervention Program (SCCIP), a single session, therapist-led intervention for families with children with cancer, suggest reductions in intrusiveness of stress symptoms for fathers and arousal symptoms for adolescents (but no effect for mothers; Kazak et al. 2004). For newly diagnosed families (SCCIP-ND) during the peri-trauma phase, the intervention includes parents only;

research suggested reductions in anxiety and PTSS in parents (though reductions were not statistically significant; Kazak et al. 2005). In addition, a number of other universal, early interventions in medical settings have been found to "do no harm" and are reported by families as helpful in navigating the challenges of medical care. These interventions focus on providing basic psychoeducation about emotional reactions during peri-trauma and acute trauma phases, promoting the child's current adaptive coping strategies, and including the parent as a part of recovery. Examples of these interventions include AfterTheInjury.org (Marsac et al. 2013) and the Cellie Coping Kit (Marsac et al. 2012, 2014).

For children demonstrating PTSS and needing services, evidence of current interventions is stronger. For example, Coping Coach is a web-based intervention designed for children following acute trauma. The intervention is designed to be initiated during the peri-trauma or acute trauma phase (e.g., the hospital or doctor's office) and focuses on promoting adaptive cognitive appraisals, decreasing excessive avoidance coping, and promoting social support. Though implemented as a universal intervention in the pilot evaluation study (and meeting the "do no harm" criteria), results suggested the greatest impact on PTSS for at-risk children. Additionally, during the early ongoing phase of trauma, Berkowitz et al. (2011) found promising results for children who participated in the Child and Family Traumatic Stress Intervention (CFTSI) following a PTE resulting in visit to a pediatric ED, a forensic sexual abuse program, or a police department's victim services (see Chap. 7).

For children in medical settings rising to the indicated level of need, evidence to support specific treatment approaches varies based on the trauma identified. For example, if primary care or other medical settings determine that a child has PTSS related to a past trauma (e.g., violence, sexual abuse), trauma-focused CBT has a strong evidence base. For children presenting in medical settings with behavior or adherence difficulties, behavioral and cognitive-behavioral interventions are well-established treatments. However, while we expect that CBT/ TF-CBT would be efficacious for children with significant medical traumatic stress or PTSD related to medical care, no RCTs have been conducted to examine the effectiveness of TF-CBT on reducing medical traumatic stress; more research is needed to determine which treatments are most effective for these pediatric populations. These interventions are most often implemented during the ongoing/discharge phase of treatment but may be initiated earlier if a child's distress and/or impairment are high.

Conclusions

Medical settings are ideal settings to identify and support children exposed to PTEs. Children presenting to healthcare networks, especially those from underserved populations, may not come to the attention of MH providers in other ways. PTSS affect children's physical health and functional outcomes (Landolt et al. 2009; Zatzick et al. 2008). The implementation of trauma-informed care, including regular screening for psychological symptoms, is recommended across all phases of medical care (Marsac et al. 2015a; Price et al. 2016). Evidence suggests that psychoeducation about normative emotional reactions and when to get help, supporting adaptive coping, and behavioral or cognitive-behavioral treatments may be helpful to children with challenging injuries, illnesses, and/or medical treatments. More research is necessary to establish the most efficacious treatments for children with significant PTSS related to medical events, though theory suggests that adapting effective CBT/TF-CBT interventions should be relevant and effective for children with medical traumatic stress.

References

Alderfer MA, Mougianis I, Barakat LP, Beele D, DiTaranto S, Hwang WT, Kazak AE (2009) Family psychosocial risk, distress, and service utilization in pediatric cancer. Cancer 115(S18):4339–4349. doi:10.1002/cncr.24587

Alisic E, Jongmans MJ, van Wesel F, Kleber RJ (2011) Building child trauma theory from longitudinal studies: a meta-analysis. Clin Psychol Rev 31(5):736–747. doi:10.1016/j.cpr.2011.03.001

Alisic E, Zalta AK, van Wesel F, Larsen SE, Hafstad GS, Hassanpour K, Smid GE (2014) Rates of post-traumatic stress disorder in trauma-exposed children and adolescents: meta-analysis. Br J Psychiatry 204:335–340. doi:10.1192/bjp.bp.113.131227

Banh MK, Saxe G, Mangione T, Horton NJ (2008) Physician-reported practice of managing childhood posttraumatic stress in pediatric primary care. Gen Hosp Psychiatry 30(6):536–545. doi:10.1016/j.genhosppsych.2008.07.008

Berkowitz SJ, Stover CS, Marans SR (2011) The child and family traumatic stress intervention: secondary prevention for youth at risk of developing PTSD. J child psychol psychiatry,allied disciplines 52(6):676–685. doi:10.1111/j.1469-7610.2010.02321.x

Center for Pediatric Traumatic Stress (2009) HealthCareToolBox.org. Retrieved 1 Dec 2015, from http://www.HealthCareToolbox.org

Center for Pediatric Traumatic Stress (2015) Working with children and familes experiencing medical traumatic stress: a resource guide for mental health professionals. Retrieved 25 Nov 2015 from http://www.HealthCareToolBox.org

Chavira DA, Stein MB, Bailey K, Stein MT (2004) Child anxiety in primary care: prevalent but untreated. Depress anxiety 20(4):155–164. doi:10.1002/da.20039

Cluxton-Keller F, Riley AW, Noazin S, Umoren MV (2015) Clinical effectiveness of family therapeutic interventions embedded in general pediatric primary care settings for parental mental health: a systematic review and meta-analysis. Clin Child Fam Psychol Rev 18(4):395–412. doi:10.1007/s10567-015-0190-x

Copeland W, Keeler G, Angold A, Costello E (2007) Traumatic events and posttraumatic stress in childhood. Arch Gel Psychiatry 64(5):577–584. doi:10.1001/archpsyc.64.5.577

Cox C, Kenardy J (2010) A randomised controlled trial of a web-based early intervention for children and their parents following accidental injury. J Pediatric Psychol 35:581–592. doi:10.1093/jpepsy/jsp095

Cox C, Kenardy J, Hendrikz J (2008) A meta-analysis of risk factors that predict psychopathology following accidental trauma. J Spec Pediatr Nurs 13(2):98–110. doi:10.1111/j.1744-6155.2008.00141.x

Hildenbrand AK, Marsac ML, Daly BP, Chute D, Kassam-Adams N (2015) Acute pain and post-traumatic stress after pediatric injury. J Pediatr Psychol. doi:10.1093/jpepsy/jsv026

Husky MM, Miller K, McGuire L, Flynn L, Olfson M (2011) Mental health screening of adolescents in pediatric practice. J Behav Health Serv Res 38(2):159–169. doi:10.1007/s11414-009-9207-x

Kahana S, Feeny N, Youngstrom E, Drotar D (2006) Posttraumatic stress in youth experiencing illnesses and injuries: an exploratory meta-analysis. Traumatology 12(2):148–161. doi:10.1177/1534765606294562

Kassam-Adams N (2014) Design, delivery, and evaluation of early interventions for children exposed to acute trauma. Eur J Psychotraumatol 5. doi:10.3402/ejpt.v5.22757

Kassam-Adams N, Garcia-Espana J, Marsac ML, Kohser K, Baxt C, Nance M, Winston FK (2011) A pilot randomized controlled trial assessing secondary prevention of traumatic stress integrated into pediatric trauma care. J Trauma Stress 24(3):252–259. doi:10.1002/jts.20640

Kassam-Adams N, Marsac ML Brief practical screeners for acute posttraumatic stress symptoms in children in English and Spanish, Journal of Traumatic Stress, in press

Kassam-Adams N, Marsac ML, Hildenbrand AK, Winston FK (2013) Posttraumatic stress following pediatric injury: update on diagnosis, risk factors, and intervention. JAMA Pediatr 167(12):1158–1165. doi:10.1001/jamapediatrics.2013.2741

Kassam-Adams N, Marsac ML, Kohser K, Kenardy J, March S, Winston FK (2015a) Pilot randomized controlled trial of a novel web-based intervention to prevent posttraumatic stress in children following medical events. J Pediatr Psychol. doi:10.1093/jpepsy/jsv057

Kassam-Adams N, Marsc M, García-España J, Winston F (2015b) Evaluating predictive screening for children's post-injury mental health: new data and a replication. Eur J Psychotraumatol 6:29313

Kazak A, Alderfer M, Streisand R, Simms S, Rourke M, Barakat L, Cnaan A (2004) Treatment of posttraumatic stress symptoms in adolescent survivors of childhood cancer and their families: a randomized clinical trial. J Fam Psychol 18:493–504. doi:10.1037/0893-3200.18.3.493

Kazak A, Kassam-Adams N, Schneider S, Zelikovsky N, Alderfer M, Rourke M (2006) An integrative model of pediatric medical traumatic stress. J Pediatr Psychol 44:343–355. doi:10.1093/jpepsy/jsj054

Kazak A, Struber M, Barakat L, Meeske K (1996) Assessing posttraumatic stress related to medical illness and treatment: the Impact of Traumatic Stressors Interview Schedule (ITSIS). Fam Sys Health 14:365–380. doi:10.1037/h0089795

Kazak AE, Rourke MT, Alderfer MA, Pai A, Reilly AF, Meadows AT (2007) Evidence-based assessment, intervention and psychosocial care in pediatric oncology: a blueprint for comprehensive services across treatment. J Pediatr Psychol 32(9):1099–1110. doi:10.1093/jpepsy/jsm031

Kazak AE, Schneider S, Didonato S, Pai AL (2015) Family psychosocial risk screening guided by the Pediatric Psychosocial Preventative Health Model (PPPHM) using the Psychosocial Assessment Tool (PAT). Acta oncologica 54(5):574–580. doi:10.3109/0284186X.2014.995774

Kazak AE, Simms S, Alderfer MA, Rourke MT, Crump T, McClure K et al (2005) Feasibility and preliminary outcomes from a pilot study of a brief psychological intervention for families of children newly diagnosed with cancer. J Pediatr Psychol 30(8):644–655. doi:10.1093/jpepsy/jsi051

Kenardy J, Cobham V, Nixon RD, McDermott B, March S (2010) Protocol for a randomised controlled trial of risk screening and early intervention comparing child- and family-focused cognitive-behavioural therapy for PTSD in children following accidental injury. Bio Med Central Psychiatry 10:92–101. doi:10.1186/1471-244X-10-92

Kenardy J, Thompson K, Le Brocque R, Olsson K (2008) Information provision intervention for children and their parents following pediatric accidental injury. Eur Child Adolesc Psychol 17(5):316–325. doi:10.1007/s00787-007-0673-5

Kramer DN, Hertli M, Landolt MA (2013) Evaluation of an early risk screener for PTSD in preschool children after accidental injury. Pediatrics 132:945–951

Landolt MA, Buehlmann C, Maag T, Schiestl C (2009) Brief Report: quality of life is impaired in pediatric burn survivors with posttraumatic stress disorder. J Pediatr Psychol 34(1):14–21. doi:10.1093/jpepsy/jsm088

Landolt MA, Vollrath M, Ribi K, Gnehm H, Sennhauser F (2003) Incidence and associations of parental and child posttraumatic stress symptoms in pediatric patients. J Child Psycho Psychiatry 44:1199–1207. doi:10.1111/1469-7610.00201

Marsac ML, Hildenbrand A, Kohser K, Winston F, Li Y, Kassam-Adams N (2013) Preventing posttraumatic stress following pediatric injury: A randomized controlled trial of a web-based psycho-educational intervention for parents. J Pediatr Psychol. doi:10.1093/jpepsy/jst053

Marsac ML, Kassam-Adams N, Hildenbrand AK, Nicholls E, Winston FK, Leff SS, Fein J (2015a) Implementing a trauma-informed approach in pediatric health care networks. JAMA Pediatr 170(1):1–8. doi:10.1001/jamapediatrics.2015.2206

Marsac ML, Winston F, Hildenbrand A, Kohser K, March S, Kenardy J, Kassam-Adams N (2015b) Systematic, theoretically grounded development and feasibility testing of an innovative, preventive web-based game for children exposed to acute trauma. Clin PractPediatr Psychol 3(1):12–24. doi:10.1037/cpp0000080

Marsac ML, Hildenbrand AK, Clawson K, Jackson L, Kohser K, Barakat L, Alderfer MA (2012) Acceptability and feasibility of family use of The Cellie Cancer Coping Kit. Support Care Cancer 20(12):3315–3324. doi:10.1007/s00520-012-1475-y

Marsac ML, Klingbeil OG, Hildenbrand AK, Alderfer MA, Kassam-Adams N, Smith-Whitley K, Barakat LP (2014) The Cellie Coping Kit for Sickle Cell Disease: initial acceptability and feasibility. Clin Pract Pediatr Psychol 4(2):10

Murray C, Lopez A (1996) The global burden of disease: a comprehensive assessment of mortality and disability from diseases, injuries, and risk factors in 1990 and projected to 2020. Harvard University Press, Cambridge, MA

Kassam-Adams N, Marsac ML (2009) Brief practical screeners for acute posttraumatic stress symptoms in children in English and Spanish (under review)

Najjar N, Davis LW, Beck-Coon K, Carney Doebbeling C (2009) Compassion fatigue: a review of the research to date and relevance to cancer-care providers. J health psychol 14(2):267–277. doi:10.1177/1359105308100211

Price J, Kassam-Adams N, Alderfer MA, Christofferson J, Kazak AE (2016) Systematic review: a reevaluation and update of the integrative (Trajectory) model of pediatric medical traumatic stress. J Pediatr Psychol 41:86–97. doi:10.1093/jpepsy/jsv074

Roberts, N.P., Kitchiner, N.J., Kenardy, J., & Bisson, J. (2009). Multiple session early psychological interventions for the prevention of post-traumatic stress disorder. Cochrane Database Syst Rev (3), CD006869. doi: 10.1002/14651858.CD006869.pub2

Robins PM, Meltzer L, Zelikovsky N (2009) The experience of secondary traumatic stress upon care providers working within a children's hospital. J Pediatr Nurs 24(4):270–279. doi:10.1016/j.pedn.2008.03.007

Salloum A, Scheeringa MS, Cohen JA, Storch EA (2014) Development of stepped care traumafocused cognitive-behavioral therapy for young children. Cogn Behav Pract 21(1):97–108. doi:10.1016/j.cbpra.2013.07.004

Schappert SM, Rechsteiner EA (2008) Ambulatory medical care utlization estimates for 2006. National health statistics reports; no 8. Hyattsville, MD: National Center for Health Statistics. 2008

Shemesh E, Lurie S, Stuber M, Emre S, Patel Y, Vohra P, Shneider B (2000) A pilot study of posttraumatic stress and nonadherence in pediatric liver transplant recipients. Pediatrics 105(2):29–36

Stoddard FJ, Luthra R, Sorrentino EA, Saxe GN, Drake J, Chang Y, Levine JB, Sheridan RL (2011) A randomized controlled trial of sertraline to prevent posttraumatic stress disorder in burned children. J Child Adolesc Psychopharmacol 21(5):469–477. doi:10.1089/cap.2010.0133

Substance Abuse and Mental Health Services Administration. (2015). Trauma-informed approach and trauma-specific interventions. Retrieved 25 Nov 2015 from http://www.samhsa.gov/nctic/trauma-interventions

Trickey D, Siddaway AP, Meiser-Stedman R, Serpell L, Field AP (2012) A meta-analysis of risk factors for post-traumatic stress disorder in children and adolescents. Clin Psychol Rev 32:122–138. doi:10.1016/j.cpr.2011.12.001

Van Meijel EP, Gigengack MR, Verlinden E, Opmeer BC, Heij HA, Goslings JC et al (2015) Predicting posttraumatic stress disorder in children and parents following accidental child injury: evaluation of the screening tool for early predictors of posttraumatic stress disorder (STEPP). BMC Psychiatr 15:113. doi:10.1186/s12888-015-0492-z

Zatzick D, Jurkovich G, Fan M, Grossman D, Russo J, Katon W, Rivara F (2008) Association between posttraumatic stress and depressive symptoms and functional outcomes in adolescents followed up longitudinally after injury hospitalization. Arch Pediatr Adolesc Med 162(7):642–648. doi:10.1001/archpedi.162.7.642

Zehnder D, Meuli M, Landolt MA (2010) Effectiveness of a single-session early psychological intervention for children after road traffic accidents: a randomised controlled trial. Child Adolesc Psychiatry Ment Health 4:7–17. doi:10.1186/1753-2000-4-7

Trauma-Informed Care in Inpatient and Residential Settings

Jennifer F. Havens and Mollie Marr

20.1 Principles of Trauma-Informed Care in Inpatient and Residential Settings

A history of exposure to traumatic events is the norm in youth utilizing residential care, whether it be acute or subacute inpatient care or longer-term residential placement. Studies of youth in inpatient psychiatric settings reveal traumatic exposures in over 90 % of admitted youth and rates of post-traumatic stress disorder (PTSD) from 25 to 33 % (Adam et al. 1992; Craine et al. 1988; Gold 2008; Havens et al. 2012b; Allwood et al. 2008; Lipschitz et al. 1999). By definition, youth placed within the child welfare system have been exposed to abuse and/or neglect. Studies in this population reveal rates of PTSD from 19 to 40 % (Kolko et al. 2010; Famularo et al. 1996).

Despite the ubiquity of traumatic exposure of youth in these settings, many systems fail to adequately identify and address the clinical and behavioral issues related to traumatic exposure (Havens et al. 2012a; Giaconia et al. 1995; Mueser and Taub 2008; Hawke et al. 2009; Deters et al. 2006; Jaycox et al. 2004; Lipschitz et al. 2000; Grasso et al. 2009; Keeshin et al. 2014). When lack of recognition of trauma

---

J.F. Havens, MD (✉)
Department of Child and Adolescent Psychiatry, New York University School of Medicine, New York, NY, USA

Department of Child and Adolescent Psychiatry, Bellevue Hospital Center, New York, NY, USA
e-mail: jennifer.havens@nyumc.org

M. Marr, BFA
Department of Child and Adolescent Psychiatry, New York University School of Medicine, New York, NY, USA

Oregon Health & Science University, Portland, OR, USA
e-mail: mollie.marr@nyumc.org

exposure and PTSD extends to high-risk populations of adolescents, it has serious implications both for mental health treatment planning and their safe management in residential settings (Ford and Blaustein 2013; Ford et al. 2012a; Havens et al. 2012a). Clinicians may find these youths to be refractory, or only partially and transiently responsive, to a wide range of pharmacotherapy regimens if traumatic stress reactions are not addressed in treatment (Opler et al. 2009). Evidence-based psychotherapies for a range of other internalizing and externalizing problems may prove similarly ineffective (Ford and Cloitre 2009), and it is impossible to prescribe the appropriate trauma-focused therapies in the absence of a PTSD diagnosis. On the management side, intrusive reexperiencing and hyperarousal symptoms may precipitate crises that place the adolescent and treatment providers at risk (Ford et al. 2009, 2012a). Providers and program staff may become frustrated and reluctant to continue to attempt to engage with and actively treat or conduct rehabilitative interventions with these adolescents. Stigmatizing labeling may occur, both on an informal (e.g., "incorrigible," "unreachable") and diagnostic (e.g., "borderline or antisocial personality traits," intermittent explosive disorder, bipolar, conduct, or psychotic disorders) level. The adolescent may be alternately pressured to act appropriately and engage in prosocial activities or isolated from the therapeutic or rehabilitative program and peers—either of which can trigger significant clinical deterioration (Havens et al. 2012a).

Therefore it is essential that inpatient and residential care settings implement interventions to identify and address the impact of trauma on youth in their care. Fortunately, over the last 20 years, significant progress has been made in the development and implementation of practices and policies that support the development of trauma-informed care systems. For example, in the USA, the Substance Abuse and Mental Health Services Administration (SAMHSA) of the Department of Health and Human Services has supported multiple efforts to create trauma-informed care (TIC) systems. This national-level organization has been instrumental in explicating definitions of trauma-informed care systems in the USA, with substantial amount of federal and state funding allocated to promoting the development of approaches and principles of such systems. SAMHSA has defined a trauma-informed approach as follows:

"A program, organization or system that is trauma-informed:

1. Realizes the widespread impact of trauma and understands potential paths for recovery;
2. Recognizes the signs and symptoms of trauma in clients, families, staff, and others involved with the system;
3. Responds by fully integrating knowledge about trauma into policies, procedures, and practices; and
4. Seeks to actively resist re-traumatization." (SAMHSA 2015)

SAMHSA has also identified key principles of a trauma-informed approach, which include safety, trustworthiness and transparency, peer support, collaboration and mutuality, empowerment, voice, and choice (SAMHSA 2014). In addition, SAMHSA has identified well-known trauma-specific interventions that have been implemented in public settings in the USA (SAMHSA 2015) that can be applied in a range of settings to help staff and clients effectively address the consequences of traumatic exposure. In Canada, the Manitoba Trauma Information and Education Centre (MTIEC) built on the key principles defined by SAMHSA and created a trauma toolkit to help organizations and providers adapt, develop, and deliver trauma-informed services (MTIEC 2016). As part of this toolkit, they adapted an organizational checklist which can be used to identify and guide the integration of trauma-informed practices. The toolkit also includes chapters on the experience of immigrants and refugees as well as the impact of colonization and residential schools on First Nations and Inuit communities highlighting the importance of incorporating cultural awareness and competence in the development and delivery of trauma-informed programming.

Unlike specific psychotherapeutic interventions for trauma, which have been rigorously tested in randomized controlled trials (Cohen 2010; Silverman et al. 2008), there is a limited evidence base in support of the effectiveness of trauma-informed care (Hanson and Lang 2014). A small number of primarily adult studies and one adolescent study have shown a reduction in the use of seclusion and restraints following trauma-informed staff education and the introduction of trauma-informed practices (Muskett 2014; Azeem et al. 2011). The implementation of trauma-informed care is a complex and fluid organizational change intervention; it is not surprising that there is no clear consensus about what trauma-informed care actually consists of as well as no clear empirical support for any one systematic approach to implementing trauma-informed care systems.

The most extensively implemented and described whole system intervention is Sanctuary. The Sanctuary Model is an evidence-supported intervention (Rivard et al. 2005), initially developed for use on adult inpatient psychiatric units, and has been adapted for use in residential, outpatient, welfare, and prison settings (Bloom 1997). It incorporates tools to guide organizations and providers in creating and implementing trauma-informed policies and procedures, interventions, and trauma-focused treatment. The Sanctuary Model defines seven commitments to: "Nonviolence, Emotional Intelligence, Social Learning, Open Communication, Democracy, Social Responsibility, Growth and Change" (Sanctuaryweb 2016). The commitments are part of a shared language and approach consistent across organizations despite diverse settings and unique populations served and represent shared organizational values.

Another whole system approach is Trauma Affect Regulation: Guide for Education and Therapy (TARGET), a manualized, evidence-based intervention designed for individuals who have been impacted by trauma that can be delivered in multiple modalities (individual, group, family milieu) (Ford 2006). While TARGET was originally developed as a treatment intervention for high-risk youth which focused on emotional and behavioral regulation skills, and problem-solving strategies, it was revised as a milieu program and incorporates trauma-informed training to staff.

TARGET as a milieu intervention aims to increase the skill and ability of frontline staff to work effectively with youth that have experienced trauma. This adaptation is known as *TARGET 1,2,3,4* or T4. Staff can use T4 to help reinforce youth use of core TARGET skills, de-escalate challenging situations, engage youth in problem-solving discussions, and manage their own stress reactions. Providing staff with T4 training will enhance their skill in de-escalating potential conflicts with or between detained youth, which is expected to contribute to reductions in youth aggression toward staff and other youth. Two studies evaluated the impact of implementing T4 and TARGET groups for youth in secure juvenile detention facilities and found significant reductions in youth disciplinary infractions, aggression toward staff, and use of seclusion (Ford et al. 2012b; Marrow et al. 2012b).

20.2 Implementing Trauma-Informed Care in Inpatient Acute Psychiatric Settings

Despite the ubiquity of traumatic exposure and trauma-related symptomatology in acute inpatient settings (Havens et al. 2012a, b; Fehon et al. 2001; Lipschitz et al. 1999), there has been little systematic work done on the implementation of trauma-informed care in these settings. At Bellevue Hospital Center, a tertiary care public hospital located in New York City, we operate three inpatient child and adolescent psychiatric units (45 beds) serving youth between 2 and 18 years of age. The current model of inpatient psychiatric care in the USA is an acute stabilization model; youth are admitted when they present a danger to themselves or others or when their psychiatric illness impairs their ability to be safe in less intensive settings. The average length of stay is 13 days.

Systematic screening for trauma exposure and PTSD on the Bellevue Hospital Center inpatient psychiatric child and adolescent services over the last 6 years reveals consistently high rates of PTSD, with 23 % of children and adolescents over the age of 7 screening above the clinical cutoff for PTSD. Youth who screen positive for PTSD usually present a constellation of internalizing and externalizing symptoms and have often been misdiagnosed prior to admission due to a lack of proper identification of trauma-related symptoms (Havens et al. 2012a, b).

The search for appropriate trauma-informed interventions for short-stay intensive inpatient settings (average length of stay 13 days) yielded nothing other than the Sanctuary Model and TARGET, which was prohibitive in terms of intensity of training and cost. What follows describes the implementation of our model of trauma-informed care for inpatient psychiatric settings, with a focus on practicality, feasibility, and maintenance. Implementation includes four essential elements:

1. Systematic trauma screening
2. Staff trauma training
3. Trauma skills groups for children and adolescents
4. Ongoing monitoring of trauma-informed care implementation

20.2.1 Systematic Trauma Screening

PTSD is consistently under-identified in clinical practice (Havens et al. 2012a, b; Giaconia et al. 1995; Mueser and Taub 2008; Hawke et al. 2009; Deters et al. 2006; Jaycox et al. 2004; Lipschitz et al. 2000), particularly in the presence of high-risk behaviors such as aggression, emotional volatility, and suicide ideation and attempts (Havens et al. 2012a, b). The integration of systematic trauma screening into standard practice insures that the impact of trauma on present symptoms and behaviors will not be overlooked even when present as part of a complex clinical picture. Systematic screening also identifies trauma in children and adolescents presenting with primarily avoidance and numbing or dissociative symptoms. Trauma is frequently overlooked in these children because their symptoms are less apparent and external, despite continuing to have a significant impact on quality of life. In addition to identifying trauma exposure, many trauma screening tools also include a symptom checklist which matches symptoms to DSM-5 criteria and can provide a provisional PTSD diagnosis and be used to track the severity of symptoms over time. In addition to identifying PTSD and trauma-related symptoms in patients, the process of screening also serves to maintain a trauma-informed culture. The trauma screen is completed early in the admission, and patients learn that staff are interested in hearing about what happened to them and are willing and capable of listening to their most painful experiences. Screening results are discussed as part of clinical care planning, used to inform treatment and disposition planning, and included in discharge summaries. Systematic integration of the screening process normalizes the discussion of trauma for both patients and staff and alleviates the commonly held belief that talking about traumatic events in a hospital setting will cause greater harm than good.

At Bellevue Hospital Center in New York City, we use the UCLA PTSD Reaction Index (Steinberg et al. 2004) to screen all patients 7 years of age and older at admission and discharge (age range for screening determined by measure). All patients over seven are screened for depression with the Children's Depression Inventory (the most common comorbidity in traumatized youth and frequently missed, particularly in aggressive youth) (Kovacs 1992). Youth over 10 years old are also screened for problematic substance use with the CRAFFT (Knight et al. 2002). Screens are completed through one-on-one verbal administration to insure that problems related to literacy or comprehension will not hinder the accuracy of the screen and to provide patients the opportunity to ask questions and take breaks. The first part of the UCLA PTSD Reaction Index is a trauma exposure checklist beginning with natural disasters and gradually moving to interpersonal traumas and abuse. The checklist responses are yes/no; therefore, the child is not required to provide details about the trauma. At the conclusion of the checklist, the most "bothersome" trauma is identified and briefly described as well as any traumas the patient might wish to add. Additional screens for post-traumatic stress symptoms include the Trauma Symptom Checklist for Children (TSCC) (Briere 1996) and the Child PTSD Symptom Scale (Foa et al. 2001). For depression, the Patient Health Questionnaire-9 (PHQ-9) has been used for adolescents (Kroenke et al. 2001), while the Beck Depression Inventory for Youth (BDI-Y) (Beck et al. 2001) and the Center for Epidemiological Studies Depression Scale Modified for Children (CES-DC) (Weissman et al. 1980; Faulstich et al. 1986) are available for children 7–14 years and 6–18 years, respectively.

During the training on the administration of screens, staff are provided with scripts and guidance on how to discuss the screening process and trauma with patients.

Clinician Hi, I'm Mary, a doctor here. If it is okay with you, I'd like to ask you some questions. I'm going to ask about scary things that happen to people. We ask everyone who comes to the hospital these questions, because we know that scary things happen sometimes and that it can be hard to talk about. The answers are yes or no and you don't have to discuss anything if you don't want to.

For many patients, the completion of the trauma screen is the first time they have acknowledged everything that has happened to them directly to another person. Patients often comment that no one has asked these questions before or that they did not know how to talk about "being hit at home" as a scary thing. Patients sometimes deny all traumas during the screening process and then discuss traumatic events later with their clinician. Likely, the process of completing the screen and listing possible traumatic events helped enable the patient to discuss her experiences at a later time. Trauma screening is repeated at discharge. In some cases, patients report additional traumas at discharge; this is especially common for patients who identified significant symptoms of avoidance and numbing during their admission screen.

20.2.2 Staff Training

A fundamental understanding of the impact of trauma on behavior, the relationship between traumatic exposure and mental illness, and the nature of coping skills utilized by traumatized youth is essential for all staff interfacing with youth in inpatient settings. This is particularly important for frontline milieu staff, who spend the most time with youth in these settings and usually have the least access to training and support around working with these often challenging youth. Thoughtful and accessible training that deepens the staff's understanding of the impact of trauma on behavior and self-concept allows staff to understand aggressive and self-destructive behavior within the context of what these youth have experienced. Importantly, this understanding increases staff empathy for and reduces staff judgment of challenging behaviors. Switching queries and lines of conversation from "what are you doing" or "why are you doing this" to "what happened to you" allows staff to approach difficult behaviors with an attitude of curiosity rather than a need for control or a punitive approach, both of which tend to exaggerate rather than reduce challenging trauma-related behaviors. For example, frontline staff whose responsibility includes maintaining order often react to the agitation of youth triggered by traumatic reminders by providing directives to stop such behavior. When delivered in an authoritarian and threatening manner, these directives can actually increase a sense of a lack of safety in youth, leading to an increase in agitation. Staff knowledge of the presentation of both dissociation and flashbacks in youth are key to successful work with traumatized youth. When working with individual youth, it is essential that staff are aware of particular triggers for that child (e.g., yelling, invading personal space, physical contact). With such knowledge staff can avoid re-traumatizing the youth as well as help the youth develop more effective coping skills when triggered.

In order to cultivate that understanding and curiosity, inpatient staff need solid foundational grounding in the following areas:

- The relationship between trauma and behavior and mental illness
- The effect of trauma on the developing brain
- Common nonoptimal coping strategies used by traumatized youth
- Supporting traumatized youth to develop more effective coping skills
- Vicarious trauma and organizational stress associated with working with traumatized youth

In developing staff training, we have worked with experts in the field of childhood trauma who had experience with adult education and training. In order to facilitate a shared language across disciplines, we have chosen a train-the-trainer model, where staff across multiple disciplines, including frontline milieu staff, are trained together as trainers. This approach helps break down hierarchical structures that are often barriers to shared learning. It also serves to empower the frontline staff by acknowledging the special contributions they make in minute-by-minute interactions with youth. This train-the-trainer model involves an initial 2 days of training in the modular curriculum, followed by three to 6 weeks of weekly practice sessions in delivering the training. This is important when training staff as trainers who had little to no experience in public speaking and training. These multidisciplinary staff trainers then go on to train their peers which also enhances learning over trainings delivered by "expert outsiders."

Our current iteration of staff trauma training is based on an adaptation of "Think Trauma," a four-module training designed for frontline staff working with adolescents in juvenile justice settings (Marrow et al. 2012a). This is a cased-based, interactive adult education tool, which we have found to be accessible to both frontline and clinical staff. We are in the process of adapting this for use with mental health providers which involves changes to the case material and expansion of the sections of children and trauma. The training will be expanded to include coverage of differential diagnosis in traumatized youth important to mental health providers.

The modular training will be delivered in 90-minute sessions to all staff working on our inpatient units. Our experience in other settings implementing "Think Trauma" has shown us that this takes four to 5 weeks to get through the basic modules and several more weeks to provide makeup sessions for missed sessions. Annual booster sessions are provided to maintain skills, and the full training will be incorporated into the orientation for all new nursing staff.

When training inpatient staff, it is necessary that training sessions be short (hours rather than days) as staff coverage is also an issue in these settings. It is also important that booster sessions be built in particularly early in the implementation of trauma-informed care. We have also found that sensitivity and awareness to staff reactions during training are essential. Given how common traumatic exposure is and how traumatizing working with these youth can be, staff are sometimes triggered by the material presented during trauma trainings. Explicit or graphic video or written description of youth trauma exposure can trigger adult staff who have experienced similar traumas. It is important to orient staff before training that such reactions are common and to provide self-care tips. Just as in the trauma screening of youth, staff training can often be the first time an adult trainee connects their own trauma exposures and symptoms. Trainers need to be vigilant to trainees struggling with traumatic reminders and support those trainees both in the training session and, if necessary, outside the session.

Effective trauma training serves as the foundation for the reinforcement of new knowledge in the day-to-day milieu work and must be integrated into the ongoing interactions with youth. This is done through multidisciplinary communication about youth's trauma status that includes frontline milieu staff. This can be done without violating confidential communications about the nature of the trauma by using a shared vocabulary that speaks in general terms about trauma and focuses on real-time triggers for the youth (i.e., being yelled at by adult males, staff getting too physically close to a youth, arguments in the milieu, etc.). This kind of shared communication and knowledge among staff is very helpful in containing traumatic reactions and avoiding re-traumatization.

It must be remembered that staff trauma training, while essential, must be followed by ongoing communication and supervision around the effect of trauma on individual youth. We have also found the implementation of trauma-related skills groups into the ongoing milieu programming keeps the trauma knowledge alive and shared (see skills groups below).

20.2.3 Trauma Skills Groups

Trauma-related skills groups are an essential component of trauma-informed care programming. Skills groups cover topics such as the identification and management of emotions, understanding the impact of trauma, coping and relaxation skills, creating and maintaining safety, and future planning and establishing relationships. On the inpatient units at Bellevue Hospital Center, structured and manualized trauma skills groups are integrated into unit programming for all patients. Interdisciplinary teams of staff members colead skills groups on the child and adolescent units. These interdisciplinary teams include physicians, psychologists, nurses, social workers, creative arts therapists, and child life specialists. As described above, these skills groups provide a common knowledge and language among staff and youth that allow them to continuously integrate supports for traumatized youth into the milieu work. It must be remembered that these groups are not venues for individual processing of their own trauma history; this work should generally be confined to individual psychotherapy. Rather these groups provide the foundational knowledge and skills to children and adolescents, increased capacity to understand their emotions and behavior, and groundwork for longer-term trauma processing work.

While all staff receive the milieu training, training for the trauma treatment groups is specific to the clinical staff. Trainers providing group instruction led brief courses over several weeks on the topics described above in a classroom setting during regularly scheduled shifts, while staff not involved in the training provided coverage. The trainings were co-led by staff from different disciplines and delivered to staff representing all disciplines present on the unit. Group facilitation training and trauma skills group content training were incorporated into this initial training. Incorporation of the concepts and skills covered in the trauma skills groups ensured that all staff not only understood the material covered in the groups but were capable of supporting patients in learning the concepts or practicing and applying new skills. Following the introductory training, staff participated in weekly supervision with unit group leaders. Over time, these weekly supervision sessions were expanded to include discussion of trauma skills in group sessions.

When new clinical staff join the unit, they participate in interdisciplinary peer-led trainings as part of their orientation. Once on the unit, they join the weekly supervision sessions and are paired with a senior trainer who mentors them in applying the new skills and ultimately in leading trauma skills groups. We found that participation in the trauma skills groups as a leader reinforces the key concepts introduced in the training and fosters empathy. Staff observe several groups with their assigned mentor before coleading a group and discuss group facilitation as part of their weekly supervision.

20.2.4 Skills Groups for Adolescents

There are several skills groups available for use in inpatient adolescent settings. The Sanctuary Model includes a group curriculum called S.E.L.F. which addresses four areas of healing: "safety, emotional management, loss, and future." S.E.L.F. can be used as a psychoeducational curriculum for clients as well as a model for addressing conflicts or problems within the treatment setting. There are 36 independent sessions addressing the four areas of healing. These sessions are interrelated, but can be taught in any sequence. The large number of sessions provides flexibility, allowing staff to select the session topic most relevant to the community or setting. Similarly, TARGET milieu treatment also has a group intervention which includes psychoeducation about the impact of trauma and enhancement of coping and problem-solving skills. TARGET addresses not only PTSD symptoms but also interpersonal and emotional regulation difficulties common to chronically traumatized populations like justice-involved youth.

Case Example: Skills Training in Affective and Interpersonal Regulation for Adolescents We chose to implement and test Skills Training in Affective and Interpersonal Regulation for Adolescents (STAIR-A), an evidence-based individual intervention shown to improve affect regulation and interpersonal skills in traumatized adolescents because we were able to adapt the treatment by consolidating and shorten the intervention ("Brief STAIR-A") to the needs of an acute treatment (13-day) stay in collaboration with the developers. The treatment was also a good fit because it was developed and validated with multiple traumatized children and addresses not only symptoms related to trauma but also social and interpersonal deficits resulting from trauma and abuse. Given that the average length of stay on the adolescent unit is 13 days, therefore three sessions were created with a focus on skills. Adolescents can enter the program at any session and continue through multiple program cycles. The skills groups focus on (1) affect recognition and trauma psychoeducation, (2) emotion regulation and coping skills, and (3) communication skills, especially in difficult situations. The group aspect of these sessions allows for peer education and structured social interactions. Adolescents practice discussing tough emotions with peers and relate to shared experiences. Groups are co-led by members of the clinical team, and all adolescents are invited to join the group, even if not diagnosed with PTSD. At the conclusion of each session, adolescents work on an individualized safety plan for use on the unit and after discharge. Initial evaluation of the program indicates positive benefits for the youth at discharge including both decrease in symptoms and increase in coping skills self-efficacy (Gudiño et al. 2014) An example of some of the topics discussed in STAIR-A Session 2 (emotion regulation and coping skills) follows.

Brief STAIR-A Emotion and Coping Skills Session

Group Leader: Remember we were talking before about how our mind, body, and behavior gives us clues when we are angry. We all also have our own ways that we cope with anger and other strong emotions. We're going to go around the room and each person will list one way you already cope. As we go around, we are going to write the ideas on the board.

Markus: I dunno. I try to work off steam, I guess.

Group Leader: What do you do to work off steam?

Markus: I work out. Pump, run, shoot hoops.

Group Leader: Great example. I'm going to write "Work Out." What about you Ellie?

Ellie: I like to draw.

Group Leader: Art is a great way to express what you are feeling and to get it out.

Kay: I watch TV or listen to music. I don't want to think, just make everything quiet.

Group Leader: Distraction can be really helpful sometimes. What you'll find is that there is a time and place for different types of coping skills. Some will work better for one thing than for another.

Rick: I like listening to music too or sleeping!

Group Leader: Some coping skills might work for some people more than others, and sometimes the same coping skills work for a lot of people. When you look at this list we have just made, which coping skills do you think work best for you? Keep in mind there are no right or wrong answers! Did you get any ideas from someone else that you hadn't considered in the past?

Kay: I like the idea of working out. Normally I just want to get away, ya know? Hide behind noise or zone out in front of the TV or computer. But running sounds good.

Group Leader:	Has anyone ever tried a coping skill that didn't work out for them? How about any coping skills that worked in the moment but backfired later on?
Mary:	I have one that's helpful, but no one let's me do it.
Group Leader:	What is that?
Mary:	Smoking pot. It really helps with I'm nervous, calms me down every time.
Group Leader:	Okay, I hear you. Your natural response to feeling anxious is to smoke pot. So, let's fast forward 10 years, you're on a job interview and you're feeling anxious. Do you think you'll get hired if you pull out that coping skill?
Mary:	No.
Group Leader:	It's always good to have several coping skills that you know help you. You can't use every coping skill in every situation. Markus said that his favorite coping skill was to work out or go for a run, but he couldn't do that in the middle of class. That's another good reason why it helps to have a bunch of different coping skills so that you can match the coping skill to how you feel and also where you are. Let's work on expanding your list! Safety plans are updated with new coping skills or triggers at the end of each group. Staff have access to the safety plans throughout the adolescent's stay and can refer to them to help an adolescent practice coping.
Clinician:	Markus, I can see you're upset about not getting enough time to play basketball. We can't go back and play more now, but we have other things planned this afternoon, and you'll be able to go to the gym tomorrow. Let's look at your Safety Plan.
Markus:	It's not going to help.
Clinician:	Some of things you wrote down worked before, let's take a look.
Markus:	Those won't work.
Clinician:	I know you like basketball, that's on here. What if you bounced one of the balls in the comfort room?
Markus:	Could try.
Clinician:	Let's try! If it doesn't work we can try something else from your list. Sometimes the first thing you try doesn't work, so you just try something else.

Skills Groups for Children

The Israel Center for the Treatment of Psychotrauma developed an intervention for children called Building Emotional and Affect Regulation (BEAR) (Pat-Horenczyk et al. 2004). BEAR is a six-session group for children ages 7–12 and addresses physical and emotional regulation, interpersonal regulation, cognitive-emotional regulation, and social support. BEAR incorporates "mindfulness techniques, cognitive behavioral strategies and narrative interventions" (METIV 2016).

Children's Awareness Regarding Emotional Stress (CARES), an inpatient, structured skills trauma group for children ages 7–11, was developed by a multidisciplinary team at Bellevue based on existing principles and modules from trauma-focused cognitive-behavioral therapy (Cohen and Mannarino 1996) and cognitive-behavioral intervention for trauma in schools (Jaycox et al. 2004). Similar to Brief STAIR-A on the adolescent inpatient units, the concepts introduced in CARES are also used to orient staff to the impact of trauma on children and behavior and to reinforce their trauma training in an ongoing way. There are five CARES sessions which introduce children to feelings and psychoeducation about trauma, relaxation and coping skills, breathing, yoga, and basic cognitive-behavioral skills. Children practice coping skills during each session, and yoga and sensorimotor activities developed in collaboration with occupational therapists are incorporated into unit programming outside of the session to enhance sensorimotor skills development. Groups are led by a single leader, but each child has a staff member or volunteer to help them complete the exercises and guide them through the activities. All staff members participate in the group, modeling behaviors and skills for the children.

CARES Relaxation and Coping Skills Example

Group Leader: Now we've learned about feelings and behaviors. If we learn skills to manage our emotions we can feel better and behave better. The skills we're going to work on now can help us when we're feeling strong emotions.

Everyone in this room has an *important power*—the power of your mind, the power of your imagination. We are going to use this power to help us feel better and braver.

We're going to learn about a skill using *happy imagery*. That is when we change bad thoughts or bad images in our mind to happy thoughts or happy images so we feel better. What is something that makes you happy?

Devon: Pizza!
Kim: Skittles!
Alex: Recess.
Group Leader: Great examples! Thank you for sharing. How many people like pizza? Wow, that looks like everyone. Ok, we're going to practice using our power. Close your eyes or look down and picture pizza in your mind. What does it smell like? What does it taste like? Is there cheese? Pepperoni? Is the bread soft? Is it warm? Does it warm your hand? Imagine taking a bite. Does it taste good? Now open your eyes. How do you feel?
Devon: Hungry!
Group Leader: That can happen! It means you were really imagining the pizza. Good work! How many of you could picture the pizza? When we think and picture something happy in our mind, we call it happy imagery. If you weren't able to imagine the pizza, don't worry, it

Group Leader: takes practice and you'll be able to do it. We can use different happy images to help us when we are feeling bad or scared. We can take a little break from what is upsetting us and think about something that makes us happy.

Group Leader: What should we do if we have tried happy imagery and still don't feel better? Now, it's time to learn some relaxation skills to help us further. These skills are helpful when we are feeling strong emotions in our body. Maybe our neck or shoulders are tense, maybe we are clenching our fists, or maybe our body feels stiff and tense. Take a moment to see how your body feels right now. Does anything feel tense or stiff?

Alex: My head hurts.

Kim: My shoulders and arms feel hard.

Group Leader: OK, let's learn some new skills.
The first one is called: *Reach for Skittles* (Arm Stretching): Look! You see a rainbow of skittles across the ceiling and you want to get them. Stretch your right arm ... stretch it hard, stretch it up over your head ... you almost get the skittles ... almost ... stretch ... Oh, you've got one, yummy, drop your arm, feel how relaxed it is. Oh, look! There are some more skittles on your left side, stretch out your left arm, stretch ... stretch, stretch it up over your head ... Whoa, you've got one ... drop your arm, yummy!
How does your body feel now after we have stretched and relaxed? Does it feel different in any way?

Kim: My arms feel more floppy.

Group Leader: Kim, before we tried this stretch, you said your shoulders and arms felt hard, do they feel better when they are floppy?

Kim: Yes, I think they do. They don't hurt as much.

Group Leader: That's good. That means they are more relaxed. You might find that stretching during the day or when you are upset helps you feel better. You will find that different stretches may work better at different times, so if one doesn't seem like it works immediately, try another one!
If you find one that makes you feel better or that you really like, let one of us know.
We can add it to your Safety Card. That way, if you get really upset and have trouble thinking about what will help you feel better, we can look at your Safety Card together and then help guide you through that stretch. This is true for all of the skills we practice together. Any of the skills you find helpful can be added to your personal Safety Card. When you leave, you'll have a whole list of things you can do when you're upset or need to deal with something tough.

Brief STAIR-A and CARES represent the trauma skills group component of trauma-informed programming on the child and adolescent inpatient units. Since implementing trauma-informed programming in 2008, a noticeable shift in culture has occurred. Child's behaviors are more frequently understood in the context of trauma and development, and staff are better able to integrate the identification and practice of coping skills in response to emotional volatility and during de-escalation.

20.2.5 Ongoing Monitoring of Trauma-Informed Care Implementation

One of the common pitfalls in the implementation of trauma-informed care is the assumption that ongoing monitoring is not necessary once training and programming have been implemented. First, staff turnover is the norm in many inpatient and residential settings; therefore, trauma-informed training for new staff should be incorporated into the orientation training. Regular assessment of the staff's trauma knowledge and skills level is helpful in creating a framework for booster training. Booster training or ongoing trauma-informed education should be built into staff development and training in a consistent and ongoing way.

Second, we have found that ongoing monitoring of the individualized care helps keep staff on track in dealing with traumatized youth. We have achieved this through weekly treatment rounds where senior clinical leadership briefly reviews the case loads on all our inpatient units with the treatment teams. The clinical leader has the trauma screening results available for all inpatients and makes sure all staff on the team has integrated that knowledge into their treatment planning.

The program elements described above have been in place on our inpatient service for the last 6 years and have helped us create a trauma-informed care system that helps both staff and youth effectively manage the behavioral consequences of traumatic exposure. Of course it is not possible to deliver the complete effective treatment for traumatized youth in a brief inpatient hospital stay. However, there is no excuse for ignoring the central role traumatic exposure plays in the behavioral challenges of hospitalized children and adolescents. This only contributes to misdiagnosis and inappropriate treatment planning and does a tremendous disservice to young people who must be helped to see the relationship between their life experiences and their emotions and behavior. The thorough implementation of trauma-informed care in inpatient and residential settings provides staff with the knowledge and skills to work effectively with challenging youth, reducing the level of violence and tension in these settings. It is a keystone to the creation of a safe and therapeutic environment, the most basic and essential element of healing.

References

Adam BS, Everett BL, O'Neal E (1992) PTSD in physically and sexually abused psychiatrically hospitalized children. Child Psychiatry Hum Dev 23(1):3–8

Allwood MA, Dyl J, Hunt JI, Spirito A (2008) Comorbidity and service utilization among psychiatrically hospitalized adolescents with posttraumatic stress disorder. J Psychol Trauma 7(2):104–121

Azeem MW, Aujla A, Rammerth M, Binsfeld G, Jones RB (2011) Effectiveness of six core strategies based on trauma informed care in reducing seclusions and restraints at a child and adolescent psychiatric hospital. J Child Adolesc Psychiatr Nurs 24(1):11–15

Beck JS, Beck AT, Jolly JB (2001) Beck youth inventories. San Antonio, TX: Psychological Corporation

Bloom SL (1997) Creating sanctuary: toward the evolution of sane societies. Routledge, New York

Briere, J. (1996) Trauma symptom checklist for children. Psychological Assessment Resources, Odessa, pp 00253–00258

Cohen JA (2010) Practice parameter for the assessment and treatment of children and adolescents with posttraumatic stress disorder (AACAP official action). J Am Acad Child Adolesc Psychiatry 49:414–430

Cohen JA, Mannarino AP (1996) A treatment outcome study for sexually abused preschool children: Initial findings. J Am Acad Child Adolesc Psychiatry 35(1):42–50

Craine LS, Henson CE, Colliver JA, MacLean DG (1988) Prevalence of a history of sexual abuse among female psychiatric patients is a state hospital system. Hosp Community Psychiatry 39:300–304

Deters PB, Novins DK, Fickenscher A, Beals J (2006) Trauma and posttraumatic stress disorder symptomatology: patterns among American Indian adolescents in substance abuse treatment. Am J Orthopsychiatry 76:335–345

Famularo R, Fenton T, Kinscherff R, Augustyn M (1996) Psychiatric comorbidity in childhood post traumatic stress disorder. Child Abuse Negl 20(10):953–961

Faulstich ME, Carey MP, Ruggiero L, Enyart P, Gresham F (1986) Assessment of depression in childhood and adolescence: an evaluation of the Center for Epidemiological Studies Depression Scale for Children (CES-DC). Am J Psychiatry 143(8):1024–1027

Fehon DC, Grilo CM, Lipschitz DS (2001) Correlates of community violence exposure in hospitalized adolescents. Compr Psychiatry 42(4):283–290

Foa EB, Johnson KM, Feeny NC, Treadwell KR (2001) The child PTSD symptom scale: a preliminary examination of its psychometric properties. J Clin Child Psychol 30(3):376–384

Ford JD (2006) Trauma-focused, present-centered, emotional self-regulation approach to integrated treatment for posttraumatic stress and addiction: trauma adaptive recovery group education and therapy (TARGET). Am J Psychother 60:335–355

Ford JD, Blaustein ME (2013) Systemic self-regulation: a framework for trauma-informed services in residential juvenile justice programs. J Fam Violence 28(7):665–677

Ford JD, Cloitre M (2009) Best practices in psychotherapy for children and adolescents. In: Courtois CA, Ford JD (eds) Treating complex traumatic stress disorders: guide. Guilford, New York, pp 59–81

Ford JD, Connor DF, Hawke J (2009) Complex trauma among psychiatrically impaired children: a cross-sectional, chart-review study. J Clin Psychiatry 70(8):1155–1163

Ford JD, Chapman JC, Connor DF, Cruise KC (2012a) Complex trauma and aggression in secure juvenile justice settings. Crim Justice Behav 39:695–724

Ford JD, Steinberg KL, Hawke J, Levine J, Zhang W (2012b) Randomized trial comparison of emotion regulation and relational psychotherapies for PTSD with girls involved in delinquency. J Clin Child Adolesc Psychol 41(1):27–37

Giaconia RM, Reinherz HZ, Silverman AB, Pakiz B, Frost AK, Cohen E (1995) Traumas and posttraumatic stress disorder in a community population of older adolescents. J Am Acad Child Adolesc Psychiatry 34:1369–1380

Gold SN (2008) The relevance of trauma to general clinical practice. Psychol Trauma Theory Res Pract Pol S(1):114–124

Grasso D, Boonsiri J, Lipschitz D, Guyer AE, Houshyar S, Douglas-Palumberi H et al (2009) Posttraumatic stress disorder: the missed diagnosis. Child Welfare 88(4):157–176

Gudiño OG, Weis R, Havens JF, Biggs EA, Diamond UN, Marr M, Jackson C, Cloitre M (2014) Group trauma-informed treatment for adolescent psychiatric inpatients: a preliminary, uncontrolled trial. J Trauma Stress 27:496–500

Hanson RF, Lang J (2014) Special focus section: a critical look at trauma informed care (TIC) among agencies and systems serving maltreated youth and their families. Child Maltreat 19(3–4):275

Havens J, Ford J, Grasso D, Marr M (2012a) Opening pandora's box: the importance of trauma identification and intervention in hospitalized and incarcerated adolescent populations. Adolesc Psychiatry 2(4):309–312

Havens JF, Gudiño OG, Biggs EA, Diamond UN, Weis JR, Cloitre M (2012b) Identification of trauma exposure and PTSD in adolescent psychiatric inpatients: an exploratory study. J Trauma Stress 25(2):171–178

Hawke JM, Ford JD, Kaminer Y, Burke R (2009) Trauma and PTSD among youths in outpatient treatment for alcohol use disorders. J Child Adolesc Trauma 2:1–14

Jaycox LH, Ebener P, Damesek L, Becker K (2004) Trauma exposure and retention in adolescent substance abuse treatment. J Trauma Stress 17:113–121

Keeshin BR, Strawn JR, Luebbe AM, Saldaña SN, Wehry AM, DelBello MP, Putnam FW (2014) Hospitalized youth and child abuse: a systematic examination of psychiatric morbidity and clinical severity. Child Abuse Negl 38(1):76–83

Klinic Community Health Center, MTIEC Institute (2013) Trauma informed: the trauma toolkit. Manitoba Trauma Information and Education Centre, Winnipeg

Knight JR, Sherritt L, Shrier LA, Harris SK, Chang G (2002) Validity of the CRAFFT substance abuse screening test among adolescent clinic patients. Arch Pediatr Adolesc Med 156(6):607–614

Kolko DJ, Hurlburt MS, Zhang J, Barth RP, Leslie LK, Burns BJ (2010) Posttraumatic stress symptoms in children and adolescents referred for child welfare investigation. A national sample of in-home and out-of-home care. Child Maltreat 15(1):48–63

Kovacs M (1992) Children's depression inventory. Multi-Health System, North Tonawanda

Kroenke K, Spitzer RL, Williams JB (2001) The Phq-9. J Gen Intern Med 16(9):606–613

Lipschitz DS, Winegar RK, Hartnick E, Foote B, Southwick SM (1999) Posttraumatic stress disorder in hospitalized adolescents: psychiatric comorbidity and clinical correlates. J Am Acad Child Adolesc Psychiatry 38(4):385–392

Lipschitz DS, Rasmusson AM, Anyan W, Cromwell P, Southwick SM (2000) Clinical and functional correlates of posttraumatic stress disorder in urban adolescent girls at a primary care clinic. J Am Acad Child Adolesc Psychiatry 39:1104–1111

Manitoba Trauma Information and Education Centre (MTIEC), Klinic Community Health Centre (2013). The trauma-informed toolkit, Second edition. Retrieved from http://trauma-informed.ca/wpcontent/uploads/2013/10/Trauma-informed_Toolkit.pdf

Marrow M, Benamati J, Decker K, Griffin D, Lott DA (2012a) Think trauma: a training for staff in juvenile justice residential settings. National Center for Child Traumatic Stress, Los Angeles/Durham

Marrow MT, Knudsen KJ, Olafson E, Bucher SE (2012b) The value of implementing TARGET within a trauma-informed juvenile justice setting. J Child Adolesc Trauma 5(3):257–270

METIV, BEAR for Children (2016) Retrieved from http://traumaweb.org/bear-for-children/

Mueser KT, Taub JT (2008) Trauma and PTSD among adolescents with severe emotional disorders involved in multiple service systems. Psychiatr Serv 59(6):627–634

Muskett C (2014) Trauma-informed care in inpatient mental health settings: a review of the literature. Int J Ment Health Nurs 23(1):51–59

Opler L, Grennan M, Ford JD (2009) Psychopharmacological treatment of complex traumatic stress disorders. In: Courtois CA, Ford JD (eds) Treating complex traumatic stress disorders: an evidence-based guide. Guilford Press, New York

Pat-Horenczyk R, Berger R, Kaplinsky N, Baum N (2004) The journey to resilence: coping with ongoing stressful situations. Protocol for guidance consellors (adolescents version) Unpublished Manuscript

Rivard JC, Bloom SL, McCorkle D, Abramovitz R (2005) Preliminary results of a study examining the implementation and effects of a trauma recovery framework for youths in residential treatment. Ther Commun Int J Ther Support Organ 26(1):83–96

Silverman WK, Ortiz C, Visersvaran C, Burns BJ, Kolko DJ, Putnam FW, Amaya-Jackson L (2008) Evidence-based psychosocial treatments for children and adolescents exposed to traumatic events. J Clin Child Adolesc Psychol 37:156–183

Steinberg AM, Brymer MJ, Decker KB, Pynoos RS (2004) The University of California at Los Angeles post-traumatic stress disorder reaction index. Curr Psychiatry Rep 6:96–100

Substance Abuse and Mental Health Services Administration (2014) SAMHSA's Concept of Trauma and Guidance for a Trauma-Informed Approach. HHS Publication No. (SMA) 14–4884. Substance Abuse and Mental Health Services Administration, Rockville

Substance Abuse and Mental Health Services Administration (2015) Trauma-informed approach and trauma-specific interventions. Retrieved from http://www.samhsa.gov/nctic/trauma-interventions

The Sanctuary Model: The Sanctuary Model Components of the Sanctuary Model S.E.L.F (2016) Retrieved from http://www.sanctuaryweb.com/TheSanctuaryModel/Componentsof theSanctuaryModel/SELF.aspx

Weissman MM, Orvaschel H, Padian N (1980) Children's symptom and social functioning self-report scales comparison of mothers' and children's reports. J Nerv Ment Dis 168(12):736–740

Juvenile Justice and Forensic Settings: The TARGET Approach

21

Julian D. Ford

21.1 Introduction

More than 80 % of youth in juvenile justice or forensic settings report a lifetime history of exposure to at least one traumatic stressor, and the majority report multiple types of victimization, which places them at risk for severe and persistent behavioral and legal (e.g., recidivism) as well as emotional and developmental problems (Ford et al. 2013b). Youth also may be exposed to traumatic stressors while in juvenile justice supervision or facilities, compounding their traumatic stress symptoms and potentially leading them to engage in behavior (e.g., reactive aggression) that can endanger other youths and adults (Ford et al. 2012). Traumatized youth involved in juvenile justice also may appear to be sociopathic due to acquiring "callous and unemotional traits" as a result of emotional numbing (Kerig et al. 2012), leading them to be labeled as irredeemable and putting them at risk for lifelong incarceration or violent death (Teplin et al. 2005).

Therefore, timely and effective therapeutic intervention for youth whose functioning is impaired by traumatic stress symptoms is crucial not only for their safety, rehabilitation, and psychosocial development but also for the safety, health, and success of their peers, families, communities, schools and workplaces, and civic and recreational programs. Therapeutic intervention with justice-involved youth must address the full range of post-traumatic stress disorder (PTSD) symptoms, including severe dissociation, emotion dysregulation, reckless (including substance use) and aggressive behaviors toward self or others, and fundamental negative alterations in self-concept and expectations regarding relationships and the future. PTSD

J.D. Ford, PhD
Department of Psychiatry, University of Connecticut Schools of Medicine and Law,
263 Farmington Ave. MC1410, Farmington, CT 06030, USA
e-mail: jford@uchc.edu

© Springer International Publishing Switzerland 2017
M.A. Landolt et al. (eds.), *Evidence-Based Treatments for Trauma Related Disorders in Children and Adolescents*, DOI 10.1007/978-3-319-46138-0_21

psychotherapy for justice-involved youth also must be carefully adapted to specifically match the culture and circumstances of youth and families, the courts and legal representatives, and juvenile justice staff, and must be empirically demonstrated to be effective in this specific context.

Psychotherapy models for children and adolescents with PTSD that have established an empirical evidence base or are widely disseminated (see Section II of this book) either have not been rigorously tested with youth involved in juvenile justice settings, or have proven relatively ineffective in improving PTSD and other internalizing problems (e.g., depression) or externalizing behavior problems (e.g., aggression, delinquency) with youth who have severe externalizing behavior problems (de Arellano et al. 2014). On the other hand, interventions that have a strong evidence base with troubled youth who are behaviorally dysregulated either have not tested their effectiveness in reducing PTSD symptoms (e.g., multisystemic therapy [MST] or multidimensional family therapy [MDFT]; Henggeler and Sheidow 2012) or are designed for and have been tested with younger traumatized children but not with adolescents involved in juvenile justice systems (e.g., parent-child interaction therapy, PCIT; see Chap. 16).

One promising exception is the recent integration of trauma-focused cognitive behavior therapy with an effective therapeutic and case management program for girls who are in out-of-home child welfare placements (many of whom are juvenile justice involved), multidimensional treatment foster care (MTFC, Smith et al. 2012). MTFC provides a relational context of safety and stable adult caregiver involvement (including an individual and family therapist, case manager, mentor, and therapeutic foster parents) that is recommended—and potentially necessary (Lang et al. 2010)—for the narrative trauma memory processing component of trauma-focused cognitive behavior therapy.

However, many traumatized youth involved in delinquency and juvenile justice systems do not have a safe and stable relational support system with reliably available and emotionally responsive parents or other primary caregivers to participate in the narrative memory processing work of trauma-focused psychotherapy. Many also have never experienced secure attachment bonds with primary caregivers, or have had repeated or chronic ruptures in or losses of these crucial bonds due to neglect, caregiver death, abandonment, or mental, behavioral, or legal impairment (Ford et al. 2013b). These fundamental relational dilemmas and the combination of severe externalizing behavior and emotional numbing pose two major challenges to PTSD psychotherapy with this large subset of juvenile justice-involved youth. First, they may be unwilling to disclose, let alone to process, emotionally distressing trauma memories, and this may be a rational choice due to the absence of reliable primary caregiver support for such work. Second, they often are severely emotion dysregulated as a result of not only exposure to interpersonal traumatic stressors but also not having had the opportunity to develop emotion regulation capacities due to primary caregiving relationships that did not provide secure attachment bonds and may instead have been emotionally abusive (Spinazzola et al. 2014).

Therefore, a trauma-focused but present-centered (i.e., not requiring narrative trauma memory processing) psychotherapy, designed specifically to enhance emotion regulation and behavioral self-control as well as to ameliorate PTSD and associated internalizing symptoms, is potentially a crucial option for PTSD treatment with juvenile justice-involved youth. There is a growing empirical evidence base for skills-based emotion regulation approaches to PTSD psychotherapy with adults, including the finding that these modalities may better retain clients than trauma memory processing therapies (Ford 2016). Emotion regulation, stress management, interpersonal effectiveness, arousal regulation, mindfulness, distress tolerance, problem solving, and self-reflection skills training often are embedded in trauma memory processing therapies for PTSD. In present-centered interventions, these interventions may provide an alternative to PTSD treatment without requiring trauma memory processing. Present-focused skills-based interventions do not proscribe trauma memory processing, but instead facilitate the emotional processing of intrusive memories as they occur in vivo in daily life. TARGET is trauma-focused present-centered psychotherapy originally developed for and empirically tested in randomized clinical trials with adults with complex PTSD and chronic mental or addictive disorders (Ford 2015). The adaptation of TARGET for youth in juvenile justice settings will be described.

21.2 Trauma Affect Regulation: Guide for Education and Therapy (TARGET)

Two decades ago, as juvenile justice systems began to expand their protocols for screening youth for behavioral health needs to specifically identify unrecognized or untreated PTSD, there was no evidence-based therapeutic intervention for this population. TARGET therefore was adapted and empirically tested as an individual therapy for girls with PTSD who were involved in delinquency (Ford et al. 2012) and as a group therapy for boys and girls in juvenile detention (Ford and Hawke 2012) and high security youth incarceration facilities (Marrow et al. 2012).

TARGET begins with psychoeducation that explains PTSD symptoms as the result of a shift in the brain's stress response systems. In order to provide a nontechnical but scientifically based meta-model (a framework for understanding specific treatment models) for youth, families, line staff, administrators, and judges, TARGET uses nontechnical language and graphics that are comprehensible at a fifth grade reading level to describe how traumatic stress reactions represent the brain's shift into survival mode. First, there is the "alarm" in the brain (i.e., the amygdala, primarily the basolateral nucleus, which activates the body's peripheral autonomic nervous system and stress hormone system). Closely adjacent in the brain is the hippocampus, which serves as a "memory filing center" and search engine for the storage and retrieval of contextual memories and related experiential information. Thirdly, there is the medial, orbital, and dorsolateral prefrontal cortex, which constitutes the brain's "thinking center," overseeing the integration and translation of information about stressors and how to respond to them in conscious thoughts, emotions, goals, and plans (Teicher and Samson 2013). This biological meta-model provides a transparent and destigmatizing explanation of how the brain adapts to enable a person to survive exposure to traumatic stressors: the brain's alarm gets hyperactivated to signal that a life-threatening emergency is occurring, and this burst of alarm signals floods the brain's filing center and creates an information overload that often exceeds the filing center's processing capacities. As a result, the filing center cannot convert the immediate sensory/perceptual input into memories that are organized, contextualized, useful, and informed by information files from previous experiences. Memories of traumatic stressors thus inherently are fragmented, disorganized, and flooded with shock and distress or disconnected from emotion. PTSD can be understood as occurring when the brain's alarm center—and along with it, the rest of the body including the brain's filing and thinking centers—are stuck in survival mode.

This biologically informed (Ford, 2009) educational meta-model translates directly into the skill set that TARGET teaches for recovery from PTSD. Because PTSD involves biologically based and affectively supercharged implicit cognitions associated with persistent intrusive reexperiencing, hypervigilance, and avoidance, awareness of those implicit threat-based filters or biases is a vital prerequisite to the explicit processing that is the basis for regaining adaptive functioning as well as for successful trauma memory processing (e.g., approach rather than avoidance, reappraisal rather than passive reexperiencing, problem solving rather than hypervigilance). TARGET therefore teaches a seven-step sequence for reflective self-awareness of "alarm reactions" that is summarized in an easily accessible acronym of relevance to trauma survivors, "FREEDOM":

- *F*ocusing on one thought that you choose based on your core values and self
- *R*ecognizing micro-momentary triggers for post-traumatic "alarm" reactions
- Distinguishing alarm-driven ("reactive") versus adaptive ("main") *E*motions
- Distinguishing alarm-driven ("reactive") versus adaptive ("main") *E*valuations
- *D*efining and distinguishing adaptive ("main") goals versus alarm-driven ("reactive") goals
- Distinguishing alarm-driven ("reactive") versus adaptive ("main") *O*ptions, and
- *M*aking a positive contribution by using these steps to reset the brain's alarm

The seven-step sequence is designed to facilitate self-monitoring, non-avoidant experiential awareness, and behavior analytic chain analyses (Follette et al. 2009), in order to enhance awareness of the otherwise implicit sequential links between in vivo triggers and the cascade of emotions, thoughts, goals, and actions that comprise trauma-related stress reactions. The FREEDOM sequence facilitates reprocessing (i.e., reappraisal, problem solving) and adaptive behavioral activation (i.e., initiation and sustained completion of goal-directed action) by drawing attention to the dialectical interplay between post-traumatic stress reactions that are "reactive" (i.e., alarm-based) and the person's "main" (i.e., based on core values, relational investments, and sense of self) emotions, beliefs, goals, and behavioral options.

Focusing is the meta-skill (the core skill that provides a template for all other skills) in TARGET that underlies all of the remaining FREEDOM skills. Focusing involves making the shift from hypervigilant hyper- or hyporeactivity (i.e., trauma-related alarm reactions) to proactive reflective self-awareness and self-control. A widely known mnemonic for seeking help in the face of danger, *SOS*, is used to operationalize focusing:

- *S*low down: Notice and sweep your mind clear of all perceptions and thoughts.
- *O*rient yourself by choosing one thought (using words, imagery, sound, or any sensory modality) that represents what is most important to you right now based on what you value and believe in and who you are as a person.
- *S*elf-check by rating (on a scale from 1 to 10) your levels of (a) stress (from none at all to worst ever) and (b) personal control (from none to most ever).

The FREEDOM and SOS sequences provide a toolkit and checklist for the therapist and client to simplify, organize, and flexibly deploy a complex array of psychosocial tactics for recognizing the signs of being stuck in trauma-related survival mode and drawing upon core emotions, values, and relational and self-related resources to restore a sense of personal agency. The FREEDOM steps are learned and practiced incrementally through dialogue with a therapist, or in guided interactions in therapy groups or milieu programs. A handout outlining how to apply the FREEDOM steps (the "practice exercise for FREEDOM") is used by the client to review recent (or past) experiences both in session and independently as homework between sessions or as an experiential activity in milieu settings (e.g., detention or incarceration facilities, residential treatment or foster programs). The practice exercise is designed to enable clients to distinguish "alarm reactions" from focused self-regulation, in order to enhance their ability to use their innate skills for focused self-regulation while experiencing PTSD symptoms. The goal is not to attempt to eliminate symptoms (which may paradoxically increase their severity) but to encourage mindful awareness and acceptance by recognizing PTSD symptoms' alarm origins and adaptive intent, and choosing to focus on and utilize more self-congruent ("main") inner resources and behavioral choices: emotions, thoughts, goals, actions, and criteria for self-evaluation.

TARGET also has a creative arts activity designed to enhance positive and negative emotion recognition skills by having participants create personalized "lifelines" via collage, drawing, poetry, and writing. The lifeline provides a way to apply the SOS and FREEDOM steps to constructing a life narrative that includes traumatic and stressful events but does not involve repeated retelling of them. TARGET does not require trauma memory processing, but instead engages clients in a process of learning how to systematically reconstruct narratives describing current or past stressful events. The lifeline's premise is that knowing how to reconstruct memories that are predominantly dysphoric, fragmented, and incomplete in order to make them more emotionally and cognitively coherent and complete and will enhance the client's ability to regulate distressing emotions related either to past traumatic stressors or current stressful events.

Thus, the FREEDOM sequence is compatible with narrative trauma memory processing—in fact, it is designed as a systematic guide to the sequential dialectical information processing that is necessary for successful memory processing. However, by highlighting the possibility of accessing the individual's core values and sense of self (the "main" component in every emotion, beliefs, goal, and behavioral choice), the FREEDOM sequence is designed to enhance present-centered self-reflection and self-efficacy that is empathic (i.e., grounded in the recognition of the fundamental uniqueness and worth of oneself and other persons). This is particularly relevant with adolescents and young adults involved in the justice system due to their common dual role as victims as well as perpetrators of psychological trauma (Haufle and Wolter 2015; Spenser et al. 2015). The FREEDOM sequence was designed to increase self-reflective awareness of morally grounded emotions, which has been specifically associated with the inhibition of violence (Bowes and McMurran 2013) and which has been shown to be a deficit for many youth who become involved in juvenile justice (Palmer and Begum 2006).

21.3 Case Examples

An example of a TARGET group with each gender will be provided, highlighting group interaction at the beginning of a boys group and how traumatogenic dynamics (Finkelhor and Browne 1985) of powerlessness, stigmatization, betrayal, and sexualization were addressed with the girls. Due to the often brief length of stay in juvenile detention facilities, a four-session TARGET adaptation (T4) has been designed and conducted with more than 3000 boys and girls (in gender-specific groups) in juvenile detention and secure residential centers over the past 10 years. Groups are led by Masters- and Bachelors-level counselors and juvenile justice staff who have been trained by and receive ongoing on-site clinical consultation (with direct observation and structured feedback based on a TARGET group fidelity checklist) from certified TARGET trainers. Groups typically are held twice weekly and are attended on a rolling enrollment basis in order to include as many youth as possible. Group leaders meet with youths individually whenever possible to give them a summary of key take-home points if they enter a TARGET group on the second or third session, and the fourth session is generally closed (i.e., only ongoing group members may attend) because it is a closure session. TARGET group sessions start with a brief overview of the group rules and the session's topic by the group leader, followed by a check-in by each group member using the ten-point rating scales for current "stress level" and "personal control" from the SOS. After the SOS is introduced in session 3, group members lead the entire group in doing a two-minute SOS at least three times (the beginning, middle, end of session) in order to set a tone of focused attention. In community settings (e.g., diversion or mental health clinics), the FREEDOM skill set is taught in 10- to 12-session group or individual therapy, but the briefer T4 adaptation will be used to illustrate how TARGET is delivered with juvenile justice-involved youth in groups. To preserve privacy and confidentiality, pseudonyms are used and all personal details have been disguised with the youths represented by composites rather than actual individuals.

21.3.1 Boys T4 Group in Juvenile Detention

Five boys attended T4 group for the first time (Alok, Carlos, Levon, Rahim, Tomas), and one (Michal) was repeating the group after having attended a T4 group in a previous stay in detention. The dialogue illustrates how T4 begins.

Leader: Welcome to TARGET group; let's all sit down and get focused. I think everyone knows everyone here [addresses each member by name]. The group has four sessions and this is the first. Today we'll look at how stress affects the brain, so you can use your brain to be in control instead of letting your brain's stress reactions control you. To do that, you have to be able to focus, which means paying attention to what's most important in a situation.

Rahim: Like to where the party is, and the girls, which my man Tomas excels at (laughs).

Tomas: Don't be messin' with me homes, I'm not in the mood for your BS.

Leader: That's a good example of focusing Tomas; I appreciate your reminder that we're here for a serious purpose and not to trigger anyone else—humor is fine if we're all laughing together and being respectful, but not when it's disrespectful and distracting, okay, Rahim?

Rahim: Okay, whatever ... all right, I get it!

Leader: To get back in focus, let's do a quick check-in. Michal, you've done TARGET group before, so I don't want to put you on the spot but would you walk us through the stress and personal control scales (points to a SOS poster on the wall with the two self-check scales)?

Michal: Yeah, I can do that. Okay so first you rate your stress level, from one to ten. One is no stress and 10 is extreme. So my stress right now is a 7 'cause I'm not happy to be here but I'm not freaking out. And then you rate your control: 1 is really low, right, like not in control, and 10 is totally in control—that always gets me turned around some. But my control is an 8 right now; I'm dealing with things so I can get out of here as soon as possible.

Leader: Exactly, Michal, thanks, and I'm glad your personal control is high—you're not totally focused, which would be a 10, but you're handling the stress—which is pretty high too, understandably, but not the worst ever which would be a 10 on stress. Let's go around and get everyone's stress and control ratings right now, okay, Levon what about you?

Levon: I don't know, I'm never really stressed so I guess I'm a zero on stress. Nothing's interfering with my control so I'm a 10 on that.

Leader: Thanks Levon, you can't go below 1, so I'll check you in as a 1 and 10. Alok?

Alok: Stress 5, control 9. I'm here, doing okay, good control.

Tomas: I was a 1 on stress ... but I'm still only a 2 on stress, 9 on control.

Carlos: No stress, totally in control ... okay, that's a 1 and 10.

Rahim: I have a lot of stress being here, I'm a 10. I do not want to be here!

Leader:	Being in detention is stressful for everyone, Rahim, thanks for being willing to say that directly. But I want to check with you, did you mean this place, detention, or this group, or both? We're going to do our best to make this group helpful to each of you, not more stress.
Rahim:	I meant detention; I don't like being locked up with people I don't know. I don't really want to be in this group either; it's not gonna help me 'cause I've been in a lot of groups, and it's all pretty lame. Getting out is the only thing that's gonna lower my stress.
Leader:	I think you're probably saying something that others are thinking about groups like this, you're smart to be skeptical if groups or counseling hasn't seemed very helpful so far. Am I right, is Rahim saying something true for others? (Looks around, sees general nodding of heads indicating agreement). Let's see if this group can do anything different that's actually helpful, I can't promise that but all I'm asking is that you all give this a fair chance, okay?
Carlos:	I don't like groups where you just have to sit and listen to a lot of phony talk about how to be a better person, or a bunch of stories about being stressed out and f__ed up.
Tomas:	Exactly. We all know why we're here, so just deal with it and don't be making it worse by doing guilt trips or whining about how unfair everything is.
Michal:	I did this group the last time I was here: no preaching, no sob stories. It's not mad tope and it's not a ticket outta here, but you might learn something if you give it a chance.
Tomas:	Yeah, yeah, yeah, polish that apple. What did *you* learn, you're back here again?
Michal:	Just like you, man, I was all, this is stupid: only geeks or emos would go for this. But truth, I'm back here 'cause I made all the mistakes that I didn't pay attention to in the group.
Leader:	Sounds like that alarm in your brain kept you in reactive mode, Michal, but now you're doing some things to focus your brain—which really is all this group is about. After we finish the check-in, we'll look at what's going on in our brains, and you can add your perspective.
Rahim:	My brain is just fine; I don't want anyone messin' with it here! (Laughs.)
Leader:	No problem, Rahim, no one's messing with your, or anyone else's, brain. We're just going to look at what goes on in everyone's brain when they're stressed so that even if you have a lot of stress—like you said you do now—you can use your brain to handle the stress and achieve your goals, like getting out of detention, and not coming back, and your positive goals for what you want to accomplish in life too. The brain is a complicated machine, very high tech, so you have to know how it works in order to use it effectively and get the most out of it. I think you're already using your brain because I see you listening and you made a serious point with good humor. Is your stress level still the worst ever, a 10? And what's your personal control?

21 Juvenile Justice and Forensic Settings: The TARGET Approach   453

Rahim: Hey, this isn't the worst ever stress, I've seen a lot worse for sure. Yeah, I'm only about a 6 or 7 on stress. I'm fine with control, like an 8 or 9, since I can't control everything yet!

Leader: Okay, that's good to know. If anyone does get up to a 9 or even 10 on stress and your personal control is lower than a 5 while we're meeting, or between group sessions, that's when the brain skills from this group might help you regain personal control so you can handle whatever is stressing you in a way that achieves your goals. And if there's anything that I or the group members can do to help you have positive control, check in and let us know. I know you guys mostly handle stress on your own, or with the support of people you know and trust, so I'm not saying this group is better than that. The group, and any skills you're open to learning here that you think are worth using, are just an addition to skills you already have for handling stress. Is everyone okay with that, at least giving the group a chance despite being skeptical about it?

Levon: That's okay with me, like I said my stress is low and my control is high. So what is it about my awesome brain that I still need to learn, 'cause I think I already got it handled.

Leader: Good question. Did you know that you have an alarm in your brain, and when you—or me, or any of us—act without thinking and do something we regret or get into trouble it's because we didn't use the rest of our brain to make smart choices and re-set the alarm? Let me show you what I mean; here are pictures of how the brain works when you're under stress and how the alarm in your brain can take over and hijack you if you don't know how to reset it.

21.3.2 Girls T4 Group in Juvenile Detention

Three girls participated in a TARGET group in the girl's detention program: Arianna, a 16-year-old of mixed Caucasian and Latina/African-Caribbean ethnicity from an intact urban upper middle-class family; Ronnie, a 15-year-old of Caucasian ethnicity from a low-income single-parent rural family; and Tisha, a 16-year-old of African-American ethnicity who was adopted from birth by a Caucasian lesbian couple.

Arianna was arrested for repeated shoplifting 6 months after being sexually assaulted by a former boyfriend. In the detention center's intake interview, Arianna told that she had been sexually molested by an uncle when visiting cousins for several weeks during the summer at age 11. She'd felt afraid to tell anyone until she returned home to her parents, and then she felt ashamed and guilty when her parents reported the molestation to the police, and he was sent to jail after she had to testify for the trial. She said that her parents had been so angry and upset that, even though they tried to comfort her and reassured her that it wasn't her fault, she worried that she'd hurt them and the rest of her family—and she felt sure that her cousins hated her because her parents would never allow to visit or talk to them or their family again. Arianna recalled being taken to a therapist for several months afterward and described learning mental and relaxation coping skills, which had helped her "not cry all the time" and feel calmer when she felt upset. She also wrote a story about what had happened, with the therapist's help, and when she read it to her parents, she said they all started crying, but she felt better because she saw that her parents believed and weren't mad at her, so it felt like it was past and over and done. After the recent assault by her former boyfriend, she'd tried to use those skills and write a story about it, but her mind would go blank or she'd start sobbing or get so angry that she would punch the walls. Then she started to find herself stealing things without realizing it. She said therapy couldn't help, because something was really wrong with her, and the writing and coping skills wouldn't work anymore.

Ronnie grew up with no contact with her biological father (who had been incarcerated for drug and violent crimes, including domestic violence, since Ronnie was 2 years old), living with her mother and a series of male partners who frequently drank and used drugs to excess. She had five half-siblings, including an older sister who she viewed as a surrogate mother (but who was repeating their mother's pattern of unstable relationships and heavy substance use) and four younger sisters and brothers toward whom she felt a maternal sense of protectiveness (but with whom she was unable to have regular contact due to all being placed in foster homes). She remembers rarely feeling safe in her mother's home, fearful for her mother as well as herself due to recurrent physical battering by male partners, two of whom sexually molested her at ages 12 and 14. Ronnie had difficulty fitting in with peers and in doing schoolwork, feeling as though she was always too suspicious of others and unable to concentrate on school (despite being an avid reader). She turned to drinking and drugs for an escape from feelings of hopelessness and worthlessness.

Tisha grew up in an extended family with grandparents as primary caregivers, but after her grandfather died of a heart attack, her grandmother became harshly punitive, telling Tisha that she was "no good, a ho just like your ma" and beating her for imagined or real infractions. Tisha tried to earn her grandmother's acceptance by passively accepting the punishment and became determined to fight anyone else who disrespected her. She was inducted into a gang in a violent initiation ceremony and used by the gang as a sentry during robberies and a gladiator-like fighter in showdowns with other gangs. Tisha was forced to have sex by male members of the gang, which she considered simply a price of membership. She acknowledged large gaps in memory when she would "lose it" fighting or when she was being sexually victimized.

Session 1 After introductions, the leader (a female social worker) reviewed group rules and expectations, emphasizing that no one would be required to talk about past traumatic experiences or sensitive private personal information. The leader described the group as a chance to learn about how extreme stress changes the brain and practical ways to get the brain reset when stress reactions otherwise lead to confusion and trouble. She added the caveat that this might not be anything new for them, but that most people had never learned how the brain works under stress, beginning with the fact that there is an alarm in the brain that can become stuck in crisis mode.

Using examples derived from but not specific to each girl's history, she described how feeling confused or frustrated and having meltdowns or going on automatic pilot and doing things on impulse or while spaced out can result when a healthy crisis/survival reaction by the brain's alarm mode during traumatic experiences becomes a chronic state of extreme reactivity (or shutdown) when you don't know how to reset the alarm. The leader also used examples similar to the girls' histories to show how, despite not knowing about the alarm, they may still have succeeded in temporarily re-setting their brains' alarms by activating their thinking centers and focusing on memory files based on their core values (e.g., respect, honesty, loyalty, success). She showed the girls handouts with pictures of the key brain areas so they could visualize what was happening in their brain when a stress reaction occurred and when they reset the alarm.

The girls' unanimous response was: "How come nobody ever told me about this alarm before!?" They quickly made the connection between reactive emotions and behaviors and not knowing how to use their brain's thinking center to focus on what was most important to them, so their brains' trauma-reactive alarms never got reset. Arianna understood why the writing and coping skills had worked in the past but now seemed not to work, as a result of her brain's alarm becoming supercharged in survival mode as a result of the added stress of the recent assault. Ronnie recognized that skipping school and getting high were ways to try to turn off the alarm reactions she had when she was bullied and told she was worthless both at school and at home, but that these coping tactics actually turned on her alarm even more because they reduced rather than increased her ability to focus and have personal control. Tisha was more skeptical, but grudgingly acknowledged that "maybe" fighting girls from other gangs and letting her own gang members physically and sexually assault her were turning up her inner alarm and not resetting it.

Session 2 In an initial check-in, Tisha responded to the leader's question of whether anything from the first session had been useful, by describing how she had stopped herself from physically assaulting another girl who was talking to other girls and "gave me the look." When asked how she had chosen not to fight, Tisha said usually she would assault a potential enemy instantly, "I'd look at her and the next thing I know I'm beating her," but before she went into that "zone" this time "I heard that alarm goin' off in my brain, and I said to myself, 'she ain't worth it,' so I just stared her down until she stopped looking at me, 'cause I have a real evil look and no one can outlast me." The leader commented that it appeared that Tisha's mind was even more powerful than her strong body, and Arianna and Ronnie expressed admiration: "awesome!"

The leader elicited an example from each other girl of how they could use their "mind power" if an alarm signal was triggered in their brain. She highlighted their shared ability to both recognize signs of an alarm reaction and focus mentally on achieving their primary goal—instead of reacting without thinking (i.e., on impulse or in a dissociative state). The group reviewed handouts designed to help them be aware of the triggers that could set off their brains' alarms and brainstormed ways they could use their "mind power" to handle the trigger situations and alarm reactions and achieve their goals. Ronnie talked about how she shuts down when triggered by an adult or peer bully, and how she feels "like a loser, just trash," when she lets that happen. The leader invited the other girls to say if they'd ever felt that way, even if they were able to hide it—and both Arianna and Tisha acknowledged this, which shocked Ronnie because "I thought you both always had it together; you're not weak like me." The leader reframed the girls' honest admissions as a sign that all of them, including Ronnie, are "strong, not weak, because you have the strength to acknowledge painful feelings and to take responsibility for not letting bullies beat you down even if you feel like you haven't always stood up for yourself the way you want to." She added, "when other people try to intimidate you or make you feel bad about yourself, now you know that they are just letting their alarms run their lives because they don't have the power to turn down their alarms and stop hurting or mistreating others. You stand up to them when you use your mind power to make choices that you think are right, and don't let your alarm—or their alarm—control what you do, what you think, or who you are." Arianna and Tisha added, "You aren't the loser; it's the abuser and bully who's weak and they can't drag you down anymore!" Without explicitly referring to stigmatization and betrayal, this session's work on alarm triggers helped each of the girls to acknowledge and begin to feel able to overcome these traumatogenic dynamics.

Session 3 The leader used the girls' prior and current examples of successes in recognizing and handling alarm reactions to teach the SOS. Rather than making the SOS a rote exercise, the leader helped the girls see how they were doing the SOS whenever they tapped into their "mind power" by stopping and thinking about "what's really important in your life to *you*, and *who you are as a person*" when a trigger elicited a stress reaction. Using the analogy of physical exercise, she explained how the SOS could be a way to build the strength of their minds if they used it on a regular basis to focus their brain's thinking and memory filing centers and reset their alarms. "I like that better than the relaxation skills I learned in therapy as a kid," said Arianna, "because it's better to be strong than to be relaxed. I really only relax when I feel strong and know I'm safe."

The session was spent brainstorming "orienting thoughts" that the girls could (or already did) use to access their core values before, during, or after having stress reactions. They found it helpful to learn that an orienting thought didn't have to be just words, but could be visualizing a person, place, or activity that represented the healthy relationships, safe places, and interests or talents that meant the most to them—or music, poetry, or stories that expressed their core values. Arianna took this one step further by coming up with the idea of writing fiction based on her own life as a way to harness the power of her brain's thinking and memory centers. She recognized that keeping a journal had helped her to preserve some personal control after the sexual traumas and decided that being a writer was an important part of being true to the part of the SOS referring to "who I am as a person—I'm not a victim or a thief, that's what my alarm pushes me to act like, but when I'm a writer I take back my personal control. I used to use writing just to feel sorry for myself or like I needed to take things to make up for what they took from me, but now I focus first and then write both sides of the story, the stress alarm and focus for personal control. When my characters get all messed up, I help them do an SOS so they can reset their alarms!"

Session Four The leader again drew on examples from the girls' lives to explain how focusing on core values and positive sense of self is not just a mental exercise but can lead to taking actions that express those values and their true self. She cautioned that even if a person is highly mentally focused and has great "mind power," the brain's alarm can still take control if the thinking and memory centers aren't used to translate orienting thoughts into practical goals. The group discussed differences between "reactive" (i.e., alarm-driven) and "main" (i.e., based on core values and one's true self) goals, and how the most effective goals often combined both perspectives in order to be, in Ronnie's words, "real, not pretending everything is okay or that I don't have to watch out for myself, but also not just doing whatever I have to get by."

All three girls had experienced sexual trauma, and having sexuality tainted by betrayal, stigmatization, and powerlessness (i.e., sexualization) was addressed in the closure discussion at the end of this session. In response to the leader's asking what problems the girls might face when using T4 to strengthen and use their "mind power," Tisha replied: "What good is it if I'm focused and have my main goals, but other people use me when their alarms tell them they can f__ with me? They don't know they have an alarm in their brain, and they surely don't know to reset it. Next thing you know, they're f__ing with me, or really f__ing me and using me like their sex toy. I don't think they *have* a thinking center in their brains, they think they can treat me and other girls like such garbage." The other girls resonated with this dilemma, saying that being treated that way wasn't right. But, as Tisha put it, "what can we do about it, they gonna use us, and if we try to stop them they hurt us worse!" The leader responded by acknowledging the very serious dilemma and highlighted the combination of reactive (alarm-based) goals ("to protect yourself from being victimized")—which made complete sense given the harm and danger the girls had experienced (or were currently, in Tisha's case, experiencing) as a result of sexual exploitation—and main goals which reflected their valuing of themselves and of having sexuality as a healthy and safe part of their lives ("to be with people who treat you with the respect and appreciation that you deserve, and who join you in honoring your body and who you are as the beautiful person you truly are"). The girls were somewhat skeptical that main goal was possible, but strongly endorsed it and expressed determination to support each other and other "people with thinking centers" in pursuing it.

21.4 Special Challenges when PTSD Psychotherapy Is Provided in Juvenile Justice Settings

Youth in the juvenile justice system, and their families and peers, often face ongoing or new sources of danger or harm (e.g., family, peer, or community violence; emotional, verbal, or sexual abuse; bullying; neglect; inadequate protection from accidental or interpersonal victimization). When exposure to traumatic stressors leads to symptoms that are peri-traumatic rather than only post-traumatic, the FREEDOM self-regulation skills are of particular relevance and value. Youth in secure juvenile justice facilities, in law enforcement or judicial processing procedures, or in community or peer group settings, where violence is condoned or encouraged (e.g., gangs), also may be exposed to verbal or physical aggression from adults or peers that may not be explicitly traumatic but which can reactivate traumatic stress reactions, including hypervigilance, hyperarousal, or intrusions of traumatic images (Ford and Blaustein 2013). As illustrated in the case example, the FREEDOM skill set can provide a structure to facilitate processing of reactions to, and developing options for effective coping with and recovery from, current traumatic stressors or other major life stressors (e.g., family breakup, out-of-home placements, arrest and detainment or incarceration). This includes helping youths advocate constructively for themselves with potential or actual perpetrators and fulfilling mandated reporter responsibilities to advocate directly for youths' safety when they are in danger.

Cultural sensitivity is a crucial challenge for PTSD psychotherapists working with youth in juvenile justice settings. They must be cognizant of the disproportionate sanctions placed by law enforcement and the judicial system on youth of ethnoracial minority backgrounds and those whose sexual orientation is non-heterosexual (Feierman and Ford 2015). In addition to differences in language (colloquial or formal) and cultural norms, values, and expectations, these youth and their families and their ethnocultural and identity-based communities, as well as those of formerly or currently oppressed religious backgrounds, may experience intergenerational stress reactivity due to historical trauma (e.g., youth of African-American, Native American, Middle Eastern, or South American backgrounds or religious groups whose ancestral predecessors were subject to genocide or racially based political violence; McGregor et al. 2015; Pole et al. 2008). The developmental tasks, goals, and culture of adolescence also result in expectancies, norms, and language that differ substantially from those of adults regardless of their ethnocultural identification. As illustrated in the case examples, the language, activities, and interpersonal etiquette with which PTSD therapy is delivered can, and must, be adapted to be meaningful and respectful to youth and families of very diverse backgrounds.

Youth in the juvenile justice system also range in age from middle childhood (e.g., as young as 9 or 10 years old) to adolescence and early adulthood (e.g., early 20s in some jurisdictions). Preteen or latency-age youth are developmentally much younger physically and psychosocially than the majority of their peers in the system and, along with older youth who have developmental or learning disabilities, are vulnerable to victimization and socialization into delinquency by older youths who have acquired a callous and unemotional persona and use violence and hypervigilance as tools for physical or psychosocial dominance as a result of adverse social learning or their own past traumatic victimization. On the other hand, older or more mature youth often are admired by their younger peers and can be positive role models and protectors for younger youth if they (the older youths) have achieved the advances in cognitive and moral development that can occur in the transition from adolescence to young adulthood. Therefore, having a mix of ages in PTSD therapy groups can be beneficial so long as all forms of overt or subtle bullying, coercion, and victimization are carefully monitored and prohibited by the therapist.

Girls are a unique, and unfortunately growing, subpopulation in juvenile justice (Kerig and Becker 2012). Girls often end up in the law enforcement and juvenile justice system as a result of domestic or community conflict or violence and sexual trauma in which they are victims, witnesses, or secondary/incidental contributors (e.g., committing assault, theft, or prostitution as a means of self-protection). Several studies have found that girls in juvenile justice settings are three times more likely than boys to report direct exposure to or witnessing of family violence, and five to ten times more likely to have been sexually abused (with as many as one in three girls disclosing sexual abuse). Sexually abused girls experience an accelerated onset of puberty neurohormonally (e.g., developing secondary sexual characteristics and libido as early as age 9 or 10) and correspondingly are at risk for further sexual victimization in adolescence (Noll et al. 2003), including becoming entrapped in sexual slavery by human traffickers. The very intimate nature of such prevalent sexual traumatization, as well as the developmental importance of supporting girls in defining an identity and life goals that do not place them in the traditional stereotypic role of dependence upon males, are among several strong reasons for conducting gender-specific PTSD therapy groups.

An additional challenge is systemic rather than related to the characteristics of the youth: PTSD psychotherapy will reach the large subpopulation of youth in juvenile justice systems who are experiencing post-traumatic impairment only if they are implemented systematically on a sustained basis. TARGET therefore has a dissemination infrastructure for exportation of the model to large organizations and service systems. TARGET has been implemented in several large juvenile (and adult criminal) justice systems in the United States, and in multi-program agencies and organizations in North America and Europe providing mental health, child welfare, juvenile justice, substance abuse treatment, and homelessness services. The implementation program is overseen by a small business established by the University of Connecticut Research and Development Office and involves an intensive organizational readiness assessment, multiday trainings for clinicians and staff who directly implement the intervention, overview presentations for all other agency/organization administrators and staff to support consistent implementation, and a multiyear protocol for quality assurance (including independent rating by the trainers of videotape recordings of TARGET sessions); ongoing consultation to ensure fidelity and enhance competence of implementation; assistance with implementation and analysis of data from outcome, alliance and satisfaction measures; and a certification process for both TARGET providers and TARGET trainer/consultants. The implementation infrastructure and process was rated as 4.0 on a 4.0 scale by the US Department of Health and Human Services Substance Abuse and Mental Health Services Administration's (SAMHSA) peer-reviewed National Registry of Evidence-Based Programs and Practices (see www.nrepp.samhsa.gov). Dissemination projects testing adapted versions of TARGET and a train-the-trainer program for line staff as well as clinicians in the child welfare and juvenile justice systems are conducted by the Center for Trauma Recovery and Juvenile Justice, which is a Treatment and Services Adaptation Center in the SAMHSA National Child Traumatic Stress Network (www.nctsn.org).

21.5 The Evidence Base for the TARGET Intervention

TARGET was developed and tested clinically and scientifically first with adults with psychiatric and/or substance abuse disorders comorbid with complex PTSD. Four published randomized clinical trial studies and two published quasi-experimental field studies have reported empirical evaluations of the TARGET intervention. In a randomized controlled trial comparing outpatient group therapy with or without TARGET, the TARGET condition was shown to be effective in this format in reducing PTSD-related beliefs and significantly more effective than treatment as usual in sustaining sobriety self-efficacy with adults in substance abuse treatment (Frisman et al. 2008). In a subsequent randomized controlled trial comparing TARGET versus a manualized supportive group psychotherapy with incarcerated women with complex PTSD, both interventions achieved statistically significant reductions in PTSD and associated symptom severity and increased self-efficacy, with low dropout rates (<5 %) (Ford et al. 2013a). However, TARGET was significantly more effective in increasing sense of forgiveness toward others who have caused harm in the past.

TARGET also has been tested as a one-to-one psychotherapy for PTSD. A randomized controlled trial included low-income mothers with PTSD who were caring for a young child (and often for several children ranging from infants to adolescents). Compared to an efficacious social problem solving therapy for PTSD, present-centered therapy (Frost et al. 2014), TARGET was shown to have incremental efficacy in achieving sustained (at 3- and 6-month follow-up assessments) reductions in PTSD severity and enhanced affect regulation capacities (Ford et al. 2011). TARGET and PCT both were associated with significant reductions in symptoms of depression, dissociation, anger, and anxiety, and improvements in interpersonal functioning and relationships.

In juvenile justice and forensic settings, one randomized clinical trial with girls involved in delinquency and two field trials with adolescents in juvenile justice residential programs provided evidence of TARGET's effectiveness. In the randomized clinical trial study, TARGET delivered as a one-to-one therapy was more effective than a relational therapy in reducing PTSD (intrusive reexperiencing and avoidance) and anxiety symptoms and improving post-traumatic cognitions and emotion regulation (Ford et al. 2012). Relational therapy was an active treatment rather than a minimal contact control: while TARGET reduced girls' self-reported anger and increased their sense of hope, those effects were even stronger in the relational therapy.

In the two quasi-experimental design juvenile justice field trial studies, TARGET was delivered as a group and milieu intervention. Compared to matched groups of detained or incarcerated youth receiving services as usual, TARGET was associated with greater reductions in violent incidents and punitive disciplinary sanctions (e.g., restraints, seclusion) (Ford and Hawke 2012; Marrow et al. 2012), in recidivism

(Ford and Hawke 2012). With incarcerated youth diagnosed with severe emotional disturbance, TARGET was associated with reductions in depression and anxiety and improvement in optimism, self-efficacy, and engagement in rehabilitation (Marrow et al. 2012). In the juvenile detention setting, where short stays often limit the number of sessions that could be provided before youths were released back to the community, each session of TARGET group was associated with 54 % fewer disciplinary incidents and 72 fewer minutes of disciplinary seclusion for each youth during the modal (14-day) stay in detention. TARGET's effectiveness as a group and individual therapeutic intervention thus has been supported with girls and boys involved in juvenile justice. TARGET's effectiveness with women parenting young children and women in prison also suggests that it can contribute to interrupting the intergenerational transmission of traumatic victimization (Widom et al. 2015) and thereby reduce youth involvement in juvenile justice (Ford et al. 2006). Therefore, research is needed to test the model's effectiveness with parents and families of youth who are involved in (or at risk for future contact with) juvenile justice. TARGET's association with increased safety and reduced coercive sanctions in juvenile justice facilities suggests that it may improve not only youth's behavior and functioning but also the correctional milieu in which they are placed for rehabilitation; how TARGET leads to change in juvenile justice program milieus (e.g., change in staff attitudes or institutional practices and culture), and whether this translates to increased community safety (e.g., reduced youth recidivism) and to the healthy and productive development of high-risk youth as they transition developmentally into adulthood, will require lengthy prospective research studies as well as treatment outcome trials.

Research establishing and enhancing the effectiveness of interventions for post-traumatic stress such as TARGET is crucial in order to assist victimized youths such as Arianna, Ronnie, and Tisha. Effective interventions are needed not only to assist these youths recover from post-traumatic stress but also to enable them to develop the skills and attributes that they need to navigate successfully through the juvenile justice system—and to avoid future involvement in the justice systems. With systematic studies of the impact of interventions such as TARGET over many years and decades, we can learn whether (and how) such interventions enable vulnerable youth to successfully meet the challenges of adolescence and adulthood. Moreover, research is needed to determine if, and how, interventions for post-traumatic stress can contribute to preparing youths such as Arianna, Ronnie, and Tisha—and their male peers—to become adults who are able to protect the next generation of children from becoming caught in the tragic intergenerational cycle of victimization and involvement juvenile justice system.

References

Bowes N, McMurran M (2013) Cognitions supportive of violence and violent behavior. Aggress Violent Behav 18(6):660–665. doi:10.1016/j.avb.2013.07.015

de Arellano MA, Lyman DR, Jobe-Shields L, George P, Dougherty RH, Daniels AS, Ghose SS, Huang L, Delphin-Rittmon ME (2014) Trauma-focused cognitive-behavioral therapy for children and adolescents: assessing the evidence. Psychiatr Serv 65(5):591–602. doi:10.1176/appi.ps.201300255

Feierman J, Ford JD (2015) Trauma-informed juvenile justice systems and approaches. In: Heilbrun K, DeMatteo D, Goldstein N (eds) Handbook of psychology and juvenile justice. American Psychological Association, Washington, DC

Finkelhor D, Browne A (1985) The traumatic impact of child sexual abuse: a conceptualization. Am J Orthopsychiatry 55(4):530–541

Follette V, Iverson K, Ford JD (2009) Contextual behavior trauma therapy. In C Courtois, JD Ford (Eds.), Treating complex traumatic stress disorders: An evidence-based guide (pp. 264–285). New York: Guilford

Ford JD (2009) Neurobiological and developmental research: Clinical implications. In C Courtois, JD. Ford (Eds.), Treating complex traumatic stress disorders: An evidence-based guide (pp. 31–58). New York: Gilford

Ford JD (2015) An affective cognitive neuroscience-based approach to PTSD psychotherapy: The TARGET model. J Cog Psychother, 29:69–91

Ford JD (2016) Emotion regulation and skills-based interventions. In: Cook J, Gold S, Dalenberg C (eds) Handbook of trauma psychology. American Psychological Association, Washington, DC

Ford JD, Blaustein ME (2013) Systemic self-regulation: a framework for trauma-informed services in residential juvenile justice programs. J Fam Violence 28:665–677. doi:10.1007/s10896-013-9538-5

Ford JD, Chapman J, Mack M, Pearson G. (2006) Pathway from traumatic child victimization to delinquency: implications for juvenile and permanency court proceedings and decisions. Juv Fam Court J 57(1):13–26

Ford JD, Hawke J (2012) Trauma affect regulation psychoeducation group and milieu intervention outcomes in juvenile detention facilities. J Aggression Maltreat Trauma 21(4):365–384. doi:10.1080/10926771.2012.673538

Ford JD, Steinberg KL, Zhang W (2011) A randomized clinical trial comparing affect regulation and social problem-solving psychotherapies for mothers with victimization-related PTSD. Behav Ther 42(4), 560–578. doi:10.1016/j.beth.2010.12.005. S0005-7894(11)00048-7 [pii]

Ford JD, Chapman JC, Connor DF, Cruise KC (2012) Complex trauma and aggression in secure juvenile justice settings. Crim Justice Behav 39(5):695–724

Ford JD, Chang R, Levine J, Zhang W (2013a). Randomized clinical trial comparing affect regulation and supportive group therapies for victimization-related PTSD with incarcerated women. Behav Ther 44(2):262–276. doi:10.1016/j.beth.2012.10.003

Ford JD, Grasso DJ, Hawke J, Chapman, JF (2013b). Poly-victimization among juvenile justice-involved youths. Child Abuse Negl 37:788–800. doi:10.1016/j.chiabu.2013.01.005

Frisman LK, Ford JD, Lin H, Mallon S., Chang R (2008) Outcomes of trauma treatment using the TARGET model. J Groups Addict Recovery 3:285–303

Frost ND, Laska KM, Wampold BE (2014) The evidence for present-centered therapy as a treatment for posttraumatic stress disorder. J Trauma Stress 27(1):1–8. doi:10.1002/jts.21881

Haufle J, Wolter D (2015) The interrelation between victimization and bullying inside young offender institutions. Aggress Behav 41(4):335–345. doi:10.1002/ab.21545

Henggeler SW, Sheidow AJ (2012) Empirically supported family-based treatments for conduct disorder and delinquency in adolescents. J Marital Fam Ther 38(1):30–58. doi:10.1111/j.1752-0606.2011.00244.x

Kerig PK, Becker SP (2012) Trauma and girls' delinquency. In: Miller S, Leve LD, Kerig PK (eds) Delinquent girls: contexts, relationships, and adaptation. Springer, New York, pp 119–143

Kerig PK, Bennett DC, Thompson M, Becker SP (2012) "Nothing really matters": emotional numbing as a link between trauma exposure and callousness in delinquent youth. J Trauma Stress 25(3):272–279. doi:10.1002/jts.21700

Lang JM, Ford JD, Fitzgerald MM (2010) An algorithm for determining use of trauma-focused cognitive-behavioral therapy. Psychotherapy 47:554–569. doi:10.1037/a0021184

Marrow M, Knudsen K, Olafson E, Bucher S (2012) The value of implementing TARGET within a trauma-informed juvenile justice setting. J Child Adolesc Trauma 5:257–270

McGregor LS, Melvin GA, Newman LK (2015) Differential accounts of refugee and resettlement experiences in youth with high and low levels of posttraumatic stress disorder (PTSD) symptomatology: a mixed-methods investigation. Am J Orthopsychiatry. 85(4):371–381. doi: 10.1037/ort0000076

Noll JG, Trickett PK, Putnam FW (2003) A prospective investigation of the impact of childhood sexual abuse on the development of sexuality. J Consult Clin Psychol 71(3):575–586.

Palmer EJ., Begum A (2006) The relationship between moral reasoning, provictim attitudes, and interpersonal aggression among imprisoned young offenders. Int J Offender Ther Comp Criminol 50(4):446–457. doi:10.1177/0306624X05281907

Pole N, Gone JP, Kulkarni M (2008) Posttraumatic stress disorder among ethno-racial minorities in the United States. Clin Psychol Sci Pract 15(1):35–61

Smith DK, Chamberlain P, Deblinger E (2012) Adapting Multidimensional Treatment Foster Care for the treatment of co-occurring trauma and delinquency in adolescent girls. J Child Adolesc Trauma 5(3), 224–238

Spenser K, Betts LR, Gupta MD (2015) Deficits in theory of mind, empathic understanding and moral reasoning: a comparison between young offenders and non-offenders. Psychol Crime Law 21(7):1–16

Spinazzola J, Hodgdon H, Liang L, Ford JD, Layne C, Pynoos R, Briggs E, Stolbach B, Kisiel C (2014) Unseen wounds: the contribution of psychological maltreatment child and adolescent mental health and risk outcomes. Psychol Trauma Theory Res Pract Policy 6:518–528

Teicher MH, Samson JA (2013) Childhood maltreatment and psychopathology: a case for ecophenotypic variants as clinically and neurobiologically distinct subtypes. Am J Psychiatr 170(10):1114–1133. doi:10.1176/appi.ajp.2013.12070957

Teplin LA, McClelland GM, Abram KM, Mileusnic D (2005) Early violent death among delinquent youth: a prospective longitudinal study. Pediatrics. 115(6):1586–1593. doi:10.1542/peds.2004-1459

Widom CS, Czaja SJ, DuMont KA (2015) Intergenerational transmission of child abuse and neglect: real or detection bias? Science 347(6229):1480–1485. doi: 10.1126/science.1259917

School-Based Interventions

22

Thormod Idsoe, Atle Dyregrov, and Kari Dyregrov

At least nine people were wounded, and ten others were killed when a man opened fire on a campus in Southwest Oregon in October 2015 (NBCnews 2015). In Littleton, Colorado, in 1999, two boys aged 17 and 18 opened fire at Columbine High School, killing 12 students and one teacher, before committing suicide (Leary et al. 2003). In October 2015, a 21-year-old man, dressed as Darth Vader from the Star Wars movies, walked into a Swedish primary school with a long knife and killed a 15-year-old student and a 21-year-old teaching assistant. These are tragic examples, among several from around the world, of traumas affecting school children. Childhood traumatic stress can have a huge impact on almost every kind of developmental process, and the high number of traumatic events experienced by children has added to calls for schools to serve as healing agents for childhood trauma (e.g., Jaycox et al. 2014). Schools are an optimal arena for mental health interventions because they provide access to all children on a regular basis and over time.

In this chapter, we will first discuss some of the underlying concepts related to school-based interventions, before considering the particular challenges for schools in their meeting with children who have experienced traumatic events. We then consider an example of effective practice and finally give a brief overview of the evidence base for interventions.

T. Idsoe, PhD (✉)
Norwegian Center for Child Behavioral Development, Oslo, Norway
e-mail: thormod.idsoe@uis.no

A. Dyregrov
Center for Crisis Psychology, Bergen, Norway
e-mail: atle@krisepsyk.no

K. Dyregrov
Bergen University College, Bergen, Norway

Center for Crisis Psychology, Bergen, Norway
e-mail: Kari.Dyregrov@hib.no

© Springer International Publishing Switzerland 2017
M.A. Landolt et al. (eds.), *Evidence-Based Treatments for Trauma Related Disorders in Children and Adolescents*, DOI 10.1007/978-3-319-46138-0_22

22.1 Background

Childhood trauma is associated with educational consequences and a decline in academic performance. Abused children have been found to have significantly lower school performance than comparable non-abused children (Veltman and Browne 2001). In some studies, exposure to violence has been associated with decreased grade point averages (Boyraz et al. 2016; Hurt et al. 2001; Mathews et al. 2009).

As many as 15–20 % of adolescents report clinical range mental health problems (Mathiesen et al. 2009; Rones and Hoagwood 2000), but only a small percentage ever receive help in the form of targeted interventions or treatment services (Helland and Mathiesen 2009; Rones and Hoagwood 2000; Sund et al. 2011). This means that a large group of young people in need of help does not receive it, which again may cause additional challenges for schools in supporting this large group of "unhelped" students all the way from start of school through graduation. Finding better ways of supporting students at risk of mental health problems is likely to be beneficial for their school motivation because of the relationship between mental health and academic achievement (Gustavsson et al. 2010; Masten et al. 2005).

More traumatized students could be reached if supportive interventions were provided closer to the school context because schools provide access to all children on a regular basis and over time. Immigrant students, who as a group underuse mental health services, may gain particular advantage from school-based interventions. Group-based approaches could be used in schools, either by the educational psychological service, school nurses, or counselors/special educators at school. Such interventions could improve equitable access to treatment, which is currently overly related to social status. However, mental health interventions in school demand expertise from both mental health and education.

22.2 Characteristics of School Settings and Special Challenges

Schools are probably the place where children and adolescents spend most of their organized time outside their families. They are also, for many, a primary social context where students meet many of their friends. This places schools in an exceptional position for providing social support for children who have been exposed to traumatic events. Concomitantly, teachers can facilitate and customize the learning environment to provide individual students with the best help possible (Dyregrov and Dyregrov 2008; Dyregrov et al. 2014). Therapists, healthcare professionals, and educational personnel need to be aware of the huge potential schools have for helping children and adolescents who have been exposed to traumatic events.

The nature of the trauma (e.g., collective versus individual) will have implications for the level of the intervention and who it is targeted at. Possible scenarios could be large-scale traumas affecting the whole school (shootings, fires, death of a student), large events that indirectly affect the school (e.g., disasters in the community, events that are exposed through the media), events that affect the class (student or teacher in the class is seriously wounded or killed), individual events (student losing parent or sibling), and other events (sexual abuse, bullying, victimization). No matter what, it is important that schools make plans for how to intervene if such events occur. These plans must involve all staff and students, but the amount of involvement at different organizational levels will depend on the kind of trauma. If necessary, large meetings must be established in order to get a collective understanding of the situation and to secure standardized procedures at all levels of the organization. Parent meetings can also be necessary. Strong leadership at the highest levels is required in order to ensure the best practice for interventions.

Schools' potential for providing support related to childhood trauma can have multiple phases. First, a general foundation of empathy and support is necessary in order to provide a framework for all other efforts in the school context. School climate has been found to be a resilience factor in crises (Yablon 2015). Second, schools must have crisis intervention plans in place for events that demand immediate attention. Third, schools can serve as providers of therapeutic strategies through intervention programs in order to secure early intervention but also provide strategies for long-term recovery (Jaycox et al. 2014). Schools may also be in a position to discover problems that are slow to arise.

For these reasons, schools need crisis management plans for catastrophic events or other traumatic incidents. The plans should contain both early intervention and long-term follow-up strategies for all those who are identified as in need of help and should involve peers, families, teachers, school administrators, and other members of the school society. It is important that the plans have been discussed and evaluated in meetings with all employees at the school in order to anchor the plans. This is a key feature to allow the plans to work.

22.2.1 Teacher Empathy and Involvement

Regardless of the type of trauma, teachers are very important for exposed students because of the influence and position that follows from the teacher's role. First, an important task which teachers are well placed to take on is to help the child/adolescent back to school after a trauma as soon as possible. This may allow children to experience the continuity and stability of the school routine and may reduce the adverse consequences of a possible chaotic and/or sad atmosphere at home. Of course, the schools must make demands, but students should know that they can take a break if they are exhausted. In accordance with a country's laws for school, the schools must be quick to decide how absence should be recorded, and these procedures should be synchronized for the whole staff. Teachers need to talk to the students and adjust teaching and requirements for what each individual student is capable of at the time. Such conversations need to be repeated periodically. In addition to the fact that the schools can be a "safe haven," providing "mental time-out," teachers and peers can give support that may be helpful. Students will differ when it comes to how much and what kind of support they need and from whom. It is therefore important to adjust the situation to the individual needs of the children and their families. In addition to individual adjustments and concerns, schools can also create frameworks for collective processing if many or all of their students have been exposed to the traumatic event. We discuss an example of this below.

The objective of supporting young people in crisis should therefore be twofold: to provide individual attention and consideration and to create a good framework for the collective processing of the event, which also can enable social support to emerge for those more adversely affected. The main premise for remedial measures to be effective is that trust, empathy, and contact are present between the student and teacher – as well as other key adults. In addition, it is important that there is cooperation between home and school (Dyregrov and Dyregrov 2008).

To facilitate support in the best way possible for a traumatized child, it is important that teachers and staff signal a caring and understanding attitude through exploring how the situation is for the student. After this "mapping process," efforts can be adjusted according to individual needs. Schools need to involve the student and their family in planning individual adjustments as part of a reciprocal process among school, parents, and student. If the traumatic event affected one or several students in the class, it may be beneficial to discuss the incident with the class and facilitate discussion and education related to grief, loss, and crisis responses. Informing students and the school community about the event should be done in cooperation and through mutual understanding with the family of the pupil(s) that are most personally affected.

Teachers need to be aware that following a traumatic event, children may be vulnerable and hypersensitive. The interaction between teacher and students in crisis can be very challenging, and it can be difficult for the teacher to determine whether the care is perceived as good or intrusive. Whether it is perceived as good will depend on the existing relationship between the student and the teacher and how the student feels at the moment. It is important for teachers to move forward gently and show that they understand the child's situation. While young people want true empathy from teachers, it must be such that they can accept it. It is important to sit down, talk with the student, and take adequate time in undisturbed surroundings. Teachers must not "raid" the child with empathy and physical contact. Unless a teacher has been in a very similar situation at the same age, it is not wise to say that you understand how it feels, but rather listen, be present, and show that you care. If the teacher implicitly and explicitly signals that he or she is there for the student when he or she is ready to talk or to receive support and repeats this over time, those who need support will more readily accept it (Dyregrov 2006). Some of the best support happens when teachers show that they care by asking how the child is doing regularly, over time, and in a caring manner. However, it should be noted that the teacher's role is difficult (Alisic et al. 2012; Dyregrov et al. 2013, 2014) in that they have to balance the role of a teacher and of a carer.

It is crucial for the young person that the teacher cares with a genuine commitment to their particular situation. The student needs to understand that the teacher will do their utmost to prevent the traumatic event from adversely affecting the student's achievements at school. This must be stated explicitly by the teachers. Teachers can state that they will be there for the student over time and together they can agree on a process to keep the teachers informed with updated information about how the child is doing academically and adjustments can be made as necessary. Commitment to the individual needs of the students must be linked to knowledge about and competence regarding what happens to children and adolescents who experience loss or trauma in general. Teachers should be well informed about the common reactions in crisis situations, what symptoms are normally seen, and how the individual child may be affected in terms of crisis reactions, grief, concentration problems, and learning difficulties. Such knowledge takes away misunderstandings that the child is being "lazy" or that the child should be "over what happened" in a brief or specific period of time. Symptoms may last for months and way beyond any time limits that teachers and other professionals working with children may expect or wish. Teachers can be informed about such issues through teacher education and through whole-school approaches like HEARTS (Healthy Environments and Response to Trauma in Schools) (Dorado et al. 2016).

22.2.2 Adjustments for Individual Traumatized Students

It is important to provide accurate and appropriate information to the school community about what has happened in order to provide effective social support as well as adjust the academic activities for students. It is important that teachers take the initiative to identify the student(s) who has experienced the traumatic event and may need additional support and adjustments. But of course, the student and his/her family must agree. When something has happened to a child, the teacher can ask the child and the family how they would like the information to be provided to the other children. It could be done by the teacher or in cooperation between the teacher and the child. Younger children may prefer the teacher or the parents to inform their peers. Such information gives pupils an opportunity to ask questions and express their own reactions together with adults. In this way, schools can prevent misunderstandings, spreading of rumors, and too intimate and intense questioning from classmates. Teachers can facilitate schoolmates' understanding the situation and elicit support in a way that is accepted, tolerated, and desired by the exposed child. For younger children, it may be necessary that teachers protect them against peer exclusion, rude comments, or intrusive questions in relation to what happened. The teacher must also inform other teachers about what has happened and what strategies are being put into place so that they can provide support in ways acceptable to the child and family. It will be helpful and strengthen a sense of security and safety in the exposed child if he or she knows who has been told about the situation. The same should be done if the child changes school. The new school and staff should be informed about the same issues.

22.2.3 General Adjustments

Children exposed to trauma may experience reading and learning difficulties. Many are tired and have problems with concentration, while some react by trying to do better at school than before. However, after a while, the efforts to maintain or exceed past performance can be exhausting. One strategy by which to respond to this circumstance is for schools to establish a room where students can rest if they are tired. This may also have the benefit of keeping students at school and allowing them to return as quickly as possible to their studies.

It is very important to inform adolescents that they should relax their perceived obligations in the aftermath of the event and let them know that they have some flexibility regarding absence from school. Time-out is acceptable, although it can be good to return to regular school routines and try to follow their regular school plan. It is very important for students to know that the rules for absence can be relaxed during the first period and for some students this flexibility may need to be in place for a long time.

We also believe that traumatized children who have difficulties sleeping will do better if they are allowed to arrive at school a bit later rather than being extremely tired all day. Children with concentration and/or learning difficulties during school hours can be flexibly provided with "time-out" where they are allowed to go out of class or simply be more passive in class without grades being affected. In some instances, it may be better to propose that the student participate in an outplacement doing practical work (i.e., as an apprentice) instead of academic work or a leave of absence from school for short periods. Some young people may be so bothered by what has happened that they may benefit from sitting in a separate room or diverting their minds from school learning, for example, by playing computer games. Others may need waivers from (some) examinations or extended time for examinations or may need to change the type of examinations depending on whether they are able to concentrate best on written or oral tests.

22.3　How to Do School-Based Interventions[1]

Most school-based interventions are group based, are provided in the early aftermath after a trauma, and consist of CBT techniques that have proven to be helpful in the treatment of child PTSD, so evidence-based practices for treating child PTSD within school are largely built on CBT techniques (Jaycox et al. 2009; Rolfsnes and Idsoe, 2011).

Based on the framework described in the previous section which emphasizes the importance of supportive interventions, schools can provide interventions to assist children in coping with the traumatic stress that they have experienced. In the following section, we will provide an example of a procedure that was developed by the Children and War Foundation (http://www.childrenandwar.org) in which one of the authors (AD) took part. This procedure (see Table 22.1 for an overview) can be used within schools following situations that have affected many children. The manual has been used successfully among children following different traumatic exposures around the world and included routine and systematic assessment of the children

---

[1] The following presentation is largely based on Smith et al. (2013).

Table 22.1 A procedure for techniques for traumatized children developed by the Children and War Foundation (http://www.childrenandwar.org) that can be used within schools following situations that have affected many children

Section 1: Intrusion
Session 1
Getting to know each other, introducing the group, normalizing and educating, establishing a safe place
Session 2
Imagery techniques; auditory, olfactory, and kinesthetic techniques; dual-attention tasks; dream work; distraction; bothering thoughts or worries; closing the group; homework tasks
Section 2: Arousal
Session 3
Getting started, homework review, introducing the topic, muscle relaxation, breath control, guided imagery, coping self-statements, using a fear thermometer, short form of relaxation and skills to practice in the session, sleep hygiene, activity scheduling, homework, closing the group
Section 3: Avoidance
Session 4
Getting started, homework review, introducing avoidance and exposure, brainstorming traumatic reminders as a group, individual list of reminders, graded exposure, constructing a personalized fear hierarchy, planning for real-life exposure, helpful and unhelpful avoidance
Session 5
Exposure to traumatic memories: drawing, writing, and talking, looking to the future, homework, closing the group

Largely based on Smith et al. (2013)

with well-known measures before and after the intervention. Evidence shows improvement among children taking part (for a review of the results, see Yule et al. (2013). The focus is on early intervention by teaching children how to cope with their stress in order to prevent later problems from developing. The procedure is described in detail in the manual called "Children and Disaster: Teaching Recovery Techniques" (Smith et al. 2013). The aim is to teach children, in a step-by-step procedure, skills and techniques which are helpful in coping with symptoms following traumatic events. Even though depression and other problems like headaches and stomachaches may also be present, the focus of this manual is on posttraumatic stress reactions. This is because they are the most common, the most distressing, and the most developmentally disruptive problems (e.g., Thienkrua et al. 2006).

The intervention consists of five weekly two-hour group sessions with up to 15 children from 8 years and older. Sessions 1 and 2 address intrusive thoughts and feelings, such as bad memories, nightmares, and flashbacks. Session 3 addresses arousal, such as difficulties in relaxing, concentrating, and sleeping. Sessions 4 and 5 address avoidance, such as children's fears, and difficulties in facing up to reminders of the traumatic event. Each of the five sessions starts with a review of the principles and ideas behind the techniques, and then it proceeds with a set of practical instructions and activities to be carried out. Finally, tasks for children to carry out as homework are provided. The intervention is also accompanied by two parent sessions.

The manual is designed to reduce the need for later treatment. Since sessions aim to equip children with the tools to master different common posttraumatic reactions, it can be started within the first month after the disaster/trauma. However, following disasters, it may take time before a program can be set up, and the start of sessions may be several months after the event. Even after completing the sessions, severely affected children will continue to need further help, and some guidelines on how to identify these children are also provided.

In some disaster situations, i.e., earthquakes, all children are affected and can make use of the tools they learn in the sessions. The formation of the group will reflect the type of situation. It may be students from the same class or students from different classes at the same school (i.e., after a school event affecting some but not all children at the school). One parent session is scheduled at the start of the sessions and one at the end. The parent sessions inform parents about what the children will learn, briefly explains the content of each session, and motivates the parents to support the children in their homework between sessions. A new parent module is currently being developed and tested.

The group leaders do not have to be mental health professionals, other professions such as teachers can successfully lead groups (see Yule et al. 2013). The two leaders have equal roles in the groups. The groups are not intended to be similar to didactic classroom teaching. Nor are they treatment groups, which entail a good deal of difficult and heavy emotional expression. The groups are proactive and encourage self-help and mutual support. The role of the two co-leaders is crucial in setting the pace and tone of the group. They act as models for children in showing respect and understanding of others, listening attentively, demonstrating empathy, initiating a sense of optimism, active coping and self-efficacy without undermining children's problems, and using humor where appropriate.

Section 1 Intrusion

Session 1
Intrusive memories come unexpectedly, often triggered by reminders in the environment that children can be unaware of. They may also come as nightmares. Because these memories can be very vivid and frightening, they can be overwhelming, and many children fear that they are going crazy or that they are out of control. The main aims of the first sessions are to show that such reactions are normal and to give children the skills to regain control over their memories. Even though the children will not be able to forget these memories, they can learn how to remember without being overwhelmed by emotion and to be in charge of them.

There are five session goals:

- *Children to get to know each other.* The children should sit in a circle. The group is led by two leaders who should join the circle, but not next to each other. A few minutes are spent doing a warm-up activity (icebreaker) and getting used to being in the group together (less needed if they already know each other). The

activity could, for example, be for the children to pair up and ask each other simple questions (name, favorite food/activities) and then introduce their partner to the rest of the group.
- *Aims and structure of the groups are described.* After the introductions, the reasons for the group are explained, and children are told that this is the first of the five meetings. They are told that they will discuss the traumatic event and how it affects children. The leaders emphasize that even though it can be difficult and upsetting at times, there is also hope and optimism in coping with difficult feelings. Some core rules are established, and the leaders try to let the children participate in generating these rules. Topics like confidentiality, mutual respect, and no obligation to talk – but obligation to listen to each other, go at one's own pace, talk only about oneself but not others, listen to what the others say, do not put others down, and come to all meetings – are touched upon.
- *Education and normalization of common reactions.* Before starting on learning specific techniques, it is necessary for children to understand something about traumatic stress responses. The aims of this part are threefold: (a) to educate children about known reactions to traumatic events so that their own problems become definable and manageable, (b) to normalize their reactions so that they do not feel so alone and crazy, and (c) to share some of their stories so that they come together as a group. A list of traumatic events is generated with contributions from the group without asking for details. A flip chart is used to list the events. It is important for the group to hear that reactions to the traumatic events are common and can happen to anyone. They are called posttraumatic stress reactions, and the leaders will explain what can be done with them. A new list of reactions is compiled and written on the flip chart based on the group members' experiences but again without going into too many details. When the list has been compiled, reactions are normalized by talking about them in a general way and by telling the children that these are common reactions to traumatic events. The leaders can follow this by talking about the concept of traumatic reminders, and the group is asked what reminds them of what happened, and a new list based on this information is compiled. A connection between the reminders, the intrusive memories, and accompanying distressing emotions is made. The children are told that reminders that are partly hidden can be "discovered" and coped with, so the children can develop a sense of control. Children need to hear that help exists and are told that there are some tricks they can learn to take control over their memories. They may not be able to forget, but they will be more able to remember when they decide. Practicing the tricks is important. However, before the children learn the tricks, they need to *know how to* create a safe place in their imagination.
- *Create a safe place in their imagination.* This is achieved by asking them to imagine a place or scene that makes them feel calm and secure and happy, either a place they have been, or heard of, or a place they invent and make up themselves. Group leaders have them look for lots of good things in their scene, i.e., smell the flowers or imagine a good friend that is present. Group leaders go around and assist children when they practice. The practice is finished by asking

the group what they imagined and how they felt, and they are asked to use this when they feel the need to calm their bodies or mind, either at home or in the sessions. The session is closed by praising each child for the good work that they have done and informing that there are four more sessions to go for learning more tricks.
- *Homework.* Children are asked to practice the safe place technique at home.

Session 2

In this session, usually a week after the first, the goals are to learn a series of techniques designed to give the children more control over distressing intrusive memories. A sense of active coping should be developed, and it should be remembered that not all techniques work for all children. The techniques are thought to develop the child's ability to bring up their intrusive memories deliberately, to change them in various ways, and to switch them off. Children are advised to practice such exercises 10 min every day.

One exercise is for children to imagine their intrusive image as if on a television screen where changes to the image can be made. The children are asked to do different things with the picture such as changing the colors to black and white or to freeze the action if it is like a moving picture and finally to blur and fade the picture away. The idea is that these are first steps for the children in order to try to take control over their intrusive images or rescript them. Alternative imaginary techniques are found in the manual, as well as techniques for auditory, olfactory, and kinesthetic intrusive phenomena. We do not present the latter ones here, as visual intrusions are by far the most common.

Dual-attention tasks are also taught. They are derived from eye movement desensitization and reprocessing (EMDR) techniques (see Chap. 13) and are alternatives to the visualization techniques described above. Individual treatment protocols for EMDR employ dual-attention tasks where children deliberately recall their traumatic image with their eyes open while simultaneously tracking with their eyes the side-to-side rhythmical movement of the therapist's hand. However, research suggests that a number of alternatives to eye movements may be used with children as a dual-attention task. In the manual, when working with groups, alternate tapping of knees has been used. It is easy to administer in a group, is simple to teach, and may produce rapid spontaneous change. However, there are no studies conducted on this variation of EMDR. The basic technique involves each child tapping his or her own knee at a rhythm set by the group leader, while he or she holds the traumatic image in mind. Nothing else is required of the child, apart from noticing any changes to the image that occur spontaneously. Initially, three sets of taps for about 30 seconds each are carried out. A fourth set is then carried out while the group is told to let the picture fade. A final and fifth set is carried out while the children are told to imagine a pleasant scene instead of their trauma scene. The group is then asked for feedback before the procedure may be practiced twice more.

Intrusive memories can also come as bad dreams and nightmares. Many techniques are available for tackling this, including setting up regular evening bedtime routines; practicing relaxation techniques before going to sleep (described below); doing safe place techniques (see above); recalling dreams during the day, as well as practicing changing the dream images or applying dual-attention tasks (see above); having children draw, write down, or talk about a new and positive version of the dream (see Krakow and Zadra 2006); and other ways of restructuring or rescripting the dream.

Another technique presented for intrusive memories is distraction. This is a way of switching off the traumatic memories, although maladaptive avoidant strategies must be avoided. The group is asked what sorts of things they do when they want to forget about the traumas. A flip chart may list their suggestions, like thinking in detail about something else, taking part in favorite activities, listening to or playing music, reading a book, watching television, doing hobbies, doing sports, or playing games. The children are advised how to use such methods to establish "trauma-free zones." A final technique that can be an important adjunct to this, especially when children harbor distressing thoughts, can be to set aside a specific time like 10 min every day for the troubled thoughts and memories. Then, if these thoughts appear outside of this during the day, the child can say to himself or herself that they will not worry about this now but later in the time set aside for this.

The closing of the group follows the same procedure described for Session 1 above, and once again, they are asked to do homework. This time it is to practice one or more of the imagery techniques, to talk to a parent about dreams, and to draw a positive ending to a bothersome dream. Where children have been taught several tools, they are asked to use the tool that works best for them or try another one if the first one does not work.

Section 2 Arousal

Session 3

Children may show increased physiological arousal following exposure to traumatic events so that they may be more nervous, jumpy, and anxious and startle very easily. They may be more irritable and have problems with concentration, as well as difficulties falling or staying asleep. The third session involves training in relaxation skills.

The session can be started by using a beanbag/ball that the children throw to each other (for the youngest group, <10–11 years). The one who catches says one nice thing that has happened since the last session. After this, the homework is reviewed. They are asked for comments, and it is made sure that each child can contribute something positive. Then examples from the group about bodily sensations that accompany intrusive memories are elicited. These are written down on a flip chart. The list the group generates may include increased heart rate, heart racing, breathing quickly, shallow breathing, pain in the chest, feeling dizzy or sick, out of breath, feeling shaky, trembles, palpitations, hands shaking, hands or feet tingle, sweating, and so on. After going through these symptoms, relaxation training is commenced. Children are asked how they usually relax themselves. In this way, children's own coping strategies can be reinforced. Before starting the training, it is made sure that everyone is in a comfortable position, sitting down in a circle. Various relaxation methods can be used, but in the manual, a detailed version of the progressive relaxation method is described involving tensing and relaxing each of the major muscle groups. When finished, the participants are asked how it went, and depending on the feedback, it may be repeated.

Another technique taught is diaphragmatic breathing. They are showed by the group leader how the stomach pushes outward when inhaling and inward when exhaling. The children are asked to practice, putting one hand on their stomach just above the navel and one hand on their chest. They are shown how the muscles are used sequentially in breathing in and out, like a wave. Then children are asked to breathe in slowly through the nose counting one and then blow out slowly, saying to himself or herself "relax." They practice this several times until they have the hang of it.

A short form of relaxation that is useful for children to have at hand for sudden anxiety-provoking situations is also recommended (March et al. 1998): The child takes three or four diaphragmatic breaths and then tenses and relaxes both fists and/ or feet to the count of five to ten, followed by three to four more diaphragmatic breaths and repeats the process as needed. Children may say "relax" to themselves as they exhale. It is helpful for the child to picture himself or herself holding all the anxiety in his or her fist and letting go of all the anxiety as the fists are relaxed and the last bits of tension shaken off by shaking the hands.

It is explained to the children that the various "tricks" take practice and do not come easily at first. Breathing can be combined with the imaginary techniques described above, and normally, children will practice the muscle relaxation and breath control before they use their safe place as an additional resource. Positive self-talk can also be useful, but it is important for them to first understand the connection between thoughts and feelings. After explaining this, it gives more meaning to identifying anxiety-provoking thoughts and substituting them with positive thoughts. Using a fear thermometer is another technique for children to monitor their own fear reactions – the hotter it is, the more fearful the child. They are shown a picture of a thermometer with numbers from 1 to 10 on it and told the following: "When you're confronting your fears, you want to be able to say how scary it is. This thermometer will help you. At the bottom, number 1 means you are not scared at all, it is the most relaxed you have ever been. At the top is the most scared you've ever been." The group is asked for some emotional words that can anchor the bottom and the top of the thermometer. Each child can make her/his own thermometer to keep.

Sleep difficulties due to hyperarousal are common in children who live through disasters. The main strategies for improving sleep are establishing a regular nighttime routine (this is covered in the parallel parents' session), dream restructuring (covered in the previous session with children), and use of relaxation skills before bed (covered above). Children can use combinations of these different techniques. In addition, they may have their own tricks for falling asleep or getting back to sleep if they awaken in the night. Discussion between them is encouraged so that the children can help each other.

The homework after this session is to practice diaphragmatic breathing and muscle relaxation, as well as to check the thermometer.

Section 3 Avoidance

Session 4
Avoidance may be cognitive, which means attempting to avoid reminders of the traumatic event, or it may be behavioral, which means avoiding places and people or discussions that remind them of the traumatic event. These issues may restrict child functioning and in the end will serve to maintain the child's problems. This session starts by reviewing the homework. Then it is important to notice that the session builds on the control and relaxation techniques learned in the first two sessions.

Initially it may be helpful to talk about reminders and behavioral avoidance since this is more concrete and easier for children to relate to. Try to have the children distinguish between adaptive and maladaptive avoidance. First, it is important to be aware of what reminders are. A flip chart is used, and the group is again asked what their reminders are. These are often places and things, people, situations, sounds, and sensations. The group leader aims at getting as many reminders on the list as possible. It is made clear that avoidance can be helpful (like avoiding dangerous places) and unhelpful (e.g., places that are no longer dangerous). After brainstorming as a group, the children are asked to make their own personal list of reminders. The group leaders then introduce the idea for graded exposure by use of an example. Most children probably already know that confronting feared situations can be a way of overcoming fear and avoidance. Make it clear that exposure to the object results in a fear reaction. Avoiding the object will temporarily reduce fear; however, it also means that they will continue to be fearful in the future. The group leaders can try to make the group come up with ideas of exposure by giving them an example first. Comments from the group about similar experiences are elicited, making it an interactive session. A ladder can be used as an example of graded exposure, step-by-step, one move at the time: "We're going to do something similar with your reminders of the trauma. We need to face up to them, but we will do it step-by-step, like a ladder. To help you go up the steps, you can use all the things you want to from your toolbox. What things could you use from your toolbox to help you fight your fear as you go up the ladder?" (Smith et al. 2013). Different techniques from the toolbox can be used by the children: relaxation, breathing, safe place, fear thermometer, and coping self-statements. The children split up to make their own ladders in smaller groups, in order to cope with a feared and avoided reminder. The flip chart is used to draw a ladder, and the exposure is broken into very small steps. For example, if a child avoids a room where she/he was during an earthquake, the first step of the ladder could be looking at the building from a distance, the next step could be walking to be near the building, the next to approach the front door, and so on.

Having constructed this ladder, the children should be told that they can practice the steps themselves if they feel able and seek help from parents if necessary. Remind them of the helpfulness of the fear thermometer and the use of relaxation techniques and coping self-statements like "I can do it," "It can't really hurt me," "I know I can cope," "I'm going to beat my fear," and "My fear will go away soon." They should also write these statements down.

The basic steps for undertaking exposure are:

1. Construct a fear hierarchy.
2. Choose a target and prepare for confronting the reminder – relaxation.
3. Stay in the situation – positive self-statements.
4. Monitor fear until acceptable level – fear thermometer.
5. Self-praise and reward.
6. Repeat with a more difficult target.

One important issue is that not all avoidance behavior is maladaptive in traumatic situations. In teaching exposure skills, it is crucial that children can distinguish between functional and dysfunctional avoidance. Many places are genuinely dangerous. Children can ask themselves questions like "Can this really hurt me?" "Do grown-ups come here?" "Would my parents or elder siblings come here?" A rule could be that the children always practice a planned graded exposure with their parents before doing it.

Session 5
Even though it is important to have techniques to distract oneself from traumatic memories, it will usually be necessary to expose oneself deliberately to the traumatic memories. In this session, the intention is to engage in activities to recall traumatic experiences rather than changing them or distracting oneself from them. The intention is to enable the children to re-experience in a structured and controlled way. Several techniques can be used for this, depending on the children's level of maturity and educational experience. Writing is often a good way of processing memories, as can be drawing. Younger children will spontaneously use drawings more than writing, while adolescents make more use of writing. If one starts with drawing, each member of the group is given paper and pencils. The aim of the drawing is for the children to begin to recall their traumatic memories in a controlled way and as a basis for talking about what happened. The aim is to give children practice in recalling their memories, rather than to conduct an intense exposure session. Have the group split up and allow enough time for children to become absorbed individually in their drawing. They are asked to draw an aspect from an intrusive picture or memory. Go around the group as the children are drawing; encourage and comment on the drawings.

As with drawing, writing can be a means of imaginal exposure directly and can be used as basis for talking through the event. In the group setting, there will not be enough time for each child to produce an individual piece of writing, so the aim here is giving advice for writing activities that can be practiced later. It may be worth saying that this is not like school – things like spelling and handwriting do not matter. The point is just to get all the details of what happened out into the open. Use the flip chart. The writing should be done as a sequential story. They should write up their innermost thoughts and deepest feelings for the writing to have its optimal effect (Pennebaker 1997). See also http://www.childrenandwar.org for a writing manual developed for adolescents. In the parent sessions, parents are told to stimulate the writing but that the child writes more freely if they know that they only write for themselves.

If children get distressed, the group leader can use the group for supporting the child, but being two group leaders also allow one to take extra care of a child that needs attention. If a child becomes upset, it is also calming when the group leader just explains that it is normal to be sad or anxious following such events and that reactions will gradually be reduced. With group leaders who acknowledge and normalize what happens in the group, children feel safe, and reactions are short-lived.

This last session finishes with a proactive section on planning for the future. It means the session ends in a more positive way. Encourage discussions with open-ended questions like, "What do you hope for the future? For your families in the future? For your country? How do you see things in 5 or 10 years' time?" Review briefly the main techniques from each session. The session ends by saying that this is the last session and praising the children for coming, for working hard, and for being brave in thinking about and talking about very difficult things. Each child should be praised. At the very end, it is helpful to finish with a kind of party or celebration of their good work.

22.4 Evidence

In an extensive review of the literature that focuses specifically on school-based interventions for traumatic stress, Jaycox et al. (2009) give an overview demonstrating that much work has been accomplished within this field, but as demonstrated by Jaycox et al. (2014), the evaluation of many of the school-based programs is lagging behind their application. The intervention that we presented in the previous section can be implemented in several different settings. Even though it has not been evaluated in the school context specifically, it contains the same components as the other school-based interventions that are presented, and it has been evaluated in several other contexts. For a review of these results, see Yule et al. (2013).

In 2011, Rolfsnes and Idsoe (2011) conducted a meta-analysis of school-based treatment programs for childhood PTSD. The final number of studies that satisfied the inclusion criteria was 19. Nine of the studies used a randomized design, while ten studies used a quasi-experimental design. Sixteen studies, including six RCTs, evaluated cognitive behavioral therapy (CBT). The rest evaluated play/art therapy, eye movement desensitization and reprocessing (EMDR), and mind–body skills. Medium-to-large effects were found in 11 of the CBT evaluations and small-to-medium effects in four of the CBT studies. One very large quasi-experimental study of war-affected children in Lebanon did not find any effect of CBT on PTSD symptoms. The two school-based RCTs of play therapy and EMDR (vs. wait list control) showed medium-to-large effect sizes. Moderators were not investigated through meta-analysis; however, differences in findings could be related to factors like length, intensity of protocol training provided to the therapists, background of therapist (trained as mental health provider vs. not), severity, degree of trauma (cumulative trauma), and so on. The meta-analysis of all the 19 studies gave a mean weighted effect of medium-to-large effect. These results support the idea that school-based interventions can be effective, but further RCTs are recommended.

More recently, additional studies have been conducted on school-based interventions for childhood trauma. For example, Salloum and Overstreet (2012) evaluated the differential effects of the Grief and Trauma Intervention (GTI) with coping skills and trauma narrative processing (CN) and coping skills only (C). In this school-based approach, 70 African-American children (6–12 years old) were randomly assigned to GTI-CN or GTI-C. Both treatments consisted of a manualized 11-session intervention and a parent meeting. Children in both treatment groups demonstrated significant improvements in distress-related symptoms and social support. Wolmer et al. (2011) used a school-based approach in Israeli schools following the 2006 Lebanon War. The protocol consisted of 15 45-min manualized didactic modules delivered weekly by teachers using a coping-enhancement framework. It included topics such as "working through positive and negative experiences, stress management and control of bodily tension, affective regulation and processing (i.e., dealing with sadness and anger), attention control, identification and correction of negative thoughts, using humor as well as other coping and social-emotional competencies" (p. 312). Participating children showed a significant symptom decrease compared to a control group. The authors conclude that teachers were valuable cost-effective providers for such interventions.

Conclusions

There is no school that does not have to deal with traumatic events during a school year. However, as an arena where students spend a large part of their childhood, school is also a place where they can be helped individually or collectively. With empathic support teachers can plan for students' return after traumatic events, and they can adjust demands to facilitate the normalization of students' lives following untoward events. Teachers and mental health professionals can together implement group interventions following events that have affected groups of students or the whole school. A caring climate and tailored interventions can help fulfill students' learning potential.

Acknowledgments Thanks to Julia Norman for helping with the language.

References

Alisic E, Bus M, Dulack W, Pennings L, Splinter J (2012) Teachers' experiences supporting children after traumatic exposure. J Trauma Stress 25(1):98–101

Boyraz G, Granda R, Baker CN, Tidwell LL, Waits JB (2016) Posttraumatic stress, effort regulation, and academic outcomes among college students: a longitudinal study. J Couns Psychol 63:475–486. Retrieved from http://dx.doi.org/10.1037/cou0000102

Dorado JS, Martinez M, McArthur LE, Leibovitz T (2016) Healthy Environments and Response to Trauma in Schools (HEARTS): a whole-school, multi-level, prevention and intervention program for creating trauma-informed, safe and supportive schools. Sch Ment Health 8:163–176

Dyregrov A (2006) Sorg hos barn: en håndbok for voksne. Fagbokforl, Bergen

Dyregrov K, Dyregrov A (2008) Effective grief and bereavement support: the role of family, friends, colleagues, schools and support professionals. Jessica Kingsley Publishers, London

Dyregrov A, Dyregrov K, Idsoe T (2013) Teachers' perceptions of their role facing children in grief. Emotion Behav Diffic 18(2):125–134

Dyregrov K, Endsjø M, Idsøe T, Dyregrov A (2014) Suggestions for the ideal follow up for bereaved students as seen by school personnel. J Emotion Behav Diffic 20:289–301. http://dx.doi.org/10.1080/13632752.2014.955676

Gustavsson JE, Westling Allodi M, Alin Åkerman B, Eriksson C, Eriksson L, Fischbein S, Granlund M, Gustafsson P, Ljungdahl S, Ogden T, Persson RS (2010) School, learning and mental health: a systematic review. Stockholm: The Royal Swedish Academy of Sciences

Helland MJ, Mathiesen KS (2009) 13–15 åringer fra vanlige familier i Norge: Hverdagsliv og psykisk helse [13–15 year-olds from regular families in Norway: everyday life and mental health]. Norwegian Institute of Public Health, Oslo

Hurt H, Malmud E, Brodsky NL, Giannetta J (2001) Exposure to violence: psychological and academic correlates in child witnesses. Arch Pediatr Adolesc Med 155(12):1351–1356. doi:10.1001/archpedi.155.12.1351

Jaycox LH, Stein B, Amaya-Jackson L (2009) School-based treatment for children and adolescents. In: Foa EB, Keane TM, Friedman MJ, Cohen J (eds) Effective treatment for PTSD: practice guidelines from the International Society for Traumatic Stress Studies. Guilford Press, New York, pp. 327–345

Jaycox LH, Stein BD, Wong M (2014) School intervention related to school and community violence. Child Adolesc Psychiatr Clin N Am 23(2):281–293. doi:10.1016/j.chc.2013.12.005

Krakow B, Zadra A (2006) Clinical management of chronic nightmares: imagery rehearsal therapy. Behav Sleep Med 4(1):45–70

Leary MR, Kowalski RM, Smith L, Phillips S (2003) Teasing, rejection, and violence: case studies of the school shootings. Aggress Behav 29(3):202–214

March JS, Amaya-Jackson L, Murray MC, Schulte A (1998) Cognitive-behavioral psychotherapy for children and adolescents with posttraumatic stress disorder after a single-incident stressor. J Am Acad Child Adolesc Psychiatry 37(6):585–593. doi:10.1097/00004583-199806000-00008

Masten AS, Roisman GI, Long JD, Burt KB, Obradovic J, Riley JR et al (2005) Developmental cascades: linking academic achievement, externalizing and internalizing symptoms over 20 years. Dev Psychol 41:733–746. Retrieved from http://search.ebscohost.com/login.aspx?direct=true&db=psyhref&AN=DP.DA.GCC.MASTEN.DCLAAE&loginpage=Login.asp&site=ehost-live&scope=site

Mathews T, Dempsey M, Overstreet S (2009) Effects of exposure to community violence on school functioning: the mediating role of posttraumatic stress symptoms. Behav Res Ther 47(7):586–591

Mathiesen KS, Karevold E, Knudsen AK (2009) Psykiske lidelser blant barn og unge i Norge. Folkehelseinstituttet, Oslo

NBCnews (2015) Oregon shooting: umpqua community college gunman talked religion. Retrieved from http://www.nbcnews.com/news/us-news/officers-respond-report-shooting-umpqua-community-college-n437051

Pennebaker JW (1997) Writing about emotional experiences as a therapeutic process. Psychol Sci 8(3):162–166

Rolfsnes ES, Idsoe T (2011) School-based intervention programs for PTSD symptoms: a review and meta-analysis. J Trauma Stress 24(2):155–165. doi:10.1002/jts.20622

Rones M, Hoagwood K (2000) School-based mental health services: a research review. Clin Child Fam Psychol Rev 3:223–241

Salloum A, Overstreet S (2012) Grief and trauma intervention for children after disaster: exploring coping skills versus trauma narration. Behav Res Ther 50(3):169–179

Smith P, Dyregrov A, Yule W, Gupta L, Perrin S, Gjestad R (2013) Children and disaster: teaching recovery techniques. Bergen: Children and War Foundation. http://www.childrenandwar.org/

Sund AM, Larsson B, Wichstrom L (2011) Prevalence and characteristics of depressive disorders in early adolescents in central Norway. Child Adolesc Psychiatry Ment Health 5(1):28

Thienkrua W, Cardozo BL, Chakkraband MS, Guadamuz TE, Pengjuntr W, Tantipiwatanaskul P, Sakornsatian S, Ekassawin S, Panyayong B, Varangrat A (2006) Symptoms of posttraumatic stress disorder and depression among children in tsunami-affected areas in southern Thailand. JAMA 296(5):549–559

Veltman MW, Browne KD (2001) Three decades of child maltreatment research Implications for the school years. Trauma Violence Abuse 2(3):215–239. doi:10.1177/1524838001002003002

Wolmer L, Hamiel D, Barchas JD, Slone M, Laor N (2011) Teacher-delivered resilience-focused intervention in schools with traumatized children following the second Lebanon war. J Trauma Stress 24(3):309–316

Yablon YB (2015) Positive school climate as a resilience factor in armed conflict zones. Psychol Violence 5(4):393

Yule W, Dyregrov A, Raundalen M, Smith P (2013) Children and war: the work of the Children and War Foundation. Eur J Psychotraumatol 4:1–8. doi:10.3402/ejpt.v4i0.18424

Treating and Preventing Psychological Trauma of Children and Adolescents in Post-Conflict Settings

Anselm Crombach, Sarah Wilker, Katharin Hermenau, Elizabeth Wieling, and Tobias Hecker

23.1 The Need for Psychological Interventions in Post-Conflict Settings

In 2015, more than 60 million people worldwide were fleeing modern wars and terrorism. This is the highest number of refugees ever recorded by UNHCR. In the context of conflict and crisis, children and adolescents represent an extremely vulnerable population. Next to the consequences on physical health, children are at an increased risk to suffer from the mental health consequences of traumatic stress, most prominently post-traumatic stress disorder (PTSD), internalizing and externalizing problems. If these symptoms go untreated, they are likely to have lifelong consequences at individual, relational, and societal levels.

A. Crombach (✉) • K. Hermenau
University of Konstanz, Konstanz, Germany

NGO vivo international, Allensbach-Hegne, Germany
e-mail: anselm.crombach@uni-konstanz.de; katharin.hermenau@uni-konstanz.de

S. Wilker
University of Ulm, Ulm, Germany

NGO vivo international, Allensbach-Hegne, Germany
e-mail: sarah.wilker@uni-ulm.de

E. Wieling
University of Minnesota, Minneapolis, MN, USA

NGO vivo international, Allensbach-Hegne, Germany
e-mail: lwieling@umn.edu

T. Hecker
University of Bielefeld, Bielefeld, Germany

NGO vivo international, Allensbach-Hegne, Germany
e-mail: tobias.hecker@uni-bielefeld.de

© Springer International Publishing Switzerland 2017
M.A. Landolt et al. (eds.), *Evidence-Based Treatments for Trauma Related Disorders in Children and Adolescents*, DOI 10.1007/978-3-319-46138-0_23

23.1.1 PTSD Prevalence Rates in Children and Adolescents Exposed to War and Conflict

While PTSD prevalence rates in children and adolescents derived from epidemiological studies in Western countries vary between 0.5 and 9 % (see Chap. 2), reported prevalence rates in post-conflict settings are much higher, ranging from 25 to 44 % (Ertl et al. 2014; Schaal and Elbert 2006). The most obvious reason for these elevated rates is a higher exposure to traumatic events, as cumulative trauma exposure increases PTSD risk in a dose-dependent manner (Catani et al. 2008). However, children and adolescents in post-conflict settings are exposed to additional risk factors. These include forced displacement, poverty, parental loss and family disruption, ongoing political and community violence, and stigmatization. A central risk factor for children is family violence, which can aggravate the vulnerability toward adverse consequences of war trauma (Catani et al. 2008). Ongoing conflicts and adverse life conditions impair psychological recovery. Further, the presence of severe mental health symptoms is associated with difficulties in daily functioning, as well as increased feelings of revenge, which prevent young adults from actively participating in rebuilding, reconciliation, and peace-building processes. Therefore, the effective treatment of trauma-spectrum disorders in post-conflict settings is of utmost importance for enabling children to develop their potential and to allow for sustainable reconciliation and peace.

23.2 Psychological Interventions in Post-Conflict Settings

Mental health interventions in post-conflict settings must address several challenges. First, extremely high numbers of traumatized children and adolescents are met by a very small number of mental health professionals raising the question of how mental health treatments can be effectively disseminated. Second, a high level of daily stressors, such as insecure socioeconomic situations, may aggravate mental health symptoms. Third, traumatized parents might struggle to implement positive parenting practices and provide a caring environment to their children, alongside ongoing domestic violence and parental alcohol abuse, often resulting in further exposure to traumatic experiences within the family. Children living in institutional care are also at a high risk of being neglected and exposed to harsh discipline and violence. Accordingly, sustainable psychological intervention programs need to consider both treatment of individual post-traumatic psychopathology and the prevention of familial/institutional violence in order to promote mental health, successful integration, and societal participation of children and adolescents. In this manner, programs addressing child-rearing practices interrupt the detrimental cycle of family violence and psychological maladjustment, while individual treatment increases the child's functionality in dealing with upcoming stressful circumstances (Catani et al. 2008; Saile et al. 2014). Finally, children and adolescents might not only be survivors of violence, but may have committed offenses themselves in order to survive as child soldiers or on the street. Therefore, the successful reintegration of child perpetrators might require specialized mental health interventions.

23.2.1 Disseminating Mental Health Interventions in Post-Conflict Settings

23.2.1.1 Integration of Psychosocial and Mental Health Interventions

The most pressing question regarding mental health interventions in post-conflict settings is how to respond to the high demand for treatment with the scarcity of local mental health professionals. Indeed, many psychosocial programs prioritize a reduction in daily stressors because they are known to exacerbate mental health symptoms. Subsequently, mental health interventions could be reserved for individuals who do not recover even when psychosocial conditions are improved. Yet, prioritizing psychosocial conditions over mental health problems might not be an adequate strategy for several reasons: (1) individuals suffering from PTSD are more likely to perceive situations as stressful; (2) mental health disorders could produce further daily stressors such as poverty because of an inability to work (Neuner 2010); and (3) children and adolescents might not benefit from psychosocial interventions (e.g., educational programs aimed at reducing poverty) as mental health symptoms impair their ability to concentrate, learn, and integrate with their peers. In light of the aforementioned reasons, mental health interventions need to form an integral part of humanitarian programs in post-conflict settings. In order to achieve this "paradigm shift," mental health interventions should (1) be short term; (2) be easy to train and disseminate to local paraprofessionals; (3) be sensitive to the local circumstances and cultural belief systems; (4) be implemented in cooperation with existing local structures such as reintegration centers, local nongovernmental organizations (NGOs), and primary health care; (5) include trauma-focused modules; and (6) involve a rigorous scientific evaluation (Schauer and Schauer 2010). Unfortunately, very little research has been devoted to outcome evaluation of mental health interventions in post-conflict settings in general (Neuner and Elbert 2007) and for children and adolescents in particular.

23.2.1.2 Mental Health Interventions for the Treatment of Post-Traumatic Psychopathology in Post-Conflict Settings

As resources in post-conflict settings are limited, one approach that has been utilized previously is to deliver mental health interventions in a group-based setting. For the treatment of children and adolescents, many interventions have utilized the natural environment of the children and applied mental health interventions in the school classrooms. School-based interventions aim at both promoting stress resilience and reducing post-traumatic psychopathology. They include elements of psychoeducation, cognitive behavioral therapy, skills training and emotion regulation techniques, creative and expressive elements such as arts or dance therapy, as well as limited trauma exposure in some interventions (Fazel et al. 2014). In general, the evidence for school-based interventions in post-conflict settings is mixed, with some studies reporting positive effects on mental health outcomes, while others find beneficial effects only in subgroups, or even report null and negative effects. A recent systematic review reported that only half of the included school-based mental health interventions showed beneficial effects (Fazel et al. 2014). One reason for this inconsistent effect might be the presence or absence of trauma-focused elements in school-based interventions. In general, effective treatments for children with PTSD involve exposure to the traumatic experiences (Landolt and Kenardy 2015). However, this trauma-focused component might have negative effects in a group setting, as the trauma narrative of one survivor could trigger intrusive memories of other group members (Litwack et al. 2015). Furthermore, the heterogeneity of participants (including children with and without mental health problems), and delivered interventions, is problematic, as it is difficult to determine which intervention modules are beneficial or risky for which recipient. Hence, according to the current state of research, school-based interventions cannot be recommended as a treatment for trauma-related mental health disorders in post-conflict settings (e.g., Ertl and Neuner 2014).

Ertl and Neuner (2014) proposed the screen-and-treat approach as an effective alternative to school-based interventions. According to this strategy, the prevalence of mental health disorders would first be determined in systematic diagnostic interviews. In a second step, a specific mental health intervention would be delivered to those who display clinically relevant symptoms in an individual setting. Trauma-focused interventions that have been successfully implemented and scientifically evaluated for the treatment of traumatized children in post-conflict settings are Narrative Exposure Therapy (NET; Schauer et al. 2011) for Children (KIDNET, see Chap. 11; application in post-conflict setting, see Catani et al. 2009) and Trauma-Focused Cognitive Behavioral Therapy (TF-CBT, see Chap. 8; application in post-conflict setting, see McMullen et al. 2013). NET is an individual therapy approach that has been especially developed for the needs of survivors of multiple traumatic experiences. NET was designed to incorporate a simple training model to be used with lay counselors and to be further disseminated in a train-the-trainer approach (Jacob et al. 2014). Accordingly, NET might be especially suited to fill the mental health gap in post-conflict settings. The TF-CBT treatments that have been successfully applied in post-conflict settings were delivered in groups; however, the trauma exposure modules were implemented as individual sessions (McMullen et al. 2013). As such, general emotion regulation skills and psychoeducation can be communicated in groups, while the trauma-focused treatment takes place on an individual basis. This can also represent a time- and cost-effective strategy in post-conflict settings. Table 23.1 provides an overview of selected research-based PTSD treatments and prevention approaches in conflict settings. TF-CBT and NET will not be discussed further, as they are extensively described in Chaps. 8 and 11 of this book.

23.2.1.3 Preventing Further Violent Experiences in Child Survivors of Conflict

The sole implementation of trauma-focused psychotherapy for children neglects the fact that children might suffer from continuing traumatization resulting from harsh parenting and familial or institutional violence. This increases the risk of child psychopathology, aggressive behavior, and academic difficulties (e.g., Hermenau et al. 2011; Saile et al. 2014). As a result, increased attention has been given to the importance of parenting interventions in post-conflict settings, as parents are the most

23 Treating and Preventing Psychological Trauma of Children

Table 23.1 Scientifically evaluated interventions for treatment and prevention of trauma and violence in children and adolescents in post-conflict settings

Focus	Target group	Treatment approach	Further reading
Trauma treatment	Individual child survivors of conflict or violence	Trauma-Focused Cognitive Behavioral Therapy (TF-CBT)	Chapter 8 of this book
Trauma treatment	Individual child survivors of conflict or violence	Narrative Exposure Therapy for Children (KIDNET)	Chapter 11 of this book
Prevention of child maltreatment	Parents	Adapted Parent Management Training Oregon (PMTO)	Section 23.3.1
Prevention of child maltreatment	Caretakers in institutional care	Interaction Competences with Children (ICC)	Section 23.3.2
Trauma treatment and reintegration/violence prevention	Traumatized child perpetrators	Narrative Exposure Therapy for Forensic Offender Rehabilitation (FORNET)	Section 23.4

proximal resources to intervene and prevent adverse child outcomes (Gewirtz et al. 2008). The application of a parenting training, the adapted *Parent Management Training Oregon* model, in post-conflict Northern Uganda will be introduced in Sect. 23.3.1. In addition, many children in post-conflict settings are raised in institutional care. The trying working conditions and excessive demands on caregivers, limited training in childcare, and accepted social norms about child-rearing all culminate in promoting harsh discipline in institutional care settings. Therefore, interventions promoting positive discipline in institutional care are of utmost importance to preventing children from experiencing further harm. Hence, we will introduce the intervention program *Interaction Competences with Children* in Sect. 23.3.2.

23.2.1.4 Effective Treatments of Traumatized Offenders in Post-Conflict Settings

In addition to surviving multiple traumatic experiences, child soldiers and street children might perpetrate violent acts because they are forced or misled by their environments and are fighting for survival. A significant number adapt by developing positive feelings (e.g., pride, power, and joy) toward aggressive behavior (termed *appetitive aggression*), which can be crucial for survival and might be reinforced by material gain or admiration and comradeship (Crombach and Elbert 2014). Understandably, it might become difficult for those children to reintegrate into a peaceful society and leave behind violent behavior due to their struggle with both trauma-related disorders and violence-associated feelings of thrill and power (Hermenau et al. 2013a). Striving for positive emotions in an otherwise adverse environment, they might seek for opportunities to experience control and success through acts of aggression. Hence, not only traumatic events but also events in which the child survivor acted as a perpetrator need to be addressed in psychotherapy to allow for successful rehabilitation. An adaption of NET for the needs of traumatized perpetrators of violence termed *Narrative Exposure Therapy for Forensic Offender Rehabilitation* will be introduced in Sect. 23.4.

23.3 Preventive Interventions Targeting Child Maltreatment and Family Violence

23.3.1 Adapted Parent Management Training Oregon Model: A Systemic Approach for Preventing Family Violence in Post-Conflict Settings

23.3.1.1 Theoretical Underpinnings

The adapted intervention for a post-conflict community in Northern Uganda was based on the *Parent Management Training Oregon* (PMTO) model that uses an indirect approach to influencing child outcomes with an explicit focus on testing the social interaction learning theoretical model. The program takes place with mothers, fathers, both parents, or adult caregivers. No direct intervention is conducted with the children. Thus, changes in child adjustment can be more directly attributed to benefits of the parents' parenting practices. Changes in coercive discipline (negative reinforcement, negative reciprocity, and ineffective discipline) and positive parenting (skill encouragement, monitoring, positive involvement, and problem solving) have consistently shown classic prevention effects with the control group deteriorating and the experimental group showing no decrement. Core PMTO components include *positive reinforcement* to promote prosocial behavior, effective *limit setting* to decrease deviant behavior, *monitoring* to ensure that behavior is consistent, family *problem solving* to provide skills to prevent and manage stress and conflict, and *positive involvement* to emphasize the importance of spending time together in pleasant activity (Forgatch et al. 2013). The evidence in support of PMTO with various family structures and difficult family contexts has been replicated in numerous studies worldwide and, more recently, disseminated to populations that include families affected by psychological trauma in post-conflict settings (Wieling et al. 2015a).

23.3.1.2 Enhancing Family Connection: Content and Implementation

Adapted PMTO was first piloted in Northern Uganda in 2012 to test the feasibility of implementing a parenting intervention in a post-conflict setting. A brief overview of the training components and parenting modality is included in this section.

Training: The standard PMTO facilitator training program requires participation in five workshops over approximately 12–18 months with the inclusion of observed practice with fictional and real cases and extensive coaching. Certified specialists, coaches, and mentors using a set of manuals conduct training and continuously assess the implementation fidelity. Individual and group coaching is provided live by phone/videoconferencing or in written format until trainees meet proficiency for certification. Tracking adherence to the model and competent delivery emphasizes fidelity (for details see Knutson et al. 2009).

PMTO sessions: Over several decades multiple studies have used slightly adapted PMTO manuals with a range of session numbers (typically 10–14 sessions) to fit their populations of interest. The standard content and order of PMTO sessions incorporating core and supporting dimensions are identifying family strengths and goals using proactive (what to do) language, teaching clear communication strategies, the use of social and instrumental reinforcers to develop and strengthen skills of the children, how to identify specific emotions and regulation strategies, and using effective discipline (e.g., time-out, privilege loss, and work chores). Specifically, PMTO session titles include *encouraging cooperation, teaching new behavior, observing and regulating emotions, setting limits, communicating with children, problem solving, managing conflict, monitoring children's activities, and promoting school success* (see Forgatch and Domench Rodriguez 2015, for a detailed elaboration of PMTO session content).

PMTO sessions typically last for 90 min and follow a specific structure that includes starting each session with debriefing homework and introduction of new content area (using active teaching, various differentiating role-plays, and transition activities) and ends with new homework assignment. Participants are given a parent manual and receive between-session phone calls for support with homework assignments. Maintaining a strong 5:1 ratio of support, praise, and encouragement relative to negative interactions for parents participating in groups is central in this model that emphasizes isomorphic processes between what parents experience from PMTO facilitators and what children experience from their parents at home. A unique emphasis of PMTO relative to other parenting interventions is an emphasis on clinical and teaching processes to reduce resistance to change. Findings from studies using direct observations of therapy sessions indicated that in addition to client characteristics (e.g., poverty, depression, antisocial qualities), therapist behavior emphasizing confront–teach strategies often elicits resistance. PMTO was designed to incorporate active teaching, such as role-play and problem solving, and to strengthen supportive clinical processes (Forgatch et al. 2013).

Adapted PMTO: The abbreviated nine-session manual used for feasibility testing of the model focused on PMTO core components and emphasized emotional regulation. It also included a session focusing on the intergenerational transmission of various family dynamics (a multigeneration genogram was used to explore family legacies as well as maladaptive coping and relational patterns), and trauma-focused psychoeducation and topics relevant to local family contexts (e.g., couple and family dynamics, violence, substance abuse, poverty, ongoing fear of war) were incorporated throughout all sessions. A complete adapted PMTO facilitator manual was comprised of instructions on session materials, start-up activities, debriefing home

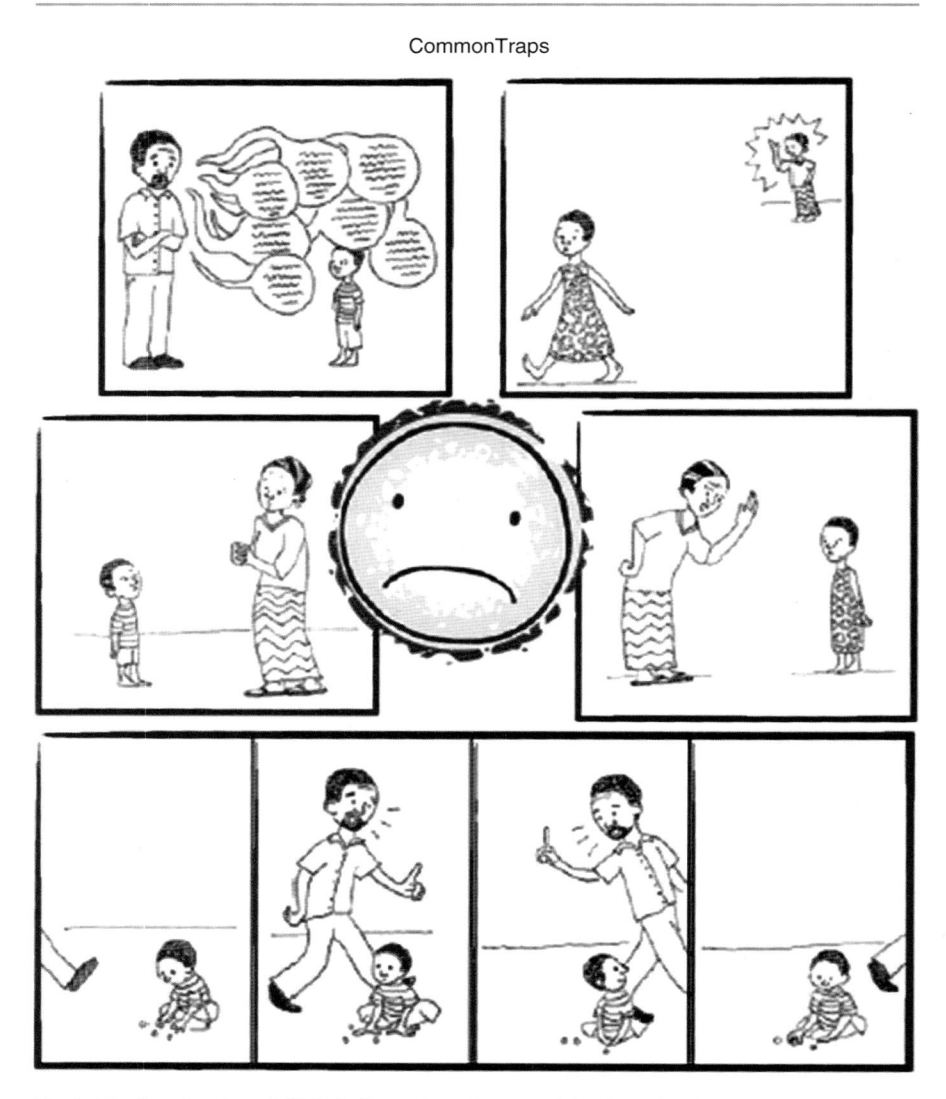

Fig. 23.1 Sample adapted PMTO illustration of parent giving bad directions

practice, session content, special games and role-plays, home practice assignment, and time allocation for each activity. An accompanying parent guide illustrated key content themes and home practice assignments (see Figs. 23.1 and 23.2 for sample illustrations). We were purposeful to include Uganda-based art and photos of African families with the intent of instilling pride and celebrating cultural heritage. Future adapted PMTO intervention trials will be expanded to more closely approximate the 14-session model and include fathers and/or additional caregivers in the parenting group intervention.

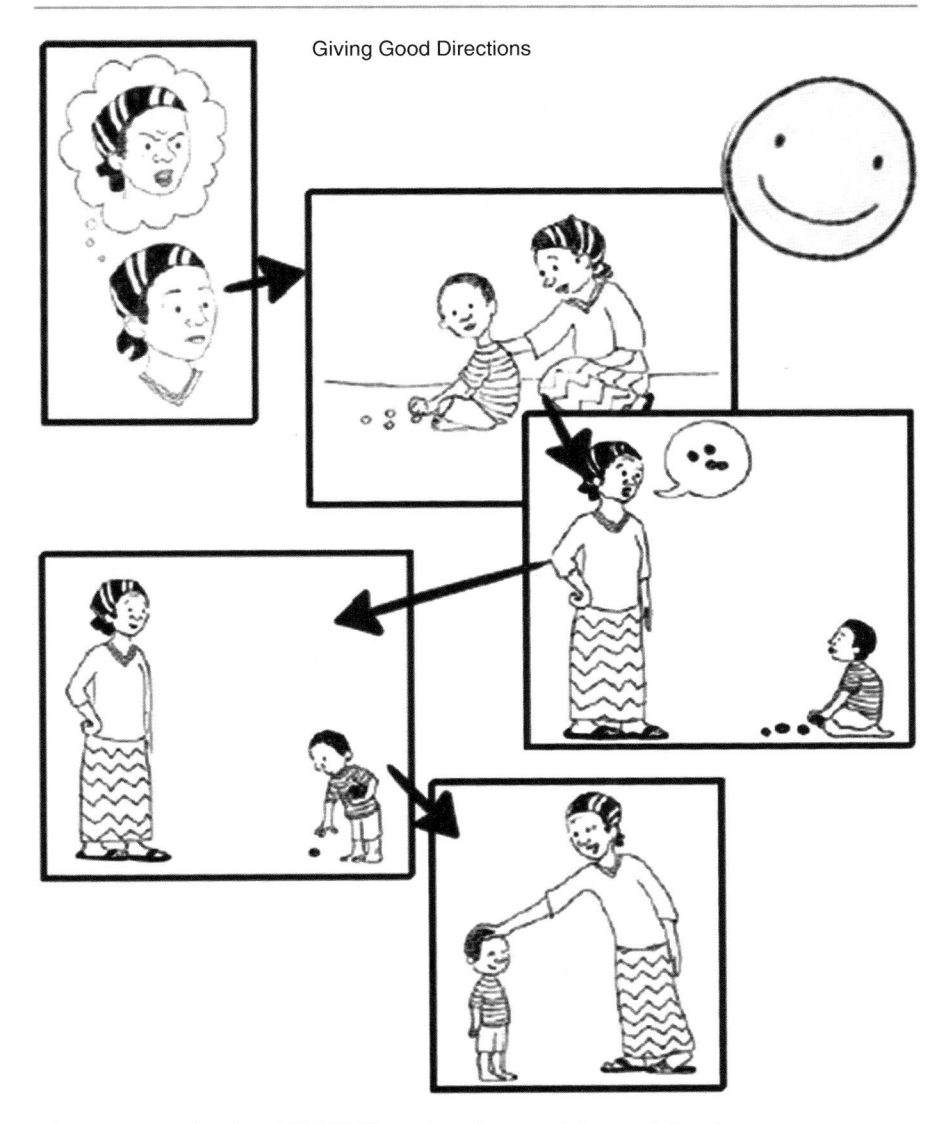

Fig. 23.2 Sample adapted PMTO illustration of parent giving good directions

23.3.1.3 Common Challenges During Implementation

The challenges of translational science, including implementation and dissemination of evidence-based interventions, raise myriad challenges in post-conflict societies. These challenges cut across ecosystemic levels with complex implications at every level – micro-, meso-, exo-, and macro-system. In addition to the necessity of demonstrating cultural relevance and effectiveness in the transfer of evidence-based interventions for at-risk populations, evaluating the success of an implementation is distinct from assessing clinical treatment outcomes (e.g., Fixsen et al. 2009; Proctor et al. 2009). Much recent emphasis has been placed on the importance of building translational research, which encompasses implementation and dissemination efforts. Several phased and interlocking stage models have been proposed to advance this science. Forgatch et al. (2013) proposed a four-stage dynamic implementation process that takes into account the adopting community and purveyor collaborations through (1) preparation, (2) early adoption, (3) implementation, and (4) sustainability. Curran et al. (2012) go a step further in making the case for "hybrid effectiveness-implementation" designs, which test the intervention and implementation strategies. The adapted PMTO feasibility project described in this chapter was positioned as an early phase preparation and adoption study that will now inform a larger hybrid effectiveness-implementation study with that same community.

Opportunities and challenges: The project was conceptualized in response to local requests for support with parenting needs and soon resulted in the first pilot with a group of mothers. The project benefited from having a stable location, support of the locally well-established NGO vivo, invested local counselors who were already trained trauma counselors when the project started and who were trained to interpret and co-facilitate parenting intervention sessions, culturally adapted measures and parenting protocol, and a team of PMTO-trained therapists and researchers to conduct the intervention. Despite the many challenges along the way (e.g., language, cultural gaps, poverty, illiteracy, norms and values regarding parenting practices, substance use, domestic violence), there was a great degree of local acceptance of the intervention (e.g., mothers were open to learning and trying new skills with their children). Ongoing challenges include the development of training and dissemination strategies that can be more easily transferred to local post-conflict communities while maintaining model fidelity, which has shown to be directly associated with sustained changes in parenting practices and child outcomes.

23.3.1.4 Feasibility and First Empirical Evidence

In 2012, a nine-session adapted PMTO intervention was conducted with 14 mothers in Uganda to assess three integrated components of feasibility: (1) usability, logistics and process of running the intervention; (2) limited efficacy, preliminary evaluation of outcomes; and (3) acceptability, degree to which the intervention is suitable and satisfying to the recipients. Participants were recruited because all mothers were affected by the war and reported experiencing parenting difficulties with at least one child between the ages of 7 and 13 years.

All mothers attended all nine parenting sessions. Detailed descriptions regarding *usability* components of the feasibility study support the use of a culturally adapted visual manual to communicate core ingredients of the model, the successful integration of interpreters to assist in co-facilitating the groups, and the inclusion of small food and transportation incentives to encourage group attendance (see Wieling et al. 2015b for full description). Regarding implications for *limited efficacy*, mothers and children showed evidence of changes regarding (1) the use of positive reinforcement, encouragement, and praise (mothers reported noticing and giving praise for prosocial behaviors in unprecedented ways and children reported changes in their mothers' and in their own behaviors), (2) discipline behavior (mothers and children reported less use of harsh punishment and beatings and greater use of alternative discipline strategies such as removal of privileges), and (3) parental involvement (mothers reported more love and calm in the family that was often related to learning how to regulate their emotions and having acquired the skills to communicate more effectively with their children) (see Wieling et al. 2015b for full description of findings).

At the 5-month qualitative follow-up interview, 13 mothers reported a number of changes in themselves and their families that speak further to the *acceptability* and relative sustainability of the intervention. The primary themes distilled from follow-up interviews included statements about (a) spreading the model to others, (b) increased use of encouragement, (c) less use of beatings for discipline, (d) talking effectively with children, and (e) increased love in the family. The feasibility results of this study are modest and must be further tested in randomized controlled studies that also evaluate dissemination strategies of preventive interventions in post-conflict settings. However, this work represents early promise for improving mental health and family functioning for some of the most affected populations worldwide.

23.3.2 Interaction Competences with Children: A Preventive Intervention for Caregivers Improving Care Quality and Preventing Maltreatment in Institutional Care

23.3.2.1 Theoretical Underpinnings

The preventive intervention approach *Interaction Competences with Children* (ICC) aims to improve adult–child relationships and prevent maltreatment. Following *chronic stress theory*, the typical care environment in an institutional care setting is stressful for children because of the lack of a consistent, warm, sensitive, contingent caregiver, which otherwise would reduce the stressful nature of an insecure post-conflict environment. Furthermore, ICC is based on *attachment theory*. As a consequence of parental loss, and the many and varying caregivers, institutionalized children often lack a secure, stable attachment to a caregiver. Interventions aiming to improve care quality in institutional care have shown promising results (McCall 2013). Nevertheless, interventions focusing on both improving care quality and preventing further maltreatment are scarce. Therefore, we expanded the theoretical foundation to elements from social learning, cognitive behavioral, and developmental theory to additionally focus on prevention of harsh discipline and other forms of maltreatment. ICC for caregivers (ICC-C) in institutional care has been informed by the FairstartGlobal[1] training concept and the parenting guidelines of the American Academy of Pediatrics.

---

[1] http://www.fairstartglobal.com/

23.3.2.2 ICC Training Workshop for Caregivers in Institutional Care

ICC-C has been designed as a 2-week training workshop (12 full days) for caregivers working in institutional care settings. ICC-C offers a basic introduction to the essential interaction competencies in the work with children focusing mainly on warm, sensitive, and reliable caregiver–child relationship and nonviolent, warm, and sensitive caregiving strategies. ICC-C is guided by the following key principles:

- Participative approach: Trainees are invited to participate actively, to tailor the program, and to develop their own strategies on how to implement the training content in their daily work.
- Practice orientation: Practice units follow the theoretical input aiming to enable the trainees to use the acquired skills in their daily work.
- Trustful atmosphere: Trainees are encouraged to talk openly about work problems and their own experiences of harsh punishment and maltreatment, with the aim of creating a trusting and open atmosphere assuring confidentiality.
- Sustainability: Sustainability of the training is ensured through intensive practicing, repetition of the new knowledge, self-reflection, and the training component *teamwork and supervision*, described below.
- Team building and new ideas for games: To facilitate team building and to exchange ideas that caregivers can use in their daily work with children, trainers and trainees suggest and play games, sing songs, or dance together.

ICC-C begins with a welcome session in which the expectations, wishes, and concerns of the trainees are explored. Seven core components form the content of ICC-C. They are conducted in the following order:

1. *Child development (three sessions at 90 min)*: The aim of the first component is fostering empathy and understanding toward the children and enabling trainees to better assess the children's abilities, thus forming age-appropriate expectations. In the beginning, the trainees discuss the needs of children of different ages in a small-group exercise. A short presentation of topics that came up in the small groups is followed by theoretical input about important steps in the development of children. The subsequent discussion relates the knowledge about child development to implications for the daily work with children of various ages. A small-group exercise helps trainees to practice forming age-appropriate expectations and caring approaches.
2. *Caregiver–child relationship (four sessions at 90 min)*: This component aims to point out the importance of secure attachment and bonding as well as elements of how to establish and improve a caregiver–child relationship. During a theoretical input, the importance of secure attachment and bonding for children is emphasized. Subsequently, trainees in small groups elaborate on the implications of being a parental figure and role model for children living in institutional care (e.g., whose parents have died or are unable to care for them). Communication skills in a warm, understanding, and sensitive manner are developed together

with the trainees and practiced in role-plays. Subsequently, the trainees discuss and practice communicating clear and age-appropriate instructions in small-group discussions and role-plays.

3. *Effective caregiving strategies (eight sessions at 90 min)*: This component seeks to provide alternative caregiving strategies in place of harsh and injurious discipline and to reduce feelings of helplessness. It starts with a discussion about which caregiving strategies trainees consider useful and effective. Subsequently, different strategies to maintain good behavior and to change misbehavior (e.g., reinforcement systems, privilege removal, contracts) are introduced and practiced in small groups using interactive elements such as role-plays. Trainees' ideas about challenges that may occur when implementing new skills in daily routine are discussed. This component encompasses several sessions as nonviolent caregiving strategies are developed and adapted to the specific contexts together with the trainees, practiced, and repeated a number of times to include them in the active action repertoire of the trainees.

4. *Maltreatment prevention (seven sessions at 90 min)*: The aim of this component is to raise awareness of the detrimental consequences of harsh punishment and other forms of child maltreatment. This component is closely linked to the newly learned effective caregiving strategies. ICC-C emphasizes action alternatives as many caregivers use harsh punishment because they lack nonviolent techniques. Developing nonviolent caregiving strategies beforehand, trainees may be more open to question commonly used strategies. At the start of this unit, all trainees are invited to reflect on and share their own experiences of harsh punishment and maltreatment during childhood. To create a trustful atmosphere, all trainees agree that all information that is shared during self-reflection will be confidential and will not be shared with anybody outside of the workshop. In the following discussion, common caregiving and discipline strategies in the country and culture are discussed. Self-reflection often helps to allow a personal discussion about potential risks and consequences of harsh punishment and other forms of maltreatment that are not so much influenced by societal attitudes. Furthermore, through self-reflection trainees are less likely to feel offended, which will reduce resistance. A theoretical input points out potential consequences of harsh punishment and other forms of maltreatment. Subsequently, common myths about corporal punishment are explored and discussed in small groups. To reinforce a change in attitude, the trainees are invited to reflect on their own use of harsh punishment toward children and their feelings when using harsh punishment. In small groups, trainees develop and discuss ideas, opportunities, and challenges for implementing nonviolent caregiving strategies in their daily work.

5. *Supporting burdened children (seven sessions at 90 min)*: This component seeks to provide knowledge of common emotional and behavioral problems that children in institutional care may face. It also communicates that burdened children may not misbehave purposely, but rather that it is an expression of psychological problems. Furthermore, this component also aims to reduce the fears and helplessness of caregivers. Common emotional and behavioral problems, such as (traumatic) stress reactions, depression, oppositional and aggressive behavior,

bed-wetting, delayed development, and being HIV positive, are explained. Strategies for handling such challenges are introduced and discussed. In small groups the trainees develop ideas and strategies to support particularly burdened children within their institutions. This component also asks the caregivers to describe other common difficulties of at-risk children and to discuss strategies to support these children.

6. *Child-centered institutional care (seven sessions at 90 min)*: The aim of this component is to enable the trainees to realize changes that are possible in their own workplace which improve the living conditions for children and working conditions for caregivers. Although structural changes are not generally implemented when conducting ICC-C, the importance of an adequate caregiver–child ratio; warm, sensitive, and stable caregiver–child relationship; and family-like groups is explained. In small groups, trainees compare the situation of children in families and in institutional care settings. Next, a theoretical input emphasizes key elements of institutional care settings that impact children's development, physical, and mental health. Further, the importance of play for a healthy development is stressed. In small groups trainees discuss ideas, challenges, and strategies to introduce these key elements into their particular workplace. Aspects like safety, structures, rituals, and rules are also introduced and discussed. In small groups trainees develop ideas and strategies on how to implement the discussed aspects in their work environment.

7. *Teamwork and supervision (two sessions at 90 min)*: This component covers improving immediate working conditions and ensuring the implementation of the training contents in the workplace. The importance of a good work atmosphere and supporting colleagues is discussed. Possibilities for supervision and where to seek help are discussed together with the trainees.

In the end of the first and second week, one session of 90 min should be used to repeat and highlight what the caregivers have learned and to discuss open questions. The intervention ends with a feedback and farewell session including a farewell ritual.

23.3.2.3 Common Challenges During Implementation

ICC-C is designed to be applicable in post-conflict regions and other low- and middle-income countries. However, due to limited resources in post-conflict countries, institutional care settings are often limited to offering only basic provisions of food and shelter and face major difficulties providing sensitive and child-oriented care. For example, unfavorable caregiver–child ratios (e.g., one caregiver caring for 20 or more children) and poorly trained, overburdened personnel rarely allow for sensitive care to meet the various needs of children. Where it is not possible to secure funds necessary to hire more staff, ICC-C can enable caregivers to implement structural changes within the limited opportunities of the particular setting (e.g., creating family-like groups, assigning each child to a primary caregiver, introducing regular meetings within family-like groups, etc.). However, the particular circumstances of the institutional care setting determine which and how many of the suggested changes can be implemented.

Many caregivers lack training in childcare as it is often assumed that everyone can raise children. Nevertheless, being a caregiver in institutional care means raising children who are often burdened with various psychological problems. ICC-C may raise awareness of children's needs and may contribute to improve the caregiver–child relationship. However, it does not replace proper training in effective child-rearing practices. Rather ICC-C reduces the gap in knowledge between what is required and what exists.

It may be that the management of an institution chooses to implement ICC-C without consulting the caregivers. This could result in resistance to active involvement in the training workshop. Caregivers may experience a threat to their self-esteem when outsiders wish to educate them about how to deal with "their" children. Therefore, it is highly important to build trust. It is crucial that trainers adopt an open attitude that acknowledges the difficult work conditions of the trainees and to collaborate with the trainees. Team building activities and involving the caregivers and their feedback in the program design help to create an open and trusting atmosphere.

Changing long-standing norms is challenging, especially because the use of corporal punishment and other harsh discipline measures is very common, socially accepted, and generally regarded as effective in many regions throughout the world. Hence, it may happen that one is confronted with strong resistance by the trainees to rethink disciplinary measures. However, involving the trainees in creating the change and formulating their own training may help to promote engagement in the process. Reflections about the caregivers' own experiences of harsh punishment and maltreatment, discussions about consequences of maltreatment for children, and intensive practicing of effective nonviolent caregiving strategies may facilitate a change of attitude regarding harmful discipline and maltreatment.

The support of the management staff of the childcare institution is crucial for achieving long-term sustainability. The management needs to support the ideas that are developed during the intervention and should provide room for peer supervision. It also may happen that trainees become aware of their poor working conditions during ICC-C training. If the management is unwilling or unable to contribute to changes in working conditions, this may reduce the motivation to implement the newly learned strategies and potential structural changes. So involving the management as well as the caregivers and promoting a dialogue between the different interests are essential to ensure long-term changes.

23.3.2.4 Feasibility and First Empirical Evidence

In a recent feasibility study with caregivers in Tanzania (Hermenau et al. 2015), the participating caregivers rated the feasibility and efficacy of ICC-C immediately before, directly after, and 3 months following the intervention. The trainers showed high satisfaction with the implementation of the units, the caregivers' participation, comprehension, and motivation. Consistently, caregivers reported a high demand, good feasibility, high motivation, and acceptance of the intervention. They reported improvements in caregiver–child relationships, as well as in child behavior. Furthermore, we assessed exposure to harsh punishment, maltreatment, and mental health of all children living in one institution from which all caregivers had been trained. The children were interviewed 20 months before, 1 month before, and 3 months after the training. Children reported a decrease in harsh punishment and physical maltreatment and a decrease in mental health problems. As such, ICC-C seems feasible under challenging circumstances and research provides the first glimpses of its effectiveness.

23.4 Treating Traumatized Violent Offenders by Means of Narrative Exposure

23.4.1 Theoretical Underpinnings

The *Narrative Exposure Therapy for Forensic Offender Rehabilitation* (FORNET; Hecker et al. 2015) has been adapted from (KID)NET (for details, see Chap. 11) to account for the fact that conflict and war experiences might not only lead to trauma symptoms but also to feelings of appetitive aggression (i.e., positive emotions linked to aggressive behavior). The principal idea of this approach is inspired by the observation that the highly elevated emotional arousal experienced during traumatic events prevents the genesis of a comprehensive autobiographic memory representation: Trauma-related cognitions, (negative) emotions, physiological reactions, and sensory cues (e.g., blood, screams, the sound of gunshots) are not embedded in contextual information (when, where, and how the events happened) but build up to a so-called *fear network*. Consequently, lacking the contextual association with the past, one gets easily triggered and feelings of imminent threat in the present are evoked. As perpetrating violence is usually also related to a highly elevated emotional arousal, a similar memory process is thought to explain the phenomenon of appetitive aggression: Perpetrating violent acts while feeling in control and experiencing the admiration of others might lead to the buildup of a *hunting network* consisting of (positive) emotions, cognitions, and physiological reactions associated with sensory cues. The perpetration of different kinds of violence results in the hunting network becoming increasingly detached from specific contexts. Subsequently, appetitive aggression becomes easily triggered by cues such as blood and causes the individual to enjoy the perpetration of violence.

Following the logic of (KID)NET, FORNET aims to dissolve the fear and the hunting network by anchoring cognitions, emotions, physiological reactions, and sensory impressions in the context of a particular event. By means of narrative exposure, trauma memories and appetitive aggressive memories are reactivated and elaborated to form a coherent narrative integrating both emotional-sensory elements and the corresponding autobiographical context information. The additional detailed elaboration of perpetrated violent acts allows offenders to regain control of their aggressive impulses.

23.4.2 Implementation of FORNET with Children and Adolescents

In this chapter we limit the presentation of FORNET to a brief overview addressing aggressive and violent behavior (for the core principles of (KID)NET, see Chap. 11, and for further details of FORNET, see Hecker et al. 2015) and focusing on particular challenges when implementing FORNET with minors. FORNET was designed and adapted to different settings to facilitate the reintegration process of former child soldiers and street children. While some of them are young adults when entering the reintegration process, a significant number return as children and adolescents. Thus far, the youngest person to receive FORNET was 11 years old.

Objectives and key principles: FORNET aims to reintegrate negative emotions related to traumatic experiences (e.g., fear, anger, shame, guilt) and positive emotions related to the perpetration of violent acts (e.g., excitement, satisfaction, dominance) to past contexts, thereby integrating them into the autobiographical memory. The objective is to help the client structure his/her memories by creating a chronological narration of his/her life. The therapist assists the client during the process in an authentic, empathic, validating, and understanding manner. For the therapy process, it is essential that the therapist does not judge the client for his/her deeds.

Considerations prior to implementation: FORNET is a short-term intervention that consists of several sessions (usually between 5 and 10) lasting 60–90 min each. As offenses are discussed in detail, the therapist needs to be aware of the law regulations of the specific country that might affect the therapeutic confidentiality and inform the client as well as the guardian about those. Furthermore, the guardian and the child/adolescent need to make an informed decision about the participation in the therapy process. While (KID)NET hands over a written narration of the clients' personal history elaborating the traumatic experiences in detail, FORNET often has to be conducted without a written narration in order to ensure the safety of the client. Prior to the intervention, a detailed diagnostic assessment including the assessment of appetitive aggression has to be conducted.

First session: In this session the client receives psychoeducation during which the rationale of the therapy is explained. In addition to the psychoeducation conducted in (KID)NET, explaining/providing a rationale for the perpetration of violent acts and emphasizing the need for talking about these experiences are crucial. Many children/adolescents can relate to the following statement: "In new situations, particularly in stressful moments when we do not have much time to think, we often react in a similar way to what we were used to in the past. Sometimes our reaction might cause future conflicts and/or we might regret it later. We may attack somebody because we are not aware of how our past experiences shape us. By exploring the violent experiences in your past, you will be more aware of your emotions and thereby be better able to influence your reaction." Then, the therapist and the client gain an overview of all significant emotional events throughout the client's life by conducting the lifeline exercise: The client arranges his/her emotionally significant life events in chronological order by putting symbols on a rope which represents the course of his/her life from birth until the present day. Flowers represent positive events, while stones symbolize negative events including traumatic experiences. The perpetration of violence is represented by an additional symbol – a stick – to avoid forcing the client to assign a specific valence to such events. Subsequently, the therapist needs to identify together with the client the most significant traumatic events and violent acts related to elevated (negative and positive) emotional arousal for further elaboration.

Session narrations: Throughout the following sessions, the therapist guides the client in talking in detail and in chronological order about the life events with the highest emotional arousal (including both stones and sticks). This therapy process closely follows the procedure of (KID)NET. Ideally each important event is addressed during one session. Similar to the narrative exposure of traumatic events, the therapist slows the narration down when the client starts the narration of a perpetrated violent act. The therapist ensures that the context of the event (e.g., when, where, in which life period it had happened) is sufficiently established. Then, the client is encouraged to talk about his/her experience from the beginning (i.e., what happened prior to the event) via the moment of highest arousal until the end of the story when he/she is not excited/afraid anymore. Throughout the narration the therapist ensures the explicit perception and verbalization of sensations, cognitions, emotions, and physiological reactions at the appropriate part of the story. In particular the client needs to realize that telling the story in great detail evokes emotional and physiological reactions in the present. In order to achieve this objective, the therapist has to guide the client through his/her bodily reactions and emotions in the *here and now*, connecting and contrasting them to the emotions of *back then*. Key element of success during the narration of violent acts is the unconditional and non-judging acceptance and expression of any emotion. At the end of the story, the therapist needs to ensure that the elevated arousal, in particular the arousal related to appetitive aggression, is not present anymore before ending the narrative exposure. Finally, the client will be asked how he/she evaluates committing the violent act from a today's point of view. The therapist contextualizes once again the particular emotions: "I understand that you are still proud of having beaten the enemy severely back then because you became suddenly respected among your peers." If the client points out that today he/she is not proud anymore, the therapist emphasizes why the client has changed his/her point of view. Throughout the sessions the therapist assists the client in expressing, contextualizing, understanding, and thereby appropriately regulating his/her emotions.

Last session(s): After the narration has reached the present day, the therapist and the client review the lifeline, reorder events if necessary, and evaluate the impact of the narration on the client's current well-being. In addition, the last session aims to assist the client to develop (realistic) perspectives for the future, to boost self-esteem, and to facilitate access to positive emotions related to socially accepted activities. During this session the therapist discusses the client's aims and wishes for the future, potential obstacles, and personal strengths, which might foster success. The therapist emphasizes the client's resources and strengths and encourages the client in his/her future plans and wishes. In order to boost self-esteem, the client is encouraged to tell an event in which he/she experienced positive emotions during a socially accepted activity. The therapist guides the client until he/she experiences the most exciting and arousing moment of this event, then stops the narration, and lets the client revel in these positive emotions. After their individual treatment, clients are invited to participate in group sessions that focus on the challenges that go along with changes of role and identity (e.g., from being child soldier to becoming a member of the civil society). In the group sessions, clients have the opportunity to exchange stories about the adaption processes to their new role, including social status, stigmatization, and how to support each other.

23.4.3 Special Challenges of Implementing FORNET

In post-conflict settings, PTSD symptomatology in children and adolescents who have suffered childhood maltreatment, loss of attachment figures, and severe violence is often associated with trust issues toward adults. Opening up to therapists about perpetrated violent offenses requires trust due to legal issues, fear of punishment, and fear of being rejected. An open, nonjudgmental, and unconditionally accepting attitude of the therapist is absolutely essential to assist them in understanding their own emotions. While therapists certainly do not have to approve violent acts, they need to show an understanding for the individual who committed those offenses in particular circumstances and support him/her in the reintegration process.

Sometimes, former child soldiers and street children tend to evaluate their past violent behavior as useful and remain proud of it. Such an evaluation during the therapy process might be difficult to accept because social norms would expect feelings such as shame and guilt. However, arguing with the client might affect the trusting relationship that is necessary to talk openly about the active involvement in violence. The therapist might need to restrain him-/herself in order to be nonjudgmental and contextualize the emotions in the past. Grief, shame, and guilt are often more strongly related to traumatic experiences than to appetitive aggressive violent acts and have to be addressed according to the logic of (KID)NET (see Chap. 11).

The lack of mental health structures and affordable assistance often confronts therapists with difficult decisions when clients report suicidal and homicidal ideations. Such cases demonstrate the importance of integrating FORNET in existing structures assisting these vulnerable children. Lacking the option for referrals, the therapists should conduct suicidal and homicidal preventions and create close session-to-session contact. A good therapeutic alliance may be the best prevention possible. Throughout the course of FORNET, emotions related to suicide or revenge usually get successfully reduced but need to be addressed throughout the whole process and particularly during the final session.

23.4.4 Empirical Evidence

To date three randomized clinical trials indicate that FORNET is a promising approach to treat former child soldiers and street children in post-conflict settings. In all these trials, FORNET was compared to treatment as usual either in demobilization or in reintegration centers that also included psychosocial support. Two of these studies were conducted in the DR Congo with former combatants including former child soldiers (age range 16–25 years). Results showed that FORNET successfully reduced symptoms of PTSD and comorbid disorders and enhanced integration into civil society (Hermenau et al. 2013b; Köbach et al. 2015). Furthermore, Köbach et al. (2015) provided evidence that the dissemination of FORNET is possible via train-the-trainer models with local lay counselors. In a trial with Burundian former street children (age range 11–23 years), FORNET successfully reduced their involvement in everyday violence (Crombach and Elbert 2015). The beneficial effects of FORNET seem to be long-lasting as they were observed up to 12 months after treatment completion.

23.5 Research-Based Mental Health Interventions in Post-Conflict Settings: A Way Forward

The reviewed literature and the interventions presented in this chapter highlight the potential of research-based mental health interventions for children and adolescents in post-conflict settings. Rigorous scientific evaluation may guide practitioners in the field to implement promising treatment approaches for trauma-related disorders. The treatment gap between the high percentage of affected children and adolescents and available mental health professionals highlights the need to train local lay counselors in the implementation and dissemination of effective treatment approaches and to strengthen mental health capacities in conflict-affected countries. In addition to treating children and adolescents affected by trauma-related disorders, high levels of childhood maltreatment in families and institutional facilities have to be addressed. Reducing maltreatment will prevent children and adolescents from suffering mental health disorders, diminishing the treatment gap and intergenerational traumatization that may result in ongoing cycles of violence. The implementation of scientifically based rigorous research is possible in post-conflict settings. Yet, more research is needed to derive sound treatment recommendations and guidelines that are necessary to overcome the burden of past conflicts for future generations.

References

Catani C, Jacob N, Schauer E, Kohila M, Neuner F (2008) Family violence, war, and natural disaster: a study of the effect of extreme stress on children's mental health in Sri Lanka. BMC Psychiatry 8:33. doi:10.1186/1471-244X-8-33

Catani C, Kohiladevy M, Ruf M, Schauer E, Elbert T, Neuner F (2009) Treating children traumatized by war and Tsunami: a comparison between exposure therapy and meditation-relaxation in North-East Sri Lanka. BMC Psychiatry 9:22. doi:10.1186/1471-244x-9-22

Crombach A, Elbert T (2014) The benefits of aggressive traits: a study with current and former street children in Burundi. Child Abuse Negl 38(6):1041–1050. doi:10.1016/j.chiabu.2013.12.003

Crombach A, Elbert T (2015) Controlling offensive behavior using narrative exposure therapy: a randomized controlled trial of former street children. Clin Psychol Sci 3:270–282. doi:10.1177/21677026145 34239

Curran GM, Bauer M, Mittman B, Pyne JM, Stetler C (2012) Effectiveness-implementation hybrid designs: combining elements of clinical effectiveness and implementation research to enhance public health impact. Med Care 50(3):217–226. doi:10.1097/MLR.0b013e3182408812

Ertl V, Neuner F (2014) Are school-based mental health interventions for war-affected children effective and harmless? BMC Med 12:84. doi:10.1186/1741-7015-12-84

Ertl V, Pfeiffer A, Schauer-Kaiser E, Elbert T, Neuner F (2014) The challenge of living on: psychopathology and its mediating influence on the readjustment of former child soldiers. PLoS One 9(7):e102786. doi:10.1371/journal.pone.0102786

Fazel M, Patel V, Thomas S, Tol W (2014) Mental health interventions in schools in low-income and middle-income countries. Lancet Psychiatry 1(5):388–398. doi:10.1016/S2215-0366(14)70357-8

Fixsen DL, Blase K, Naoom S, Wallace F (2009) Core implementation components. Res Soc Work Pract 19(5):531–540. doi:10.1177/1049731509335549

Forgatch MS, Patterson GR, Gewirtz AH (2013) Looking forward: The promise of widespread implementation of parent training programs. Perspect Psychol Sci 8(6):682–694. doi:10.1177/174569161350347

Forgatch MS, Domench Rodriguez M (2015) Interrupting coercion: the interative loops among theory, science, and practice. In: Dishion T, Snyder J (eds) The oxford handbook of coercive relationship dynamics. University Press, Oxford

Gewirtz A, Forgatch M, Wieling E (2008) Parenting practices as potential mechanisms for children's adjustment following mass trauma: literature review and prevention research framework. J Marital Fam Ther 34(2):177–192. doi:10.1111/j.1752-0606.2008.00063.x

Hecker T, Hermenau K, Crombach A, Elbert T (2015) Treating traumatized offenders and veterans by means of narrative exposure therapy. Front Psych 6:80. doi:10.3389/fpsyt.2015.00080

Hermenau K, Hecker T, Mädl A, Schauer M, Elbert T (2013a) Growing up in armed groups: trauma and aggression among child soldiers in DR Congo. Eur J Psychotraumatol 4:21408. doi:10.3402/ejpt.v4i0.21408

Hermenau K, Hecker T, Schaal S, Maedl A, Elbert T (2013b) Addressing post-traumatic stress and aggression by means of narrative exposure – a randomized controlled trial with ex-combatants in the eastern DRC. J Aggress Maltreat Trauma 22(8):916–934. doi:10.1080/10926771.2013.824057

Hermenau K, Hecker T, Ruf M, Schauer E, Elbert T, Schauer M (2011) Childhood adversity, mental ill-health and aggressive behavior in an African orphanage: Changes in response to trauma-focused therapy and the implementation of a new instructional system. Child Adolesc Psychiatry Ment Health 5(1):29. doi:10.1186/1753-2000-5-29

Hermenau K, Kaltenbach E, Mkinga G, Hecker T (2015) Improving care quality and preventing maltreatment in institutional care – a feasibility study with caregivers. Front Psych 6:937. doi:10.3389/fpsyg.2015.00937

Jacob N, Neuner F, Maedl A, Schaal S, Elbert T (2014) Dissemination of psychotherapy for trauma spectrum disorders in postconflict settings: a randomized controlled trial in rwanda. Psychother Psychosom 83(6):354–363. doi:10.1159/000365114

Knutson NM, Forgatch MS, Rains LA, Sigmarsdóttir M (2009) Fidelity of Implementation Rating System (FIMP):the manual for PMTO. Implementation Sciences International, Inc., Eugene

Köbach A, Schaal S, Hecker T, Elbert T (2015) Effectiveness and dissemination of narrative exposure therapy for Forensic Offenders Rehabilitation (FORNET). Clin Psychol Psychother. doi:10.1002/cpp.1986 Advance online publication

Landolt MA, Kenardy JA (2015) Evidence-based treatments for children and adolescents. In: Schnyder U, Cloitre M (eds) Evidence based treatments for trauma-related psychological disorders. Springer, Heidelberg, pp 363–380

Litwack SD, Beck JG, Sloan DM (2015) Group treatment for trauma-related psychological disorders. In: Schnyder U, Cloitre M (eds) Evidence based treatments for trauma-related psychological disorders. Springer, Heidelberg, pp 443–447

McCall RB (2013) The consequences of early institutionalization: Can institutions be improved? – Should they? Child Adolesc Ment Health 18(4):193–201. doi:10.1111/camh.12025

McMullen J, O'Callaghan P, Shannon C, Black A, Eakin J (2013) Group trauma-focused cognitive-behavioural therapy with former child soldiers and other war-affected boys in the DR Congo: a randomised controlled trial. J Child Psychol Psychiatry 54(11):1231–1241. doi:10.1111/jcpp.12094

Neuner F (2010) Assisting war-torn populations – should we prioritize reducing daily stressors to improve mental health? Comment on Miller and Rasmussen (2010). Soc Sci Med 71(8):1381–1384. doi:10.1016/j.socscimed.2010.06.030

Neuner F, Elbert T (2007) The mental health disaster in conflict settings: Can scientific research help? BMC Public Health 7:275. doi:10.1186/1471-2458-7-275

Proctor E, Landsverk J, Aarons G, Chambers D, Glisson C, Mittman B (2009) Implementation research in mental health services: an emerging science with conceptual, methodological, and training challenges. Adm Policy Ment Health 36(1):24–34. doi:10.1007/s10488-008-0197-4

Saile R, Ertl V, Neuner F, Catani C (2014) Does war contribute to family violence against children? Findings from a two-generational multi-informant study in northern uganda. Child Abuse Negl 38(1):135–146. doi:10.1016/j.chiabu.2013.10.007

Schaal S, Elbert T (2006) Ten years after the genocide: trauma confrontation and posttraumatic stress in Rwandan adolescents. J Trauma Stress 19(1):95–105. doi:10.1002/jts.20104

Schauer M, Schauer E (2010) Trauma-focused public mental-health interventions: a paradigm shift in humanitarian assistance and aid work. In: Martz E (ed) Trauma rehabilitation after war and conflict. Springer, New York, pp 389–428

Schauer M, Neuner F, Elbert T (2011) Narrative exposure therapy: a short-term treatment for traumatic stress disorders. Hogrefe & Huber, Toronto

Wieling E, Mehus C, Möllerherm J, Neuner F, Achan L, Catani C (2015a) Assessing the feasibility of providing a parenting intervention for war-affected families in Northern Uganda. Fam Community Health 38(3):253–268. doi:10.1097/FCH.0000000000000064

Wieling E, Mehus C, Yumbul C, Möllerherm J, Ertl V, Laura A, Forgatch M, Neuner F, Catani C (2015b) Preparing the field for feasibility testing of a parenting intervention for war-affected mothers in Northern Uganda. Fam Process. doi:10.1111/famp.12189

Part IV

Summary and Conclusions

How to Treat Children and Adolescents with Trauma-Related Disorders

24

Markus A. Landolt, Marylène Cloitre, and Ulrich Schnyder

At the end of this volume, after having reviewed the basic concepts of child trauma, the currently available evidence-based or evidence-informed treatment approaches, and the various settings in which traumatized children are treated, we will summarize the current knowledge on assessment and treatment of trauma-related psychological disorders among children and adolescents. The first section of this book, specifically the chapters on epidemiology and public health issues, has clearly shown that childhood trauma and its effects are a major issue across the globe. The variety of events that can lead to trauma-related disorders in children and adolescents is large and includes all forms of child maltreatment, war, terrorism, natural disasters, accidents, and learning about the sudden death or severe injury of a loved one. Children's and adolescents' exposure to potentially traumatic events is not only much more common than has previously been believed but can also have large negative effects on development in physical, psychological, and social domains across the lifespan, especially when trauma happens in early childhood and when it is interpersonal, chronic, and the result of an accumulation of multiple different types of events.

M.A. Landolt (✉)
Department of Psychosomatics and Psychiatry, University Children's Hospital
University of Zurich, Zurich, Switzerland
e-mail: Markus.Landolt@kispi.uzh.ch

M. Cloitre
Division of Dissemination and Training, National Center for PTSD, Palo Alto, CA, USA

Psychiatry and Behavioral Sciences, Stanford University, Palo Alto, CA, USA
e-mail: Marylene.Cloitre@nyumc.org

U. Schnyder
Department of Psychiatry and Psychotherapy, University Hospital Zurich,
Zurich, Switzerland
e-mail: ulrich.schnyder@access.uzh.ch

© Springer International Publishing Switzerland 2017
M.A. Landolt et al. (eds.), *Evidence-Based Treatments for Trauma Related Disorders in Children and Adolescents*, DOI 10.1007/978-3-319-46138-0_24

From a public health perspective, the most important measure to reduce exposure to trauma and ensuing morbidity is primary prevention. It is beyond the scope of this book to present and discuss the interventions that are necessary on individual, family, community, and society-at-large levels to prevent trauma in childhood. However, as clinicians, we always have to keep in mind that prevention of trauma exposure is the best "treatment." We therefore should support all measures that aim at reducing the number of children exposed to any kind of trauma. If primary prevention fails, and it sadly still very often does, identification and treatment of affected children is crucial both from an individual and a public health and economic viewpoint. In the following, we will summarize the current knowledge on how to best achieve this goal.

24.1 Assessment

Providing effective treatments that are tailored to the needs of the individual child requires a thorough prior assessment of the child. Assessment should be multi-informant and should include a detailed trauma history of the child and the family (e.g., by using the "Maltreatment and Abuse Chronology of Exposure" [MACE] Scale by Teicher and Parigger 2015). Importantly, given that comorbid symptoms are very common, especially among children with chronic interpersonal trauma, assessment should be broad and not only focused on symptoms of PTSD. As described in Chap. 4 of this book, clinicians should use empirically validated measures with good psychometric properties. Descriptions and links to instruments assessing PTSD are available through the websites of the *US National Child Traumatic Stress Network* (http://www.nctsn.org/resources/online-research/measures-review) and the *International Society for Traumatic Stress Studies* (http://www.istss.org/assessing-trauma.aspx). Many of the DSM-IV measures have now been updated to meet the new DSM-5 criteria. However, these instruments focus on PTSD in school-age children. Currently, there is no DSM-5-based empirically validated instrument available to assess acute stress disorder in children and adolescents and no measure to assess the new preschool type of PTSD. Moreover, while the formulation of ICD-11 PTSD and CPTSD symptom profiles for children and adolescents have been described within the disorders, psychometrically sound measures have yet to be developed.

24.2 Secondary Preventative Interventions After Trauma Exposure

Secondary preventative measures aim at reducing acute stress symptoms and decreasing long-term psychological morbidity through interventions in the first 4 weeks after a potentially traumatic event (see Chap. 6 for an overview). We propose that interventions in the immediate aftermath of a traumatic event (*acute* interventions) differ from those provided between day 2 and 1 month after the event (*early* interventions; see Fig. 24.1). While acute interventions aim at stabilizing the

24 How to Treat Children and Adolescents with Trauma-Related Disorders

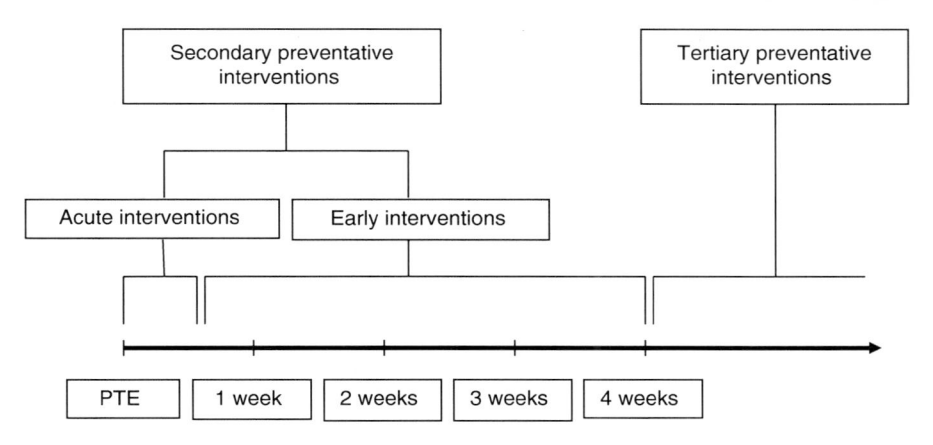

Fig. 24.1 Suggested classification of secondary preventative interventions according to time posttrauma. *PTE* potentially traumatic event

individual on-site, early interventions focus on psychoeducation, trauma processing, and coping skills to reduce acute symptoms and decrease the risk for longer-term traumatic stress symptoms.

Acute Interventions
Although there is not much evidence on interventions in the acute phase, there are currently two standardized intervention programs that are in quite wide use:

- *Psychological First Aid (PFA)* as a universal modular approach has been established for (on-site) interventions in the immediate aftermath of trauma, especially after natural disasters (Brymer et al. 2006). The PFA Field Guide has also been adapted for use in schools (Brymer et al. 2012).
- The *"D-E-F" protocol* (aiming to reduce *D*istress, provide *E*motional support, and remember *F*amily) which provides evidence-based guidelines for trauma-informed pediatric care during the acute phase of medical treatment (Stuber et al. 2006).

Notably, none of these interventions has been studied with regard to its effect in reducing acute distress and preventing long-term posttraumatic stress in children and adolescents. Therefore, the use of such acute on-site interventions is currently still not evidence based.

Early Interventions
As shown in Chaps. 6 and 7, current evidence with regard to early interventions suggests that a stepped procedure with so-called selected/targeted interventions might be the best approach to treat children in the early posttrauma phase (Fig. 24.2). There are nowadays empirically validated screeners available that allow early identification of children at risk. For school-age children the use of the *Child Trauma Screening Questionnaire* (CTSQ; Kenardy et al. 2006) or the *Screening Tool for*

Fig. 24.2 Risk-based stepwise targeted early intervention after single trauma

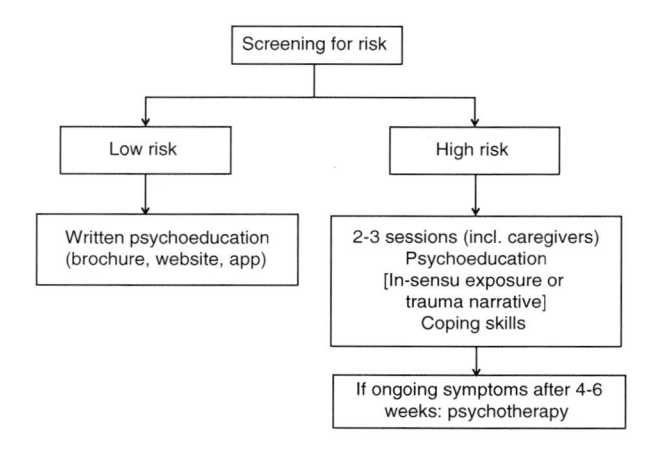

```
                    ┌─────────────────────┐
                    │ Screening for risk  │
                    └─────────┬───────────┘
                      ┌───────┴────────┐
                      ▼                ▼
               ┌──────────┐     ┌──────────┐
               │ Low risk │     │ High risk│
               └─────┬────┘     └─────┬────┘
                     ▼                ▼
         ┌────────────────────┐  ┌──────────────────────────┐
         │ Written psycho-    │  │ 2-3 sessions (incl.      │
         │ education          │  │ caregivers)              │
         │ (brochure,         │  │ Psychoeducation          │
         │ website, app)      │  │ [In-sensu exposure or    │
         └────────────────────┘  │ trauma narrative]        │
                                 │ Coping skills            │
                                 └────────────┬─────────────┘
                                              ▼
                                 ┌──────────────────────────┐
                                 │ If ongoing symptoms      │
                                 │ after 4-6 weeks:         │
                                 │ psychotherapy            │
                                 └──────────────────────────┘
```

Early Predictors of PTSD (STEPP; Winston et al. 2003) can be recommended. For preschoolers, the only available risk screener is the *Pediatric Emotional Distress Scale – Early Screener* (PEDS-ES; Kramer et al. 2013). Children at risk should then receive a standardized psychological intervention such as *Child and Family Traumatic Stress Intervention* (CFTSI, see Chap. 7). Importantly, based on the current findings, such an intervention should be provided to both the child and their primary caregivers and should include psychoeducation and discussion of coping skills that are targeted to the specific symptoms of the individual child (Kramer and Landolt 2011). It is unclear if a detailed in sensu exposure or reconstruction of the event (trauma narrative) needs to be part of such an intervention. For children at low risk for longer-term distress and their caregivers, written information (brochures, websites, apps) can be provided and should be sufficient. This stepped procedure takes into account the fact that many children are resilient after single trauma. Therefore, it seems reasonable to provide more intensive and expensive treatments only to individuals at risk for longer-term distress, while children at no or low risk and their parents are only provided with written psychoeducation.

Although the evidence on the effectiveness of early interventions in children and adolescents is still sparse (Kramer and Landolt 2011), such a stepped procedure with targeted interventions is currently the gold standard for school-age children. Importantly however, we do not have any evidence for preschool-age children at the moment. A stepped procedure in this age group is therefore not evidence based but still highly recommended – especially since we also have a validated screener for young children (Kramer et al. 2013).

24.3 Psychotherapy

As presented in this volume, PTSD and other trauma-related disorders in children and adolescents can be successfully treated. There are evidence-based or evidence-informed therapies available for all ages and many types of trauma, and the evidence clearly suggests that psychotherapy is considered the first choice of treatment. Although various guidelines (e.g., NICE guidelines, AACAP practice parameters, etc.), reviews, and meta-analyses (e.g., Gillies et al. 2012; Gutermann et al. 2016; Leenarts et al. 2013; Miller-Graff and Campion 2016; Morina et al. 2016) on effectiveness of trauma therapy in childhood are available, recommendations across these documents are quite inconsistent. This is mainly due to methodological reasons such as different definitions of evidence levels and different inclusion and exclusion criteria for selected studies. One psychotherapeutic treatment that is recommended in all guidelines and that has been found to be effective in all meta-analyses is CBT, specifically trauma-focused CBT (TF-CBT; see Chap. 8). CBT showed medium (in controlled trials) to large (in uncontrolled analyses) effect sizes with regard to symptoms of PTSD in the most recent meta-analyses by Gutermann et al. (2016) and Morina et al. (2016). Moreover, CBT proved to be effective also with regard to depression and anxiety symptoms. Since cognitive therapy (see Chap. 9), prolonged exposure therapy for adolescents (see Chap. 10), and narrative exposure therapy for children (KIDNET; see Chap. 11) are based on the same or very similar theoretical concepts, they can be recommended too, although meta-analyses on RCTs are still lacking. Eye movement desensitization and reprocessing therapy (EMDR; see Chap. 13), child–parent psychotherapy (CPP; see Chap. 15), and parent–child interaction therapy (PCIT; see Chap. 15) have a weaker evidence base than TF-CBT, but empirical support is sufficient for recommendation of use in clinical practice. However, evidence at this moment is insufficient to determine the level of effectiveness of other treatments, including Skills Training in Affective and Interpersonal Regulation (STAIR) plus Narrative Therapy – Adolescent Version (SNT-A; see Chap. 12), Attachment Self-Regulation and Competency Therapy (ARC; see Chap. 14), and Trauma Systems Therapy (TST; see Chap. 17). For these treatments, preliminary support is provided from quasi-experimental comparative studies, uncontrolled pilot studies, and case reports.

Currently, there is no evidence to conclude that children and adolescents with particular types of trauma are more or less likely to respond to certain psychological therapies versus others (Gillies et al. 2012). Many different treatment approaches and techniques are used with traumatized children and adolescents. To meet the specific needs of the individual child and to consider the severity and the degree of impairment of the child's PTSD symptoms, these approaches and techniques are very often combined by practitioners (multimodal treatment approach). Most treatments that proved to be effective employ methods such as psychoeducation, behavioral and emotional regulation, coping skills training, and cognitive processing, and they all directly address the traumatic experience (mostly through exposure and/or creation of a trauma narrative). Similar to adults (Schnyder and Cloitre 2015), there is nowadays very convincing evidence for children across all ages that treatment approaches that directly address the traumatic experiences are superior to nonspecific therapies in reducing trauma-related symptoms. In addition, and again similar to adults (Schnyder et al. 2015), the following commonalities between many evidence-based treatments can be noted and therefore seen as core components of child trauma therapy (see Table 24.1):

Table 24.1 Proposed components of child trauma therapy

Phase-based treatment approach, if needed and appropriate according to assessment
Treatment has to be age appropriate and tailored to the specific family and culture of the child
Inclusion of caregivers and other relevant systems (e.g., school) to optimize the child's recovery environment
Psychoeducation of child, caregivers, and other relevant systems
Training of emotional and behavioral regulation skills
Cognitive processing of dysfunctional trauma-related thoughts
Reconstruction and/or reconsolidation of the traumatic memories through exposure and/or creation of a trauma narrative
Address the child's competencies and future

Fig. 24.3 Phase-based approach to trauma therapy

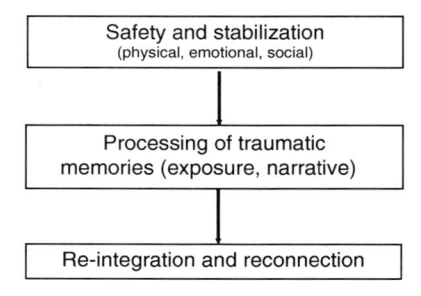

Safety and stabilization (physical, emotional, social)
↓
Processing of traumatic memories (exposure, narrative)
↓
Re-integration and reconnection

- Many therapies implicitly or explicitly use a *phase-based approach* to treat traumatized children, especially when the child has been exposed to multiple interpersonal traumatic events at a young age (Fig. 24.3). The *first step* of intervention should always be to protect the child from further exposure to traumatic events. If necessary, the child's safety needs to be ensured by implementing child protection measures. Also, if the child is emotionally very instable (e.g., acute suicidality) or severely injured (e.g., suffering great pain), appropriate stabilizing measures, including hospitalization or pharmacotherapy, need to be taken before trauma-focused treatment can begin. The *second step* of treatment includes the processing of the traumatic memories. Depending on the specific approach, this is done in a more explicit (e.g., TF-CBT, prolonged exposure, cognitive therapy, KIDNET) or more implicit way (e.g., EMDR). Finally, in a *third step*, reintegration of the child and future-related issues are the main topics of therapy. Not all treatment approaches conceptualize this last part of treatment very well.
- Trauma therapies need to consider *developmental issues*. Most treatment approaches that are currently available are specifically tailored for school-age children, and a recent meta-analysis has shown that psychological treatments are more effective in older children (Gutermann et al. 2016). There is, however, sufficient evidence showing that traumatized infants and toddlers can be successfully treated if using appropriate approaches such as child–parent psychotherapy (see Chap. 15) or parent–child interaction therapy (see Chap. 16). These treatments are quite different from the methods that are used in older children. For instance,

in CPP, the order of interventions is very flexible, and nonverbal methods such as play and physical contact are explicitly incorporated in the protocol. The fit between the therapy method and the *child's developmental stage* is very important and probably one of the most important criteria for the selection of the specific treatment method.

- Since a child, especially a younger child, is highly dependent on *caregivers*, most treatment approaches include the child's caregivers, if available. A better understanding of the child's symptoms (psychoeducation), improvement of parenting skills by helping the caregiver learn skills to manage difficult child behavior, and as a consequence improvement of the parent–child relationship are the main goals. Studies have indeed shown that inclusion of the caregivers is associated with a greater reduction of symptoms (Gutermann et al. 2016). While, for example, TF-CBT (see Chap. 8) and Trauma Systems Therapy (see Chap. 17) have conceptualized the inclusion of caregivers (and other relevant systems) into therapy in an elaborated way, other treatment approaches such as narrative exposure therapy for children (KIDNET; see Chap. 11), eye movement desensitization and reprocessing therapy (EMDR; see Chap. 13), or Skills Training in Affective and Interpersonal Regulation plus Narrative Therapy – Adolescent Version (SNT-A; see Chap. 12) are mainly provided to the individual child or youth without including the parents very much or at all.

- A crucial part of trauma therapy is *psychoeducation*. All methods presented in this volume highlight the importance of informing the child, their caregivers, and other relevant social systems about trauma and its consequences. Although different approaches provide information in a somewhat different way (based on their specific model), psychoeducation provides a map for understanding both the child's symptoms and the treatment.

- Training of the child's *emotional and behavioral regulation skills* is a fundamental part of many methods, especially the CBT approaches. As nicely shown in Chap. 17, traumatized children are often triggered by known or unknown trauma-related cues. It is important that the child becomes aware of this and learns strategies to better regulate his or her emotions and behaviors.

- As specifically highlighted by cognitive therapy, TF-CBT, and other CBT approaches, *dysfunctional cognitions* ("unhelpful thoughts") play an important role in the development and maintenance of symptoms. Children and adolescents with trauma-related disorders often have altered fundamental beliefs or schemas (e.g., seeing the world as a dangerous place, people as harmful, and oneself as helpless). It is therefore important to address these cognitions in therapy and help the child and caregivers understand how trauma has changed their views of the self, the family, the world, and the future and find new ways to think about these issues. Importantly, therapy needs to make sure that the child does not define him- or herself as a trauma victim but as a survivor with a promising future.

- Many treatment approaches focus on the *disturbance* or even *failure of the memory system* which is typical for trauma-related disorders. Reconstruction and reconsolidation of the traumatic memory are seen to be necessary parts of successful treatment. Research has shown that retrieval of traumatic memories induces a transient and instable state during which memories can be updated, modified, or even deleted. This process is called reconsolidation (Lane et al. 2015). The need to reconstruct traumatic memories, to put them into a context, and to reinstall a sense of mastery is well founded on neuroscience research showing that in traumatized children, the amygdala is overreactive and the hippocampus and medial prefrontal cortex are downregulated (see Chap. 5). Notably, the different treatment approaches use quite different techniques to address this failure of memory and to modify reactivated traumatic memories. While creation of a trauma narrative ("to put the traumatic experience into words") and in sensu or in vivo exposure is essential for CBT approaches, it is, for example, not the case in EMDR where in sensu exposure is performed but the processing of the traumatic memories does not need to be put into words. In our view, there are probably two mechanisms that are effective in trauma treatment: (1) extinction of conditioned fear responses which is, based on learning theories, best achieved through in sensu and/or in vivo exposure (without a need to create a trauma narrative) and (2) updating of traumatic memories through a process of reconsolidation that incorporates new emotional experiences. This is probably best achieved by helping the individual create a narrative which puts the traumatic events in the correct context (place, time). As suggested by Lane et al. (2015), the essential ingredients of therapeutic change would include three steps: (a) reactivation of old memories, (b) engaging in new emotional experiences that are incorporated into these reactivated memories via the process of reconsolidation, and (c) reinforcing the integrated memory structure by practicing a new way of behaving and experiencing the world in a variety of contexts.

- Finally, although not conceptualized very well in many approaches, trauma therapy should also address the child's *competencies* and his/her *future perspectives*. Treatment approaches should not only focus on symptoms but also on enhancing daily functioning, development, and resiliency. From a patient's perspective, symptom severity may be of less interest than actual day-to-day functioning. The level of functional impairment in traumatized children may not necessarily be best captured by assessment of or change in severity of PTSD symptoms. Also, children with multiple interpersonal traumatic experiences have many negative beliefs and expectations with regard to their future. It is therefore essential to address these issues in therapy.

24.4 Pharmacotherapy

Medication may be used as second-line treatment for PTSD or other trauma-related disorders in a number of situations. In some instances, psychotherapy, and empirically supported trauma-focused psychotherapy in particular, is not available due to a lack of healthcare resources or because the child lives in a remote place or is unable to travel and see a psychotherapist for other reasons such as physical illness or handicap. Moreover, many children have comorbid psychological conditions for which safe and effective pharmacological treatments are available, for instance,

ADHD, OCD, or depression. It should be noted that there is currently no sufficient empirical support for any pharmacological compound as a treatment for pediatric PTSD. Whatever the reason may be to prescribe medication (see Chap. 18), however, this should always be done within the framework of a stable and trusting therapeutic relationship.

24.5 Treatment Contexts

This volume also addresses the fact that assessment and delivery of treatment occur in many settings other than outpatient clinics and schools. The chapters on this topic provide useful information suggesting that services in venues such as hospitals, foster care, and the judicial system require additional resources for therapies to be effective. These include the education of the support staff and the creation of "trauma-informed" environments so that the behavior of the children and youth are understood and responded to in an appropriate way. The addition of screening measures in these environments is critical as a means to identify appropriate treatments. Lastly it is important to develop procedures and devote resources to create pathways from one service to another (e.g., inpatient care to residential treatment to outpatient care) to provide a trauma-informed continuum of care that supports consistent and sustained services relevant to the child and family.

24.6 Outlook

Although many evidence-based treatments for trauma-related psychological disorders are available, there are still some significant limitations with regard to the current knowledge. First, while some promising approaches for children with complex trauma and comorbidity have been developed in the past years (e.g., ARC, SNT-A, TST), evidence regarding these treatments is still limited. Second, there is a significant lack of studies among preschool-age children, specifically below the age of 4 years. As noted in several chapters in this volume, the number of young traumatized children is very high, and the effects of trauma with regard to long-term outcomes are particularly adverse in this age group. It is therefore crucial to develop and evaluate evidence-based treatments for young children in the future. Third, as highlighted by Carrion and Kletter (2012), future treatment protocols should better integrate current findings on neurobiological mechanisms in the conceptualization of psychotherapeutic techniques. Specifically, new research on memory reconsolidation may be of particular importance (Lane et al. 2015). This may also be promising with regard to early interventions after trauma where a combination of psychological and pharmacological interventions may prove helpful in the future. Fourth, while evidence-based treatments for trauma-related disorders are available, they remain underutilized in clinical practice. Obviously, many clinicians still provide treatments that are not evidence based (e.g., pharmacotherapy as first-line treatment). Dissemination of effective treatments is therefore a crucial issue in the future. Fifth, we need more information about how to find the right approach for the individual child with his/her specific symptoms and cultural and familial background. Studies should examine factors that are relevant for an optimal fit between the individual symptomatic child and the treatment method. Specifically, the role of culture is not studied appropriately. The relative acceptability and effectiveness of treatment delivery methods (e.g., play therapy, storytelling, role playing) and format (group versus individual) are likely to depend on cultural mores and remain to be investigated. Sixth, the use of telemedical approaches, websites, apps, games, and social media in the treatment of traumatized children might be promising and should be studied in greater detail. Significant progress has been made regarding awareness of child trauma worldwide. The current wave of recognition will hopefully continue and carry forward with it additional development and dissemination of engaging, adaptable, and effective interventions for children and youth.

References

Brymer M, Taylor M, Escudero P, Jacobs A, Kronenberg M, Macy R, Vogel J (2012) Psychological first aid for schools: field operations guide. National Child Traumatic Stress Network, Los Angeles

Brymer MJ, Jacobs A, Layne C, Pynoos RS, Ruzek J, Steinberg A, Watson P (2006) Psychological first aid: field operations guide, 2nd edn: National Child Traumatic Stress Network and National Center for PTSD, Los Angeles, CA

Carrion VG, Kletter H (2012) Posttraumatic stress disorder: shifting toward a developmental framework. Child Adolesc Psychiatr Clin Am 21(3):573–591. doi:10.1016/j.chc.2012.05.004

Gillies D, Taylor F, Gray C, O'Brien L, D'Abrew N (2012) Psychological therapies for the treatment of post-traumatic stress disorder in children and adolescents. Cochrane Database of Syst Rev 12. doi:10.1002/14651858.CD006726.pub2

Gutermann J, Schreiber F, Matulis S, Schwartzkopff L, Deppe J, Steil R (2016) Psychological treatments for symptoms of posttraumatic stress disorder in children, adolescents, and young adults: a meta-analysis. Clin Child Fam Psychol Rev 19(2):77–93. doi:10.1007/s10567-016-0202-5

Kenardy JA, Spence SH, Macleod AC (2006) Screening for posttraumatic stress disorder in children after accidental injury. Pediatrics 118(3):1002–1009. doi:10.1542/peds.2006-0406

Kramer DN, Hertli MB, Landolt MA (2013) Evaluation of an early risk screener for PTSD in preschool children after accidental injury. Pediatrics. doi:10.1542/peds.2013-0713

Kramer DN, Landolt MA (2011) Characteristics and efficacy of early psychological interventions in children and adolescents after single trauma: a meta-analysis. Eur J Psychotraumatol 2:7858. doi:10.3402/ejpt.v2i0.7858

Lane RD, Ryan L, Nadel L, Greenberg L (2015) Memory reconsolidation, emotional arousal, and the process of change in psychotherapy: New insights from brain science. Behav Brain Sci 38:e1. doi:10.1017/S0140525X14000041

Leenarts LE, Diehle J, Doreleijers TA, Jansma EP, Lindauer RJ (2013) Evidence-based treatments for children with trauma-related psychopathology as a result of childhood maltreatment: a systematic review. Eur Child Adolesc Psychiatr 22(5):269–283. doi:10.1007/s00787-012-0367-5

Miller-Graff LE, Campion K (2016) Interventions for posttraumatic stress with children exposed to violence: factors associated with treatment success. J Clin Psychol 72(3):226–248. doi:10.1002/jclp.22238

Morina N, Koerssen R, Pollet TV (2016) Interventions for children and adolescents with posttraumatic stress disorder: a meta-analysis of comparative outcome studies. Clin Psychol Rev 47:41–54. doi:10.1016/j.cpr.2016.05.006

Schnyder U, Cloitre M (eds) (2015) Evidence based treatments for trauma-related psychological disorders. A practical guide for clinicians. Springer, Cham/Heidelberg/London/New York

Schnyder U, Ehlers A, Elbert T, Foa EB, Gersons BP, Resick PA et al (2015) Psychotherapies for PTSD: what do they have in common? Eur J Psychotraumatol 6:28186. doi:10.3402/ejpt.v6.28186

Stuber ML, Schneider S, Kassam-Adams N, Kazak AE, Saxe G (2006) The medical traumatic stress toolkit. CNS Spectrum 11:137–142

Teicher MH, Parigger A (2015) The 'maltreatment and abuse chronology of exposure' (MACE) scale for the retrospective assessment of abuse and neglect during development. PLoS One 10(2):e0117423. doi:10.1371/journal.pone.0117423

Winston FK, Kassam-Adams N, Garcia-Espana F, Ittenbach R, Cnaan A (2003) Screening for risk of persistent posttraumatic stress in injured children and their parents. J Am Med Assoc 290:643–649. doi:10.1001/jama.290.5.643